J. ROGAN
GENESIS ORTHOPEDICS
OCT. 94

Biomechanics in Orthopedic Trauma

Biomechanics in Orthopedic Trauma
Bone Fracture and Fixation

Allan F. Tencer, Ph.D.

Department of Orthopaedics
University of Washington
Seattle, Washington

Kenneth D. Johnson, M.D.

Department of Orthopaedic Surgery
Vanderbilt University
Nashville, Tennessee

Martin Dunitz London

J. B. Lippincott Company Philadelphia

First published in the United States of America in 1994 by J. B. Lippincott Company, Philadelphia

First published in the United Kingdom in 1994 by Martin Dunitz Ltd, London

ISBN 0-397-51462-X

Library of Congress Cataloging in Publication Data applied for

To
Annie, Signe, and Holly
and
Helen, Kelly, Karie, Kevin, and Katherine

Typeset by TecSet Ltd, Wallington, Surrey
Printed and bound in Singapore by Kyodo Printing Pte. Ltd.

CONTENTS

PREFACE

This book is an attempt to distill years of laboratory research and clinical experience in orthopedic trauma into a concise but detailed discussion of the mechanical principles underlying the stabilization of bone fractures. It is the hope of the authors that objective discussion of fixation alternatives will guide the orthopedic surgeon in selecting the most effective methods, as well as illustrating underlying concepts in the design and use of specific devices. This volume is not meant as a first text in biomechanics, of which many excellent examples abound, nor are clinical issues in fracture management addressed. There are many classic texts available that address the clinical management of fractures. Instead, this book is designed to address, in great detail, biomechanical principles as applied to fracture fixation. The reader is assumed to have a working knowledge of both basic biomechanics and orthopedic trauma surgery. However, a brief review of biomechanics as it applies to fracture fixation is provided in Chapter 1.

The primary aim of this volume is to provide a source of practical information to the orthopedic surgeon related to the underlying principles in the design and use of devices for the fixation of bone fracture. Throughout the text, emphasis is placed on conceptual understanding of basic principles, backed by data derived from experimentation when necessary. Basic principles of fracture fixation and details specific to different anatomical areas are presented. Some specific topics are based on newly generated information. These include discussions of the design factors affecting performance of screws in porous materials, the biomechanics of low contact and no contact bone plates, the stability of IM nailing in long bone fractures, percutaneous pinning techniques, the mechanical stability of pelvic fixation, including percutaneous sacral screws, and an extensive discussion of spinal fixation devices.

This book is divided into three parts. Part I addresses basic concepts related to the strength of bone and mechanisms of failure. Chapter 1 explains the basic terminology used in describing the mechanical strength and stability of fractures stabilized by internal fixation. Following this introduction, Chapter 2 summarizes the mechanical properties of bone and the factors affecting its strength both as a material and as a structure. This information is necessary when considering sites of attachment of a fixation device and in assessing its potential for resisting physiological forces. Chapter 3 describes common mechanisms of bone fracture, as a guide to understanding the mechanical aspects of the clinical problem.

Part II deals with general considerations in fracture fixation. In Chapter 4 the mechanical environment necessary for fracture healing is discussed to provide a basis for understanding the mechanical role of fixation during different phases of fracture healing. The properties of materials used in fracture fixation devices are covered in Chapter 5.

Part III provides a detailed discussion of the mechanics of fixation in various regions of the skeleton. The mechanics of commonly used devices are discussed in Chapter 6. These include the design and performance of screws in cortical and cancellous bone, and the use of bone plates and lag screws. In Chapter 7 alternatives for and fixation of upper extremity fractures are presented. Specific anatomical sites discussed include the metacarpal, the scaphoid, the distal radius, the midshaft of the forearm, and the distal and proximal humerus. Chapter 8 describes the mechanics and performance of fixation alternatives in the cervical, thoracic and lumbar spine, and the pelvis. Finally, fixation of the lower extremity, specifically the subcapital, intertrochanteric, subtrochanteric, midshaft and distal femur, and the plateau, midshaft and distal syndesmosis of the tibia are discussed in Chapter 9.

The authors would like to take this opportunity to thank a number of collaborators with whom they have been privileged to work and who patiently taught much about the functional mechanics of the skeleton; Abdul Ahmed, PhD, Robert Bucholz, MD, Berndt Claudi, MD, Sherman Coleman, MD, Vert Mooney, MD, Ralph Holmes, MD, Al Potvin, PhD, Ben Allen Jr, MD, Ron Ferguson, MD, Steve Viegas, MD, David Simmons, PhD, Wayne Daum, MD, Burke Evans, MD, ML Chip Routt, MD, Steven Benirschke, MD, Bruce

Sangeorzan, MD, Tom Trumble, MD, Jens Chapman, MD, Brad Henley, MD, Richard Harrington, MS, Randy Ching, PhD, Harold Dunn MD, and AU Dan Daniels, PhD.

PART I
BIOMECHANICS OF BONE AND FRACTURE

CHAPTER 1

Basic concepts in biomechanics of fractures and fixation

This chapter presents a short review of biomechanical principles as they relate to bone fracture and fracture/implant constructs (the load bearing structure composed of the bone fracture components and the implant). For greater detail on basic concepts in biomechanics, the reader is referred to the bibliography at the end of the chapter, which suggests further reading.

1.1 Force and moment

A *force* causes a mass to change its velocity (either accelerating or decelerating it) and/or its direction. As Figure 1.1 shows, any number of forces may act on a mass. Any force can be broken into two *components* whose vector sum equals the force. A *vector* is an entity that has both magnitude and direction. It allows the force to be represented graphically. The force components can be added graphically so that a *resultant force* can be defined. This is the net force acting on a body. The *line of action* of the resultant force defines its direction of application and the resulting direction of movement of the mass.

If a mass is fixed so that it can only rotate about one axis, such as the forearm around the elbow joint, then the force (for example, applied by a muscle) causes a *moment*, and the mass (bone)

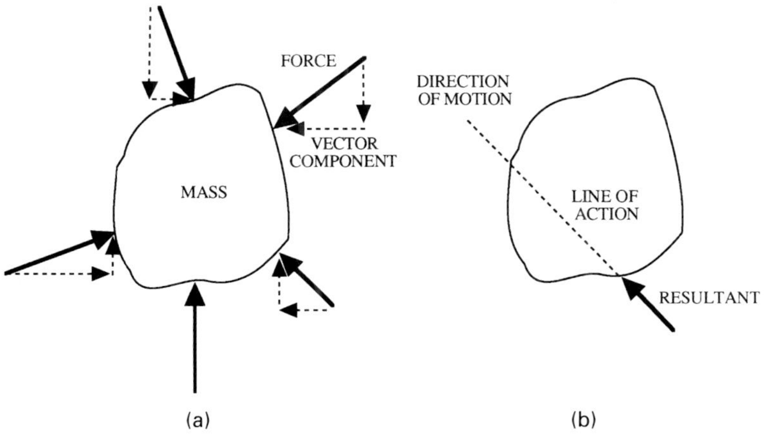

Figure 1.1

(a) A mass being acted on by several forces. By determining the magnitudes of the vector components of each force (b), a resultant force can be determined. The line of action defines the direction of motion of the mass.

will rotate about the *center of rotation* (joint axis). The moment created (Figure 1.2a) depends upon the magnitude of the force and its *perpendicular distance* from the center of rotation. Thus a muscle situated farther from the center of a joint has a larger moment, or turning force, for the same force of contraction. In order for the forces to be in *equilibrium*, there must be a *joint reaction force*, acting through the joint, which is equal in magnitude and opposite in direction to the applied force.

A *couple* or *torque* is a twisting action (Figure 1.2b) that produces no net force, or joint reaction. This might occur when two muscles on opposite sides of a joint co-contract. When a moment acts, there must be an equal and opposite force at the center of the joint, resisting the force. With a torque, only turning occurs.

1.2 Load, deformation, and work

A force acting on a material can be broken into three fundamental components. As Figure 1.3 shows, these components are *compressive*, acting inward relative to the object and perpendicular to the surface of the material (a direction sometimes referred to as *normal*), *tensile*, acting outward, and *shear*, which acts parallel to the surface of the material and tends to distort it from a rectangular into a parallelogram shape. Internal shearing also results from the application of other types of loads such as bending in a beam or twisting of a bar.

A force acting on a material causes a *deformation* (Figure 1.3). This relation of force and deformation is fundamental to the study and evaluation of fracture fixation implants, since a

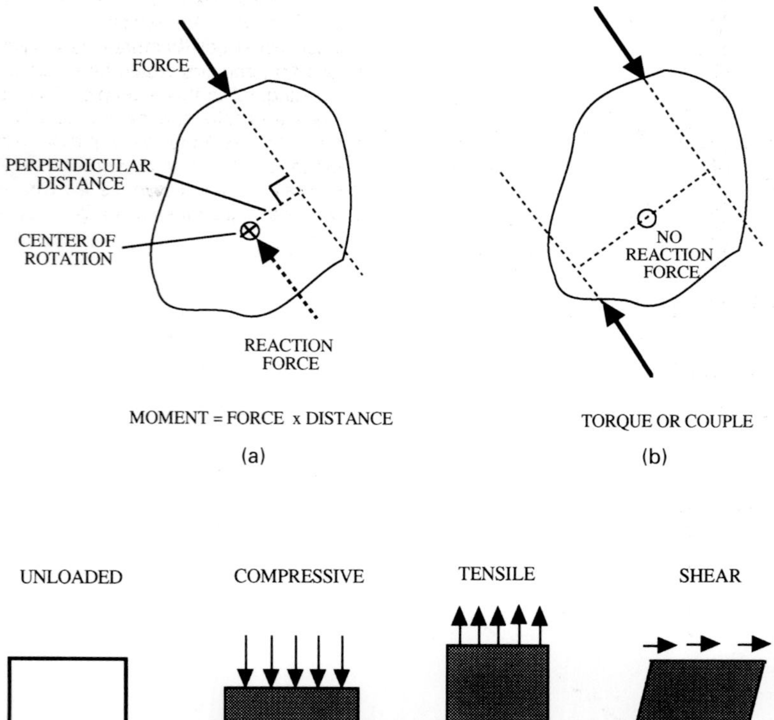

Figure 1.2

(a) The moment, or turning force, depends on the perpendicular distance of the line of action of the applied force from the center of rotation (a fixed pivot point), as well as the magnitude of the force. There must be a reaction force at the center of rotation to counteract the applied force. (b) If two equal and opposite forces act on the mass, a torque or couple is produced, with no net reaction force.

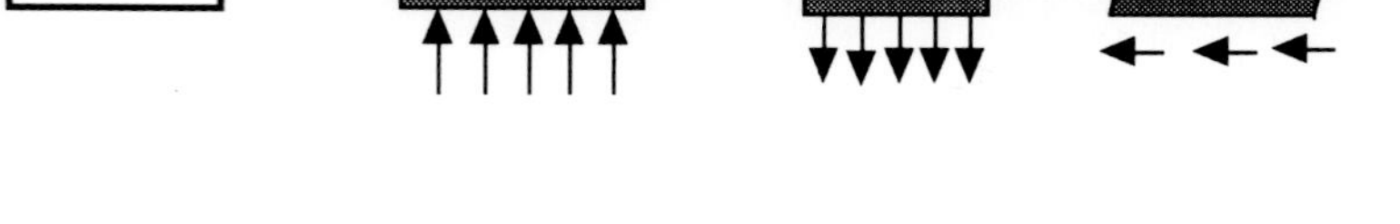

Figure 1.3

Three fundamental force components acting on a material, and the resulting deformation of the material: unloaded, compressive (normal), tensile, and shear.

primary objective is to minimize deformation (or movement) between the fracture components. Typically, as shown in Figure 1.4, a *fracture fixation construct* (i.e. a structure consisting of a fixation device mounted on a fractured bone) is mounted in a materials testing machine and the deformation of the fracture construct recorded under controlled loads. This results in a force–deformation diagram (Figure 1.5), a graphic relationship of how the construct reacts to an applied load. The *stiffness* is the slope of the curve in the *elastic* region. The slope defines a relationship between the load applied and the deformation that results. The *elastic limit* or *yield point* of the construct defines a magnitude of load below which, if the load were released, it would return exactly to its original shape.

If the force applied is increased continuously, it will at some point exceed the elastic limit of the object. At this *yield point*, some failure of the fracture construct can occur, but it may not be catastrophic. Examples are permanent bending of screws or plates, or the crushing of cancellous bone near the implant. At these load magnitudes the fracture construct has entered its *plastic region*, and release of the load will leave it

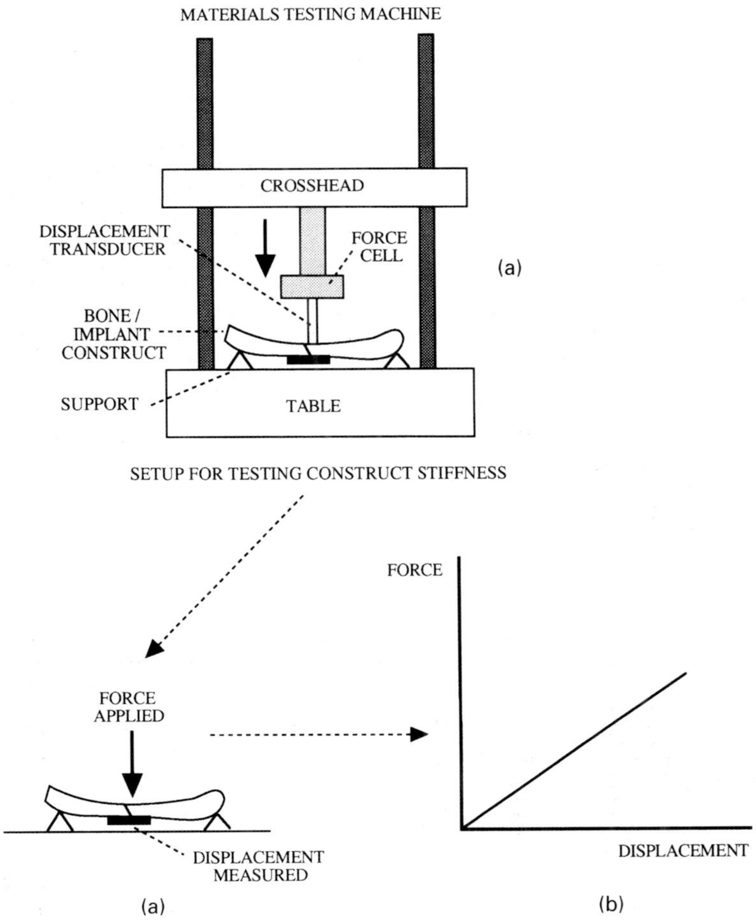

Figure 1.4

(a) Schematic diagram of a materials testing machine in which a fracture fixation construct (fractured bone with supporting implant) would be mounted for testing. (b) In this example a load is applied vertically downward, and the force and resulting deformation are measured. (c) The recorded force and deformation are shown as a plot to allow their relationship to be determined.

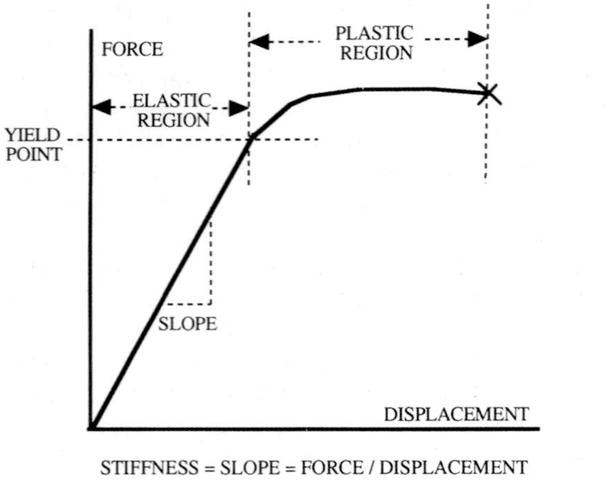

(a)

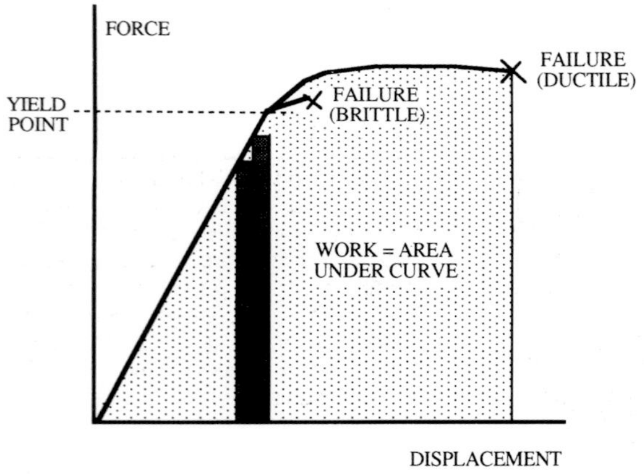

(b)

Figure 1.5

(a) Several parameters can be determined from the force/deformation plot derived from testing (shown in Figure 1.4). The slope of the elastic (linear) region is the stiffness. At the yield point the behavior changes to nonlinear, as the material or construct enters its plastic region. Typically, in this region, if the load is released, some permanent deformation will remain. At some point the utlimate load will be exceeded and the construct will fail. (b) If the plastic region is small, the material is brittle, while a large plastic region indicates a ductile material. The work (or energy) required for the material to fail is equivalent to the area under the force/deformation curve. The shaded rectangle indicates a region where the force is assumed to be approximately constant over a small displacement. Summing such regions gives the area under the curve. The area must be derived this way because the force is not constant during loading (if it were constant, the work done would simply be equal to force × displacement).

permanently deformed. Typically in this region there is considerable deformation without a large increase in load.

The area under the force–deformation curve of Figure 1.5 represents the work performed or the energy expended in loading the fracture construct. *Work* or *energy expenditure*, by definition, is the product of a force moving an object through a defined distance. Pushing a block along the ground against frictional resistance requires work. Similarly, work is performed as a fracture construct is deformed under load. If the body is purely elastic, all the work performed in deforming the object will be recovered when the load is removed. A simple example is the rebound of a spring, which stores and then releases the work of deformation. If some permanent deformation occurs, that work which went into bending screws or crushing bone will not be recovered.

The reason that the work is represented graphically by the area under the force–deformation curve is that, in the elastic region, the force increases linearly with displacment, so a simple average force cannot be defined from which to calculate work as a product of force and deformation. Instead the average force is approximated over a small displacement to calculate the approximate work over that interval. Graphically this is represented as a rectangular area whose height is the average force and base is the diplacement in that interval. Summing or integrating these small increments of work yields the area under the curve.

Knowledge of the work (or energy) to failure of a construct can be very important. Systems that allow a high degree of deformation absorb a large amount of work without catastrophic failure. Take the example of a downhill ski binding. In this system, when torque is applied through the leg, both the tibial shaft and knee joint and the movement of the binding can absorb the work applied. A properly designed and adjusted binding absorbs a large component of the work applied, thereby sparing the anatomical structures. A relatively *brittle* material such as glass may be stiffer, allowing less deformation under load, but, because it has little plastic deformation region, may not absorb as much work or energy as a *ductile* material. Rubber, which has the ability to deform significantly after yield but before failure, is therefore a more appropriate material to absorb impact than glass. Rubber has greater *fracture toughness* than glass, or the ability to absorb more work before catastrophic failure.

1.3 Stress and strain

Stress and *strain* are values derived from force and deformation that allow the properties of one material from an experimental test to be compared with another material, independent of its shape. *Stress* is defined as the force applied to a cross section of a material, divided by the area of that cross section (Figure 1.6). *Strain* is the change in length of an object divided by its original length. *Elastic modulus* is the ratio of stress to strain, which like stiffness can be derived from an experimental plot. Unlike stiffness, which is derived from the plot of force and displacement, the force must be converted to stress, and the displacement to strain, in order to derive the elastic modulus.

To understand the usefulness of these concepts, consider two engineers in different laboratories, one on the east coast and one on the west coast of North America. They both receive samples of a synthetic ligament to test. Since there are no established testing standards, each performs his/her own tensile test. East Coast

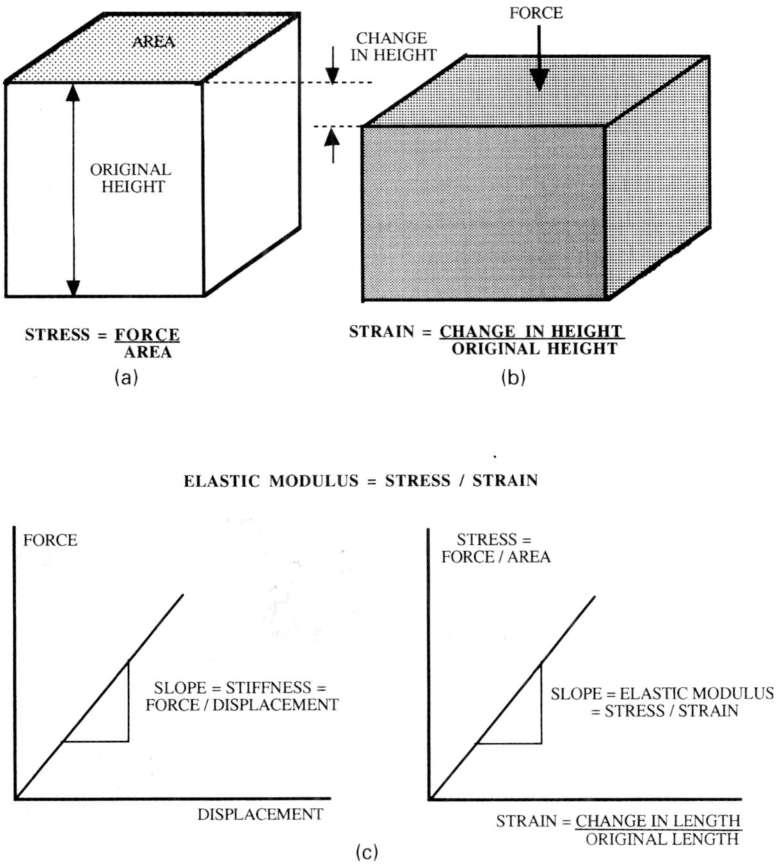

Figure 1.6

(a) The stress is defined as the force applied to a cross section divided by the area of that cross section. (b) The strain is the resulting change in height divided by the original height. (c) The stress/strain diagram can be determined from the load–deflection properties, and the slope of this line is the elastic modulus.

applies 100 N to a ligament specimen 1 cm^2 in cross section, and 5 cm long. He measures an elongation of 1 cm and calculates a modulus

$$E = \frac{\text{stress}}{\text{strain}}$$

$$E = \frac{\text{force/area}}{\text{elongation/length}}$$

$$E = \frac{100\ \text{N}/1\ \text{cm}^2}{1\ \text{cm}/5\ \text{cm}} = \frac{100\ \text{N/cm}^2}{0.2}$$

$$= 500\ \text{N/cm}^2$$

West Coast performs a similar test; however, her specimens are 0.5 cm^2 in cross section and 10 cm long. Upon loading to 100 N, she finds an elongation of 4 cm, from which she also calculates an elastic modulus

$$E = \frac{100\ \text{N}/0.5\ \text{cm}^2}{4\ \text{cm}/10\ \text{cm}}$$

$$= 500\ \text{N/cm}^2$$

Thus the results are the same, regardless of the differences in specimen geometry. (Note that actual ligament testing is more complex than that described here because of variability of the cross section of the ligament and nonuniform strain under tensile loading.)

1.4 Mechanical properties of beams

The most common objects designed to support load are a *beam, column,* or *shaft.* Implant/bone structures may act as complex beams, columns, or shafts depending upon the loads applied to them. A beam (such as an "I" beam or floor joist) is designed to support a load acting between two supports (Figure 1.7). A beam can be loaded in *three point, four point, uniform loading,* or *cantilever bending* (Figure 1.8). A cantilever has a support only at one end and has the load applied at any other point along the beam. In *three point bending* one load is applied somewhere along the beam, and there are support points at each end. In *four point bending* two loads are applied. The radius and ulna of the forearm when carrying a load with the elbow flexed, and the neck of the femur are examples of *cantilever loaded structures.*

A *bending moment* is the load that deforms a beam into a curved shape. From a biomechanical testing point of view, the bending moment in three point bending is minimum at the ends of the beam,

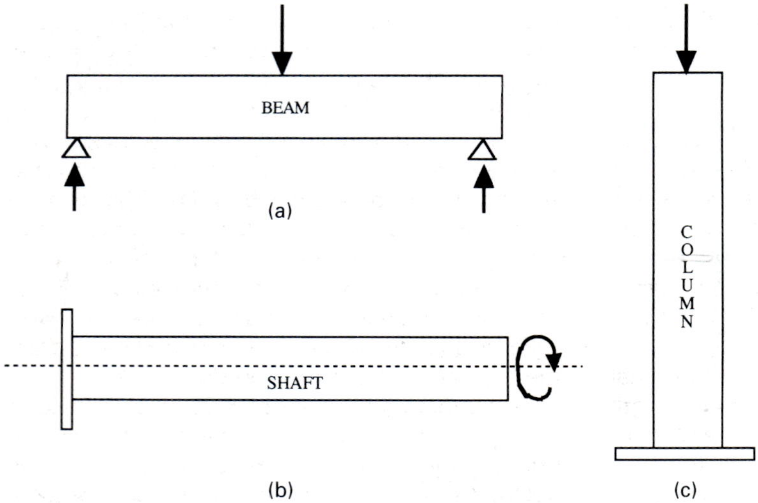

Figure 1.7

Three types of load bearing structures: (a) a beam supports loads between two supports; (b) a shaft resists torsion; (c) a column supports compressive loads.

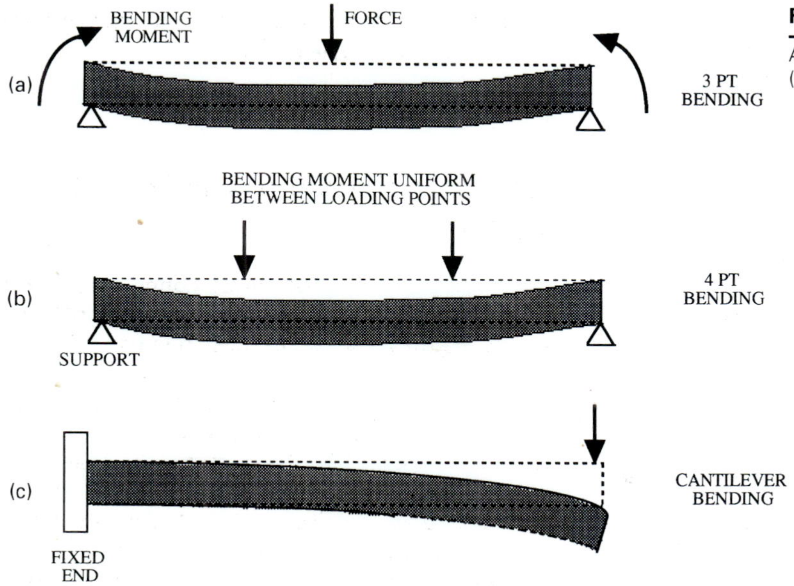

Figure 1.8

A beam can be loaded in (a) three point, (b) four point, or (c) cantilever bending.

maximum at the point of application of the load, and variable between these two locations. In four point bending of a homogeneous material the bending moment is constant between the two load points. In three point bending failure usually occurs at the point of load application, while in four point bending no particular location between the load points is predisposed to failing. It should be noted that long bones have changing cross sections, cortical thicknesses, and, near the joint surfaces, varying bone material properties. Therefore the actual bending moment magnitude in four point bending in a bone will most likely be variable.

Considering the deformation of the tibia under impact to the anterior surface, the anterior (concave) surface shortens and therefore its material must experience compressive stress. The posterior (convex) surface elongates, and thus must be in tension. At the plane in the beam where the transition from compressive to tensile stress occurs, the stress is zero. This is the *neutral axis* (Figure 1.9).

The *stiffness of a beam* (or the deflection that occurs under a given load) depends on the length of the *unsupported span* of the beam, and most importantly, its shape, which is described by the *moment of inertia* of its cross section (Figure 1.10). For a given load applied to a rectangular beam, its stiffness will decrease with the cube of its length and increase with the cube of its height. More deformation leads to greater stress and the possibility of exceeding the yield stress of the material. Thus a long slender tibia that undergoes side impact (three point bending) is more likely to fracture in bending than a short thick one.

The *moment of inertia* is a property that in effect measures the distribution of the material of the beam around the cross section. The further the material is from the neutral axis, the stiffer will be the beam under a given load. This is why structural "I" beams have their top and bottom flanges as far from each other as possible. Similarly, a hollow tube (such as a long bone) with the same amount of material in its cross section as a solid tube will be stiffer. The moment of inertia is calculated by defining a neutral axis through the cross section of the beam about which bending occurs, and then summing the products of elemental areas within the cross section and the square of their distances from the neutral axis, as shown in Figure 1.10(b).

Take for example the beam (here as a fracture fixation plate) of Figure 1.11. If this is mounted on the medial aspect of the tibia, what is the difference in resistance to bending in the anterior/posterior plane versus the medial/lateral

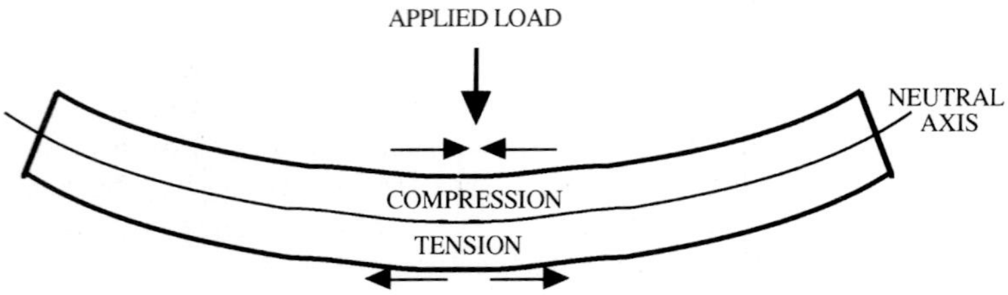

Figure 1.9

When a three point bending load is applied to a beam, the top (concave) surface shortens, resulting in compressive stress, while the bottom (convex) surface lengthens, resulting in tensile stress. At some point within the beam there is a transition between compressive and tensile stress. This is termed the *neutral axis*.

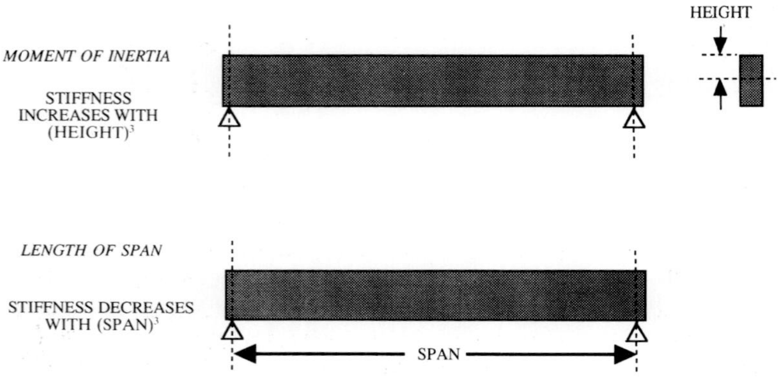

(a)

$$\text{MOMENT OF INERTIA} = \text{SUM OF } (H^2 \times d\text{AREA})$$

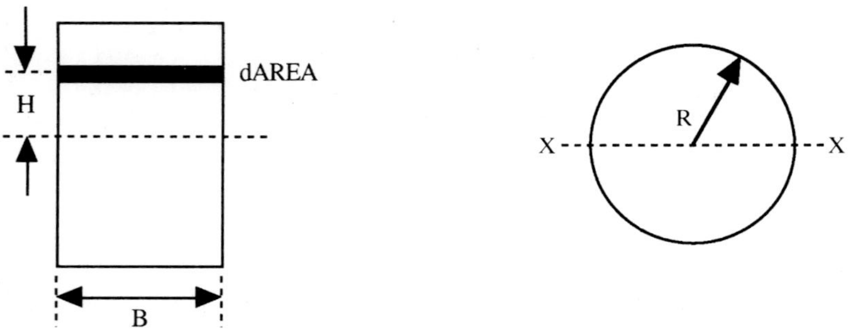

for a rectangular area:

$$\mathbf{I = B \times H^3/12}$$

for a circular area:

$$\mathbf{I = \pi R^4/4}$$

(b)

Figure 1.10

(a) Two factors that affect the stiffness of a beam are the moment of inertia and the span. (b) The moment of inertia of a cross section defines how the material of the object is distributed around the axis of bending. For the same material, a more rigid structure results if the material is further from the axis of bending. Moment of inertia is calculated by summing the products of small areas (such as that shown as a black bar) and the square of their distance from the bending axis (dotted line). For (left) rectangular and (right) circular cross sections, the method of calculating their moments of inertia are shown.

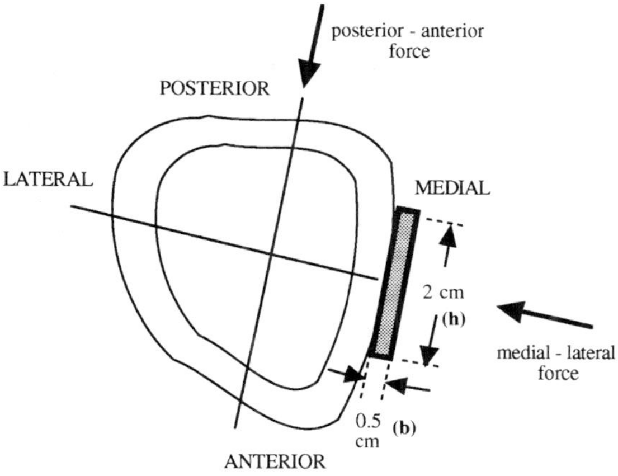

Figure 1.11

Comparison of the effect of a plate on stiffness in bending in a plane parallel or perpendicular to the surface of the plate (and neglecting any contribution from the bone).

plane (assuming that the plate supports all the load and there is no contact of the bone fracture components)?

The orientation of the plate is different relative to the direction of the applied load. Therefore the moment of inertia of the plate for a load applied anterior to posterior is (see Figure 1.11)

$$I_{AP} = \frac{bh^3}{12} = \frac{(0.5) \times (2)^3}{12} = 0.33 \text{ cm}^4$$

while if the load is applied medial to lateral, the moment of inertia is

$$I_{ML} = \frac{hb^3}{12} = \frac{(2) \times (0.5)^3}{12} = 0.0208 \text{ cm}^4$$

Therefore the difference in resistance to bending will be

$$\frac{I_{AP}}{I_{ML}} = \frac{0.33}{0.0208} = 15.9 \text{ times stiffer in AP bending}$$

A second example concerns the difference in bending stiffness between a plate and an IM nail used, for example, in fixation of a tibial fracture (again neglecting cortical contact at the fracture site) (Figure 1.12). With all other factors (such as the material from which the implant is made) being equal, the moments of inertia of the plate and rod determine the mechanical stiffness of the fixed fracture:

$$I_p = \frac{bh^3}{12} = \frac{0.5 \times 2^3}{12} = 0.33 \text{ cm}^4 \text{ (plate)}$$

or

$$= \frac{hb^3}{12} = \frac{2.0 \times 0.5^3}{12} = 0.02 \text{ cm}^4$$

$$I_r = \frac{\pi}{4} r_o^4 = \frac{3.14}{4} (0.45)^4 = 0.03 \text{ cm}^4 \text{ (solid rod)}$$

$$I_{rt} = \frac{\pi}{4}(r_o^4 - r_i^4) = \frac{3.14}{4} (0.45^4 - 0.30^4)$$

$$= 0.02 \text{ cm}^4 \text{ (tubular rod)}$$

(where r_o is the outer radius (0.45 cm) and r_i is the inner radius (0.03 cm). For typically sized implants the plate has the largest moment of inertia, depending on its orientation, followed by the solid and tubular rods .

1.5 Mechanical properties of columns and shafts

A long bone can act as a *column*, supporting a compressive load acting along its long axis, or as a *shaft*, resisting rotation. The tibia and femur act as columns, supporting the compressive load of the

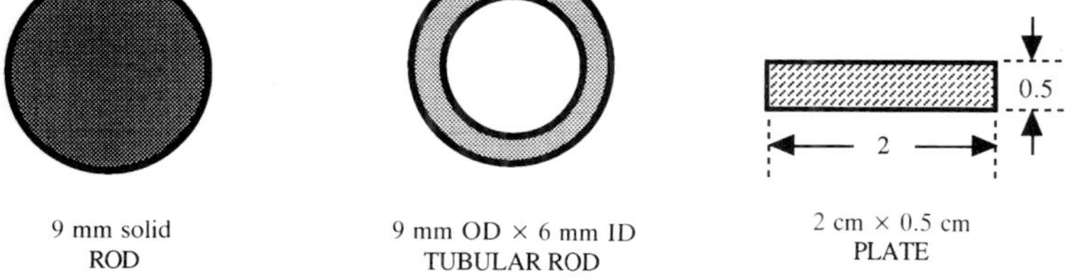

Figure 1.12

Cross sections of three typical implants that could be used to fix a tibial fracture, and their moments of inertia I (in units of cm^4, i.e. area × $distance^2$). (For calculations, see text.)

torso (and as beams resisting bending moments). Similarly, if the foot twists, these bones act as shafts, resisting torsion. The resistance of a shaft to torsion (Figure 1.13) depends upon its length, its *polar moment of inertia*, and its *shear modulus*. Polar moment of inertia is similar in concept to moment of inertia described previously (Figure 1.10b), except that it is calculated around the long axis of the shaft, instead of about an axis through its cross section. Similarly, the shear modulus is similar to elastic modulus, except of course that it describes the relationship between shear stress and shear strain.

These concepts can be illustrated by the following example. How much additional torsional stiffness is gained in fixing a femoral shaft fracture by inserting a 16 mm diameter IM nail compared with one of 14 mm diameter? Both are made of 2 mm thick stainless steel sheet, and any interdigitation of the fracture fragments is neglected. From the formula

$$T/\Theta = JG/L$$

where

T/Θ = torsional stiffness
T = torque applied to shaft
Θ = angle of twist
J = polar moment of inertia $= \frac{\pi}{2} r^4$
G = shear modulus
L = length of shaft

The torsional stiffnesses of the nails are proportional to their polar moments (J):

$$(T/\Theta)_{16} \propto J_{16} \quad \text{and} \quad (T/\Theta)_{14} \propto J_{14}$$

(both have similar length and material properties so L and G can be cancelled). Therefore the ratio of stiffnesses is:

$$\frac{(T/\Theta)_{16}}{(T/\Theta)_{14}} = \frac{J_{16}}{J_{14}}$$

$$\frac{(T/\Theta)_{16}}{(T/\Theta)_{14}} = \frac{(\pi/2)(r_o^4 - r_i^4)_{16}}{(\pi/2)(r_o^4 - r_i^4)_{14}} = \frac{8^4 - 6^4}{7^4 - 5^4} = 1.58$$

The 16 mm rod (for the material wall thickness given) is 1.58 times stiffer in torsion than a 14 mm rod of equivalent dimensions and material.

1.6 Structural stiffness

The concept of stiffness, introduced above, allows us to biomechanically compare the prcperties of different implants and techniques of fixation. In general, a known force is applied and the resulting deformation measured, either of the whole structure (i.e. the whole bone) or just across the fracture site itself. (This is clearly not the only

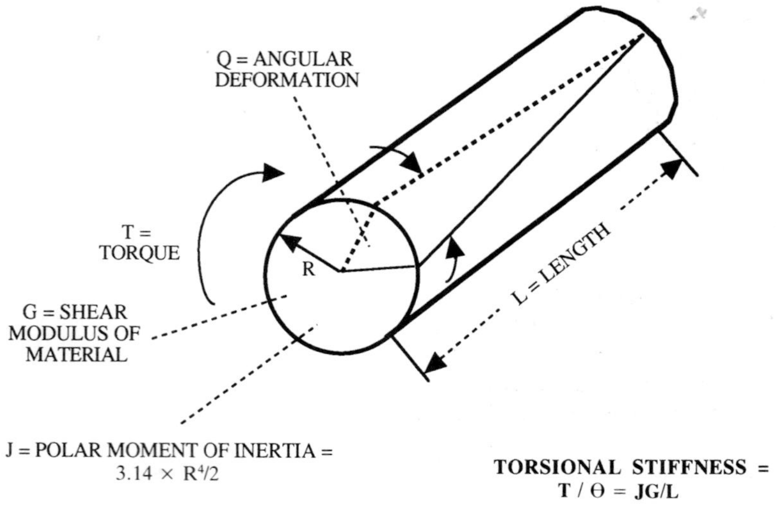

Figure 1.13

When torque is applied to a shaft or rod, angular deformation results (shown here as the difference between two lines drawn along the surface of the shaft and extending across the cross section, one before loading (dotted) and one after loading (solid)). The relationship between torsional stiffness and length, polar moment of inertia and shear modulus in a shaft is given.

consideration in selecting an implant, but does provide an indication as to the load it will bear and the resulting motion at the fracture site.)

The *axial stiffness* of a construct (Figure 1.14) is the magnitude of the applied axial load divided by the resulting linear deformation. Similarly, the *torsional stiffness* is the torque applied divided by the resulting angular deformation. The *torsional rigidity* can be found by dividing the stiffness by the length of the shaft so that it is normalized for length. *Normalization* allows the removal of additional variables in testing. *Bending stiffness* of a fracture construct is usually expressed as the bending moment divided by the resulting deformation (usually at the point of loading), or the angulation of the beam, as shown in Figure 1.14. The *flexural rigidity*, similar to the torsional rigidity, normalizes bending stiffness by the geometry of the beam, which includes the length of the span and the location of the applied forces.

These measures are very useful in comparing the performance of different implants and methods of fracture fixation. By normalizing the stiffness of constructs to the stiffness of intact bones, the rigidity of the fixation can be expressed as a *percent intact stiffness*.

1.7 Viscoelastic and nonlinear properties

Viscoelastic phenomena can affect the structural properties of a fracture fixation construct. If an implant must rely partly on loads generated in soft

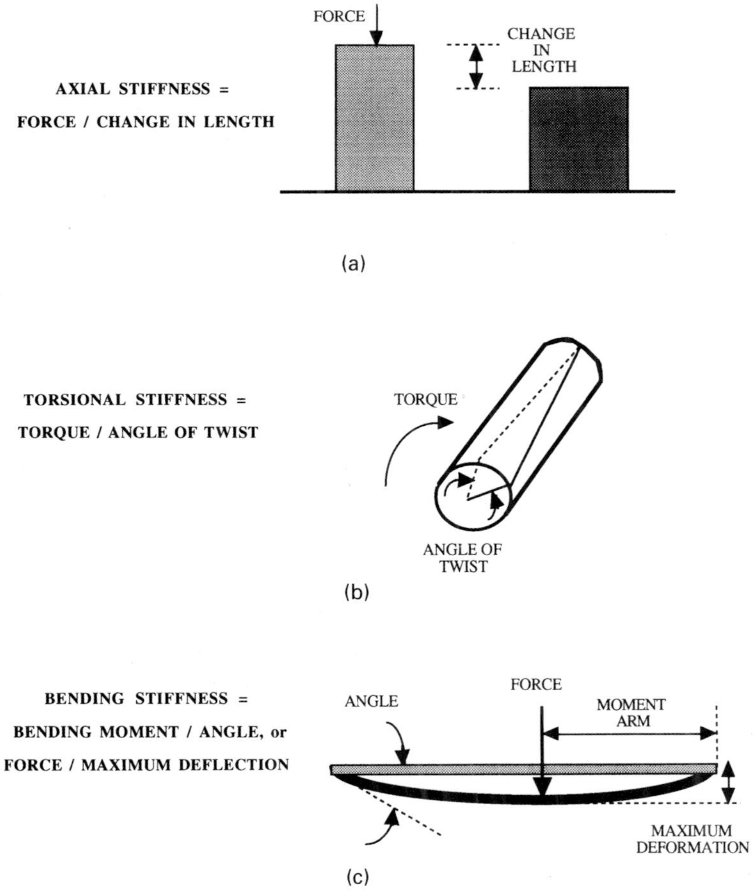

Figure 1.14

(a) Axial, (b) torsional, and (c) bending stiffnesses of a fracture-fixation construct based on measurement of deformations under known loads.

tissue, such as in a Harrington distraction rod system for spine fracture (see Chapter 8), soft tissue viscoelastic effects may need to be considered. *Viscous effects*, as opposed to a purely elastic response, result in permanent deformation under an applied load. As seen in Figure 1.15, an example of this is the (simplified) shock absorber of a car. This device allows oil to flow through a small orifice when a load is applied. When the load is released, the oil does not flow back through the orifice, so, unlike a spring, the deformation is not recovered when the load is released. In a vehicle suspension system the shock absorber lessens the movement of the suspended mass (i.e. the body of the car) in response to impacts acting against the wheels, by acting as an energy absorbing link between wheels and body. (In an actual shock absorber the fluid is pumped back and forth between chambers as the device extends and shortens.)

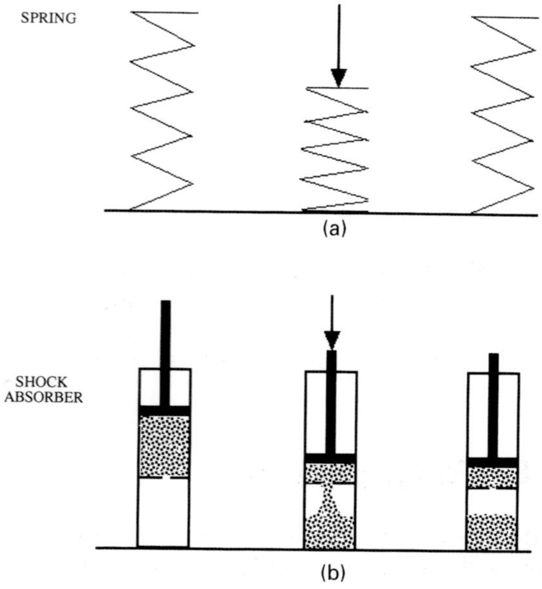

Figure 1.15

Two basic mechanical elements deforming under an applied load. (a) The spring returns to its original shape after the load is released. (b) The shock absorber (e.g. of a car) acts as a viscous element by forcing oil through an orifice, which produces a nonrecoverable deformation upon release of a load.

Viscous properties are also time dependent, as opposed to elastic properties, which are independent of the rate of the applied load. Considering the shock absorber of Figure 1.15 again, if the load is applied slowly relative to the rate at which the oil can pass through the orifice, the piston will move downward. (Note that this rate depends on the viscosity of the oil and the size of the orifice through which it must pass.) If the load is applied rapidly, there will not be sufficient time for much oil to flow through the orifice, and the piston will move very little. The compressive stiffness of the system is therefore changed.

Soft tissues have both elastic (recoverable deformation, time independent) and viscous (nonrecoverable deformation, time dependent) properties. Viscous properties are exhibited in two main forms. *Creep* is the continuous deformation under an applied load (Figure 1.16a). The best example of this is the effect of stretching one's back before exercise, which allows some of us to reach down and eventually touch our toes. In this form of viscous behavior, the applied load, the weight of the torso, is constant and the deformation unlimited. The second form of viscous behavior is *stress relaxation* (Figure 1.16b). In this case a load is applied and the initial deformation maintained. The internal force in the tissue decreases over time. Again, if one stretches (say the hamstrings) to a certain point and holds that position, the tension in muscle and tendon can be felt to decrease with time.

Viscoelastic properties can have important effects when soft tissue tension is used in the fixation of fractures. A clear example is, as mentioned above, the distraction of the spine against its own soft tissue elements for fixation of certain fracture patterns (to be discussed in detail in Chapter 8). A decrease in tension in soft tissues can change the stiffness of the fixation dramatically. Also, viscoelastic properties influence the response of bone to loading. *Strain rate* is the rate of elongation of a material, (change in length/original length)/time, which depends upon the *loading rate*. As strain rate increases, trabecular bone has been found to become stiffer in compression. The fat, marrow, and water that fill the spaces within trabecular bone may form a mechanism similar to that of the shock absorber

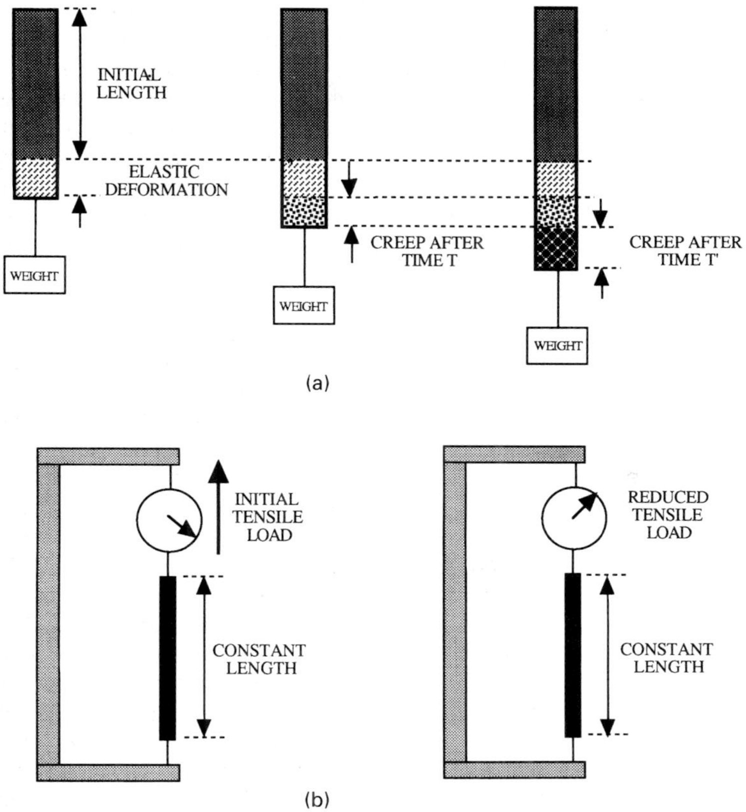

Figure 1.16

(a) Creep, or continued deformation over time under a constant load. (b) Stress relaxation, or decrease in internal load over time at a constant deformation.

discussed above. It is hypothesized that at higher loading rates, especially at load magnitudes that can cause large deformations in trabecular bone, the viscosity of fat and marrow relative to the sizes of the intertrabecular spaces and the rate at which the structure deforms, results in increases in the internal pressure and the stiffening of the structure (Figure 1.17).

A second complicating factor in fracture fixation constructs is *frictional slip. Friction* is very important in resisting motion in fractures. For example, a screw holds a plate against bone by generating a force between the plate and bone. The plate does not slip, because of its frictional contact with the bone surface. Similarly, a nonlocked intramedullary nail deforms as it is inserted into the femoral canal, and develops frictional resistance against the medullary bone, which aids in resistance to motion. A K-wire, especially one that is smooth, can only stay in place due to frictional contact with bone. Motion between surfaces with friction between them, unlike elastic deformation, is nonrecoverable.

1.8 Fatigue failure

Fatigue is a process of slow progressive failure, as opposed to catastrophic failure caused by exceeding the ultimate strength of the material. Typically, repetitive cyclic loading causes progression of a crack through a material (Figure 1.18), resulting ultimately in separation of the object into two pieces. The crack may start at a *stress concentrator* or a *stress riser*, such as at an indentation, scratch, hole, or corner (Figure 1.19). The stresses near these areas can locally be considerably

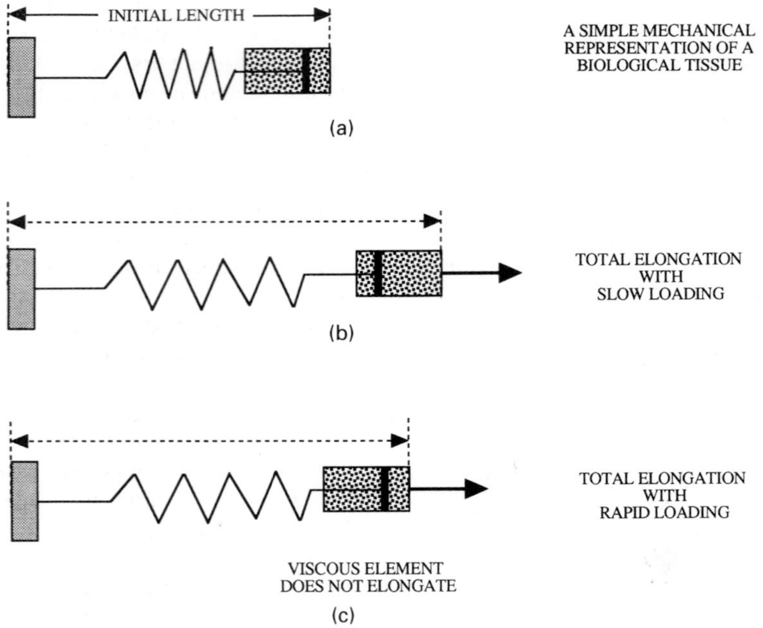

Figure 1.17

The effect of strain rate on a very simplified representation of bone having an elastic and a viscous element. (a) The unloaded system. (b) Under slow loading, the elastic and viscous elements both deform. (c) Under rapid loading, the viscous element cannot respond as quickly; therefore the total elongation is less, and the tissue appears to be stiffer.

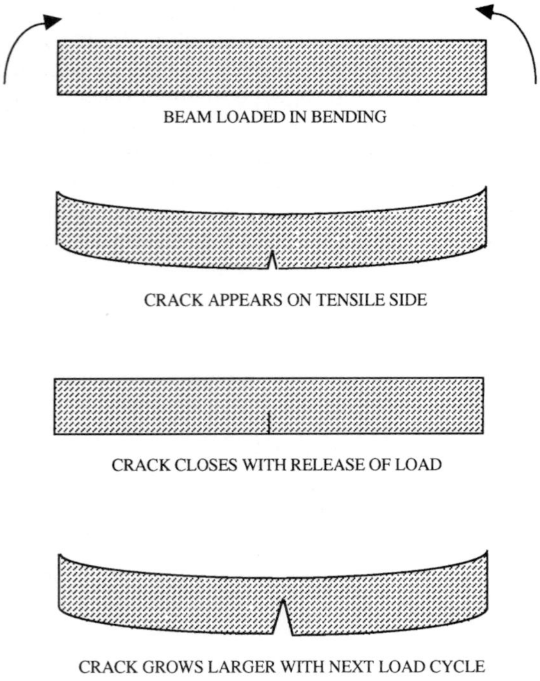

Figure 1.18

Repetitive loading, below failure load, results in the progression of a crack through the material, and ultimate separation into two pieces.

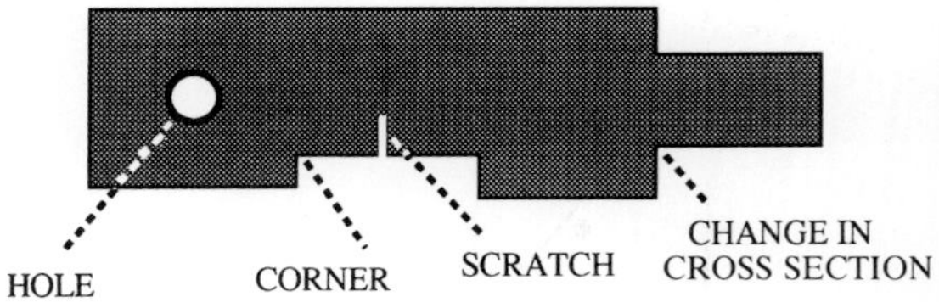

Figure 1.19

Stress concentrators (stress risers) produce increased local stresses, which may be several times higher than those in the bulk of the material, and may lead to local failure. Stress concentrators may result from corners, holes, scratches, or changes in cross section, or may be due to gouging between moving components.

greater than the average stress in the material; thus local material failure occurs in this region, and ultimately a crack progresses through the cross section.

The *stress concentration factor* (ratio of the maximum stress at the surface irregularity to the average stress in the same direction) depends on the geometry of the surface. For example, the stress concentration factor around a distal locking screw hole in an intramedullary nail subjected to bending could range from about 1.9 (hole diameter/rod diameter = 0.30) to nearly 3 (hole diameter/rod diameter < 0.01). Following this, one would be led to conclude that a larger hole in the nail is beneficial, since the stress concentration will be lessened. However, the average stress in the cross section containing the hole will increase with hole diameter because the surface area in the plane through the hole is decreased. The actual selection of hole diameter requires consideration of these factors, as well as the required strength of the screw to be placed through the hole.

The *fatigue life* of an implant in a physiological environment is complicated by at least three additional factors besides the geometry of the stress concentrator. These are motion between objects, such as a screw head on a plate, the materials used in the implant and their ability to resist corrosion, and the composition of the surrounding physiological fluids. Motion between implant components causes actual gouging of the surface, resulting in a stress concentrator, and removes the passive oxide layer on one surface, permitting *galvanic corrosion.* This type of corrosion occurs when two dissimilar materials are present in an electrolytic solution, with one acting as an anode (which gives up material) and the other as a cathode (which receives material) (see Chapter 5 for more details). Material may be removed from the tip of the crack by galvanic corrosion, further enhancing its movement across the cross section and increasing the prospect for failure.

Cyclic loading is performed to determine the resistance of a material to fatigue failure. This is typically done by applying a cyclic bending moment or tensile/compressive force to a specimen up to a predetermined stress or strain limit, and recording the number of cycles to failure. The result of these experiments is a plot of stress versus number of cycles to failure, an *S–N* plot (Figure 1.20). The *average stress range* plotted is the average of the maximum stress − minimum stress. The *S–N* plot provides a statistical estimate of the likelihood of failure at different mean stress levels.

Several important factors can influence the number of cycles to failure at a given stress level. As discussed above, these include the condition and geometry of the surface of the specimen and the surrounding environment. Also, the magnitude of the *mean stress level* of the test can influence the number of cycles to failure. As distinguished from the average stress range used to plot the *S–N* curve, which defines the range of

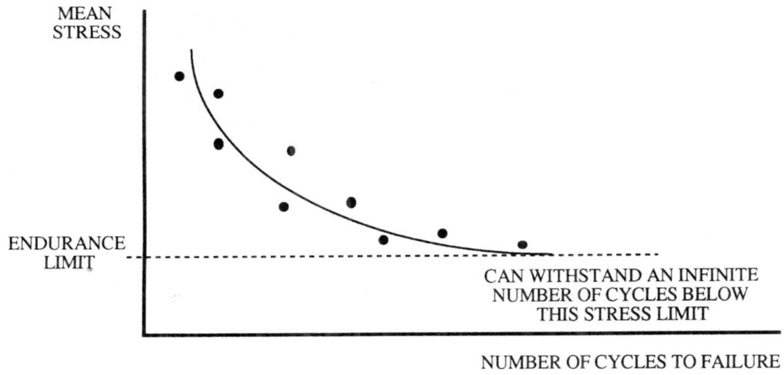

Figure 1.20

An *S–N* (mean stress versus number of cycles to failure) curve showing the endurance limit below which the material can resist an infinite number of cycles without failing.

stress, the mean stress (average of maximum stress + minimum stress) defines the average magnitude of the applied stress. The important point of this discussion is that for a higher mean applied stress, for the same stress range, the fatigue life can be considerably shortened. An implication of this discussion concerns the decision about when full weight bearing can be tolerated, say for a femur fracture fixed with an intramedullary nail. Moving from partial or non-weightbearing to weightbearing of a fracture in which load sharing by bone is not confirmed will increase both the range and the mean stress applied to the implant, and shorten its fatigue life beyond that which might be expected from benchtop fatigue testing results.

Some materials possess an *endurance or fatigue limit* (Figure 1.20), which is a stress level below which they can endure an infinite number of cycles without failing. Typically, some steels exhibit this behavior; however, nonferrous materials such as aluminium do not. Further, the testing environment can significantly influence the fatigue behavior of a material. Considering the environment, the potential for damage during insertion, and the variability of stresses applied, it is best to consider that most orthopedic implants do not have an established endurance limit, and, unless stress protected by healing bone, are ultimately prone to fatigue failure.

1.9 Principles of biomechanical testing

The testing of a fracture construct is relatively straightforward. However, as with all experimental testing, attention to detail is important in obtaining reliable, high quality results. This section is written as a guide to allow the reader to view the results of such tests with a critical eye.

Typically, questions are raised regarding the comparative rigidity and strength offered by different forms of fixation. Biomechanical testing attempts to provide an objective answer to some of these questions. Results of these experiments, as the reader will see, are prevalent throughout this volume. This testing aims to address concerns of strength and stiffness (relative motion between bone fragments) of fixation. In later chapters, others factors related to fracture healing will be addressed. Some of these include preserving blood supply to the healing area, minimizing further disruption of the injured area when implanting the fixation, offering both adequate stabilization of the fracture components and reasonable strength for load bearing, and preventing stress shielding of the underlying tissues. Biomechanical testing can obviously answer only some aspects of these questions.

All testing should be performed using accurately *calibrated* instrumentation. Calibration involves comparison of the accuracy of measurement transducers to some reproducible standard. *Reproducibility* of the test results is important to demonstrate the reliability of the methodology, and identify any unsuspected sources of error. The best determination of reproducibility is to measure values in one testing session, then refreeze, thaw, and setup specimens, repeat the test, and compare the results. This should indicate the inherent errors in the methodology and allow differentiation between real differences and experimental variation.

Consideration must be given to minimizing any changes occurring during testing. A typical example is maintaining tissue water content to minimize dehydration of bone. Loss of *tissue hydration* significantly affects the properties of bone and soft tissues. *Randomizing* the sequence of implant placement or procedures eliminates bias that could be caused by such events as bone breakdown, screw loosening, etc. Comparative testing using the same specimen as its own control usually reduces *variability* in the results. Another source of variability may involve surgical technique, particularly the placement of screws in bone of different density. This can be standardized by the use of cutting and alignment jigs, and consideration of the use of other materials that simulate the material properties of bone but are relatively uniform. An example is the use of porous foams to simulate trabecular bone.

A typical test would involve defining the directions and magnitudes of loads that a fixation system must resist in vivo, and choosing an appropriate testing model. The model most frequently chosen is a cadaver specimen of the region to be studied, which reproduces the anatomy and the properties of bony attachments. The main disadvantage of this model is the inevitable differences in properties between specimens, which creates variability that can obscure differences due to the implant or technique. After defining the loads to be applied and implants to be tested, a jig is built that will firmly attach one component of the model to the test table. The other component is fixed to the testing apparatus (see Figure 1.4), and typically compressive, torsional, and/or bending loads are applied to represent those considered to occur physiologically. Good experimental design consists of utilizing sufficient samples to obtain statistically meaningful differences. A convenient way of presenting results is to compare the stiffness of a fracture/bone construct with the intact bone. This normalizes the data to that specimen (for example, if one specimen has considerably softer bone than another), and presents the data in what may be a more clinically meaningful way, as a percent of the intact stiffness of the specimen.

1.10 Further reading

This chapter is meant to provide only a brief review of the basics of biomechanics as applied to bone fracture and fixation. The following further reading is suggested.

For basic biomechanics with clinical application:

Cochran GVB, *A primer of orthopaedic biomechanics* (Churchill Livingstone: Edinburgh and London 1982).

For basic biomechanical principles with an engineering orientation:

Ozkaya N, Nordin M, *Fundamentals of biomechanics* (Van Nostrand Reinhold: New York 1991).

For a more advanced understanding of the fundamentals of tissue properties:

Fung YC, *Biomechanics. Mechanical properties of living tissues* (Springer-Verlag: New York 1981).

For an advanced understanding of tissue properties as well as applications to prosthetics, fracture devices, gait, and other tissues in orthopedic biomechanics:

Mow VC, Hayes WC, *Basic orthopedic biomechanics* (Raven Press: New York 1991).

For a basic understanding of the engineering principles of statics:

Anand DK, Cunnif PF, *Engineering mechanics, statics and dynamics* (Allyn and Bacon: Needham Heights 1984).

For an understanding of materials in orthopedic surgery:

Black J, *Orthopaedic biomaterials in research and practice* (Churchill Livingstone: Edinburgh and London 1988).

1.11 Units

The information provided in the following chapters is quantitative; the data are therefore reported in standard units. The following are commonly used:

Force: Newton = 0.1 kilogram = 0.22 pounds force = 0.1 kilopond (kp)

Pressure or stress: force/area = Newton/metre^2. 1 N/m^2 = 1 Pascal (Pa); 10^3N/m^2 = 1 kilo Pascal (kPa); 10^6N/m^2 = 1 N/mm^2 = 1 Mega Pascal (MPa); 1 N/m^2 = $1*10^{-4}$ pounds/in^2 (psi); 10^9 N/m^2 = 1 Giga Pascal (GPa)

Moment: force * moment arm distance (Newton-meter, N-m)

Axial stiffness: force/deformation (N/mm)

Torsional stiffness: torque/angular deformation (N-m/deg)

Bending stiffness: bending load/deformation (N/mm), bending moment/angular deformation (N-m/deg)

Bending rigidity: modulus of material × moment of inertia of the beam (E × I) or (stiffness) × (geometric property of the beam, depends on type of loading, position of load, length of span) (N-m^2)

Elastic modulus: stress/strain (N/m^2), (MPa), (GPa)

Moment of inertia: m^4, mm^4.

CHAPTER 2

Factors affecting the strength of bone

This chapter deals with the basic structure of bone and how various factors affect its mechanical properties. Topics include the effects of structural parameters such as the mineral content of bone, and its collagen lamellar structure, density, and trabecular orientation. External effects such as bone age, the rate of load application, the presence of holes or defects, and the extent of use are discussed next. Mechanical property values for bone as a material as well as the strengths of whole bones are then given.

2.1 The hierarchical structure of bone

Before considering the mechanisms of fracture and the principles of stabilizing bone to allow its repair, it is important to understand the structure of bone and the factors that affect its strength. As shown in Figure 2.1, bone can be thought of as having several levels of structure. At its most fundamental level, hydroxyapatite crystals are embedded predominantly between the ends of adjoining collagen fibrils. This composite of rigid (hydroxyapatite) and flexible (collagen) components provides a material that is superior in properties to either alone. Bone is more ductile than hydroxyapatite, allowing the absorption of greater energy before failure, and more rigid than collagen, permitting greater load bearing and stiffness.

At the second level of structure, the collagen/hydroxyapatite fibrils are formed into sheets or lamellae with, in the case of mature bone, a preferred direction. The orientations of the fibers define directions of maximum and minimum strengths for a primary loading direction (Figure 2.2).

The third level of structure consists of the arrangement of the lamellae (Figure 2.2). A circular concentric structure produces a tubular haversian osteon with maximum strength along its long axis and equal but lower strength perpendicular to its circumference. Alternately, lamellae may be arranged in sheets, as found in plexiform bone, in which case the strength of the material transverse to the longitudinal axis is lower in the direction in which lamellae are being pulled apart at cement lines than in the plane of the sheets.

The fourth level of structure is the macroscopic material that results – either cortical or trabecular bone. The overriding factor governing strength at this level is the density of the material, and, for trabecular bone, its trabecular orientation. The following sections will examine the influences of these factors and others on the strength of bone in detail.

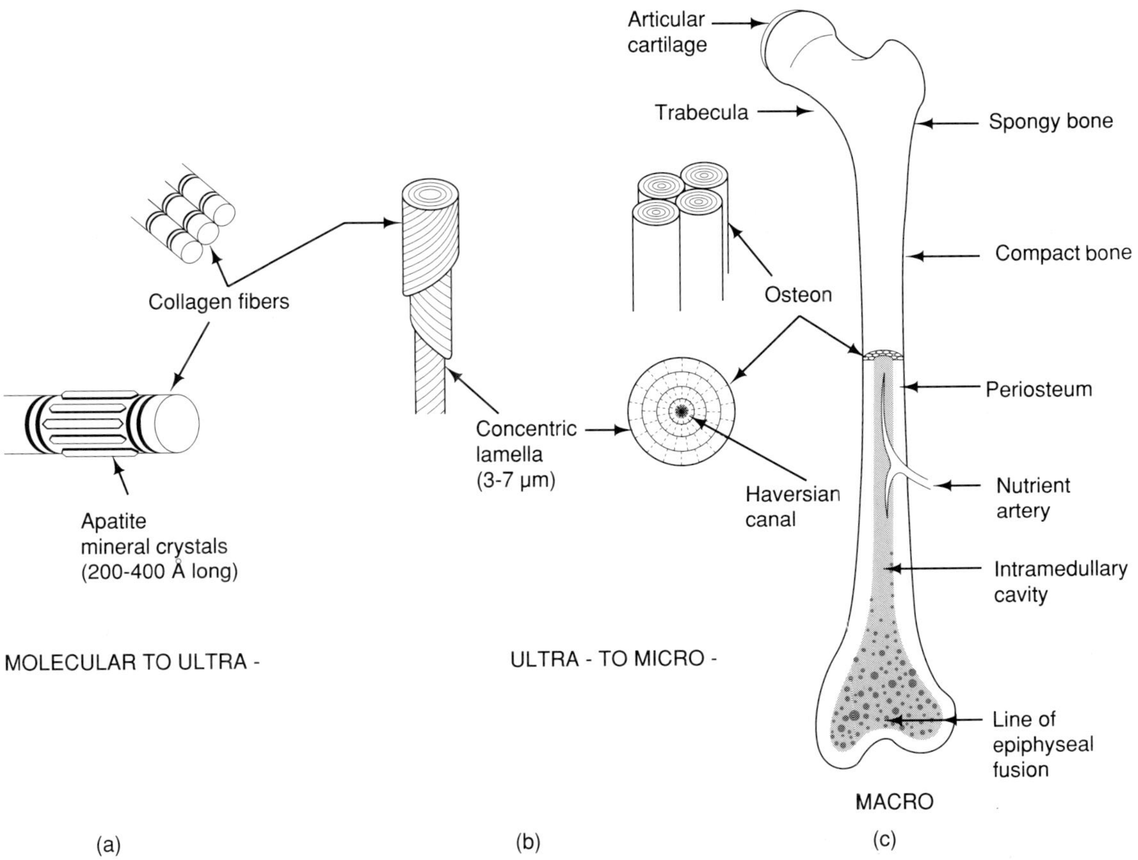

Figure 2.1

The structure of bone defining the different levels. (a) The first level is a material composed of hydroxyapatite crystals embedded between collagen fibrils. (b) The second level is an arrangement of the fibrils into sheets or lamellae with a preferred orientation. (c) In long bones, the third level consists of an arrangement of lamellae into tubular osteons (or flat sheets), which form the basic structure of cortical and trabecular bone. (Adapted from Katz JL, Composite material models for cortical bone. In: Cowin SC, ed, *Mechanical properties of bone* (Applied Mechanics Division of the American Society of Mechanical Engineers, AMD Vol 45: New York 1981) 171–84.)

2.2 The mineral/collagen ratio

At the most fundamental structural level, the ratio of mineral to collagen affects mechanical properties. Burstein et al[1] showed that progressive decalcification decreased the yield and ultimate strengths of bone in tension, as well as its modulus (Figure 2.3). Complete elimination of the mineral content reduced the behavior of bone to that similar to collagenous tissue (Figure 2.4). The transition from a stiffer elastic region to a less stiff plastic region was lost with complete removal of the mineral component, and the slope of the plastic region of the mineralized tissue was identical to the slope in the elastic region of the unmineralized tissue.[1] This shows that the collagen component is primarily responsible for deformation of bone after yield, and that the hydroxyapatite contributes significantly to increased stiffness.

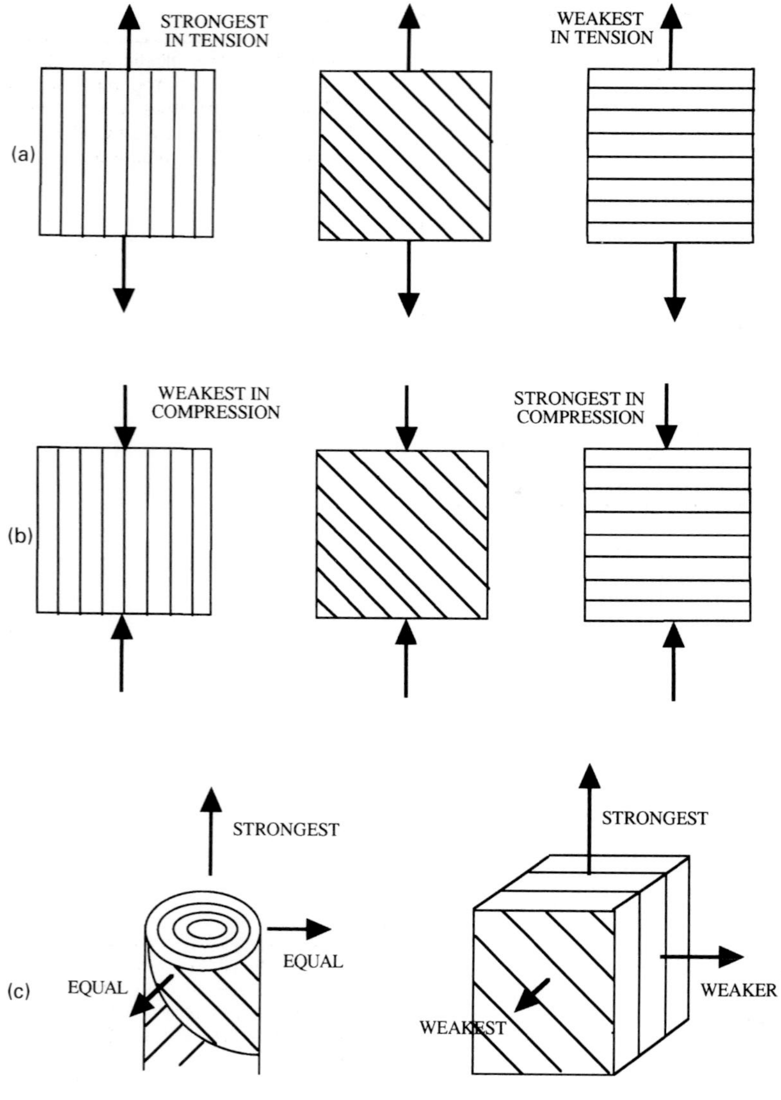

Figure 2.2

The orientation of the load with respect to the preferred direction of fibers of a lamella affects the strength of the material. (a) In tension, the strongest arrangement has fibers parallel to the applied load. (b) In compression, the strongest arrangement has fibers perpendicular to the applied load. (c) The type of packing of lamellae also affects strength transverse to the longitudinal axis. Tubular osteons have equal strength in all transverse directions. Parallel lamellae have different strengths in different transverse directions.

The role of type 1 collagen in determining the properties of bone has recently been shown, using a strain of mutant mouse, whose collagen gene was blocked.[2] Decreasing the amount of collagen in bone significantly alters its postyield behavior. Specifically, the displacement in the plastic region diminishes, and the fracture toughness (ability to absorb energy before failure) is decreased, as is the tissue strength. Thus decreasing the collagen content results in the identical effect as increasing the mineral/collagen ratio.

Small variations in the mineral content of bone (from 63% to 71%) have been shown to produce large variations in properties such as breaking stress (which increased from 6.5 kg/mm^2 to 23 kg/mm^2) and modulus of elasticity.[3] Also, increasing percent calcium from 20% to 27% has been shown

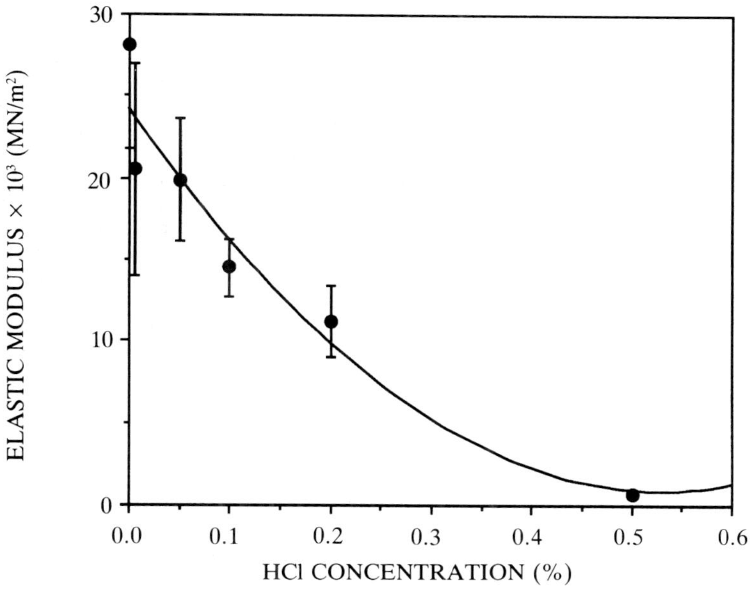

Figure 2.3

Change in tensile elastic modulus of bone samples after progressive decalcification to remove the mineral component by increasing the HCl concentration. (Data adapted from Ref 1.)

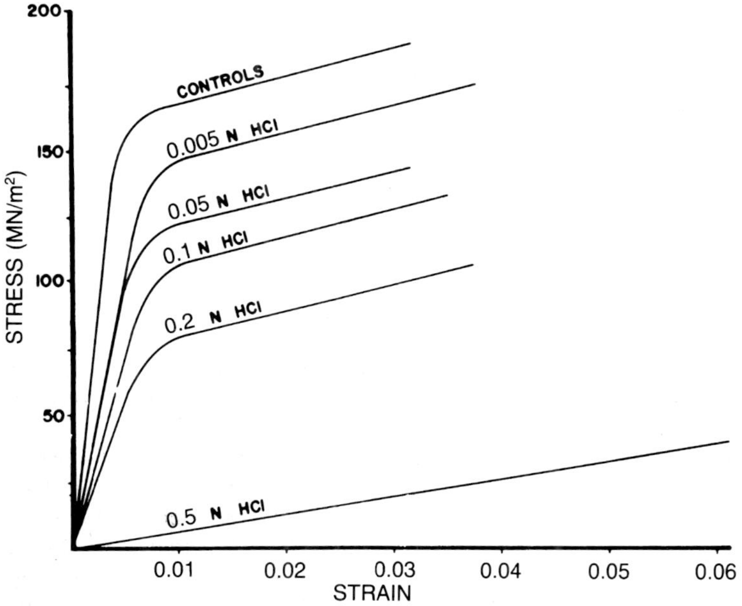

Figure 2.4

Stress/strain characteristics of bone samples in tension with progressively lower mineral content (indicated by higher concentrations of HCl decalcifying solution). With complete decalcification, the slope of the material is similar to that of the mineralized bone after yield, showing how collagen contributes to the plastic behavior of bone and hydroxyapatite to stiffening the material. (From Ref 1 with permission.)

to decrease the impact energy absorption of bone by almost a factor of 10, as demonstrated in Figure 2.5. Hypermineralized bone has reduced energy absorption capability and becomes more prone to brittle failure.[4] This fact has been proposed to explain the increased fracture incidence of bone in the elderly.

2.3 Osteon structure and organization

Considering the second level of bone structure, the effects of orientation of collagen fibers in lamellae that form osteons have been investigated. A smaller spiral angle of the collagen fibers in haversian osteons (i.e. more circumferentially oriented) results in greater osteonal compressive strength and stiffness, while a larger collagen fiber angle (more longitudinally oriented) has been shown to increase tensile strength.[5–11] This is because, as shown in Figure 2.2, the fiber orientation for optimal resistance of tension should be along the long axis of the bone for maximum strength, while for compression, fibers should be perpendicular to the applied load.

In shear, the cementitious regions between osteons have been found to be stronger than the bone lamellae.[10] The shear strength of single osteons is much lower than their tensile or compressive strengths. Understanding the structure of bone at this level helps to explain its anisotropic properties (i.e. differing strengths in different loading directions), its strength being greatest in compression, followed by tension, and finally shear (Figure 2.6).

The collagen fiber orientation has also been shown to affect the types of fractures that occur.[9] As shown in Figure 2.7, loading in compression across an osteon produces a circumferential crack in those whose lamellar fibres alternate at an angle of about 90°. This indicates that the weak links in the structure are the interlamellar bonds. In osteons whose lamellae are primarily longitudinal, cracks occur radially. The weak links in this structure are the bonds between the longitudinally oriented fibers within the lamellae.

The "packing" of haversian systems, a function of the diameter of the individual osteons, has also been demonstrated to affect the properties of bone. For example, Evans[5] found that fibular bone was stronger than femoral bone in tension, which was attributed to the fibula possessing a larger number of smaller diameter osteons than the femur, allowing for closer packing between them and an effectively denser structure.

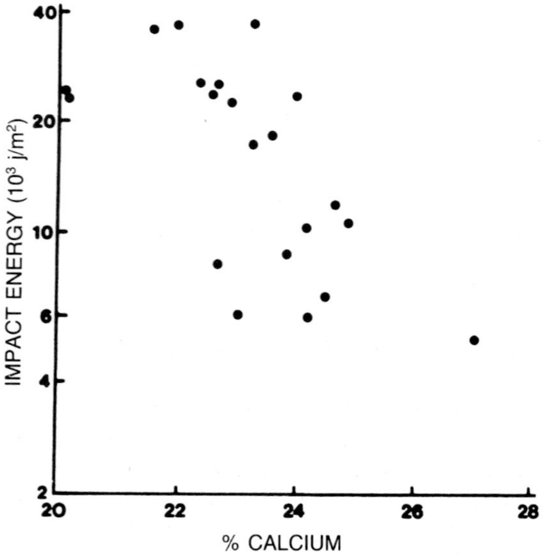

Figure 2.5

Increasing the percentage of calcium in bone significantly decreases its ability to absorb impact energy (or work). (From Ref 3 with permission.)

2.4 Bone porosity or density

Bone porosity is expressed as the percentage of mineralized tissue in a given volume. Bone density is defined as the weight of bone material per unit volume. Both have been used to determine the quantity of bone tissue in a sample. Carter and Hayes[12] as well as others[13–17] have shown a strong correlation between bone density and stiffness and strength of trabecular bone (Figure 2.8). The compressive strength of trabecular bone increases approximately with the square of its density. For example, doubling the density from

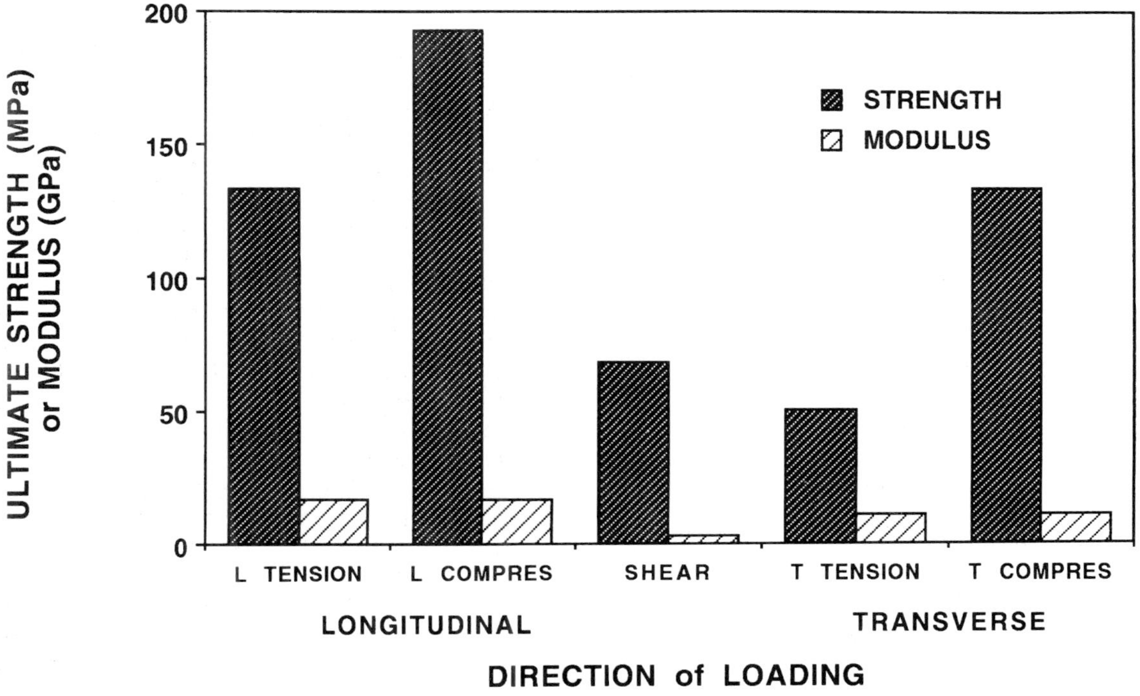

Figure 2.6

The strength of bone tissue is greatest in compression, followed by tension and then shear (data adapted from Reilly DT, Burstein AH, The elastic and ultimate properties of compact bone tissue, *J Biomech* (1975) **8:** 393–405).

0.2 to 0.4 gm/cm^3 results in a fourfold increase in strength.

Other studies have shown that the density of trabecular bone, as measured by noninvasive methods such as computed tomography (CT), is also strongly correlated with its strength (Figure 2.9).[18–22] This relationship may be very important in determining the holding power of fixation screws in trabecular bone, for example pedicle screws in lumbar vertebrae and cancellous screws in the femoral head, where the bone may be of questionable strength. Recent studies, to be described in detail later, show a significant dependence of screw pullout strength on bone porosity in cortical and cancellous bone.

Schaffler and Burr[23] found that the elastic modulus of cortical bone was also correlated with its porosity, although porosities of cortical bone are usually less than 15%, while for trabecular bone they may be as high as 70%.

2.5 Trabecular orientation

The previously discussed properties (mineral/collagen ratio, osteon structure, and bone density/porosity) are all inherent properties of bone as a material. The orientation of trabeculae influences the strength of bone as a structure in the same way as collagen fiber direction affects the strength of bone as a material. In vertebral bodies, as shown by Galante et al,[16] specimens loaded in an inferior to superior direction were more than two times as strong as those loaded lateral to medial or anterior to posterior (Figure 2.10). The

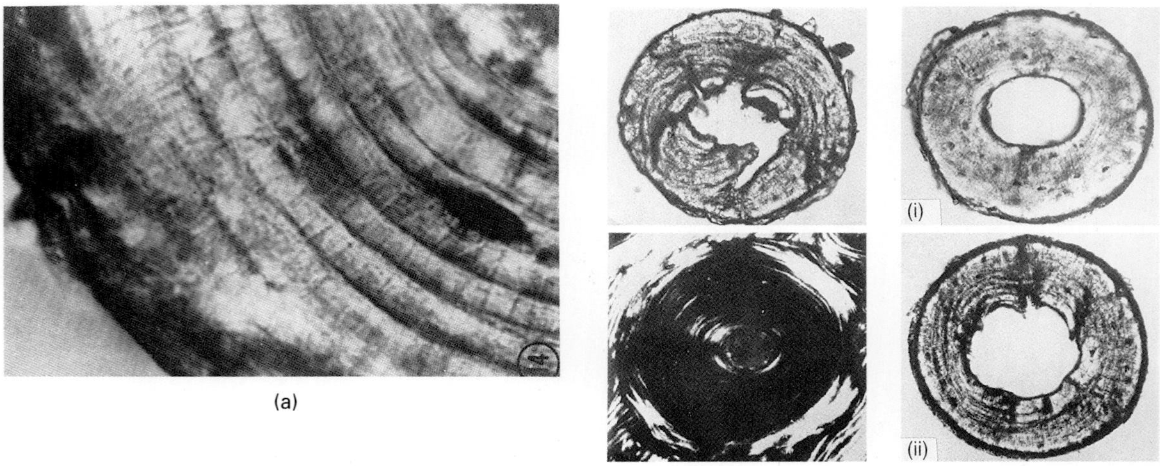

(a) (b)

Figure 2.7

(a) Loading an osteon by transverse compression shows delamination between lamellae. (b) (i) Compressive loading of an osteon with lamellae whose fibers are predominantly longitudinal results in radial cracks, indicating failure through lamellae. (ii) For an osteon loaded in compression, but having a greater fiber angle between successive lamellae (indicating that the lamellae are oriented more circumferential), cracks are circumferential, indicating that the interfaces between lamellae are the weak links. (From Ref 11 with permission.)

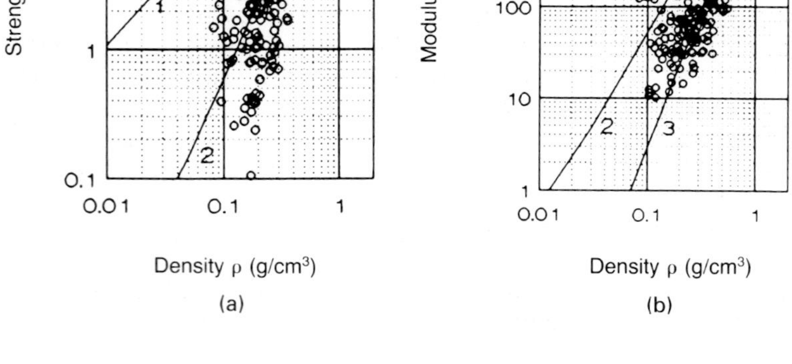

(a) (b)

Figure 2.8

(a) Power law relationship of compressive strength of trabecular bone samples and density (slope number indicates exponent). (b) Relationship between density and compressive elastic modulus. (From Hayes WC, Biomechanics of cortical and trabecular bone: implications for the assessment of fracture risk. In: Mow VC, Hayes WC, eds, *Basic orthopedic biomechanics* (Raven Press: New York 1991) 93–142, with permission.)

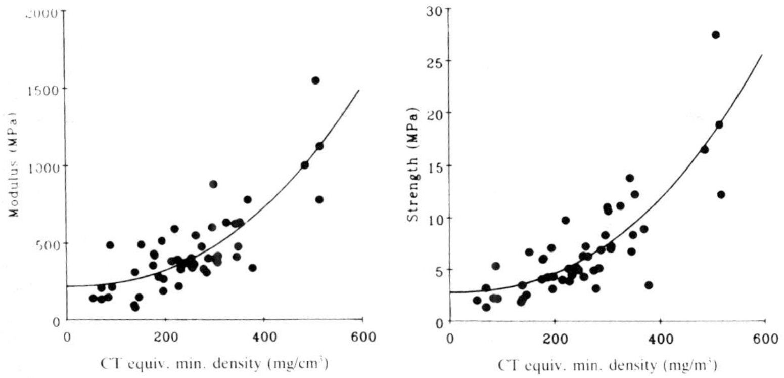

Figure 2.9

The relationship between bone density as determined noninvasively by computed tomography, and its compressive strength. (From Ref 18 with permission.)

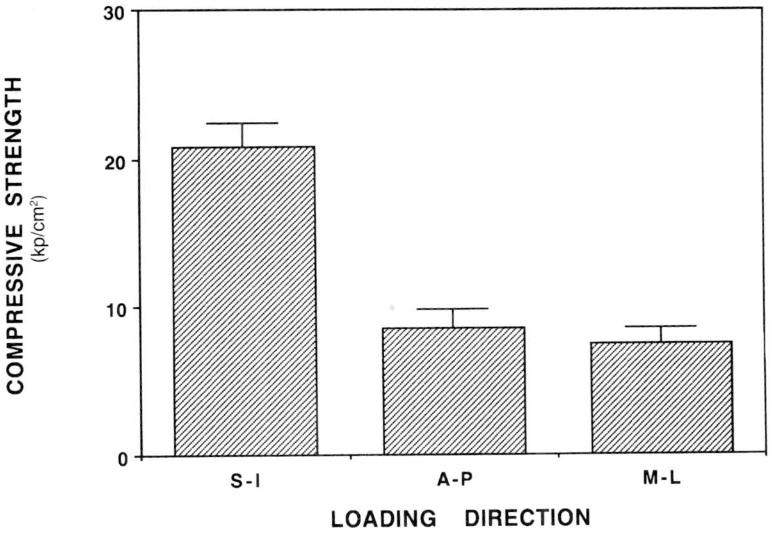

Figure 2.10

Effect of loading direction on the compressive strength of vertebral body trabecular bone. S–I, superior–inferior; A–P, anterior–posterior; M–L, medial–lateral. (Data adapted from Ref 16.)

major orientation of the trabecular architecture in the vertebra is vertical (axial), which corresponds to the major load direction–axial compression.

The laws of trabecular bone architecture were proposed by Wolff,[24] who observed similarities between the stress trajectories of a curved crane supporting a vertical load and the trabecular architecture of the proximal end of the femur. In an elegant study, Hayes and Snyder[25] compared finite element model calculations of principal stresses in the patella when loaded by the quadriceps musculature, and its trabecular architecture. They demonstrated that the trabeculae become optimally aligned so that they are oriented parallel and perpendicular to compressive loads, and at a 45° angle to shear loads (Figure 2.11). This arrangement minimizes bending of trabeculae and maximizes loading along their longitudinal axes.

2.6 Loading rate

The rate at which load is applied to bone has been shown in a number of studies[12,26–29] to be an

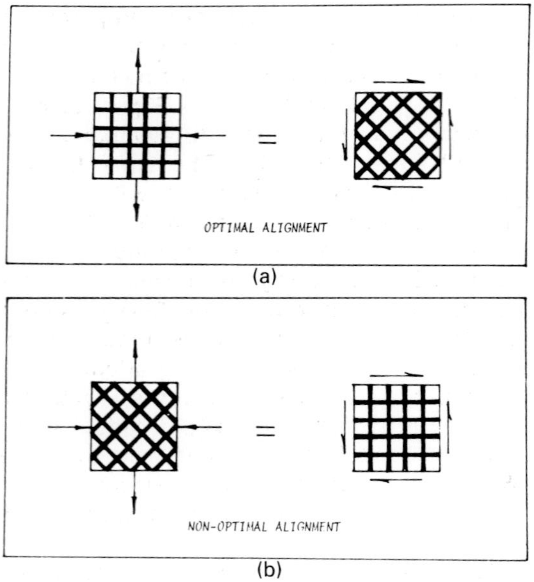

Figure 2.11

Wolff's law of trabecular architecture shows (a) optimal alignment of the trabeculae to resist compressive and tensile loads, which also produces optimal resistance to shear. This structural arrangement also minimizes bending in individual trabeculae. (b) A non-optimal arrangement of the trabeculae. (From Ref 25 with permission.)

important factor in determining the strength at which bone fails. McElhaney,[29] for example, showed a more than twofold increase in the stress to failure of human femoral samples over the range of strain rates tested, while Carter et al[50] showed similar behavior in both compact and trabecular bone (Figure 2.12). The mechanism that explains this phenomenon has been outlined in Chapter 1 (Figure 1.17); however, the specific elements contributing to this behavior are not known.

It is well known, however, that injuries involving ligaments may avulse the bony attachment in some cases and tear the ligament in others. In an injury involving a slowly applied load, the strength of bone in tension may be lower than that of the ligament, resulting in avulsion (i.e. fracture of the bone instead of the ligament). At a higher loading rate, the bone is effectively stronger, resulting in injury to the ligament (Figure 2.13).

2.7 Age

The well known clinical observation that children tend to have "greenstick" (ductile) type fractures[30]

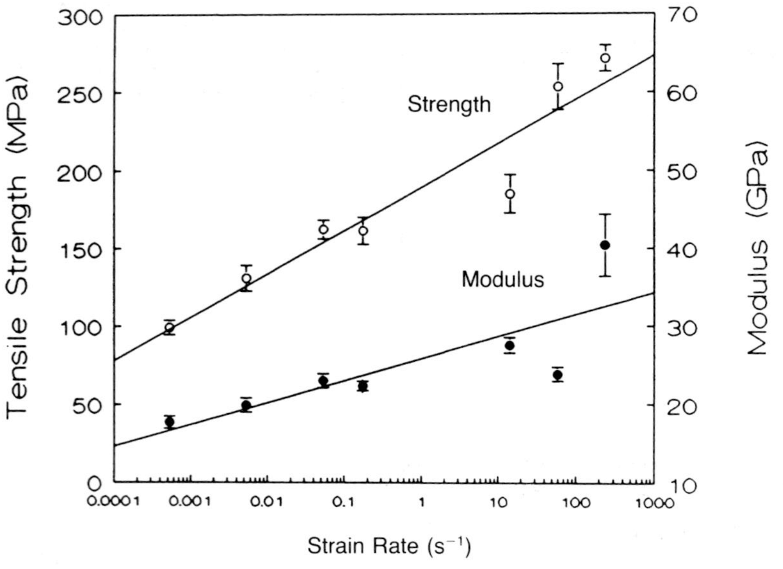

Figure 2.12

The effect of strain rate, (change in length/original length)/time (in units of s^{-1}), on compressive strength and elastic modulus of bone. (From Hayes WC, Biomechanics of cortical and trabecular bone: implications for the assessment of fracture risk. In: Mow VC, Hayes WC, eds, *Basic orthopedic biomechanics* (Raven Press: New York 1991) 93–142, with permission.)

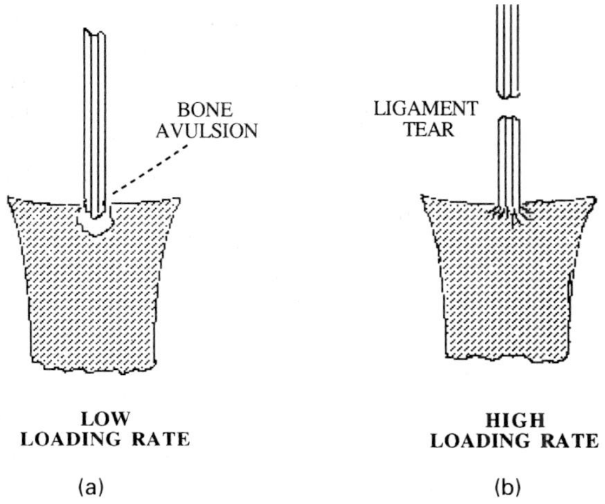

Figure 2.13

(a) Application of load at a low rate produces bone avulsion. (b) If the loading rate is higher, the bony attachment site becomes stronger and a ligament tear results.

involving considerable bending (plastic deformation) compared with adults who have more brittle failure of bone, demonstrates that significant differences exist in the mechanical properties of bone with age. This applies to the properties of bone both as a material and as a structure.

Bending strength and modulus (Figure 2.14) of bone increase from childhood to adulthood, then slowly decrease thereafter. The work (energy absorbed) to failure decreases with age in adulthood, as does the maximum deflection.[31,32] A decrease in maximum deflection indicates that the material is becoming less ductile, and as a result less able to absorb energy. Burstein et al[32] found that most of the tensile properties of femoral specimens decreased gradually with age. Most important were decreases in ultimate strain (5.1% mean decrease with decade, indicating less plastic deformation), and work to failure (6.8%), which imply that bone becomes more brittle with age and less able to absorb impact loads.[32]

At least two changes in bone can be attributed to altering the properties of bone with age. As a material, the ash content of bone, indicative of its mineral content, increases with age. As Curry[4] has shown, the energy absorbing properties of bone decrease with a rise in calcium content (Figure 2.5). Thus, in aging, bone becomes hypermineralized and as a result more brittle. A recently reported study has demonstrated that mineraliza-

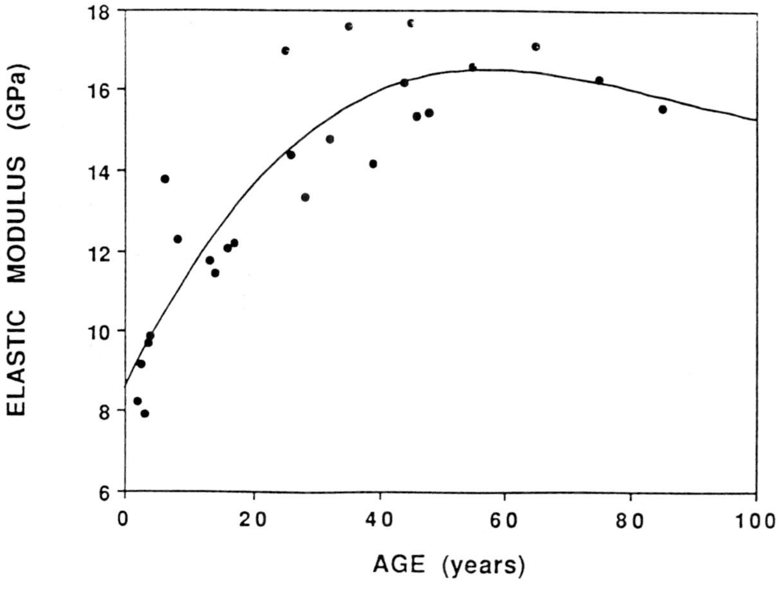

Figure 2.14

The elastic modulus of bone first increases towards adulthood, then slowly decreases with age. (Adapted from data given in Refs 31 and 32.)

tion in femoral specimens aged 60–75 years old is an average of 1.4 times higher than that in specimens aged 17–30.[33]

As a structure, bone density decreases, particularly in the trabecular bone of the vertebral bodies and femoral neck.[20–22] As shown in Figure 2.8, decreasing density significantly lowers bone strength. A further structural change affecting strength is the alteration of the cross sectional shape of the femur. While there appears to be no significant change in the geometry of the femur in males with aging, in females there is a significant enlargement of the femoral canal. Fink et al[34] have reported a mean 29% increase in the endosteal canal diameter and a concomitant 14% decrease in the periosteal diameter in femora from older (85 years) versus younger (54 years) females. This change in geometry significantly decreases the moment of inertia and the resulting strength of the bone in bending and torsion.[35]

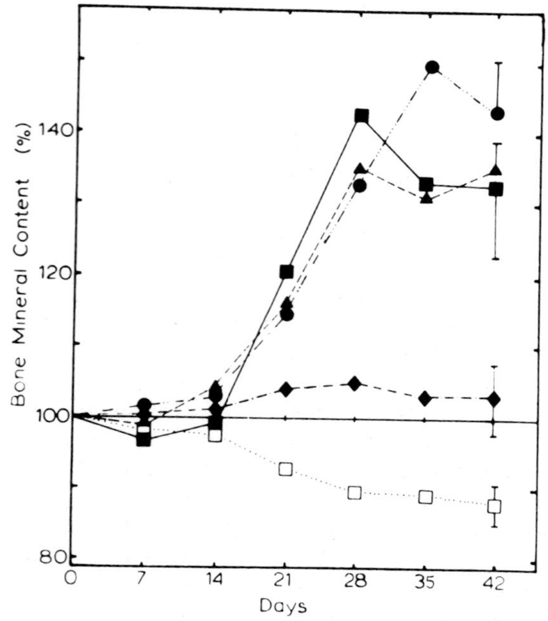

Figure 2.15

The response of bone to various loading regimens: 1800 (●), 360 (▲), 36 (■), 4 (◆), 0 (□) cycles per day of compressive strain applied to the midshaft of the turkey ulna at 0.5 Hz. (From Ref 36 with permission.)

2.8 Use and disuse

Bone responds to its functional level of use. Rubin and Laynon[36] have shown, in an avian model, that the bone mineral content decreased to 88% of normal after 42 days without functional load (Figure 2.15). This was due to thinning of the cortex, mainly by endosteal resorption. On the other hand, controlled cyclic loading, even at a rate as low as 36 cycles per day, produced a hypertrophic response, resulting in an increase of between 140% and 150% of normal bone mineral content. This new bone was deposited on the periosteal surfaces. Newer work has shown that at higher frequencies of application, smaller strain in the bone tissue is required to produce increases in bone mass.[37] In vivo correlation of this effect has been shown in the hypertrophy of the humeri in the playing arms of professional tennis players, compared with their contralateral humeri. In males, mean cross sectional changes ranged from 27% to 39%.[38]

2.9 Defects or holes

The effect of a defect or hole upon the strength of bone is well understood.[39–43] Both the size and shape of the defect affect the reduction in strength. The torsional strength of a long bone with an oval shaped defect is greater than one with a defect having sharp corners, due to the stress riser effect associated with sharper corners. The torsional strength is not greatly affected by the length of the defect.[39]

Holes drilled in bone decrease mechanical strength. McBroom et al[40] showed that the four point bending strength of long bones decreased to about 80% of normal for a hole of diameter equal to 10% of the bone cross sectional diameter. Alternatively, Edgerton et al[41] found no change in ultimate torque or energy to failure with holes of diameter less than 10% of the outer bone diameter (Figure 2.16). There was a sharp decrease in torsional strength when defect size surpassed 10%. For a hole whose diameter was 20% of bone diameter, torsional strength decreased to about 67% of normal.

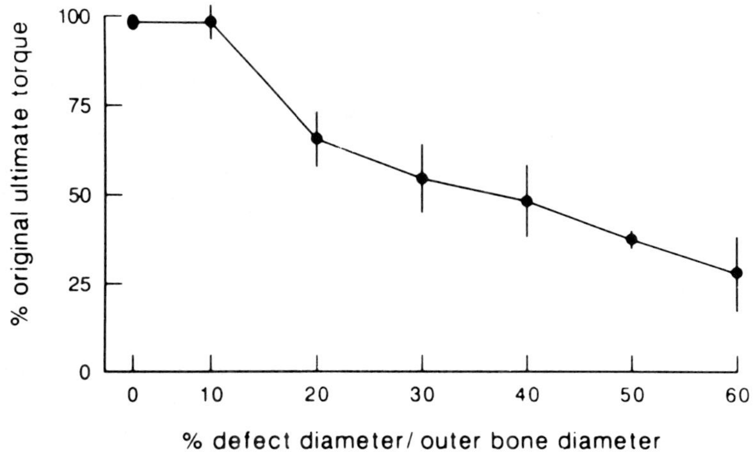

Figure 2.16

The relationship of ultimate torque, expressed as percent of intact bone to the ratio of hole diameter to bone cross sectional diameter. (From Ref 41 with permission.)

2.10 Fat and marrow

The effect of fat and marrow on bone properties is controversial. Pugh et al[44] showed that for frequencies of impact of up to 3000 Hz (normal running might result in a frequency of 3–6 Hz), trabecular bone could be considered as a purely elastic material, without any viscous effects. Swanson and Freeman[45] could detect no effect on mechanical properties of the femur due to marrow, which they simulated by filling dried bones with grease. However, more recent experiments, using intact cadaver proximal femora, have shown that stiffness in compression was greater with marrow present than when it was removed.[46]

Carter and Hayes[12] described trabecular bone as a two phase material, that is, a porous solid filled with a viscous liquid. At high strain rates only, they observed that the properties of bone were affected by the restriction of flow of marrow through intertrabecular spaces. In their experiments, both the stiffness and strength of trabecular bone increased in specimens under compression with marrow in place. In other words, as illustrated in Figure 2.17, forcing viscous fat and marrow through intertrabecular spaces at high rate relative to its viscosity and the size of the restrictions (i.e. spaces between the trabeculae) causes it to pressurize. Fluid under pressure acts as an additional load path, which increases the stiffness of the structure. As well, forcing pressurized marrow through restrictions absorbs energy. This mechanism may help to explain the observed increases in stiffness and strength of trabecular bone with increased strain rate, at least when it undergoes large deformations near failure.

2.11 The strength of bone material and whole bones

The properties of bone compared with other natural and artificial materials are shown in Figure 2.18.[47] Any material must have a compromise between stiffness and energy absorption. Higher stiffness is usually associated with lower deformation after yield and a lower capacity to absorb impact energy. Compared with other materials, as shown in Figure 2.18, bone has both intermediate strength and stiffness. Bone is unlike materials such as glass or concrete that, though very stiff, are brittle, and thus not particularly strong. Material properties for cortical and cancellous bone that are generally accepted in the literature are given in Table 2.1. In general, cortical bone is strongest in compression, followed by tension, and then shear (see also Figure 2.6). Cancellous bone as a material is both less stiff and less strong than cortical bone in compression.

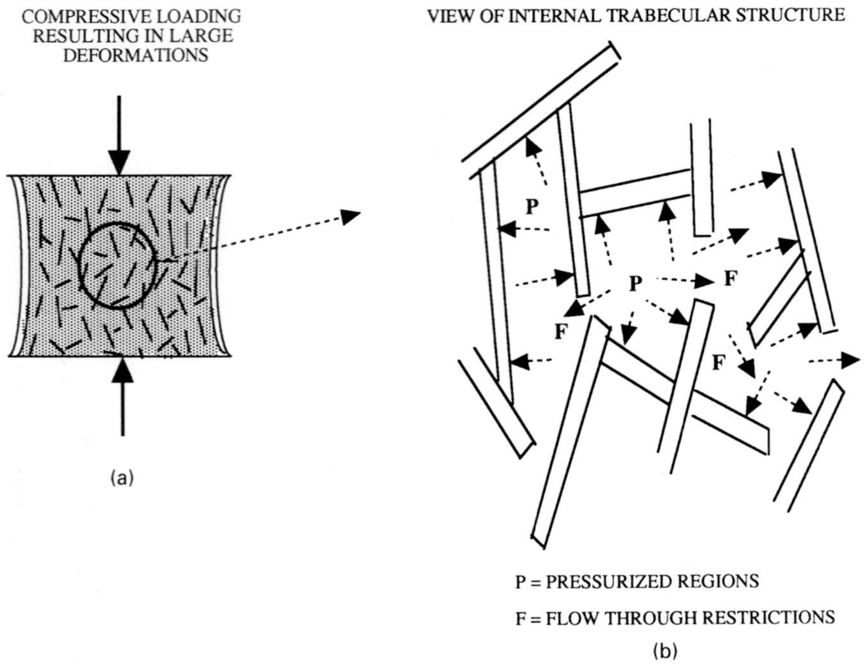

Figure 2.17

The possible role of fat and marrow in increasing the strength and stiffness of bone at high strain rates and large deformations. (a) A vertebral body under compressive load, showing trabecular architecture and marrow. (b) Enlarged view, showing pressurization of spaces between trabeculae and flow through pores.

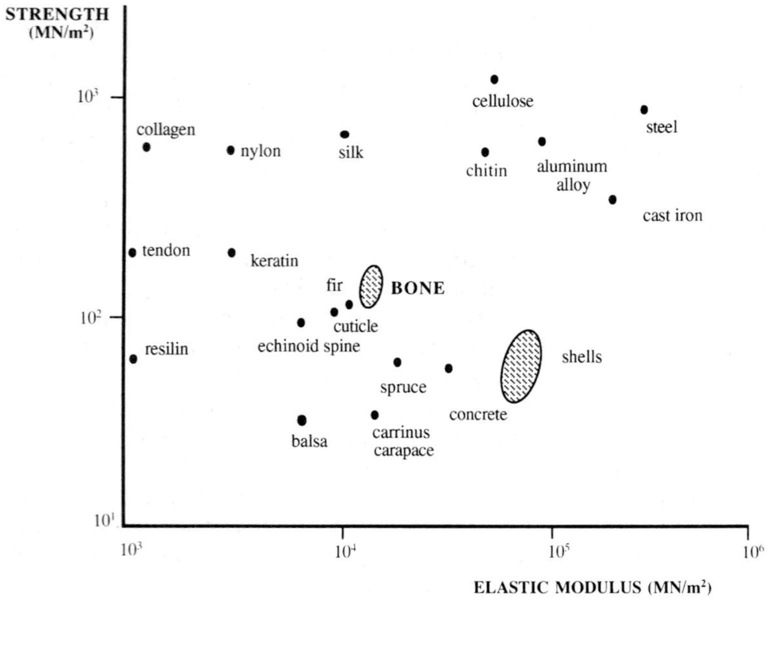

Figure 2.18

A plot of strength versus modulus for various natural and man-made materials showing the relative properties of bone. (Adapted from Ref 47.)

Table 2.1 Some properties of bone as a material.

Bone type	*Load type*	*Elastic modulus (10^9 N/m^2)*	*Ultimate stress (10^6 N/m^2)*	*Ref*
Cortical	Tension	11.4–19.1	107–146	48
	Compression	15.1–19.7	156–212	12,47
	Shear		73–82	49
Cancellous	Tension	~0.2–5	~3–20	50
	Compression	0.1–3	1.5–50	12
	Shear		6.60 ± 1.66	51

Table 2.2 The strengths of whole bones in different loading directions.

Bone type	*Loading direction and type*	*Ultimate strength*	*Ref*
Cervical spine	Axial compressive impact	980–7400 N	52–54
Lumbar spine	Axial compresive impact	1400–9000 N	19, 55–58
Sacro-iliac joints	Axial compressive impact	3450–3694 N	59
Femoral neck	Lateral to medial at greater trochanter	1000–4000 N	60, 61
Femoral neck	Vertical impact on femoral head	725–10 570 N	20,22,60
Femur	Torsion	183 N m	62
Femur	Bending from impact through the knee along the axis of the femur	6230–17 130 N	63,64
Patella	Impact perpendicular to the patella	6900–10 012 N	63
Femur	3 point posterior load at midshaft	21.2 ± 7.6–31.3 ± 14 N m[a]	65
Tibia	Torsion along long axis	101 ± 35 N m	62

[a]Energy absorbed to failure.

Apart from the variability in properties of bone material due to the factors described above, the strength of whole bones depends also upon their geometry (for example, length to diameter ratio) and material properties, such as density, and cortical thickness. Table 2.2 provides some data on the strength of various major bones of the skeleton. The wide ranges of strength values reported likely result from differences in the properties discussed above.

2.12 Summary

Bone is a complex material composed of rigid mineral crystals (hydroxyapatite) embedded within a flexible fiber (collagen) matrix. The ratio of mineral to collagen significantly affects bone material properties. Hypermineralization produces a stiffer material, but decreases impact strength. The collagen matrix provides flexibility and enhances impact tolerance. Lamellae of bone are arranged with a preferred fiber direction so as to resist the primary applied loads. In addition, in trabecular bone, the trabeculae are oriented so as to resist tension and compression and reduce bending. Apart from these structural parameters, the density of trabecular and cortical bone is also an important determinant of strength.

Changes in bone occur due to functional use and aging. Hypertrophy, due to new bone deposited on the periosteal surfaces of cortex, is the response to the application of larger loads, while bone loss from the endosteal surface is the result of disuse or aging. In addition, along with structural changes similar to those seen with disuse, aging results in hypermineralization of bone, rendering it more brittle and with reduced impact resistance.

2.13 References

1. Burstein AH, Zika IM, Heiple KG, Klein L, Contribution of collagen and mineral to the elastic–plastic properties of bone, *J Bone Jt Surg* (1975) **57A:** 956–61.
2. Jepson KJ, Mansura MK, Kuhn JL, Wu H, Jaenisch R, Bonadio JF, Goldstein SA, An in vivo assessment of the contribution of type 1 collagen to the mechanical properties of cortical bone, *Trans 38th Orthopedic Research Society Meeting* (1992) **17:** 93.
3. Currey JD, The mechanical consequences of variation in the mineral content of bone, *J Biomech* (1969) **2:** 1–11.
4. Currey JD, Changes in the impact energy absorption of bone with age, *J Biomech* (1979) **12:** 459–69.
5. Evans FG, Relations between the microscopic structure and tensile strength of human bone, *Acta Anat* (1958) **35:** 285–301.
6. Evans FG, Bang S, Differences and relationships between the physical properties and the structure of human femoral, tibial, and fibular cortical bone, *Am J Anat* (1967) **120:** 79–88.
7. Evans FG, Vincentelli R, Relation of collagen fiber orientation to some mechanical properties of human cortical bone, *J Biomech* (1969) **2:** 63–71.
8. Ascenzi A, Bonucci E, The tensile properties of single osteons, *Anat Rec* (1967) **158:** 375–86.
9. Ascenzi A, Bonucci E, The compressive properties of single osteons, *Anat Rec* (1968) **161:** 377–92.
10. Ascenzi A, Bonucci E, The shearing properties of single osteons, *Anat Rec* (1972) **172:** 499–510.
11. Ascenzi A, Bonucci E, Simkin A, An approach to the mechanical properties of single osteonic lamellae, *J Biomech* (1973) **6:** 227–35.
12. Carter DR, Hayes WC, The compressive behavior of bone as a two-phase porous structure, *J Bone Jt Surg* (1977) **59A:** 954–62.
13. Weaver JK, Chalmers J, Cancellous bone: its strength and changes with aging and an evaluation of some methods for measuring its mineral content 1. Age changes in cancellous bone, *J Bone Jt Surg* (1966) **48A:** 289–99.
14. Bartley Jr MH, Arnold JS, Haslam RK, Jee WSS, The relationship of bone strength and bone quantity in health, disease, and aging, *J Gerontol* (1966) **21:** 517–21.
15. Bell GH, Dunbar O, Beck JS, Gibb A, Variations in strength of vertebrae with age and their relation to osteoporosis, *Calcif Tissue Res* (1967) **1:** 75–86.
16. Galante J, Rostoker W, Ray RD, Physical properties of trabecular bone, *Calcif Tissue Res* (1970) **5:** 236–46.
17. McElhaney JH, Alem NM, Roberts VL, A porous block model for cancellous bone, *Am Soc Mech Eng* (1970) **70**-WA/BHF-2: 1–9.
18. Lotz JC, Gerhart TN, Hayes WC, Mechanical properties of trabecular bone from the proximal femur by single-energy quantitative computed tomography, *J Computer Assisted Tomogr* (1990) **14:** 107–14.
19. Cody DD, Goldstein SA, Flynn MJ, Brown EB, Correlations between vertebral regional bone mineral density (RBMD) and whole bone fracture load, *Spine* (1991) **16:** 146–54.
20. Alho A, Husby T, Hoiseth A, Bone mineral content and mechanical strength. An ex-vivo study on human femora at autopsy, *Clin Orthop* (1988) **227:** 292–7.
21. Dalen N, Hellstrom LG, Jacobson B, Bone mineral content and mechanical strength of the femoral neck, *Acta Orthop Scand* (1976) **47:** 503–8.
22. Leicher I, Margulies JY, Weinreb A, Mizrahi J, Robin GC, Conforty B, Makin M, Bloch B, The relationship between bone density, mineral content, and mechanical strength in the femoral neck, *Clin Orthop* (1982) **163:** 272–81.
23. Schaffler MB, Burr DB, Stiffness of compact bone. Effects of porosity and density, *J Biomech* (1988) **21:** 13–16.
24. Wolff J, Über die theorie des Knochenschwundes durch vermehrten Druck und der Knochenanbildung durch Drückenlastung, *Archiv für klinische Chirurgie (v. Langenbecks Archiv)* (1891) **42.**
25. Hayes WC, Snyder B, Toward a quantitative formulation of Wolff's Law in trabecular architecture. In: Cowin SC, ed, *Mechanical properties of bone* (Applied Mechanics Division of the American Society of Mechanical Engineers, AMD Vol 45: New York 1981) 43–69.
26. Crowninshield RD, Pope MH, The response of compact bone in tension at various strain rates, *Ann Biomed Eng* (1974) **2:** 217–25.
27. Currey JD, The effects of strain rate, reconstruction, and mineral content on some mechanical properties of bovine bone, *J Biomech* (1975) **8:** 81–6.
28. Wright TM, Hayes WC, Tensile testing of bone over a wide range of strain rates: effects of strain rate, microstructure and density, *Med Biol Eng* (1976) **14:** 671–80.
29. McElhaney JH, Dynamic response of bone and muscle tissue, *J Appl Physiol* (1966) **21:** 1231–6.
30. Borden IV S, Traumatic bowing of the forearm in children, *J Bone Jt Surg* (1974) **56A:** 611–16.
31. Currey JD, Butler G, The mechanical properties of the bone tissue in children, *J Bone Jt Surg* (1975) **57A:** 810–14.

32. Burstein AH, Reilly DL, Martens M, Aging of bone tissue: mechanical properties, *J Bone Jt Surg* (1976) **58A**: 82–6.
33. Boyce TM, Bloebaum RD, Age related hypermineralization of the femoral neck and possible fracture implications, *Trans 38th Orthopedic Research Society Meeting* (1992) **17**: 420.
34. Fink M, Noble PC, Kamaric E, Alexander JW, The effect of ageing on the shape of the proximal femur, *Trans 38th Orthopedic Research Society Meeting* (1992) **17**: 339.
35. Martin RB, Atkinson PJ, Age and sex-related changes in the structure and strength of the human femoral shaft, *J Biomech* (1977) **10**: 223–31.
36. Rubin CT, Lanyon LE, Regulation of bone formation by applied dynamic loads, *J Bone Jt Surg* (1984) **66A**: 397–402.
37. McLeod KJ, Rubin CT, Sensitivity of the bone remodeling response to the frequency of applied strain, *Trans 38th Orthopedic Research Society Meeting* (1992) **17**: 533.
38. Jones HH, Priest JD, Hayes WC, Tichenor CC, Nagel DA, Humeral hypertrophy in response to exercise, *J Bone Jt Surg* (1977) **59A**: 204–8.
39. Clark CR, Morgan C, Sonstegard DA, Matthews LS, The effect of biopsy-hole shape and size on bone strength, *J Bone Jt Surg* (1977) **59A**: 213–17.
40. McBroom, RJ, Cheal EJ, Hayes WC, Strength reductions from metastatic cortical defects in long bones, *J Orthop Res* (1988) **6**: 369–78.
41. Edgarton BC, An K-A, Morrey BF, Torsional strength reduction due to cortical defects in bone, *J Orthop Res* (1990) **8**: 851–5.
42. Leggon RE, Lindsey RW, Panjabi MM, Strength reduction and the effects of treatment of long bones with diaphyseal defects involving 50% of the cortex, *J Orthop Res* (1988) **6**: 540–6.
43. Brooks DB, Burstein AH, Frankel UH, The biomechanics of torsional fractures, *J Bone Jt Surg* (1970) **52A**: 507–14.
44. Pugh JW, Rose RM, Radin EL, Elastic and viscoelastic properties of trabecular bone: dependence on structure, *J Biomech* (1973) **6**: 475–85.
45. Swanson SAV, Freeman MAR, Is bone hydraulically strengthened? *Med Biol Eng* (1966) **4**: 433–8.
46. Ochoa JA, Sanders AP, Heck DA, Hilberry BM, Stiffening of the femoral head due to intertrabecular fluid and intraosseus pressure, *J Biomech Eng* (1991) **113**: 259–62.
47. Currey JD, *The mechanical adaption of bones* (Princeton University Press: Princeton 1984).
48. Reilly DT, Burstein AH, Frankel UH, The elastic modulus for bone, *J Biomech* (1974) **7**: 271–5.
49. Yamada H, *Strength of biological materials.* (Evans FG, ed). (Williams & Wilkins: Baltimore 1970).
50. Carter DR, Schwab GH, Spengler DM, Tensile fracture of cancellous bone, *Acta Orthop Scand* (1980) **51**: 733–41.
51. Stone JL, Beaupre GS, Hayes WC, Multiaxial strength characteristics of trabecular bone, *J Biomech* (1983) **16**: 743–52.
52. Yoganandan N, Pintar FA, Sances Jr A, Maiman D, Strength and motion analysis of the human head–neck complex, *J Spinal Disorders* (1991) **4**: 73–85.
53. McElhaney JH, Paver JG, McCrackin HJ, Maxwell GM, Cervical spine compression responses, *Society of Automotive Engineers Tech Paper* 831615 (1983).
54. Nusholtz GS, Melvin JW, Huelke DF, Alem NM, Blank JG, Response of the cervical spine to superior–inferior head impact. In: *Proceedings of the 25th Stapp Car Crash Conference* (Society of Automotive Engineers: 1981) 1197–237.
55. Bell GH, Dunbar O, Beck JS, Variations in strength of vertebrae with age and their relation to osteoporosis, *Calcif Tissue Res* (1967) **1**: 75–86.
56. Brassow F, Crone-Munzebrock W, Weh L, Kranz R, Egger-Stoeder G, Correlations between breaking load and CT absorption values of vertebral bodies, *Eur J Radiol* (1982) **2**: 99–101.
57. Hansson T, Roos B, Nachemson A, Bone mineral content and ultimate compressive strength of lumbar vertebrae, *Spine* (1980) **5**: 46–55.
58. Halton WC, Cyron MB, Stoth JRR, The compressive strength of lumbar vertebrae, *J Anat* (1979) **129**: 753–8.
59. Fasola AF, Baker RC, Hitchcock RA, Anatomical and physical effects of rapid deceleration. *WADC Tech Report, Wright–Patterson Air Force Base, Ohio* (1955).
60. Smith LD, Hip fractures, the role of muscle contraction or intrinsic forces in the causation of fractures of the femoral neck, *J Bone Jt Surg* (1953) **35A**: 367–83.
61. Melton III LJ, Riggs BL, Hip fracture: a disease and an accident. In: Uhthoff HK, Stahl E, eds, *Current concepts of bone fragility* (Springer-Verlag: Berlin 1986) 385–9.
62. Martens M, van Audekercke R, de Meester P, Mulier JC, The mechanical characteristics of the long bones of the lower extremity in torsional loading, *J Biomech* (1980) **13**: 667–76.
63. Patrick LM, Kroell CK, Martz Jr HJ, Forces on the human body in simulated crashes. In: Cragun MK, ed, *Proceedings of the Ninth Stapp Car Crash Conference* (University of Minnesota: Minneapolis 1966) 237–59.

64. Viano DC, Stalnaker RL, Mechanisms of femoral fracture, *J Biomech* (1980) **13:** 701–15.

65. Mather BS, Observations on the effects of static and impact loading on the human femur, *J Biomech* (1968) **1:** 331–5.

CHAPTER 3

The biomechanics of bone fracture

In this chapter the mechanics of bone fracture are discussed. The first topics are fatigue and impact fracture, followed by a discussion of the primary forces applied to long bones and the resulting deformations and types of fractures that occur. Details of mechanisms of fracture of bones of the upper extremity, such as the scaphoid, distal radius, and elbow, are then presented, followed by those for the spine, pelvis, and lower extremity regions such as the proximal femur, the tibial plateau, and the talus.

3.1 Fatigue fracture of bone

Fracture of bone may occur at loads below those which the material can sustain, due to a process of cumulative fatigue damage. In this process, the local stress at a stress concentrator (riser) (hole, cavity, etc) is greater than the yield stress of the material, even though the overall stress in the material does not exceed yield. In the fatigue process, a continuous series of loading and unloading cycles produces small but progressive increases in the growth of a crack starting at the stress riser. This crack continues to grow with repetitive load faster than the ability of bone to heal itself. These stress fractures are commonly seen in athletes,[1] ballet dancers,[2] military recruits,[3] or others undertaking vigorous physical activity. The fatigue properties of cortical bone specimens, given in terms of the number of load cyles that can be endured at a given stress level, are shown in Figure 3.1. The figure shows that fatigue can occur in under 10 000 load cycles at high stress. (Note that a jogger might apply over 1000 load cycles to the lower extremity in a 1 mile distance.)

In fatigue due to bending, Carter and Hayes[7] identified different mechanisms of failure on the tension and compression sides of their specimens. (In bending, as discussed in Chapter 1, the concave side undergoes compressive, and the convex side tensile, stress.) On the tension side, fracture surfaces were found to be transverse (i.e. perpendicular to the longitudinal axis of the bone specimen), as shown in Figure 3.2. A fracture plane that is transverse or perpendicular to the direction of stress indicates that the material is failing in pure tension. Local fracture was attributed to debonding of osteons at interlamellar cement bonds, the weakest part of the material.[8] The crack proceeds longitudinally along an osteon, and then traverses predominantly across a weak interface between osteons, so the transverse fracture surface is actually a series of steps across the surface, as shown in Figure 3.3. At higher strain rates, there is less longitudinal cracking, and at very high rates, pullout of osteons has been noted to occur.[8]

On the compression side, fracture surfaces are oblique to the applied load, and failure occurs by oblique cracking and longitudinal splitting (Figure

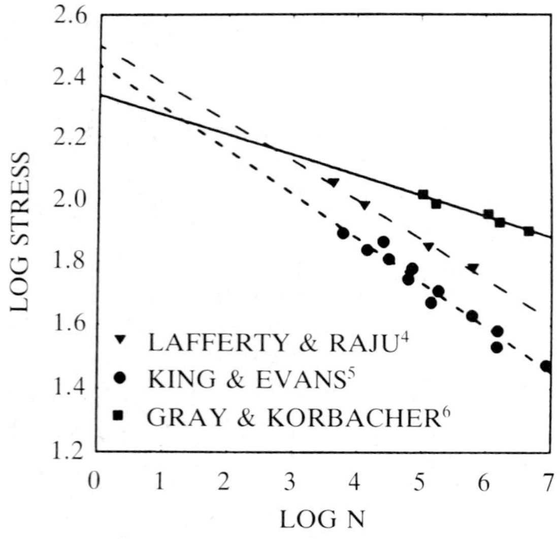

Figure 3.1

Stress versus number of cycles to failure (*S–N* curve) for bone from different experiments. Horizontal axis is logarithm of number of cycles (powers of 10) and vertical axis is logarithm of maximum stress in MPa. (From Martin B, A theory of fatigue damage and repair in cortical bone, *J Orthop Res* (1992) **10:** 818–25, with permission.)

3.2). A fracture plane that is oblique to the applied load (in this case compression) indicates that the failure occurs by shearing or slipping, as shown in Figure 3.4. Bone fracture surfaces due to compressive failure are irregular and jagged in appearance, with local crushing of bone and fragmentation. A fracture surface that is oblique to the applied load indicates that failure occurs by shearing.

3.2 Impact fracture of bone

When stresses beyond yield are applied, bone will be subjected to large deformations that generate cracks at weak interfaces and lead to failure as a load bearing structure. Saha[9] observed that mature bone in tension fails as a brittle substance. This is demonstrated by a nearly transverse fracture surface (as discussed above). However, others attribute some plastic deformation to bone after yield (Figure 3.5).[10] As discussed in Chapter 1, the degree of plastic deformation in bone depends on the collagen/mineral ratio and the orientation of collagen fibers in the lamellae. Plastic deformation may result from osteon pull-out, or from secondary microcracking, which are mechanisms that dissipate some of the energy of the impact without complete failure of the material.

Fracture cracks may initiate from a stress riser (concentrator) in bone such as an osteocyte lacuna or a blood vessel channel, an example of which is shown in Figure 3.3. Alternatively, a stress concentrator such as a lacuna may act to arrest the progress of a crack or cause it to deviate in direction.[8] Therefore the porous structure of bone has both benefits and liabilities from a structural point of view.

3.3 General mechanisms of long bone fracture

Bone is weakest in shear, followed by tension, and compression.[11] This is a very important factor to consider when determining how bone fracture occurs. Most long bone fractures are subjected to a combination of applied loads that produce a complex fracture pattern. However, if effects of specific loads are considered separately then basic mechanisms of long bone fracture can be identified.

Bending

In pure bending, the convex side is loaded in tension and the concave side in compression, as shown in Figure 3.6. The convex (tension) side will fail first, generating a crack through the bone cross section. As the crack progresses, the neutral axis shifts towards the compressive side because once part of the bone has failed in tension it has no longer any structural resistance to bending. In this way, the crack is always on the tensile side, and failure occurs in tension with a transverse fracture plane.

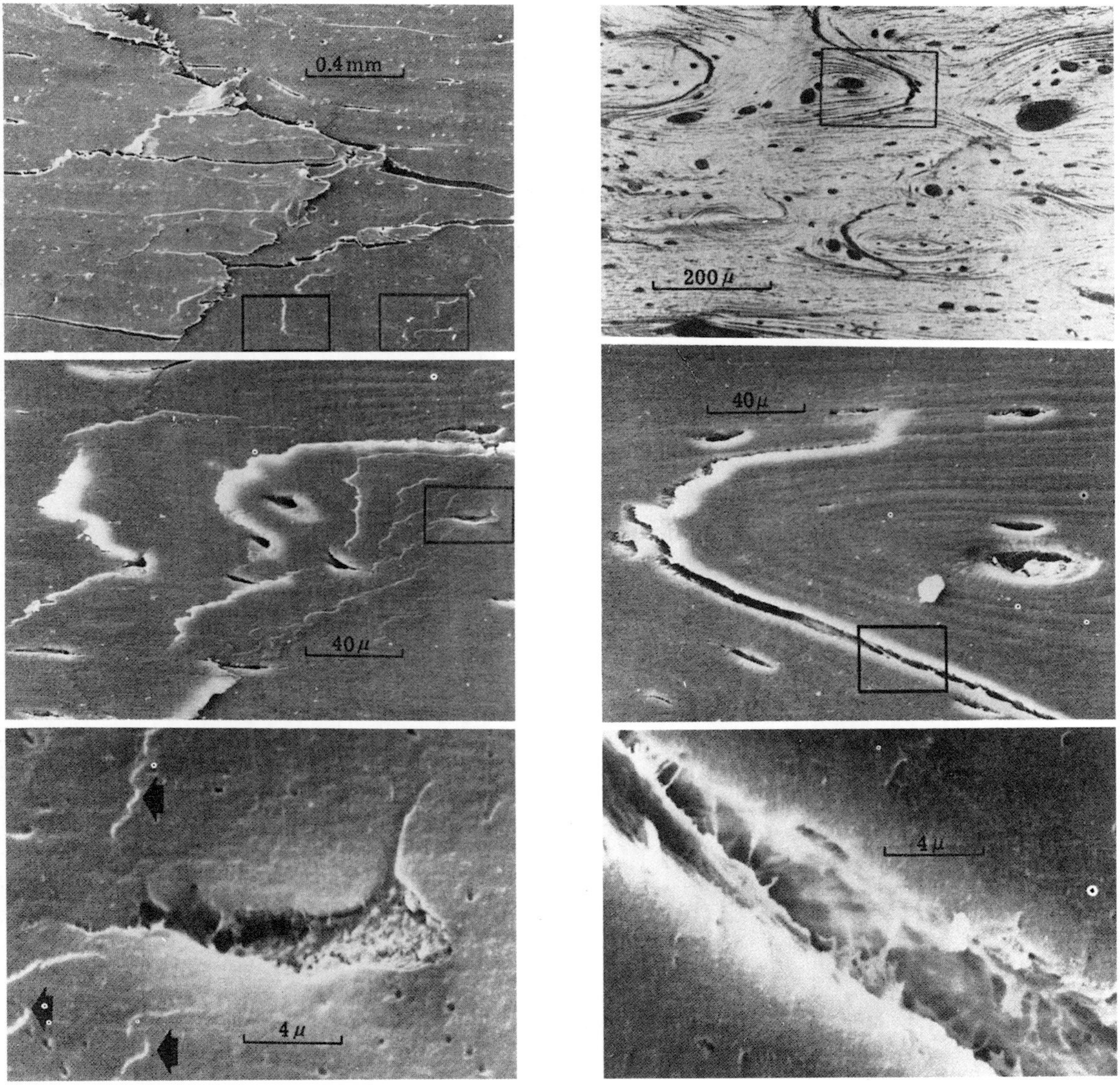

Figure 3.2

Photographs showing the mechanism of fatigue fracture in bone. *Left*: In compression (such as on the concave side in bending), progressively magnified views show the irregular pattern of the cracks formed. *Right top*: In tension (such as on the convex side in bending), cracks progress through the interfaces between osteons. *Right bottom*: Closer view of an interosteonal crack; within the crack, failure of the fibrous interface is evident. The photomicrographs from top to bottom show smaller regions (indicated by the rectangle) at increasing magnification. (From Ref 7 with permission.)

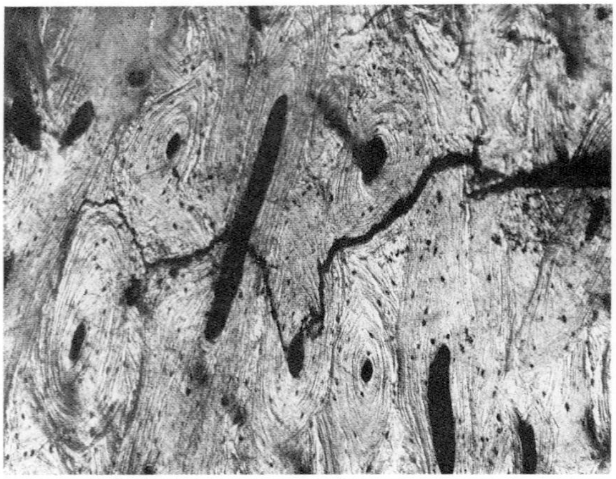

Figure 3.3

Progression of a crack across a cortical cross section. The crack progresses predominantly around the interface between osteons. (From Piekarski K, Fracture of bone, *J Appl Physiol* (1970) **41:** 1, with permission.)

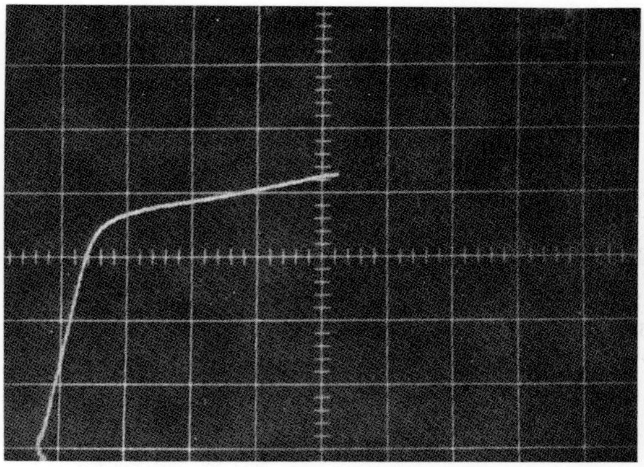

Figure 3.5

A force–deformation trace of a bone sample failing in tension. Note the large region of plastic deformation (the nearly horizontal part of the curve) that occurs before failure. (From Ref 10 with permission.)

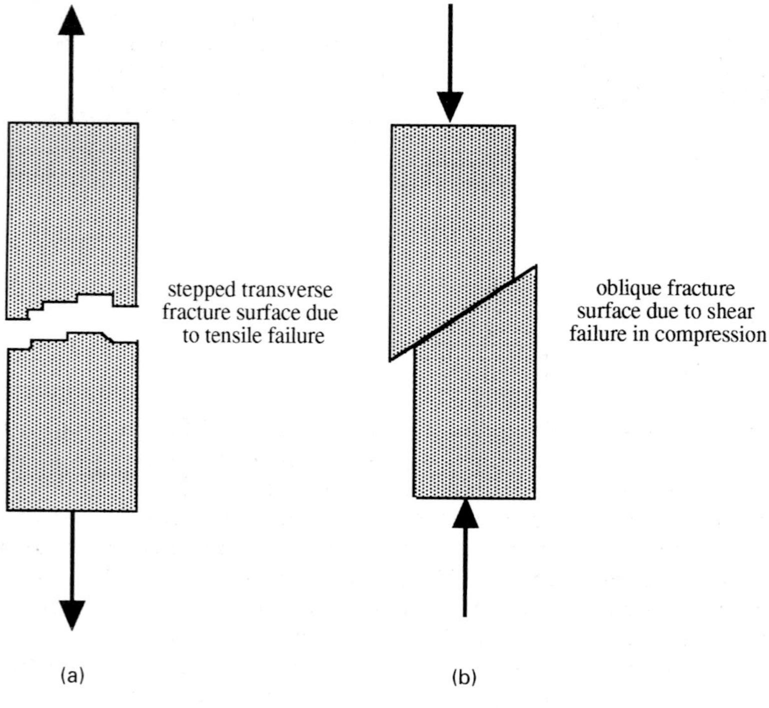

Figure 3.4

Fracture planes for tensile, and compressive failure of bone. (a) Transverse stepped fracture plane in tension. (b) Oblique fracture plane in compression, with local fragmentation of bone. Failure plane is in shear.

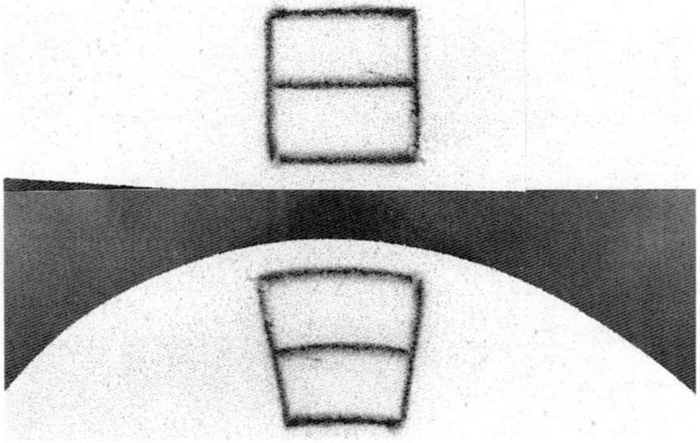

(a)

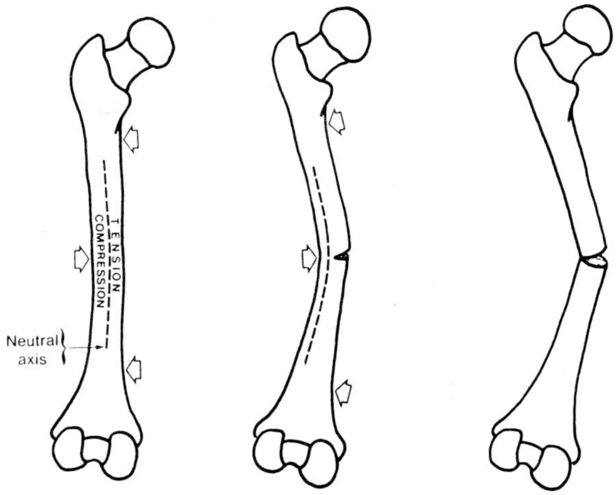

(b)

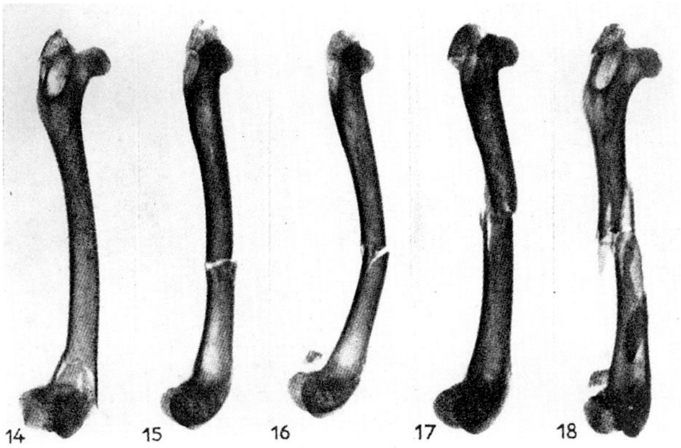

(c)

Figure 3.6

(a) Deformation of a square element inscribed in a foam beam that undergoes 3 point bending, illustrating the upper surface elongating (tension) and the bottom surface shortening (compression). (b) Schematic diagram of loading of a long bone in bending and the resulting transverse failure in tension. Note that, as the crack progresses, the neutral axis shifts to the left, so that failure continues to occur on the tension side of the bone (from Ref 12 with permission). (c) The photograph shows a series of transverse diaphyseal fractures in an experiment, which were created by bending impact loading (from Ref 13 with permission).

Bending and axial compression

When bending, which produces tension, is superimposed on axial compression, a combination of two fracture processes occurs. Bending produces a transverse crack on the tensile side of the bone, while compression results in an oblique fracture surface, as was shown in Figure 3.4. As the bone deforms, the protruding oblique surface impacts the other surface. The result is the characteristic "butterfly segment", which occurs on the concave side of the bone (Figure 3.7).[12]

Torsion

Pure torsion results in a spiral fracture with the fracture line oriented about 45° to the axis about which the torque is applied. This fracture line results from failure of the bone in tension perpendicular to the crack. As shown in the foam model of Figure 3.8, applying torsion distorts an element on the surface from the shape of a square to that of a parallelogram. The diagonal in the direction of the applied torque will elongate. Therefore the material is in tension along one

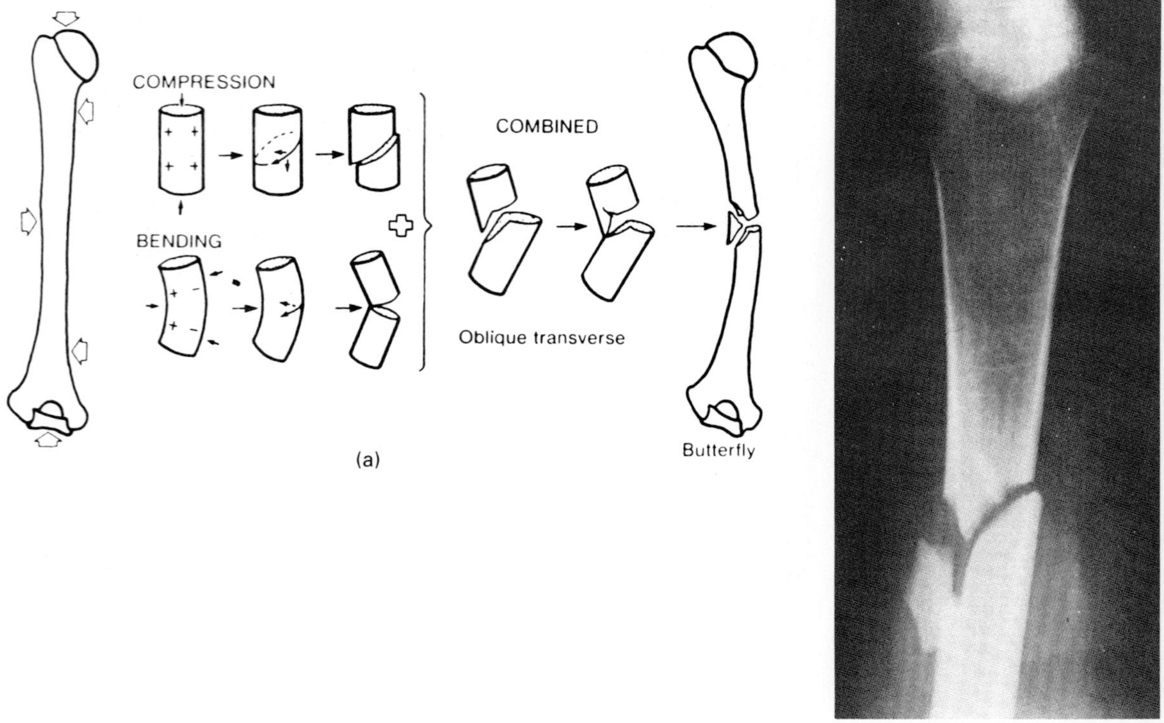

(a)

(b)

Figure 3.7

(a) A mechanism for the creation of a butterfly fracture due to combined bending and axial compression. (b) Clinical example of a butterfly fracture of the tibia. (From Ref 12 with permission.)

diagonal, and in compression along the other. Since bone is stronger in compression, tensile failure occurs perpendicular to the diagonal in tension, resulting in a crack oriented perpendicular to the diagonal that is in tension.

In pure torsion in a long bone, the material property "polar moment of inertia" (see Chapter 1) defines the strongest and weakest regions of the bone. Polar moment of inertia describes the distribution of material around the cross section. The region of a long bone with smallest polar moment of inertia is subjected to the largest deformation under load and will fail first. With this in mind, and considering Figure 3.9, which compares cross sections along the femur and tibia, it becomes clear why the distal third of the tibial shaft is a predominant location for spiral fracture.[14]

Axial compression

A pure axial compressive load creates fractures close to or within the metaphyses, as opposed to the middiaphysis, since cancellous bone is significantly weaker and will fail in compression before cortical bone. Examples of this type of long bone injury are the pilon fracture of the ankle, the distal radius fracture, and supracondylar and tibial plateau fractures about the knee, shown in Figure 3.10.

Effect of loading rate

As has been noted in Chapter 2 for bone specimens, the loading rate also affects the

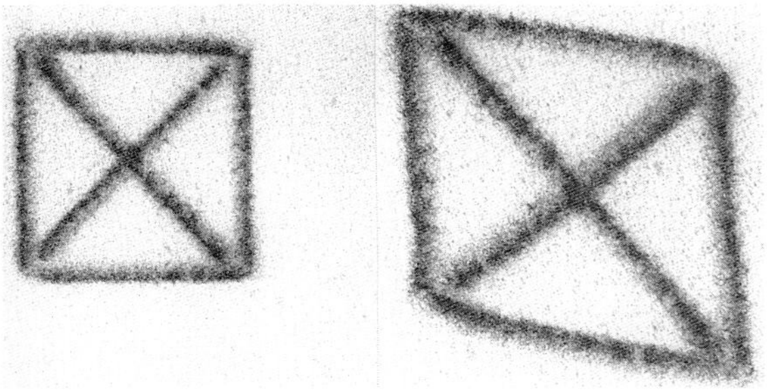

(a)

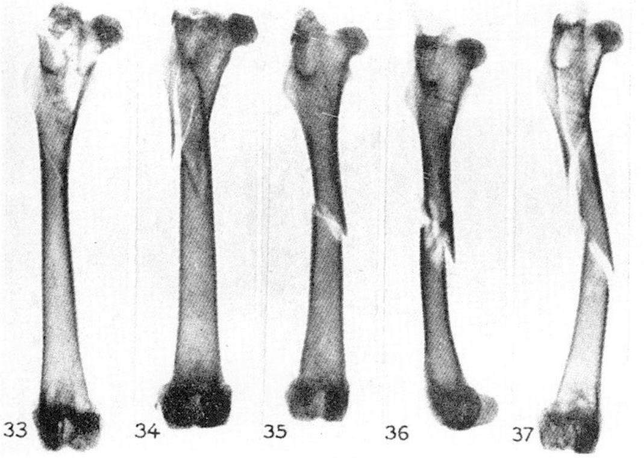

(b)

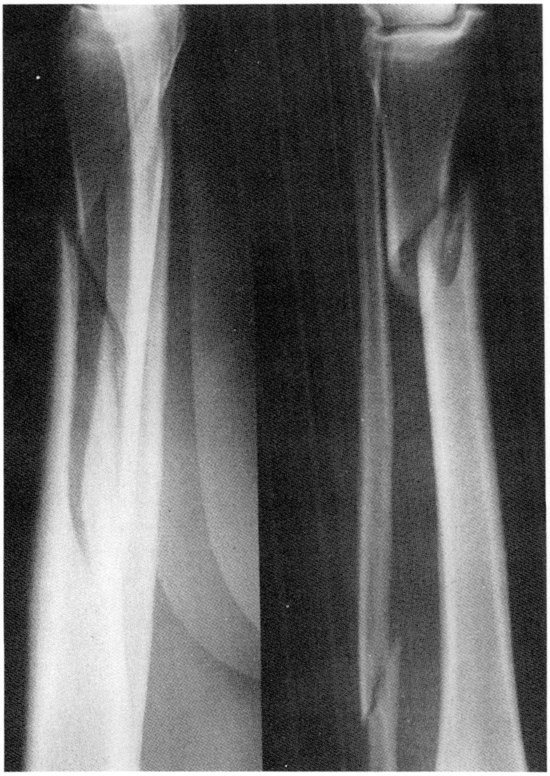

(c)

Figure 3.8

(a) In torsion, an element on the surface of the material that was initially square will distort into a parallelogram. Therefore the diagonal in the direction of the applied torque is in tension. The crack will be perpendicular to the diagonal in tension, so will spiral at 45° to the long axis, in the direction opposite to the applied torque. (b) Examples of experimental bones showing a spiral fracture pattern due to torsion (from Ref 9 with permission). (c) Clinical examples of (left) an oblique and (right) a torsional fracture. Note that these are caused by different mechanisms, the oblique fracture by a combination of bending and compression, and the spiral fracture by torsion (from Ref 12, with permission).

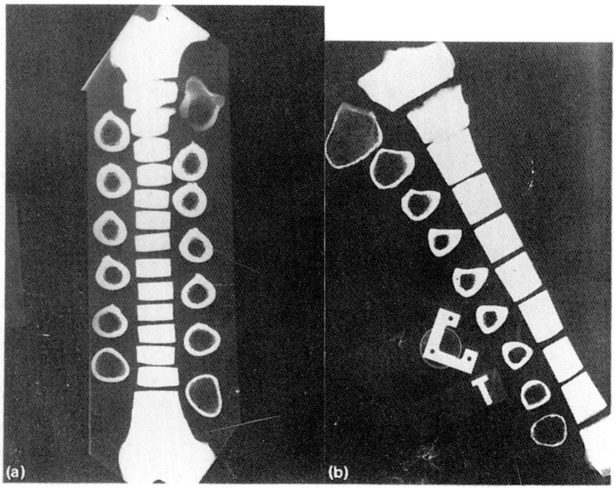

Figure 3.9

Cross sections through (left) a femur and (right) a tibia, showing cross sectional geometry at various locations along the shaft. The regions with the smallest diameters and thinnest cross sections will be the weakest. (From Ref 14 with permission.)

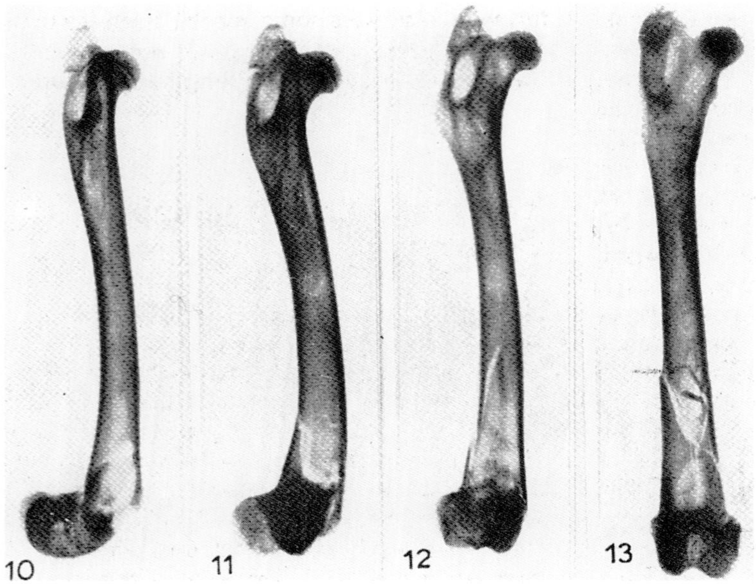

(a)

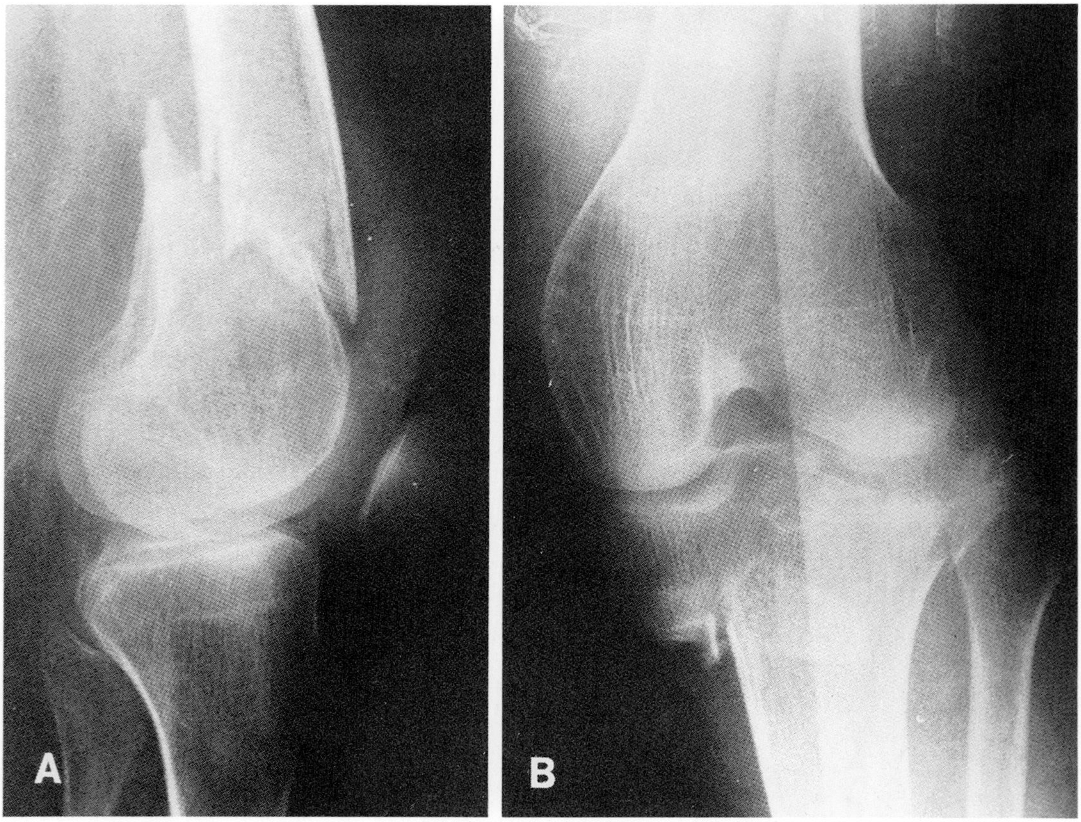

(b)

Figure 3.10

(a) Examples of the fracture pattern produced by axial loading in experimental bones (from Ref 9 with permission). (b) Clinical examples of metaphyseal compression fractures; (A) supracondylar fracture of the femur; (B) tibial plateau fracture (from Ref 12, with permission).

impact response of whole bones. For example, Mather[15] loaded femora to failure with an anteriorly directed transverse load, applied either gradually or by impact. Femora loaded by impact showed a mean 166% increase in energy absorption capacity, compared with contralaterals that were loaded slowly. Mather also found the strongest correlations to be between energy absorption and the anterior–posterior diameter of the bone, followed by its medial–lateral diameter, and the age of the specimen. (Energy absorption capacity, more than peak force, determines whether a bone will survive an impact intact or will fracture.) The reason for this may lie in the fact that a bone with larger metaphyseal regions has a larger volume of marrow that could contribute to absorbing impact energy.

An excellent summary of the general mechanisms and appearance of long bone fractures, along with the energy involved, was given by Gonza,[12] and is reproduced as Figure 3.11. The following discusses some specific fractures to the musculoskeletal system that are not covered by the previous comments on long bone fracture.

3.4 Fractures of the upper extremity

Distal radius (Colles') fracture

Impact to the outstretched hand when breaking a fall is a common mechanism in the injury to the wrist. Berg and Labosky[16] found that, experimentally, the most reliable position for producing a Colles' fracture of the distal end of the radius was 70–80° of dorsiflexion and 5° of radial deviation of the hand, and with the impact force aligned to the long axis of the radius. The result of this impact is predominantly a transverse fracture located in the distal metaphysis of the radius, due to compres-

Fracture Pattern	Appearance	Mechanism of Injury	Location Soft Tissue Hinge	Energy
Transverse	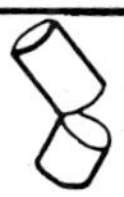	Bending	Concavity	Low
Spiral	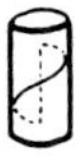	Torsion	Vertical segment	Low
Oblique-transverse or butterfly	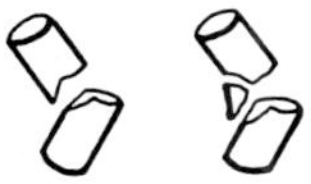	Compression + Bending	Concavity or side of butterfly	Mod
Oblique		Compression + Bending + Torsion	Concavity (often destroyed)	Mod
Comminuted	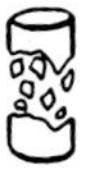	Variable	Destroyed	High
Metaphyseal compression	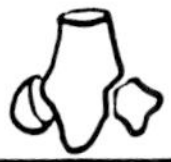	Compression	Variable	Variable

Figure 3.11

Summary of the general mechanisms and resulting appearances of long bone fractures. (From Ref 12, with permission.)

sive failure of cancellous metaphyseal bone. Associated with this fracture is either fracture of the ulnar styloid or tearing of ligaments on the ulnar side of the wrist.

Scaphoid waist fracture

Fracture of the scaphoid also occurs due to a fall on the outstretched hand. Weber and Chao[17] and Frykman[18] both showed that impact loading of the dorsiflexed hand results in distal radius fractures, except when the angle of dorsiflexion is greater than 95°, in which case the scaphoid is consistently fractured. In a scaphoid fracture (Figure 3.12), the proximal pole of the scaphoid is strongly stabilized between the radius and the capitate as well as the palmar carpal ligaments (radiocapitate and radiolunate) that attach to the proximal pole of the scaphoid. The distal pole is relatively unprotected, especially since the radial collateral ligament (which attaches to the distal pole) is lax. This results in the scaphoid being loaded as a cantilever beam with the proximal end fixed and the distal end free. The impact load directed to the distal pole of the scaphoid creates bending and fracture at the waist, its narrowest region.

Fractures about the elbow

A number of fracture mechanisms of the elbow resulting from different types of impact forces have been outlined by Harrington.[19] As shown in the schematic diagram of Figure 3.13, hyperextension causes the proximal ulna to impinge on the olecranon fossa, creating a levering effect that fractures the supercondylar region of the distal humerus. This may be combined with axial compression, causing comminution and multiple fragments. Axial compression caused by a direct fall on the elbow with the joint flexed may split the distal end of the humerus or fracture the olecranon. With an abduction moment applied along with axial loading, caused for example by a fall on the outstretched arm, fracture of the ulna and/or the distal end of the humerus can result.

3.5 Mechanisms of spine fracture

Spine fracture must be considered from the point of view of injury both to bony structures and to the interconnecting soft tissues, depending upon load application. Several authors have defined the characteristics of spine fractures resulting from

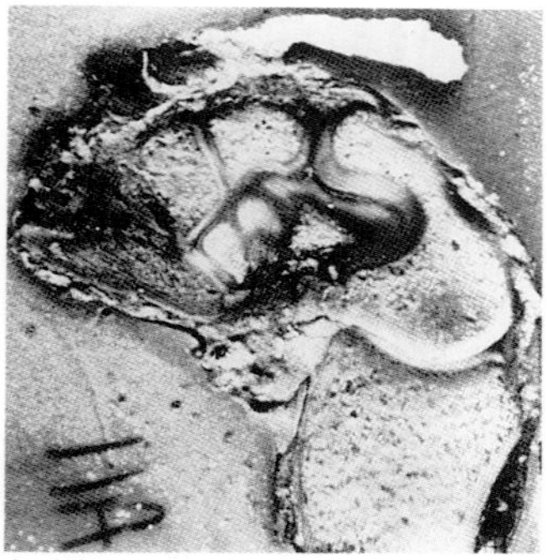

(a)

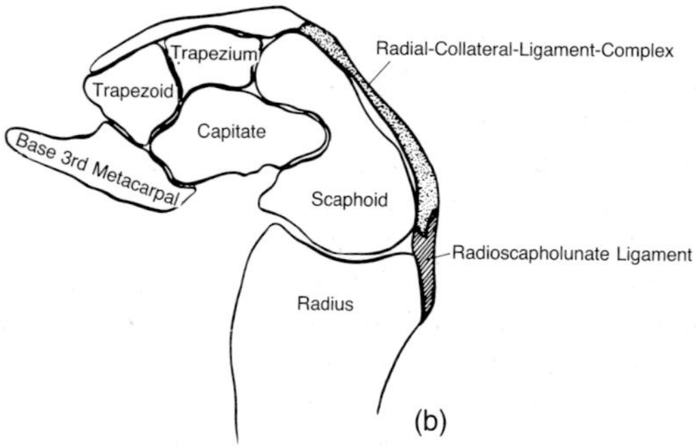

(b)

Figure 3.12

(a) Sagittal cross section through the wrist, illustrating the anatomy and orientations of the carpal bones in dorsiflexion of the hand. (b) Schematic drawing of the same cross section, showing the orientation of the scaphoid and the connecting ligaments. The proximal pole of the scaphoid is supported between the distal radius and the palmar radiolunate (RL) and radioscaphocapitate (RSC) ligaments. The distal pole is unprotected and the radial–collateral ligament is slack. With impact, the scaphoid experiences cantilever bending, and fracture occurs at the waist—the narrowest and weakest region. (From Ref 17 with permission.)

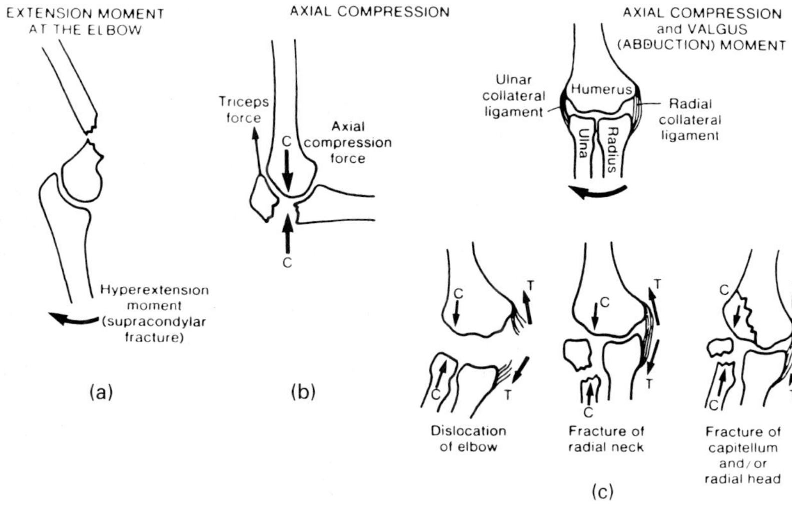

Figure 3.13

Three mechanisms of fracture about the elbow joint. (a) Hyperextension of the elbow causes supercondylar fracture of the distal humerus. (b) Axial compression produced by a fall on the elbow fractures the olecranon or may split the distal humerus. (c) An abduction moment combined with compression creates fracture of the radial neck or capitellum. (From Ref 19 with permission.)

the application of specific types of loads.[20–22] Figure 3.14 shows fundamental forces to which the spine can be subjected. The following are descriptions of fractures based on the various types of forces and moments applied to the spine.

Flexion moment

A flexion moment without significant compression results in a progression of injuries, depending on the magnitude of the moment, starting with tearing of posterior ligaments, followed by dislocation of the facet joints, tearing of capsules or fracture of the facet, pedicle or lamina, and finally progressing to damaging the disc (Figure 3.15). This occurs because the sagittal plane center of rotation in flexion is located in the posterior part of the intervertebral disc. The structures posterior to this center are loaded in tension during flexion of the spine. Although the facets are closer to the rotational axis, the lengths of the facet capsule fibers are small and the facet motion limited; therefore the actual strain that they encounter is large. For this reason, structures near the facet (i.e. capsule, pedicle) are likely to be injured in flexion.

Flexion moment and axial compression

When axial compression is combined with a flexion moment, anterior wedging of the vertebra is observed (Figure 3.16). The compressive load, which in this case is located in the anterior part of the vertebra, produces crushing of the anterior cortex of the vertebra.

Axial compression

When the load is applied closer to the middle of the vertebral body of the spine, the compressive force dominates the flexion moment, and the fracture is characterized by compression of the anterior and posterior walls of the vertebra, leading to its collapse.[23,24] The appearance of a bursting type fracture, with vertical splitting of the vertebral body and bone retropulsed into the spinal canal, may depend on the rate at which the load is applied.[25] According to Roaf,[22] bursting results from the nucleus pulposus being driven through the vertebral endplate, where it displaces fat and marrow (Figure 3.17). If the viscosity of the

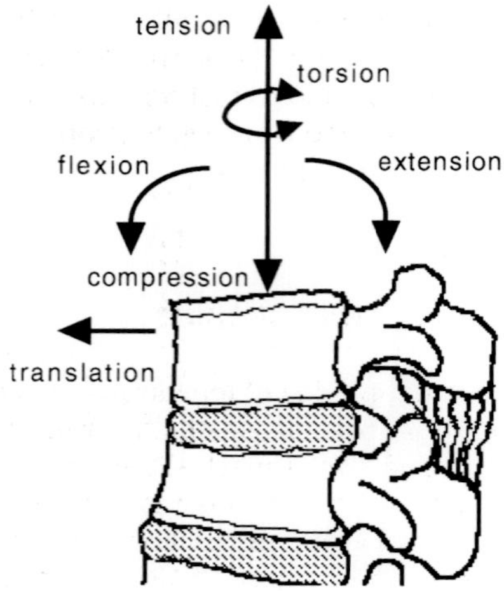

Figure 3.14

A spinal motion segment with various types of forces and moments that can cause injury. (Adapted from Ref 20.)

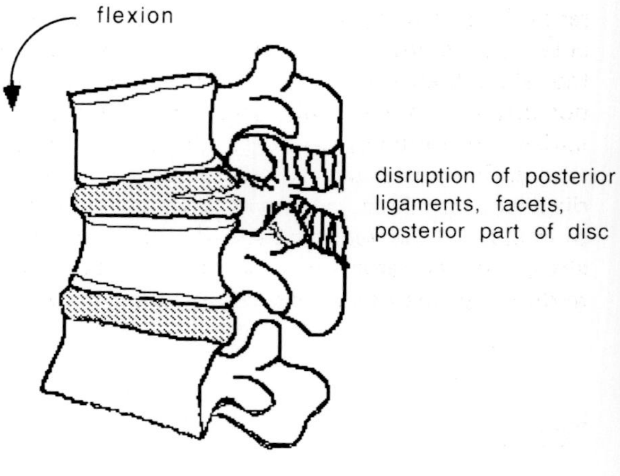

Figure 3.15

An injury resulting from a flexion moment results in progressive tearing of posterior ligaments, possible fracture of the pedicle or lamina or tearing of the facet capsules, and damage to the posterior part of the disc. (Adapted from Ref 20.)

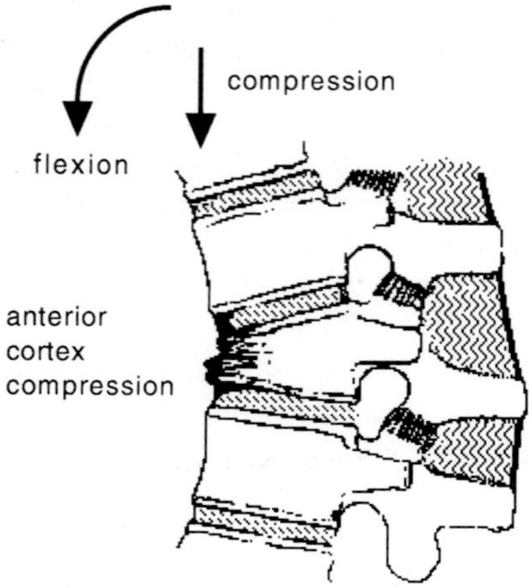

Figure 3.16

Failure of the spine due to the application of a compressive load in the anterior part of the vertebra, which causes crushing of the anterior cortex, as well as a flexion moment, which can disrupt the posterior elements. (Adapted from Ref 20.)

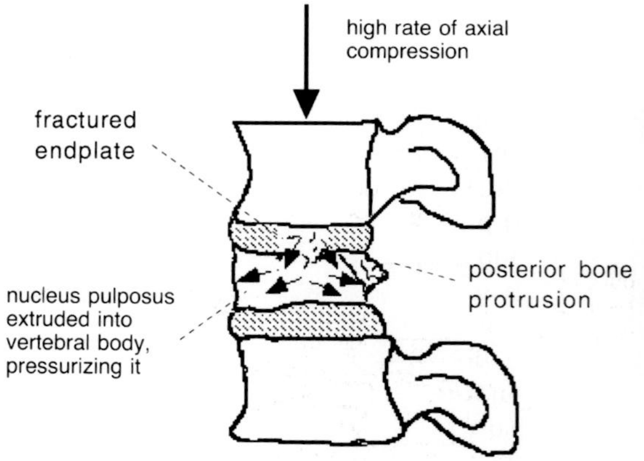

Figure 3.17

Schematic diagram of the mechanism of the compressive burst fracture of the spine, characterized by vertical cracking of the vertebra and retropulsion of bone into the spinal canal. A possible mechanism is displacement of the nucleus pulposus through the fractured endplate into the vertbral bone, which, along with deformation of the vertebra, pressurizes the fat and marrow contents. This internal pressurization may result in explosion of the vertebra and posterior retropulsion of bone into the spinal canal.

fat and marrow is great enough or the intratrabecular spaces are sufficiently restrictive relative to the rate of load application, the fluid contents may not displace immediately, and instead will pressurize the vertebra, causing it to explode from within. The posterior fragment, which commonly displaces into the canal, may result from initiation of fracture at the vertebral sinus, a large diameter stress concentrator (riser) located at about the midpoint of the posterior wall of the vertebra.

Torsion

Torsional fractures of the spine are characterized by damage to at least one of the facets, or pedicles, along with a diagonal fracture line through the vertebra (Figure 3.18). The facets are well known as key motion limiters to torsion in the thoracolumbar spine, along with the disc.[26,27] In torsion, with the center of rotation located in the posterior region of the disc, one facet experiences compressive loading, which may lead to pedicle fracture, while the other is loaded in tension by stretching of the facet capsular fibers, which may also produce fracture of the facet or tearing of the capsules. The oblique fracture line in the vertebral body is similar to the spiral fracture line that occurs in long bones, due to failure in tension in a plane oblique to the torsional axis.

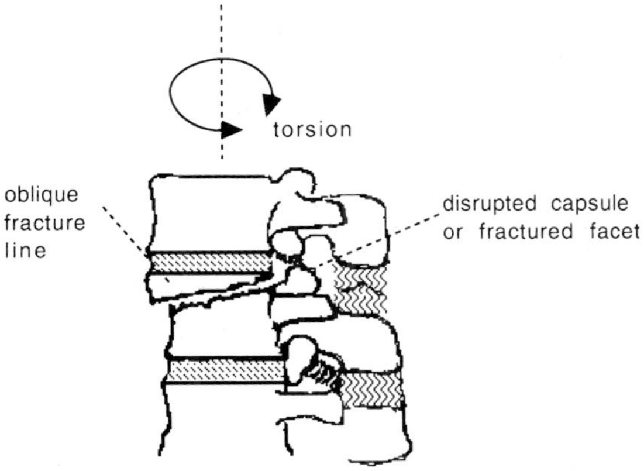

Figure 3.18

Failure of the vertebral column due to a torsional load, with characteristic fracture of a facet, and a spiral to oblique fracture line in the vertebra due to tensile failure as would occur in a long bone. (Adapted from Ref 20.)

Flexion moment and tension

Tension or distraction injuries of the lumbar spine can result from the use of seatbelts without shoulder harnesses. In an impact situation, the torso and legs of the victim are thrust towards the front of the vehicle, while the lumbar spine is restrained by the seatbelt (Figure 3.19a). Injuries due to distraction can include rupture of the posterior elements, tearing of the disc, dislocation of the facets, or a Chance fracture where the fracture line is located through the spinous process and the vertebral body bone (Figure 3.19b).[28]

Extension

A typical mechanism producing extension injuries to the spine is the whiplash injury of the neck (Figure 3.20). Because the head and neck have much smaller mass and therefore lower inertia than the torso, head movement leads that of the torso during impact and the subsequent deceleration of the victim that occurs during a rear end collision between two motor vehicles. The typical result of this extension moment is disruption of the anterior longitudinal ligament along with fracture of the spinous processes.[28]

3.6 Fracture of the pelvis

Structure

The pelvis is a complex structure, with three major bony structures and their interconnecting ligaments. Gonza[29] presented an elegant conceptual model of the pelvis, as shown in Figure 3.21(a). In order to develop a load bearing structure, he starts with a central ring to support

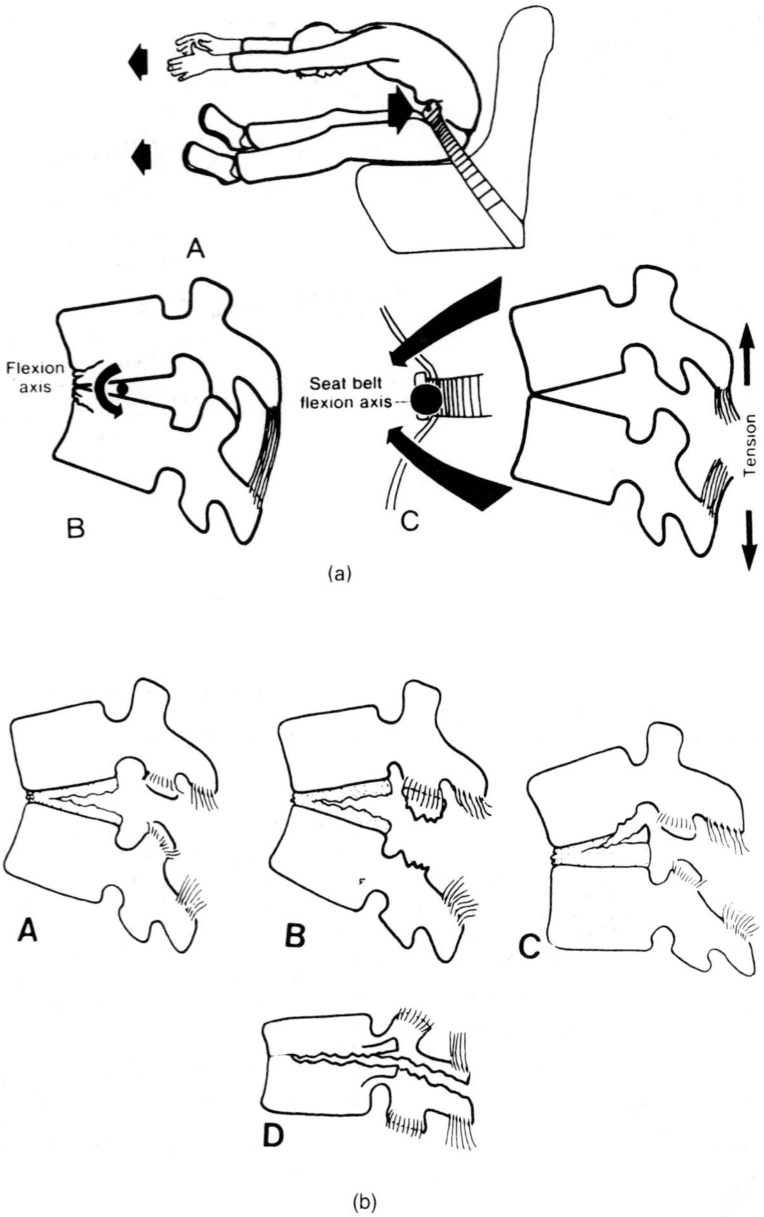

Figure 3.19

(a) A mechanism for the creation of a flexion–distraction injury to the lumbar spine due to the restraining effect of a seatbelt. (b) Various types of injuries resulting from flexion–distraction: (A) tearing of posterior elements, facet capsules, and the disc; (B) tearing of posterior ligaments and disc, and fracture of the facets; (C) disruption of posterior elements and fracture of the posterior wall of the vertebra; (D) Chance fracture through the spinous process and vertebral body. (From Ref 28 with permission.)

tension. Then pelvic wings are added to stiffen the structure to vertically oriented loads. A triangular strut is added consisting of the posterior column and the inferior pubic ramus. The acetabulum is located at the junction of the iliac wing and the triangulated inferior struts. Finally, the sacral wedge is added to complete the structure. The iliac wings are oriented so as to resist bending caused by loading through the acetabulum, as are the inferior structures. The compressive load of the torso is transformed into tension in the pelvic ring by the wedging action of the sacrum.

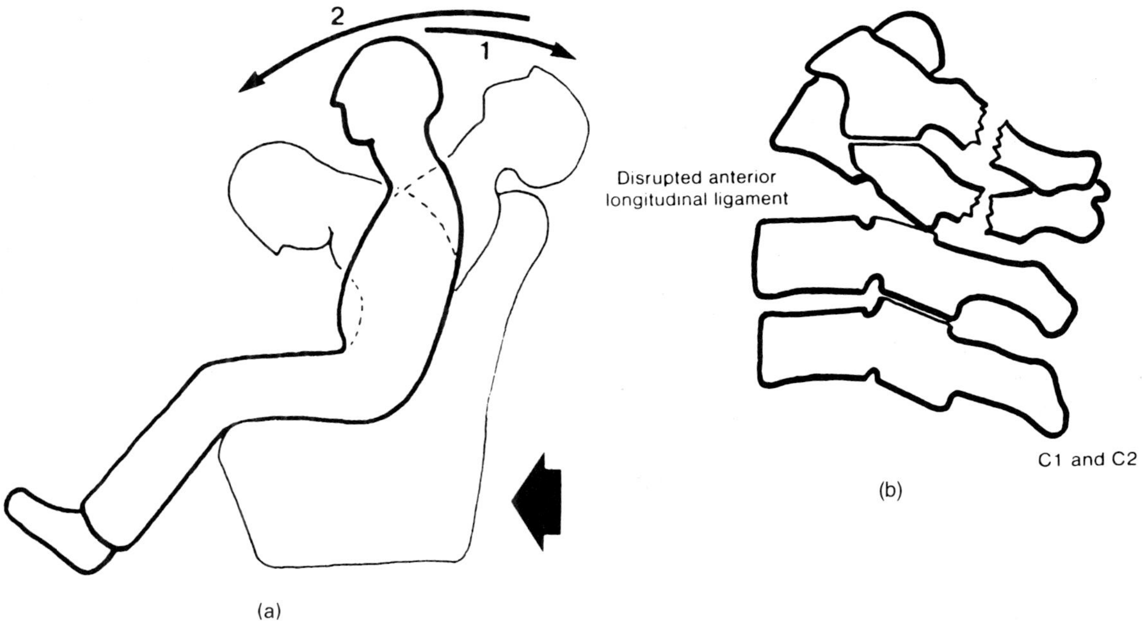

Figure 3.20

(a) Extension injuries, usually to the cervical spine, can result from the whiplash effect as the neck is hyperextended during a rear impact. (b) Typical damage to the cervical spine due to an extension injury. (From Ref 28 with permission.)

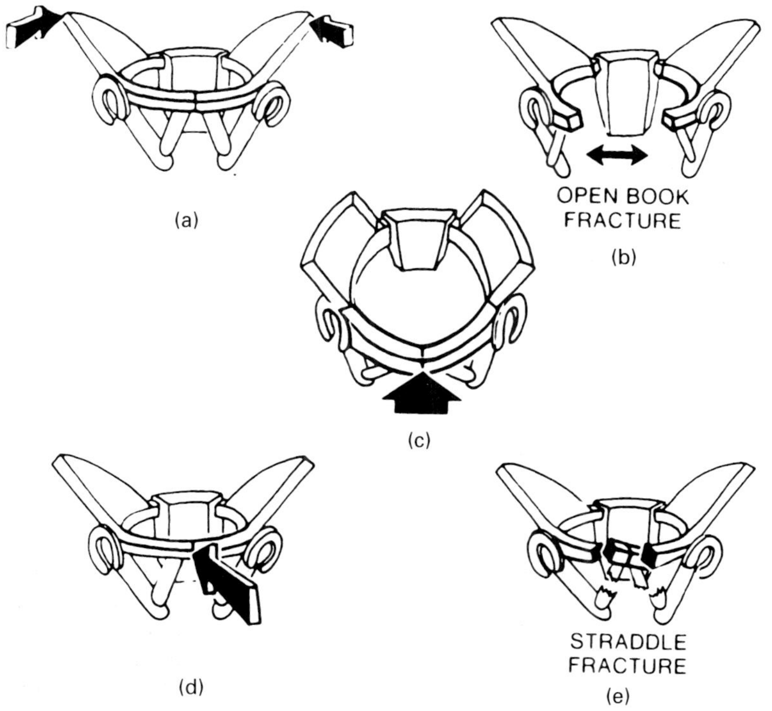

Figure 3.21

(a) A structural model of the pelvis consisting of a central ring (symphysis pubis), two vertical stiffeners (ilia), triangulated struts (inferior rami), a posterior wedge that loads the ring in tension (sacrum), and load points at the intersection of the ring, the ilia, and the rami (acetabulum). (b) A load directed posteriorly on the ilia can lead to an open book fracture, or anterior opening of the pelvis. (c,d) A direct blow to the symphysis pubis can fracture the pubic rami (e), creating a straddle fracture. (From Ref 29 with permission.)

Posterior force

A posterior force can be transmitted to the pelvis by direct impact on the iliac wings or by loading through the femora, which tends to disrupt the pelvic ring by tearing the symphysis pubis ligaments and the sacroiliac ligaments. This results in an "open book" fracture in which the two ilia are separated and rotated posteriorly (Figure 3.21b). Alternatively, a direct blow to the symphysis pubis can fracture the pubic rami, causing disruption of the anterior pelvic ring (Figure 3.21c–e).[29]

Lateral force

Lateral impacts produce different types of fractures, depending on the direction of force. A direct lateral blow causes fracture in the weaker anterior part of the pelvic ring (Figure 3.22). If the impact is directed more inferiorly, there is a component that causes rotation of the ipsilateral hemipelvis upwards, and bending of the anterior ring creates a fracture on the contralateral side.[29] The fracture occurs contralaterally because if the anterior pelvic ring is considered as a beam in cantilever bending, the highest stresses are farthest away from the point of load application, i.e. on the contralateral side.

Vertical force

A vertically upwards directed force results in shearing of the pelvic ring at its two weakest points, the bone near the symphysis pubis or its

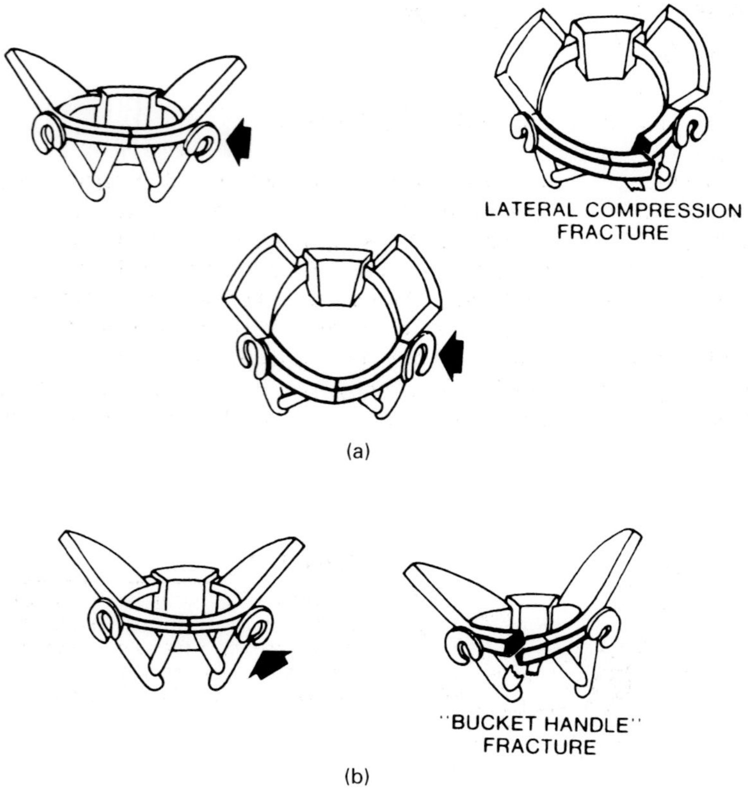

Figure 3.22

A laterally directed force creates different types of fractures, depending on the orientation of the force vector. (a) A direct lateral force results in a compression fracture of the weaker anterior part of the pelvic ring. (b) A lateral force with an inferior component produces a fracture on the contralateral side, because of the bending moment applied to the pubis symphysis as a cantilever beam. (From Ref 29 with permission.)

interconnecting ligament, and the sacroiliac joint or the sacrum (Figure 3.23).

3.7 Fractures of the lower extremity

Femoral neck fracture

A prevalent injury in the elderly is fracture of the proximal part of the hip. Considerable controversy exists as to whether reduced bone density combined with the increased brittleness of older bone results in bone failure and then a fall,[30] or whether the increased likelihood of falls in the elderly, due to poor balance or slow reaction times[31–33] is the reason for a greater number of injuries occurring in this population.

Two possible mechanisms may be responsible for this fracture, with the particular fracture pattern reflecting the forces applied. Application of vertical or nearly vertical (i.e. parallel to the axis of the femoral shaft) impact force invariably produces fracture at the base of the femoral neck with negligible comminution. This is consistent with cantilever bending fracture, where the greatest bending moment and stresses are located at the base (or supported) end of the beam (i.e. the trochanteric end of the femoral neck) (Figure 3.24a). This type of fracture would be consistent with a fracture that occurs while walking on the hip. Alternatively, Lotz and Hayes[34] have recently defined a mechanism of fracture due to fall on the greater trochanter (Figure 3.24b). The impact creates compression along the axis of the femoral neck along with bending. Recalling that combined compressive and bending loading results in oblique fracture with a butterfly component (Figure 3.11), this mechanism may explain fractures that have inferior comminution.

Femoral condyle or patellar fracture

Lower extremity injury caused by a high speed compressive force impacting the knee through the patella and acting along the axis of the femur (for example seated passengers encountering a dashboard in an automobile accident) creates measurable deformation in the knee, averaging 1.3 cm. Fracture of the patella or splitting of the femoral condyles by wedging impaction of the patella into the stiffer femoral shaft may result. An alternative occurrence due to impaction is bending fracture of the femur. The applied force acting through the femoral condyles, accentuated by the anterior bow of the femur, produces a considerable bending moment on the femoral shaft, with the potential for tensile fracture (due to bending) starting at the anterior (convex) surface of the femur.[35] These injury mechanisms are illustrated in Figure 3.25.

Gunshot fractures

Impacts caused by projectiles acting against the femur produce a different type of fracture. At high impact velocities (600–800 ft/s for 0.406–0.250 in diameter spheres; 180–244 m/s for 1–0.635 cm diameter spheres), a projectile that encounters cancellous bone imparts a radial velocity (i.e. away from the surface of the impacting sphere), moving fluid away from its path and creating a cavity in the bone. Above 1000 ft/s for 0.406 in

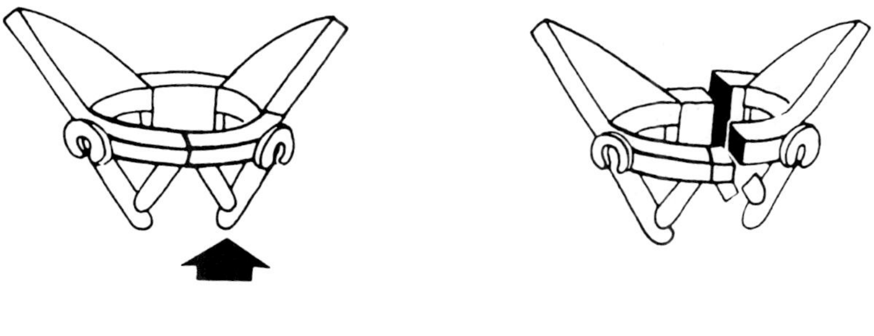

Figure 3.23

Vertical loading of the pelvis can result in shear fracture of bone and/or ligament anteriorly at the symphysis pubis, and posteriorly in the sacroiliac joint or the sacrum. (From Ref 29 with permission.)

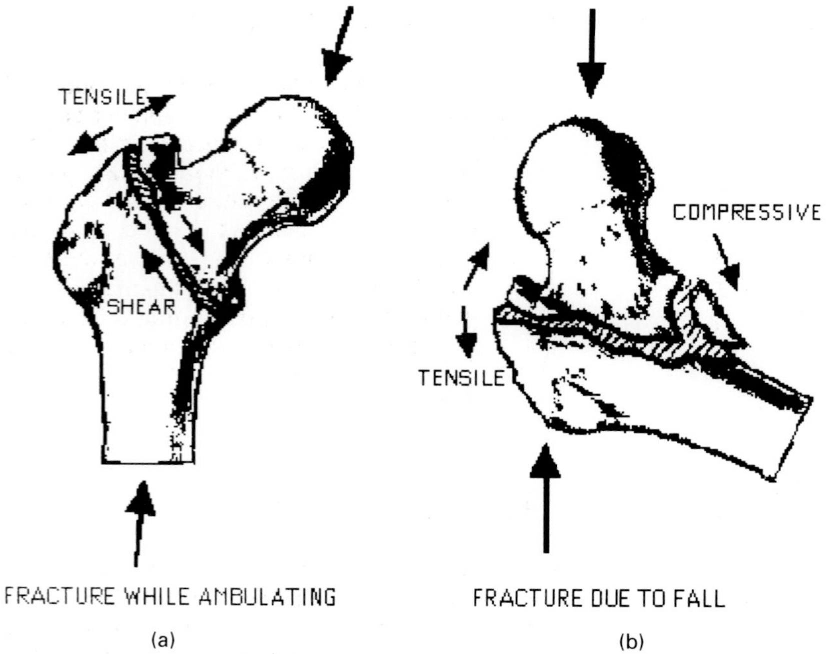

Figure 3.24

(a) Near vertical loading (parallel to the femoral shaft) results in fracture of the femoral neck at its base. (b) A fall on the greater trochanter produces compression and bending of the femoral neck, and may explain resulting inferior comminution.

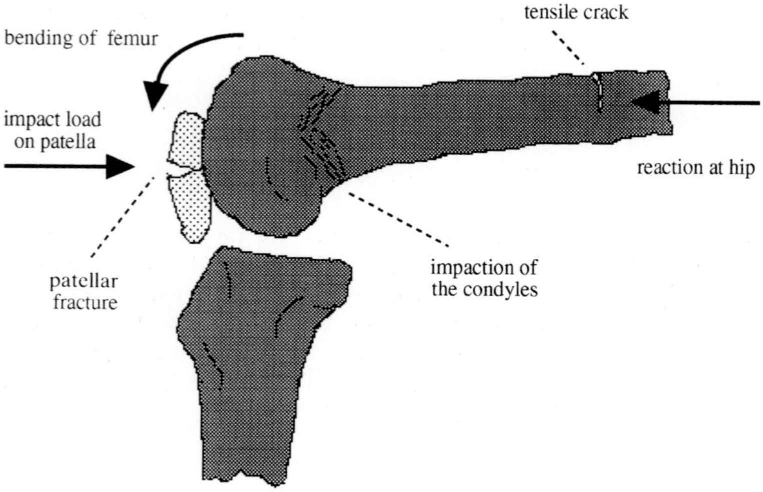

Figure 3.25

Impact to the patella with the knee flexed may create fracture of the patella, impaction of the femoral condyles, or transverse fracture in the middiaphysis of the femur due to bending.

spheres (305 m/s for 1 cm diameter spheres) or 1700 ft/s for 0.250 in spheres (520 m/s for 0.635 cm spheres), the distal femur will be completely pulverized.[36] Fragmentation without cavitation occurs in the midshaft femur with impact velocities above 600 ft/s (180 m/s).[37]

Tibial plateau fractures

Kennedy and Bailey[38] described mechanisms and resulting fracture patterns in tibial plateau injuries. As shown in Figure 3.26, a valgus (i.e. inwardly directed) force acting at the knee joint results in

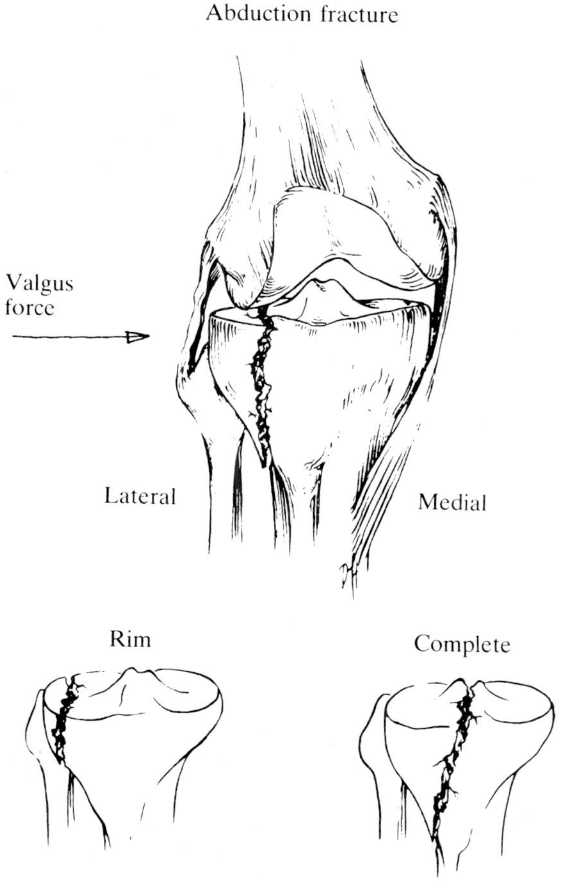

Figure 3.26

Fracture patterns resulting from a valgus (inwardly directed) force acting at the knee joint. The femur rotates and impacts the lateral condyle, resulting in compression. This creates a shear failure (vertical or oblique fracture line) in the tibial plateau with comminution. (From Ref 38 with permission.)

angulation of the femur such that impaction of the latter against the lateral condyle of the tibia occurs. The fracture is the result of compressive failure with comminution and shearing of the lateral component of the condyle. An oblique shear fracture is characteristic of failure by direct compression (see Figures 3.4 and 3.7).

Ankle malleolar fractures

Fractures due to abduction (the foot tilts outward) and external rotation of the foot result in fractures to the malleoli (which form the mortise of the ankle joint), as shown in Figure 3.27. These fractures may involve the syndesmotic ligaments between the distal tibia and the fibula or the deltoid ligaments on the medial side of the foot. The malleoli and lateral side ligaments may fracture due to the opposite motion, forced adduction (foot tilts inward) and internal rotation of the foot.[19]

Talar neck fractures

Fracture of the talar neck occurs through a mechanism similar to that of the scaphoid. Here, the body of the talus is stabilized between the tibia and the calcaneus. If the foot is then loaded in forced dorsiflexion, a large bending moment is transmitted through the neck of the talus through the talonavicular joint, creating cantilever bending and failure in the neck region, its narrowest part.

Talar dome fractures

Transchondral fractures of the talus occur during forced inversion of the foot. This motion causes the talus to rotate out of the mortise of the ankle and wedge its medial edge against the tibia. The fibular loading against the talus produces tension and shears its lateral border, which creates a chip fracture (Figure 3.28).[39]

3.8 Summary

Fracture of bone is caused by two general mechanisms: either by the failure load of the material being exceeded or by repetitive cyclic fatigue. Fatigue proceeds by the advancement of a crack, usually initiated at a stress riser (concentrator) in bone, at a stress below failure

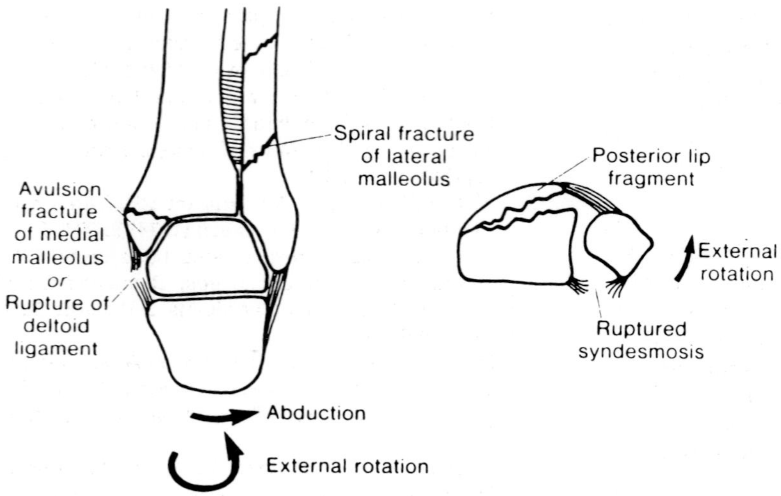

Figure 3.27

Injury to the malleoli of the ankle results from abduction and external rotation of the foot. (From Ref 19 with permission.)

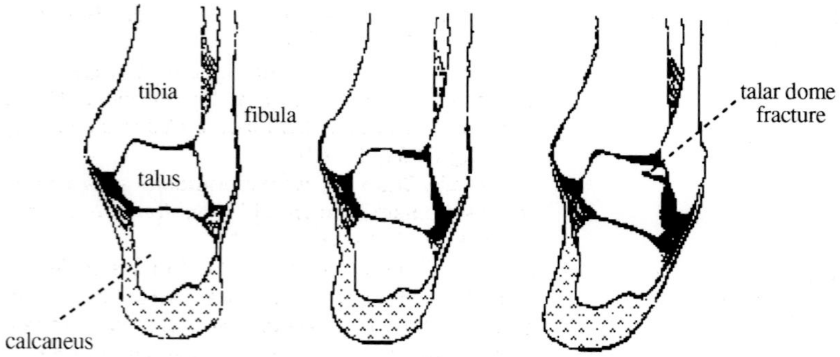

Figure 3.28

Diagram showing how forced inversion of the foot progressively wedges the lateral border of the talus against the articular facet of the fibula, creating tension and shear, and resulting in a chip fracture. (From Ref 39 with permission.)

magnitude, although it may exceed these levels locally at the stress riser (concentrator) and at the tip of the crack.

In impact fracture, long (tubular) bones exhibit fracture patterns specific to the directions of the applied loads. Axial compressive loading results in a fracture line transverse to the long axis of the bone, but located in the metaphyseal cancellous bone region. Examples are the pilon fracture of the distal tibia, fracture of the tibial plateau, and the Colles' fracture of the distal radius. A transverse fracture line seen in the middiaphysis is a result of bending that produces tensile failure on the convex side of the bone. A butterfly fragment is the result of combined axial compression and bending, applied at a high loading rate. A spiral fracture line in the midshaft indicates that torsional loading is the mechanism of failure, and should be differentiated from a short oblique fracture, which is likely due to compression combined with bending.

Several common fractures about joints occur due to specific mechanisms. For example, both scaphoid waist fractures and talar neck fractures result from the proximal end of the bone being held rigidly while the distal pole is subjected to cantilever bending. The scaphoid and talus act as cantilevers, fracturing at the neck or waist, the narrowest region. Vertebral compression and torsional fractures are similar to those occurring in long bones. The high speed spinal compression fracture that results in bursting and bone retropulsion into the canal occurs due to pressurization of the fat and marrow within the vertebral body and subsequent explosion of the latter.

Fractures of the femoral neck can occur due to loading that is nearly parallel to the femoral shaft, or by a fall onto the greater trochanter. Vertical loading results in a fracture at the base of the trochanter. Comminution may result from a fall onto the trochanter that produces predominantly compression. Fractures separating the pelvic ring result from forces that create hoop stresses (tensile stresses around the circumference of the ring) and rupture the pubic symphysis ligaments in tension. If the forces are vertical, shear fracture at the sacroiliac joint or the sacrum may result from the vertically downward weight of the torso acting through the spinal column, and the vertically upward directed force through the femora.

3.9 References

1. Devas MB, Stress fractures in the tibia in athletes or "shin soreness," *J Bone Jt Surg* (1958) **40B**: 227–43.
2. Bargren JH, Tilson DH, Prevention of displaced fractures of the femur, *J Bone Jt Surg* (1971) **53A**: 1115–17.
3. Gilbert RS, Johnson HA, Stress fractures in military recruits: a review of twelve years' experience, *Milit Med* (1966) **131**: 716–21.
4. Lafferty JF, Raju PVV, The influence of stress frequency on the fatigue strength of cortical bone, *J Biomech Eng* (1979) **101**: 112–13.
5. King AI, Evans FG, Analysis of fatigue strength of human compact bone by the Weilbull method. In Jacobson B, ed, *Digest of the 7th International Conference on Medical and Biological Engineering* (Royal Academy of Engineering Sciences: Stockholm 1967).
6. Gray RJ, Korbacher GK, Compressive behavior of bovine compact bone, *J Biomech* (1977) **7**: 287–92.
7. Carter DR, Hayes WC, Compact bone fatigue damage. A microscopic examination, *Clin Orthop* (1977) **127**: 265–73.
8. Pope MH, Outwater JO, The fracture characteristics of bone substance, *J Biomech* (1972) **5**: 457–65.
9. Saha S, The dynamic properties of bone and its relevance. In: Guista, DN, ed, *Osteoarthromechanics* (Hemisphere: Washington 1982) 1–43.
10. Burstein AH, Zika JM, Heiple KG, Klein L, Contribution of collagen and mineral to the elastic–plastic properties of bone, *J Bone Jt Surg* (1975) **57A**: 956–61.
11. Reilly DT, Burstein AH, Frankel UH, The elastic modulus for bone, *J Biomech* (1974) **7**: 271–5.
12. Gonza ER, Biomechanical long bone injuries. In: Gonza ER, Harrington IJ, eds, *Biomechanics of musculoskeletal injury* (Williams & Wilkins: Baltimore 1982) 1–30.
13. Hirsch C, Cavadies A, Nachemsen A, An attempt to explain fracture types. Experimental studies on rabbit bones, *Acta Orthop Scand* (1955) **24**: 9–29.
14. Martens M, van Audekercke R, de Meester P, Mulier JC, The mechanical characteristics of the long bones of the lower extremity in torsional loading, *J Biomech* (1980) **13**: 667–76.
15. Mather BS, Observations on the effects of static and impact loading on the human femur, *J Biomech* (1968) **1**: 331–5.
16. Berg DC, Labosky DA, Ligamentous disruptions at the wrist in an experimentally produced Colles fracture, *Trans 38th Orthopedic Research Society Meeting* (1992) **17**: 414.
17. Weber ER, Chao EY, An experimental approach to the mechanism of scaphoid waist fracture, *J Hand Surg* (1978) **3**: 142–8.
18. Frykman G, Fracture of the distal radius including sequelae–shoulder–hand–finger syndrome, disturbance in the distal radio-ulnar joint and impairment of nerve function, a clinical and experimental study, *Acta Orthop Scand* (1967) Supp 108.
19. Harrington IJ, Biomechanics of joint injuries. In: Gonza ER, Harrington IJ, eds, *Biomechanics of musculoskeletal injury* (Williams & Wilkins: Baltimore 1982) 31–86.
20. Holdsworth FA, Fractures, dislocations and fracture-dislocations of the spine, *J Bone Jt Surg* (1970) **52A**: 1534–51.
21. Ferguson RL, Allen Jr BL, A mechanistic classification of spine fractures, *Clin Orthop* (1984) **189**: 77–88.
22. Roaf R, A study of the mechanics of spinal injuries, *J Bone Jt Surg* (1960) **42B**: 810–23.
23. McElhaney JH, Paver JG, McCrackin HJ, Maxwell GM, Cervical spine compression responses, *Society of Automotive Engineers Technical Paper* 831615 (1983).
24. Nucholtz GS, Huelke DS, Luk P, Alem NM, Montalvo F, Cervical spine injury mechanisms. In: *Proceedings of the 27th STAPP Car Crash Conference* (Society of Automotive Engineers: 1983) 275.

25. Kazarian LE, Graves GA, Compressive strength characteristics of the human vertebral centrum, *Spine* (1977) **2**: 1–14.
26. Tencer AF, Ahmed AM, Burke DL, Some static mechanical properties of the lumbar intervertebral joint, intact and injured, *J Biomech Eng* (1982) **104**: 193–201.
27. Farfan HF, Cossette JW, Robertson GH, Wells RV, Kraus H, The effects of torsion on the lumbar intervertebral joints: the role of torsion in the production of disc degeneration, *J Bone Jt Surg* (1970) **52A**: 468–97.
28. Evans DC, Biomechanics of spinal injury. In: Gonza ER, Harrington IJ, eds, *Biomechanics of musculoskeletal injury* (Williams & Wilkins: Baltimore 1982) 163–228.
29. Gonza ER, Biomechanics of pelvic and acetabular fractures. In: Gonza ER, Harrington IJ, eds, *Biomechanics of musculoskeletal injury* (Williams & Wilkins: Baltimore 1982) 88–135.
30. Smith LD, Hip fractures, the role of muscle contraction or intrinsic forces in the causation of fractures of the femoral neck, *J Bone Jt Surg* (1953) **35A**: 367–83.
31. Melton III LJ, Riggs BL, Hip fracture: a disease and an accident. In: Uhthoff HK, Stahl E, eds, *Current concepts of bone fragility* (Springer-Verlag: Berlin 1986) 385–9.
32. Melton III LJ, Riggs BL, Epidemiology of age-related fractures. In: Avidoli LV, ed, *The osteoporotic syndrome: detection, prevention, and treatment* (Grune & Stratton: Orlando 1987) 1–30.
33. Melton III LJ, Wahner HW, Richelson LS, O'Fallon WM, Riggs BL, Osteoporosis and the risk of hip fracture, *Am J Epidemiol* (1986) **124**: 254–61.
34. Lotz JC, Hayes WC, Estimates of hip fracture risk from falls using quantitative computed tomography, *J Bone Jt Surg* (1990) **72A**: 689–700.
35. Viano DC, Stalmaker RL, Mechanism of femoral fracture, *J Biomech* (1980) **13**: 701–16.
36. Huelke DF, Harger JH, Buege LJ, Dingman HG, Harger DR, An experimental study in bio-ballistics. Femoral fractures produced by projectiles, *J Biomech* (1968) **1**: 97–106.
37. Huelke DF, Harger JH, Buege LJ, Dingman HG, An experimental study in bio-ballistics. Femoral fractures produced by projectiles—II shaft impacts, *J Biomech* (1968) **1**: 313–21.
38. Kennedy JC, Bailey WH, Experimental tibial plateau fractures, *J Bone Jt Surg* (1968) **50A**: 1522–34.
39. Berndt AL, Hartz M, Transchondral fractures (osteochondritis dissecans) of the talus, *J Bone Jt Surg* (1959) **41A**: 988–1018.

PART II
GENERAL CONSIDERATIONS IN FRACTURE FIXATION

CHAPTER 4

The environment for fracture healing

This chapter is intended as a basis for the design of fracture implant/bone constructs. After a brief introduction to the biological process of fracture healing, the changes in biomechanical properties of the healing fracture with time are shown. This is followed by a discussion of how the healing tissue responds to its mechanical environment, and therefore how the mechanical environment should be altered during various stages of fracture healing. Practical methods for changing the mechanical environment, specifically permitting greater load sharing as the tissue heals, are discussed. Finally, the design of implants with regard to their effects on blood flow is considered.

4.1 Biological processes in fracture healing

Cruess and Dumont[1] defined three biological stages of fracture healing: inflammatory, reparative, and remodelling. In the inflammatory stage (Figure 4.1), a hematoma accumulates within the medullary canal and beneath the periosteum, which is elevated during injury. The material within the local region of the fracture becomes necrotic due to lack of nutrition. Inflammatory cells and macrophages invade the region. Granulation tissue quickly becomes organized in the area. Vascular studies show that a blood pool forms initially, followed by occlusion, a sign of vascular obstruction with fibrous callus.[2]

As the hematoma becomes organized, a reparative phase begins. The hematoma acts as a fibrin scaffold for pluripotential mesenchymal cells from the cambium layer of the periosteum, as well as from the endosteum. These cells begin to form cartilage and fiber bone, increasing the mechanical stability of the fracture site.[1] Henricson et al[3] observed that osteoblasts in the periosteum and in the orifice of the medullary canal form trabeculae without passing through a cartilage stage. An area of crowded irregular cells (area of pluripotent cells) widens back from the fracture ends, forward to bridge the fracture, and outwards from the periosteum. Chondroblasts differentiate from this region and fill most of the free space on the muscle side of the fracture. The chondrocytes become hypertrophic, mineralized matrix appears, and vessels from the bone marrow pierce the cortical bone towards the ossification front. This stage is characterized by a marked increase in the level of type I collagen, along with the presence of TGF-β, connective tissue growth factor, and osteopontin.[4,5] At the same time, there is a proliferation of blood vessels (Figure 4.2), which are oriented perpendicular to the long axis of the bone on the periosteal side, and parallel on the medullary side. The capillaries become dilated and full of red blood cells.

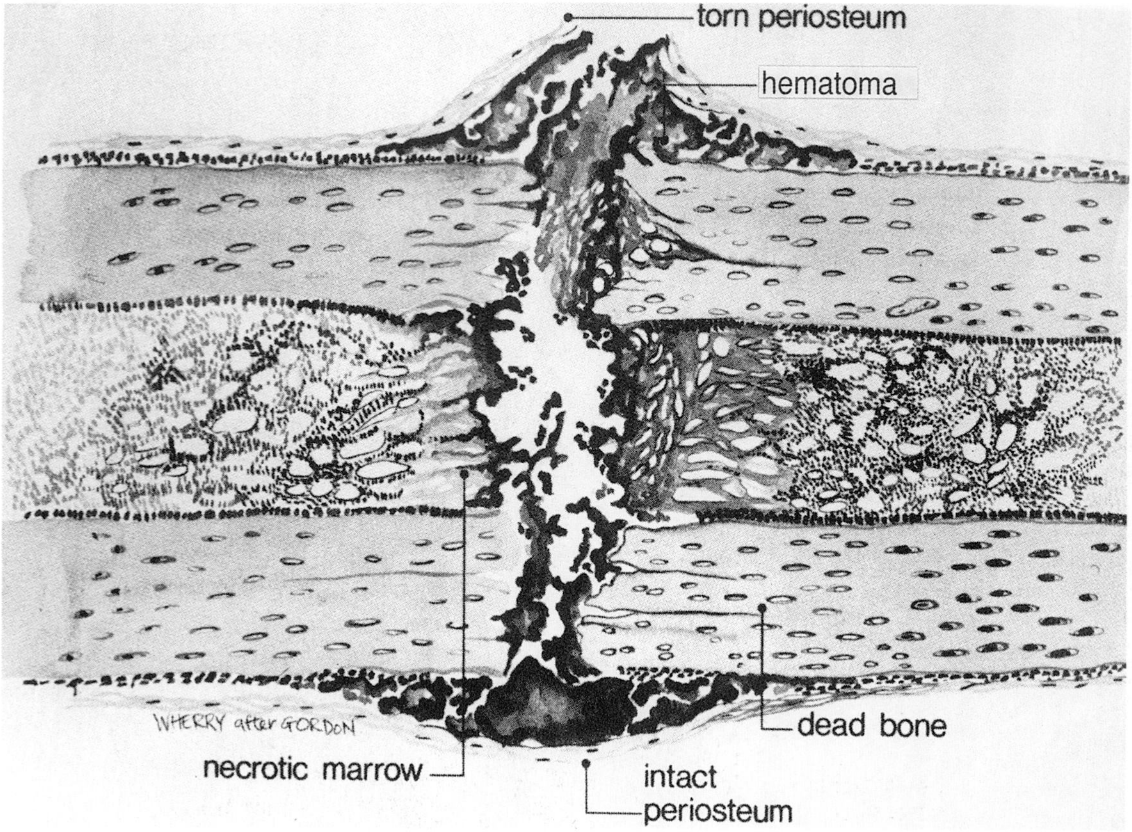

torn periosteum
hematoma
WHERRY after GORDON
dead bone
necrotic marrow
intact
periosteum

(a)

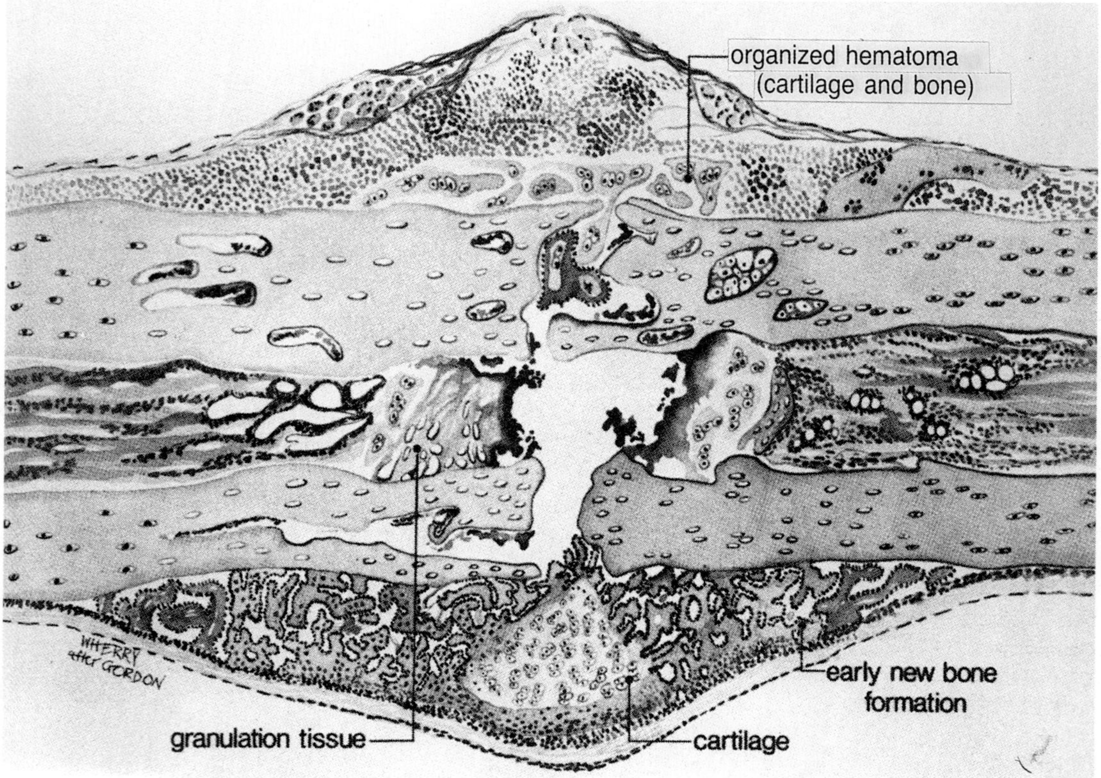

organized hematoma
(cartilage and bone)
WHERRY
after GORDON
early new bone
formation
granulation tissue
cartilage

(b)

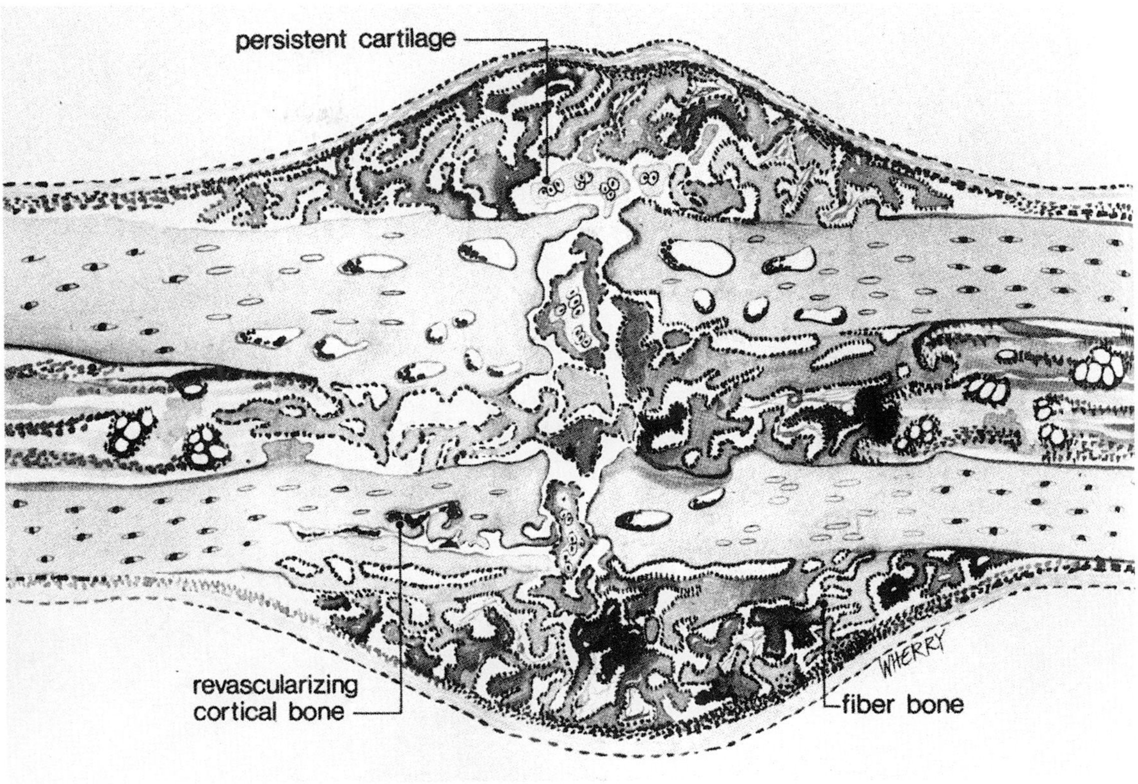

(c)

Figure 4.1

Three stages of fracture healing. (a) Formation of a hematoma and dead bone near the fracture site. (b) Organizing callus with areas of cartilage and new bone formation. (c) Fiber bone and revascularizing cortical bone. (From Ref 1 with permission.)

Biochemically, initially there exists a high concentration of glycosaminoglycans, followed by an increase in collagen and an accumulation of hydroxyapatite crystals. Osteoblasts synthesize tropocollagen, which moves extracellularly and polymerizes to form a regular organization of collagen fibrils. Crystals of calcium hydroxyapatite become clustered around the fibrils, eventually forming a rigid callus mass around the fracture. This is considered the point of clinical union. From this point, type I collagen and TFG-β levels decline.[4] Blood vessels begin to pass through the fibrous callus of one fracture fragment to reunify with those of the other component.[2]

The third stage of fracture healing occurs over a long period of time as bone remodelling removes superfluous tissue until the bone has either returned to its original shape and size, or has altered its shape to optimize the amount of material for the loads it must bear.

4.2 The biomechanics of fracture healing

Biomechanically, White et al[6] have demonstrated four distinct stages in fracture healing, characterized by differences in maximum torque and

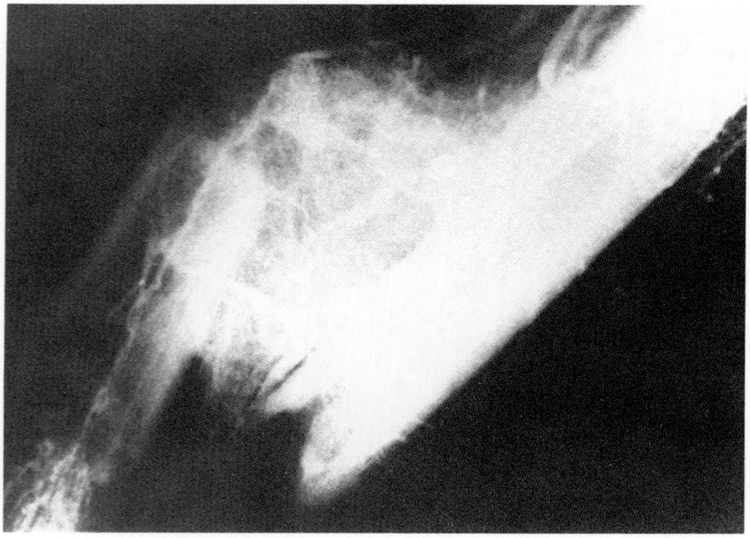

Figure 4.2

A rich vascular network reconstitutes around the site of the fracture despite the displacement of the fracture components and the short period of time since the initiation of healing ($5\frac{1}{2}$ weeks). (From Ref 2 with permission.)

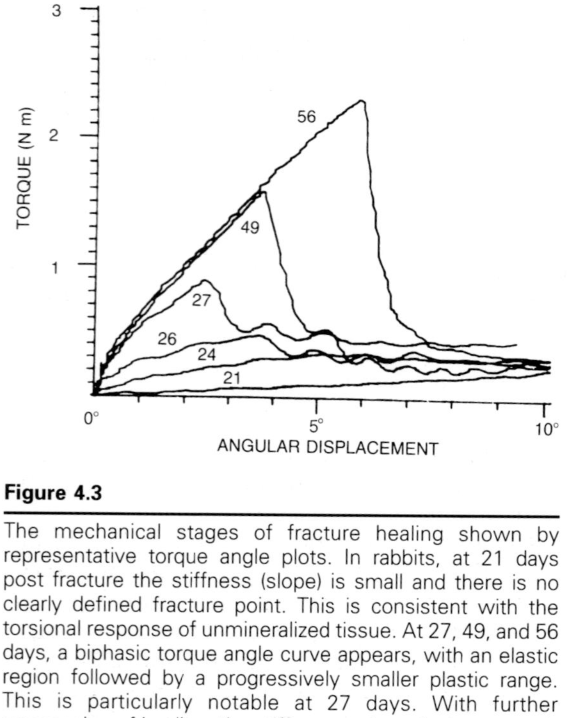

Figure 4.3

The mechanical stages of fracture healing shown by representative torque angle plots. In rabbits, at 21 days post fracture the stiffness (slope) is small and there is no clearly defined fracture point. This is consistent with the torsional response of unmineralized tissue. At 27, 49, and 56 days, a biphasic torque angle curve appears, with an elastic region followed by a progressively smaller plastic range. This is particularly notable at 27 days. With further progression of healing, the stiffness and maximum strength increase (compare 27 and 49 day curves). Also, the tolerable angular displacement before failure increases with healing time. (From Ref 6 with permission.)

energy to failure, as shown in Figure 4.3. In stage I (less than 23 days post fracture in rabbits), the bones all fail through the fracture site with low stiffness and large deformation, and have fracture site mechanical properties similar to those of collagen. In stage II, failure occurs through the injured area, but with considerably increased stiffness, and less deformation at yield. In stage III, failure occurs partly through the injured region and partly through intact bone, with significantly greater yield strength, but similar stiffness. In stage IV, failure occurs outside the region of injury, and with greater strength and energy than in stage III. The clear differences in maximum torque to failure and energy absorption between stages (which increases with greater load to failure although the deformation at failure is less) are demonstrated in Figure 4.4.

The increases in biomechanical properties during the course of normal fracture healing are related to two effects. First, there is an increase in the cross sectional area of new bone in the healing region (Figure 4.5) as a result of the enlargement of the cross section of the periosteal callus. This increases the moment of inertia of the healing region, and therefore its stiffness and

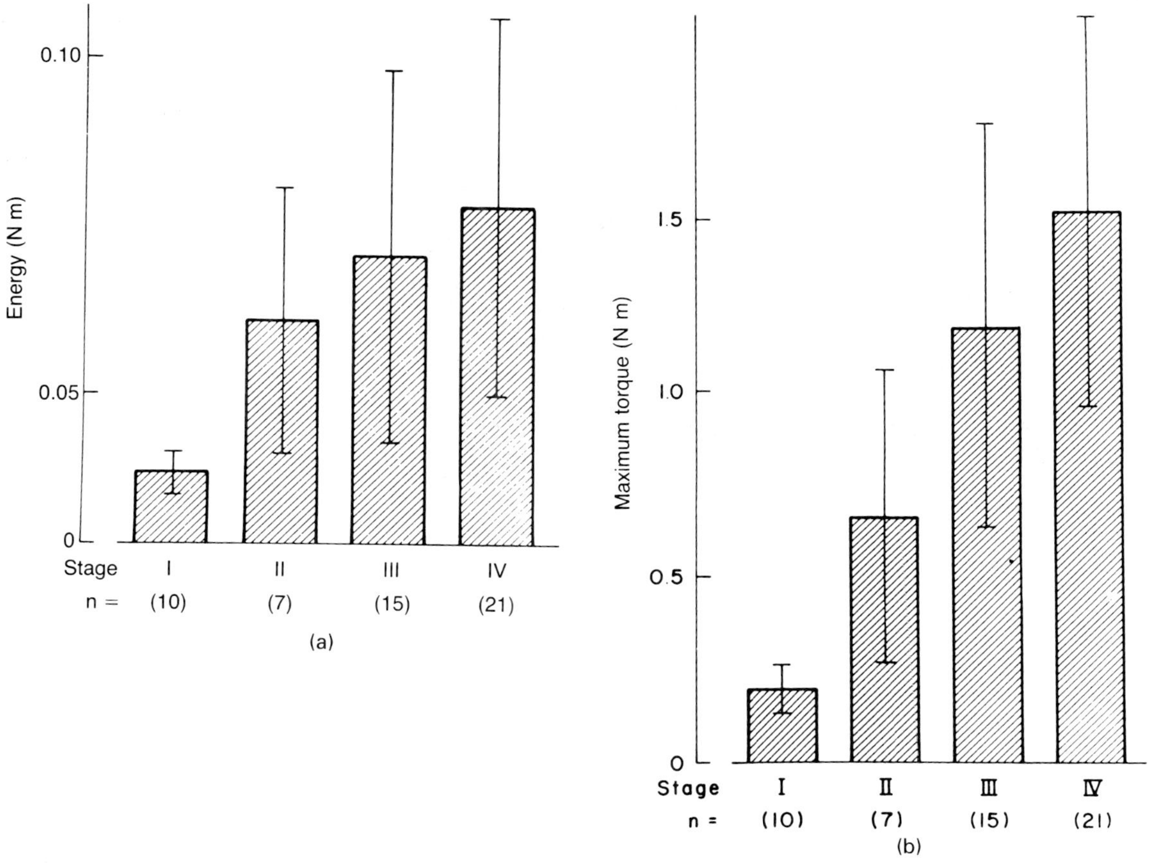

Figure 4.4

Increases in (a) the energy absorbed to failure (which is a measure of the ability of the fracture callus to absorb energy) and (b) the maximum torque to failure, for the four different biomechanical stages of fracture healing. (From Ref 6 with permission.)

strength.[8] As Figure 4.6 shows, the increase in cross section is of most benefit if the new bone is deposited as far from the central axis as possible, i.e. periosteally.

Secondly, there is a change in the material properties within the healing area. This is due partly to a decrease in porosity of the bone as it changes from a woven to a mature trabecular structure. As shown in Figure 4.7, the predominant decrease in porosity occurs in the fracture gap, followed by the periosteal region. Endosteal porosity actually increases as the bone remodels and the endosteal canal is re-established.[9] A second parameter that alters the material properties is an increase in the mineral content of the healing tissue (Figure 4.8).[7,9]

The role of vascularity in restoration of the biomechanical properties is extremely important. Chidgey et al[10] showed that the flexural (bending) rigidity of experimental fractures was only about 10% of normal bone with an avascular gap between bone ends and no medullary circulation. Rigidity increased to about 30% when vessels bridged the medullary canal and cortex, and returned to 100% with re-establishment of a normal vascular pattern (Figure 4.9).

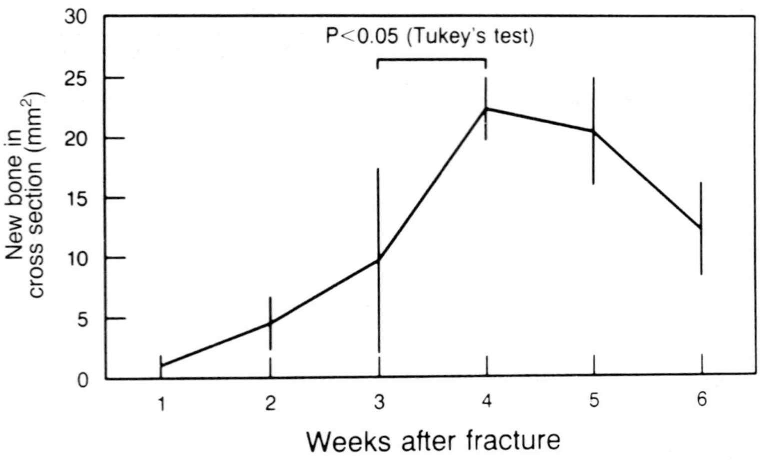

Figure 4.5

Changes in the cross sectional area of new bone in healing femoral fractures in rats with time post fracture. (From Ref 7 with permission.)

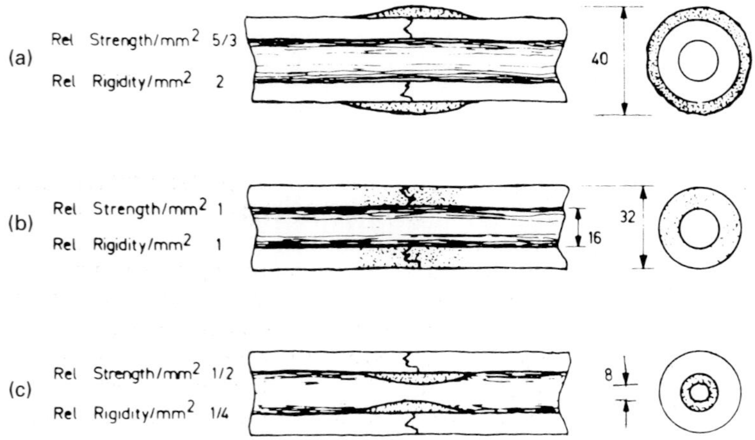

Figure 4.6

Relative to a bone that heals with (b) no fracture callus or (c) only a medullary callus, a periosteal callus (a) increases the rigidity in bending by a factor of 2 and the strength by a factor of $\frac{5}{3}$ in this example. The differences in rigidity can be calculated from the polar moments of inertia of the cross sections, assuming all have the same material properties. (From Ref 8 with permission.)

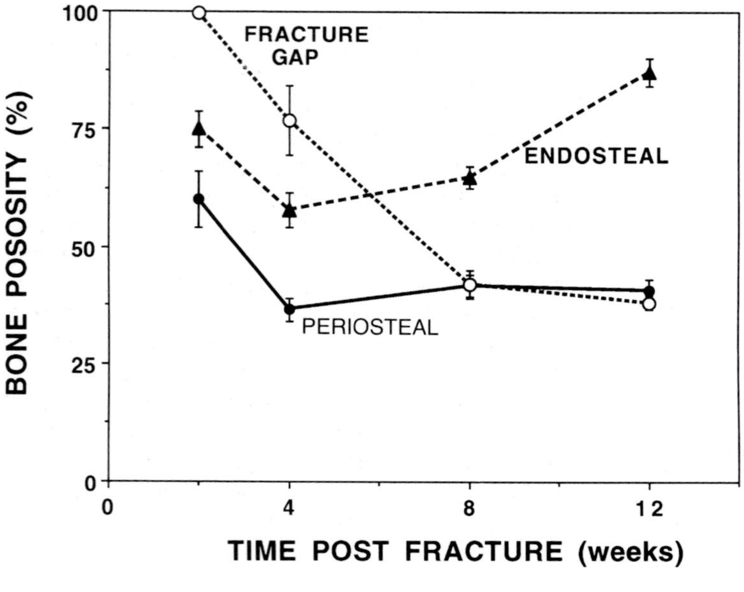

Figure 4.7

Change in porosity around healing tibial osteotomies in dogs with time post injury. Fracture gap porosity and periosteal porosity both decrease while endosteal porosity increases as the endosteal canal is re-established. (Data adapted from Ref 9.)

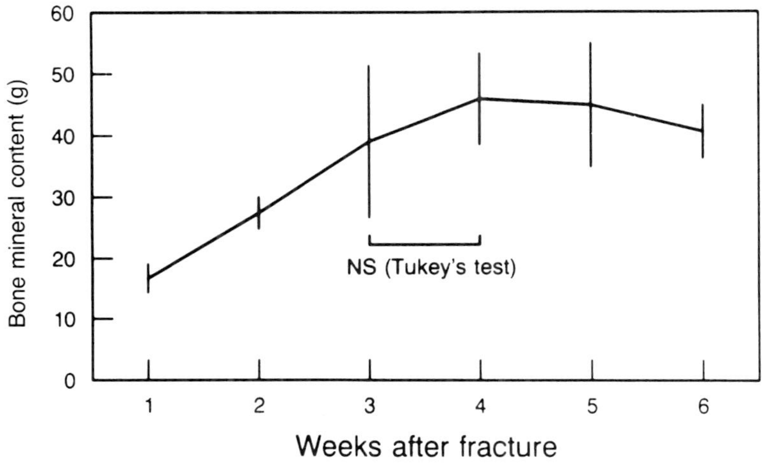

Figure 4.8

Progressive increase in the mineral content of healing fracture callus with time post fracture. (From Ref 7 with permission.)

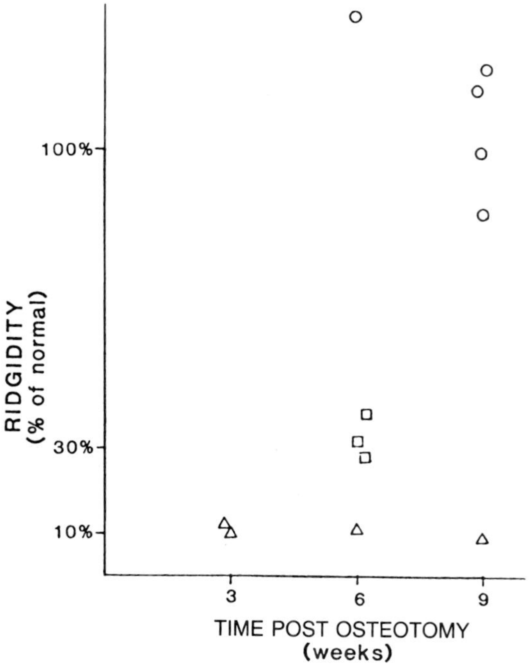

Figure 4.9

Relationship of bending rigidity of the healing fracture to its vascular properties. Symbols represent the vascular pattern: △, avascular gap between bone ends; □, vessels bridging medullary canal and cortex; ○, cortical union, returning to normal vascular pattern. (From Ref 10 with permission.)

4.3 The mechanical environment for fracture healing

Probably one of the most significant advances in the operative treatment of fractures was the incorporation of the concepts of direct apposition, rigid fixation, and axial compression of the fracture components.[8,11–15] Compression, as will be discussed in detail later with respect to the mechanics of plating, aids in creating a more rigid construct by producing friction between the fracture surfaces. If the construct is extremely rigid, the biological requirement for formation of callus to increase the rigidity of the fracture site is reduced.

In experimental osteotomies, direct healing without bridging callus occurs across a stable immobile interface at the osteotomy site (Figure 4.10). In this case, healing proceeds with minimal callus formation, and no resorption at the fracture surfaces. Instead, osteoclasts drill along the long axis of the bone shaft, crossing the fracture line. They are followed by new osteoblasts that produce osteons and restore the haversian architecture.[8] Perren[8] showed that gaps within a rigidly fixed fracture interface also heal by direct formation of lamellar bone, oriented at right angles to the fracture line, which is later remodelled (Figure 4.11). The strength at this interface is low until remodelling occurs.

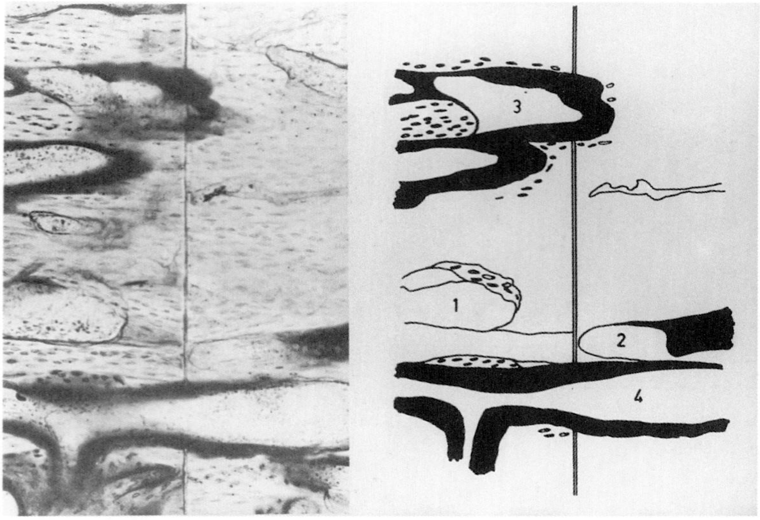

(a) (b)

Figure 4.10

Primary healing across a stable osteotomy. (a) The biological appearance of the healing osteotomy. (b) A schematic diagram corresponding to the section and identifying four stages in primary healing: (1) and (2) progression of cutting cones to the osteotomy surface; (3) crossing the osteotomy surface; (4) remodelling to a new haversian system. (From Ref 8 with permission.)

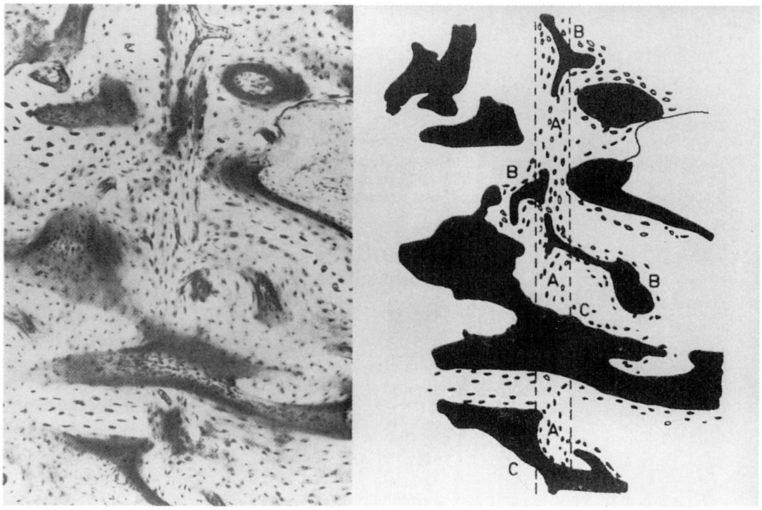

Figure 4.11

Healing of a stable but not closely approximated gap, which first fills with lamellar bone oriented parallel to the fracture surfaces, followed later by remodelling into osteons which cross the fracture surfaces. (From Ref 8 with permission.)

In actual fractures, the surfaces may be more irregular and "absolute" stability difficult to achieve. Perren[8] introduced the concept of interfragmentary strain in order to explain why different types of tissue occur in a fracture gap, and why resorption occurs. Strain is defined as the change in length that a tissue undergoes in response to an applied load, divided by its original length (see Chapter 1). A more rigid tissue such as bone can tolerate a much smaller strain before it fails ($\approx$ 2%) than can a more flexible tissue such as cartilage (failure strain $\approx$ 10–13%) or

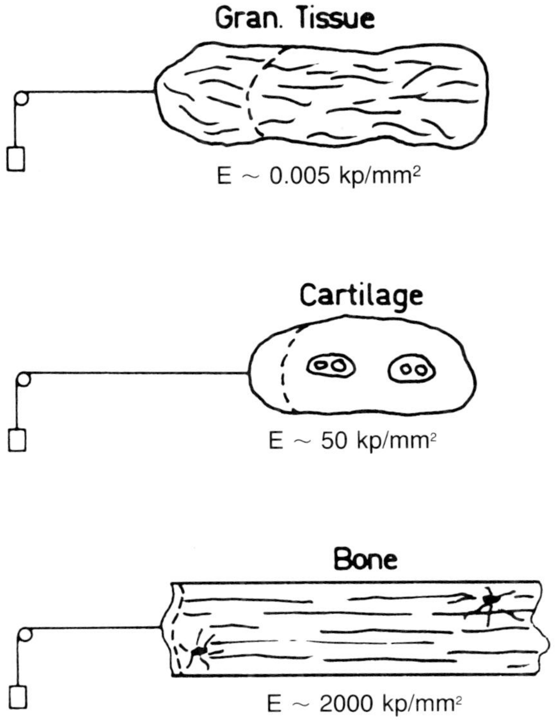

Figure 4.12

Schematic diagrams showing the relative rigidities of granulation tissue, cartilage, and bone. (From Ref 8 with permission.)

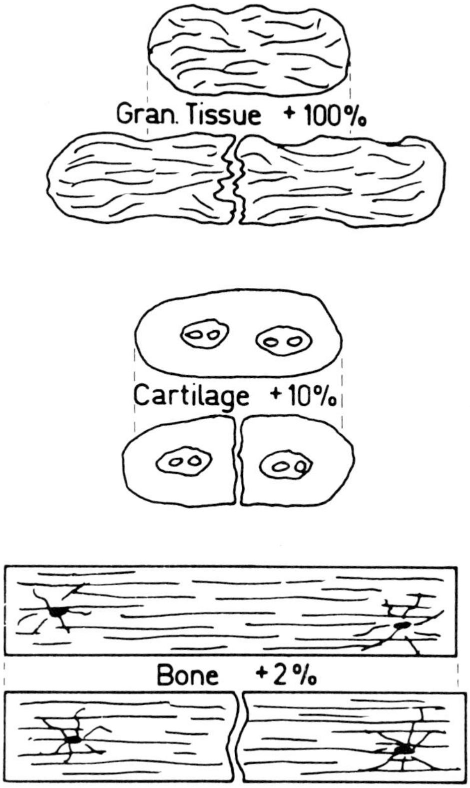

Figure 4.13

The theory of interfragmentary strain hypothesizes that the type of tissue formed in a healing gap depends upon the strain that it experiences. The strain is defined as the elongation *d* of the tissue in the gap (because of motion between the fracture components) divided by the length *G* of the tissue in the gap. Thus, for the same size of gap, *G*, if the strain *d*/*G* is between 10% and 100%, granulation tissue can be expected to form, while between 2% and 10% strain, fibrocartilage would form, and if less than 2%, bone would result in the gap. (From Ref 8 with permission.)

granulation tissue ($\approx$ 100%) (Figures 4.12 and 4.13). Therefore both the size of the gap and the motion between the ends of the gap will dictate the type of tissue that forms within it.

If the gap is very small, then for a given motion at the fracture site, the strain (elongation/original length, where original length = gap width) is large. Thus granulation tissue is most likely to be seen when the fracture gap is small but there is some longitudinal relative motion of the fracture surfaces. For the same motion, a larger fracture gap should permit cartilage formation, since the strain is smaller. Note that the tissue formed contributes to reducing fracture component motion, thus decreasing strain and allowing more rigid tissue to form. For example, considering Figure 4.13, if a gap of 1 mm exists between two fracture surfaces and the fixation allows for 0.2 mm of elongation, the strain of the tissue within the gap will be 20%, or twice the tolerable maximum of cartilage. If the tissue formed in the gap progressively decreases fracture site motion to 0.1 mm, cartilage may be able to start forming. Alternatively, if the fracture gap width is 2 mm then for the same gap motion the strain will be 10%, allowing the formation of cartilage. Cartilage is 10 000 times more rigid than granulation tissue, and will contribute to decreasing motion between the fracture ends. This further diminishes interfragmentary strain, which when it falls below 2%, according to this theory, will allow the formation of bone.[8] This theory also implies that for a given fracture gap motion, a larger gap will be more likely to permit bone formation than a smaller one.

It should be noted that the actual strains that occur within a fracture gap can be complex, even for simple longitudinal (axial compressive or tensile) stresses, because of the Poisson effect (as the tissue is elongated, its diameter decreases). This causes the tissue in the fracture gap to be largest in diameter near the bone interface, and to "neck" down in the midpart, resulting in large shear stresses, especially near the bone/gap tissue interface, where the properties of the materials are so different. Figure 4.14 shows the results of a finite element model analysis of the change in shape of a disk of fracture callus across an osteotomy gap, under tensile loading. The nonuniformity of the cross section produces shearing in the callus.[16] Considering that the fracture site is also subjected to other more complex loads, the actual strains of tissue in the fracture gap, which itself is usually variable across the fracture site, may be very difficult to predict.

As the fracture heals, the tissue in the callus begins to take on a load bearing role. As noted in Chapter 2, mechanical loading stimulates bone formation. For example, Rubin and Lanyon[17] have demonstrated that the response of bone to unloading is cortical thinning and porosity, while loading creates bone hypertrophy, especially on the periosteal surface (Figure 4.15). As shown schematically in Figure 4.16, an ideal fixation system would lose stiffness at a rate corresponding to the gain in stiffness of the healing fracture.[18] The gain in rigidity of a healing fracture, however, is not a completely uniform event. For example, Kaplan et al[19]

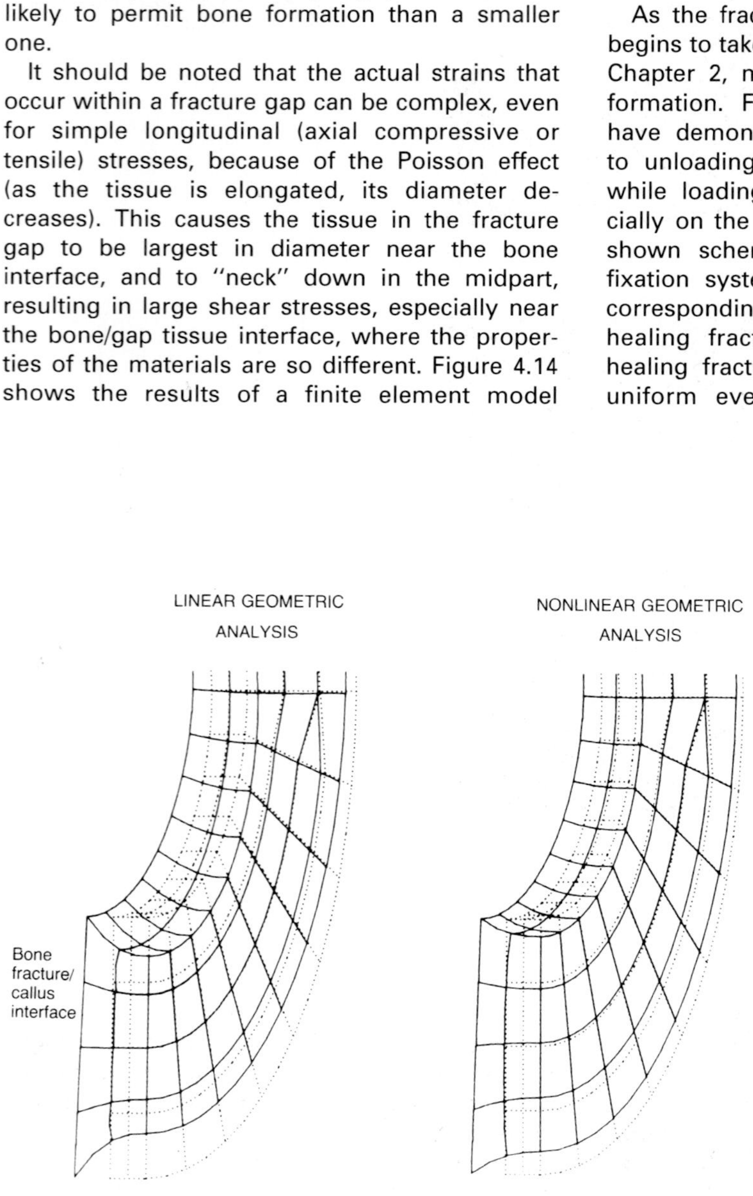

Figure 4.14

Finite element representation of the distortion of callus in an idealized osteotomy gap under an elongation stress due to the Poisson effect (the transverse diameter of a material changes as it is elongated or compressed axially). Note the "necking down" of the tissue towards the center of the gap. (The left edge in each diagram is the bone/callus interface, the dotted lines outline the shape of the unloaded callus, and the solid lines the callus under axial elongation.) Shearing occurs in elements that have distorted from their rectangular shape. (From Ref 16 with permission.)

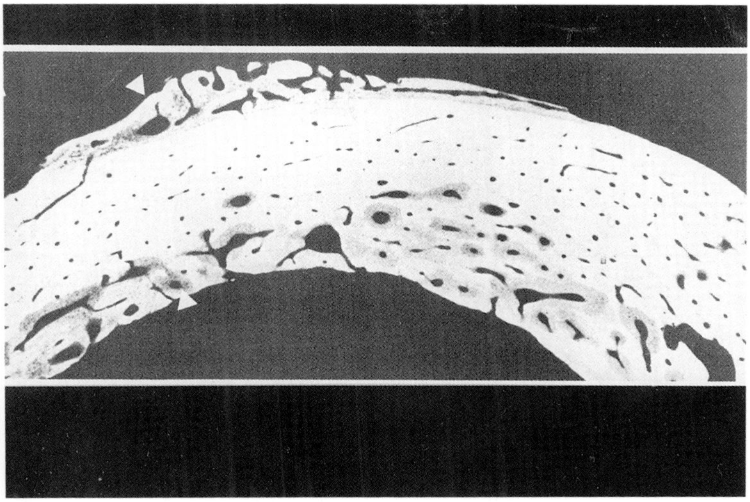

(a)

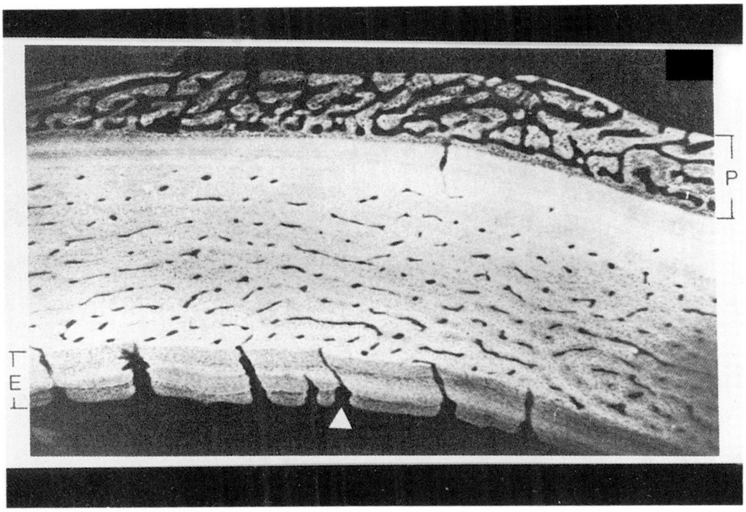

(b)

Figure 4.15

(a) A section through the cortex of the ulna of a turkey that was maintained unloaded. Thinning and porosity of the endosteal surface is evident. (b) A section through the cortex of an ulna subjected to 36 loading cycles per day for six weeks. There is no thinning of the endosteal cortex. Instead, newly deposited bone can be seen superperiosteally. (From Ref 17 with permission.)

mounted a strain gaged transducer (which measured changes in axial length) on external fixators mounted to the tibiae of rabbits with healing osteotomies. This allowed the structural rigidity of the fracture callus in axial loading to be monitored in vivo. As shown in Figure 4.17, for this animal model the actual gain in rigidity begins two weeks post surgery and rises linearly to week five, then approaches normal strength for the next three weeks. Therefore the rate of return to normal rigidity depends upon time post injury.

Based on the above discussions, a reasonable approach to producing an appropriate mechanical environment for a healing fracture would be as follows.

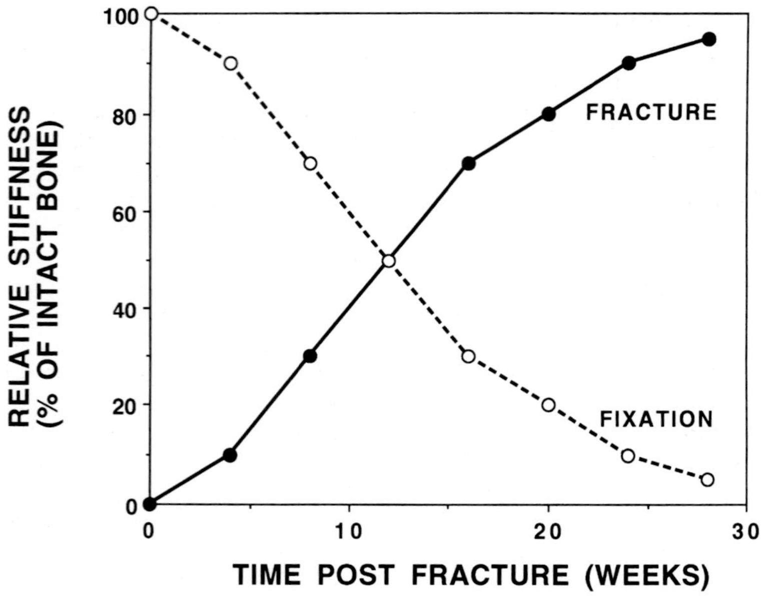

Figure 4.16

Hypothetical case in which a fracture fixation device loses stiffness at a rate corresponding to the gain in structural properties of the healing fracture, thus allowing progressive load sharing, while maintaining the stiffness of the fixation/bone construct.[18]

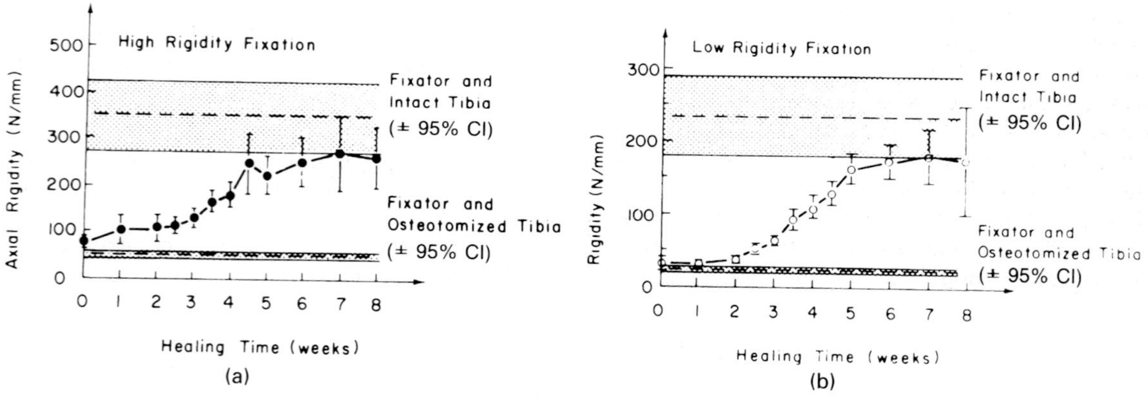

Figure 4.17

Change in the axial rigidity of the fracture callus in a healing osteotomy of a rabbit tibia fixed with (a) high rigidity and (b) low rigidity external fixation in vivo. (From Ref 19 with permission.)

- *During the early postfracture period* Maximize rigidity of the fracture region to minimize interfragmentary strain, thus promoting the formation of cartilage or bone.
- *During the middle part of the healing period* Provide progressive load sharing to the fracture.
- *During the late stage of healing* Maximize the load transferred to bone and minimize the structural role of the fixation system.

This approach is obviously quite general and vague, and probably will remain so until quantitative methods are adopted to measure the mechanical state of the healing fracture. Several methods for measuring mechanical properties have been investigated,[19–21] but are not in general use. *In the absence of quantitative measurements, it is reasonable to choose a fixation method that provides the greatest initial stability, and has some provision for permitting load sharing during the course of healing.* The next section addresses some methods that have been proposed or are used to accomplish these goals.

4.4 Alternatives for controlling the mechanical environment in fracture healing

Progressive disassembly (dynamization) of the fixation system

The change in the contribution of a fracture implant to the fracture/implant structure, from initially supporting all the load to progressively permitting load sharing, can be accomplished in several ways. A locking intramedullary rod shares a greater part of the load with bone when the distal locking screws are removed, as shown in the example of Figure 4.18.[22] Similarly, the rigidity of an external fixator can be modified by removal or repositioning of the sidebars. In the example of Figure 4.19, a triangulated half pin frame with bars on the anteromedial and posterolateral surface can be made progressively less rigid by partial disassembly.[23]

The results of dynamization of external fixation (that is, permitting some motion in the fixation, usually axial, to allow load sharing with healing bone) has been studied by Aro and Chao.[24] They found characteristics of gap healing in the fractures that were not dynamized (i.e. there was minimal load sharing), while a combination of gap and contact healing occurred on the cortex opposite the fixator. (Gap healing is defined by rough fracture ends, lamellar bone perpendicular to the fracture ends, and crossing of the gap by secondary osteons parallel to the long axis of the bone.) They concluded that early dynamization permits cortical contact, compensating for bone resorption or gaps created by imprecise reduction at the fracture surfaces.

Choosing fixation rigidity to accommodate the mechanical requirements of both early and late stages of healing

Studies have been performed to define some optimum mechanical stiffness, particularly for devices such as plates whose rigidity cannot be easily altered during the course of healing. The rigidity of a device should be great enough to

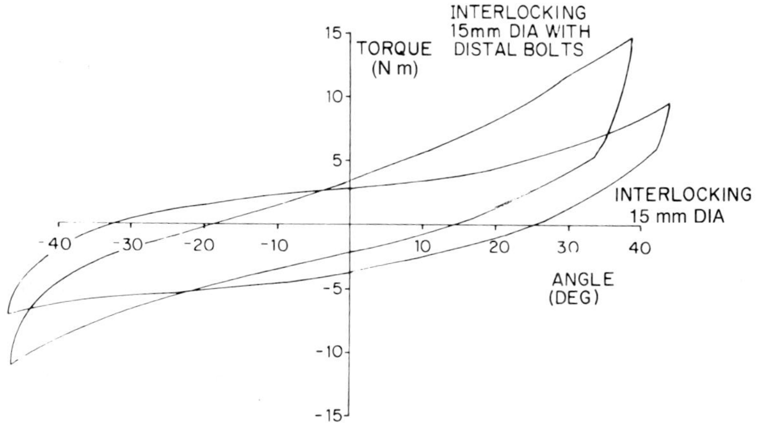

Figure 4.18

A plot of torque versus angle of a femur fixed with an intramedullary rod shows the difference in torsional stiffness with and without the distal locking screws. (From Ref 22 with permission.)

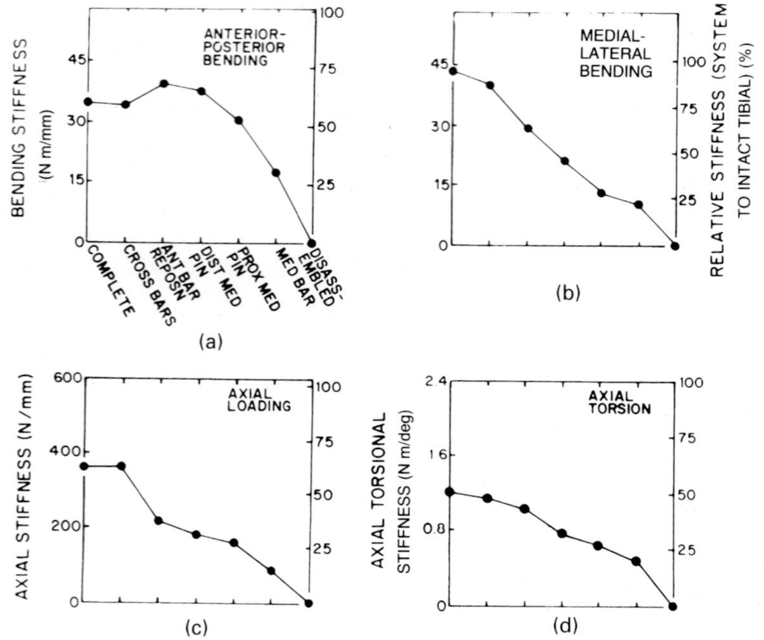

Figure 4.19

Progressive decrease in stiffnesses under different types of loads for a cadaver tibia fixed with a triangulated external fixator that is progressively dissassembled according to the steps described along the horizontal axis in (a): (a) anterior–posterior bending; (b) medial–lateral bending; (c) axial loading; (d) axial torsion. All plots are of absolute stiffness of the bone/frame construct and stiffness relative to the intact tibia. (From Ref 23 with permission.)

prevent excessive initial interfragmentary strain, yet flexible enough to allow load transfer to bone as the callus calcifies. Using plates of bending stiffness ranging from 13% to 74% of that of the intact tibia, Terjesen and Apalset[25] were able to demonstrate a decrease in callus area and strength with the stiffest plates after six weeks in the rabbit. The greatest stiffness and strength of the healing fracture were associated with the two plates of midrange stiffness. Within a range of about 20–60% of the bending stiffness of the intact bone, the strengths of the healing bones were equivalent to each other, but greater than those with either the lower or higher stiffness plate fixation (Figure 4.20).

Comparison of fracture healing with slotted (low torsional stiffness) versus closed section (high torsional stiffness) intramedullary rods has produced similar results to low versus high rigidity plates in terms of callus formation.[26] As shown in Figure 4.21, the lower stiffness IM rod produced bone healing with greater callus formation than the higher stiffness rod; however, the mechanical properties of the two groups at six months were not significantly different. These observations on the effect of fixation rigidity have been confirmed in other studies using external fixators.[27–29] It may be that the increase in the cross sectional area (and moment of inertia) of the fracture callus, in constructs with less mechanical stability, compensates for it being relatively less mature (and less mineralized), so that the same mechanical state can ultimately be reached by using either flexible or rigid fixation within the range discussed above.

After the fracture is able to support load, the requirement for rigid stabilization is replaced by the necessity of transferring load to the healing fracture. This observation was prompted by clinical reports of osteopenia and refracture of bone after removal of plates.[30–32] A number of experimental studies have addressed this problem. The placement of rigid plates on intact bone causes a transformation of the bone under the plate from cortical to cancellous and incompletely mineralized woven bone[33] with increased porosity and resorption cavities.[34,35] Woo et al[36] specifically addressed the effects of plates of different

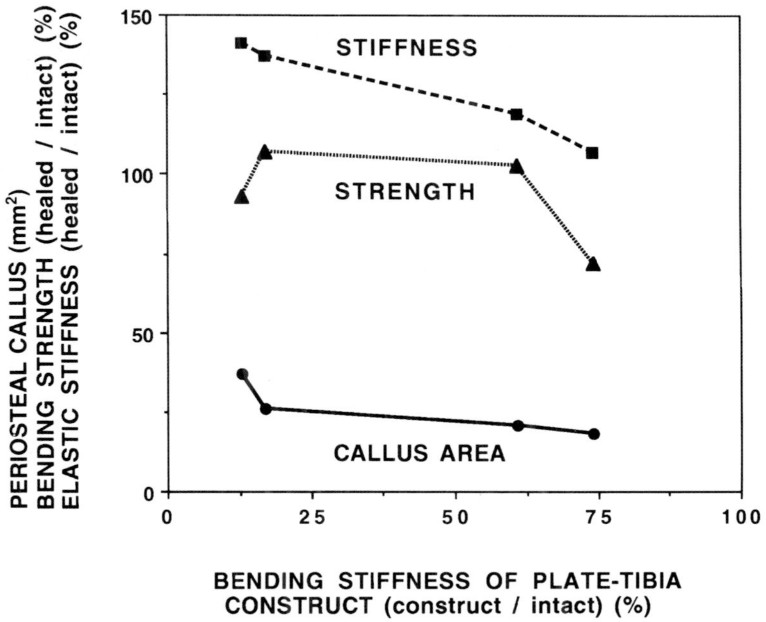

Figure 4.20

The effect of the stiffness of fixation in bending on the properties of healing tibiae at six weeks. The abscissa of the graph is the ratio (%) of the bending stiffness of the osteotomized tibia fixed with a plate of particular stiffness to that of the intact tibia. The ordinate shows callus (mm^2), and the ratio of bending strength and stiffness (%) of healed tibiae at six weeks to intact tibiae. As fixation stiffness increases, callus size decreases, along with its stiffness. The bending strength is greatest with fixation of medium stiffness. (Adapted from data of Ref 25.)

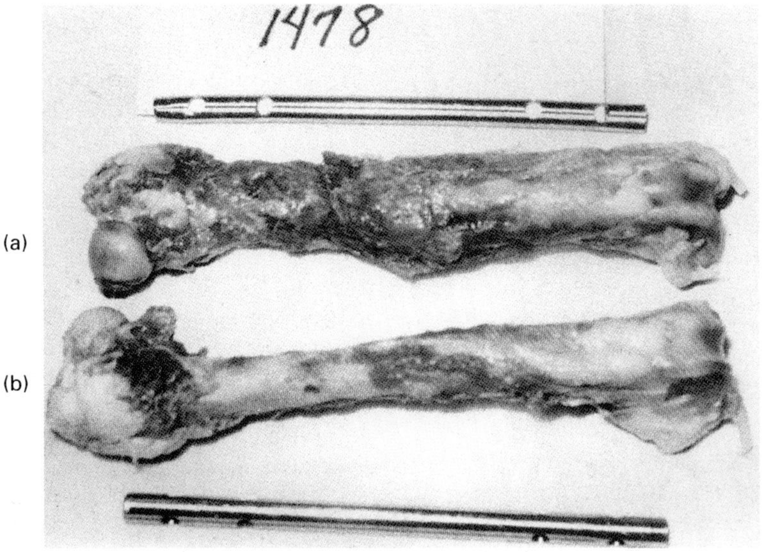

Figure 4.21

Examples of the differing healing responses in contralateral dog femora (a) fixed with a locked slotted IM rod and (b) fixed by a closed section rod of approximately 10 times the torsional rigidity, but equivalent bending and axial rigidities. (From Ref 26 with permission.)

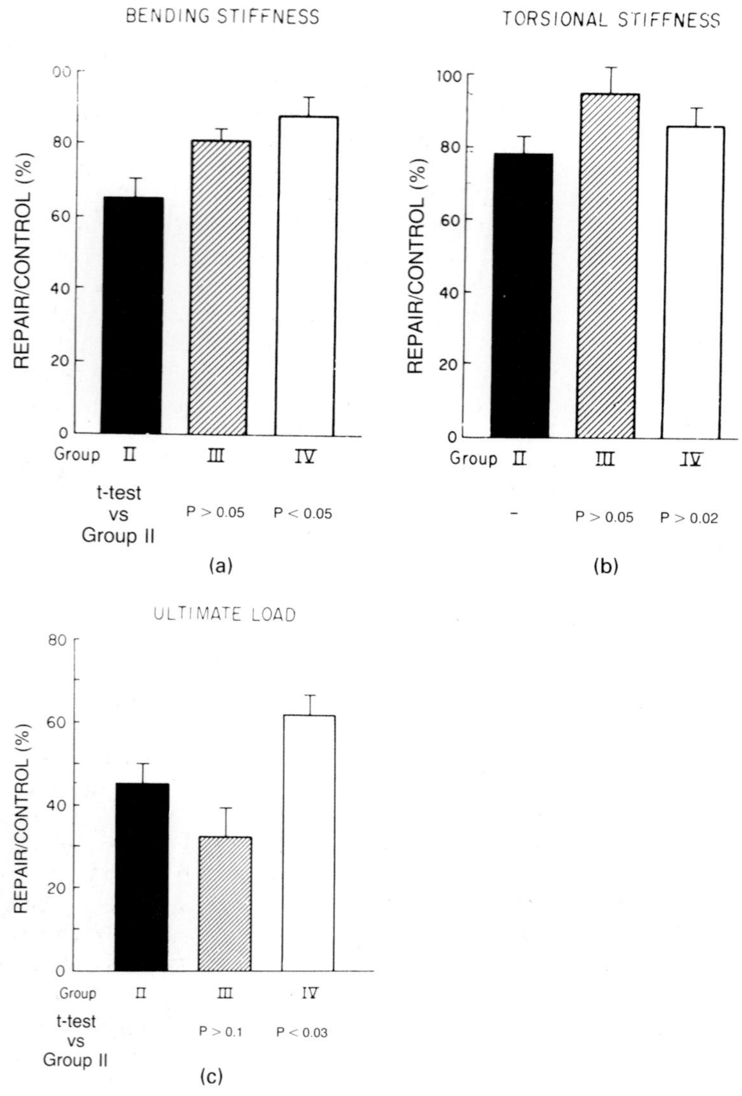

Figure 4.22

Comparisons of (a) the bending stiffness, (b) the torsional stiffness, and (c) the ultimate load of intact femora to which either solid stainless steel plates (group II, 31% bending stiffness compared with intact), tubular stainless steel plates (group III, 20%), or titanium Ti–6Al–4V plates (group IV, 3%) were fixed. Ratio is property of femur with plate removed to contralateral control. (From Ref 36 with permission.)

rigidities on bone strength. Plates equivalent to 31%, 20%, and 3% of femoral bending stiffness were placed on intact femora. The authors showed that the bending stiffness of the femora with the stiffest plates had dropped to about 65% at six months compared with 85% for the femora with the most flexible plates. Similar trends were seen in ultimate load (Figure 4.22). Carter et al[37] also have demonstrated a correlation between the added rigidity in bending due to the addition of a plate and the decrease in rigidity of the bone itself (Figure 4.23), which has been confirmed by others.[35,38–40]

Several investigators have questioned whether there is a true change in the material properties of the bone underlying the plate, or just thinning of the cortex. Woo et al[36] showed that material properties, such as elastic modulus and ultimate tensile strength of bone strips from plated intact femora decreased after six months in dogs (Figure

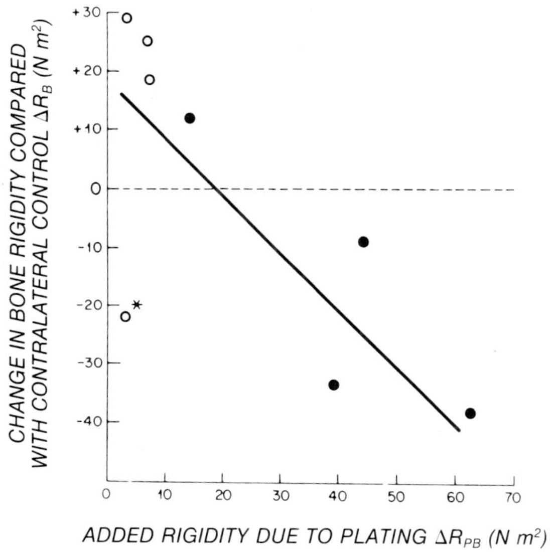

Figure 4.23

Change in bending rigidity of the femur compared to the contralateral control over time due to addition of a plate that increases the rigidity of the plate/bone construct, unloading the bone. ●, Metal-plated; ○, plastic-plated. (From Ref 37 with permission.)

4.24). After four months, there was increased labelled cortical bone (indicating remodelling) and significantly lower porosity in the corticies of femora under less rigid plates.[36] Three dimensional stress analysis has shown that this effect should occur mainly in the region of the plated femur between the innermost screws, where bone is most likely to be unloaded.[42]

The results of these investigations show that fixation within a range of about 20–60% of the intact bone results in the greatest early mechanical strength. More flexible fixation can be expected to result in more callus development than higher rigidity fixation, although fractures healing under the different conditions will ultimately have similar mechanical properties. As the fracture reaches maturity in terms of its mechanical properties, reduction of fixation rigidity, allowing loading sharing, is important to prevent further changes to the bone protected by the fixation device.

Controlled loading of the fracture site

Bone can be stimulated by controlled loading. A well known application of this concept has been to controlled distraction in limb lengthening as described by Ilizarov.[42] He showed that a separation rate of 1 mm/day applied in a progressive manner to an osteotomy gap, with intact periosteum, provided optimal bone regeneration within the gap. At a rate of 0.5 mm/day, there was premature consolidation of the osteotomy, while

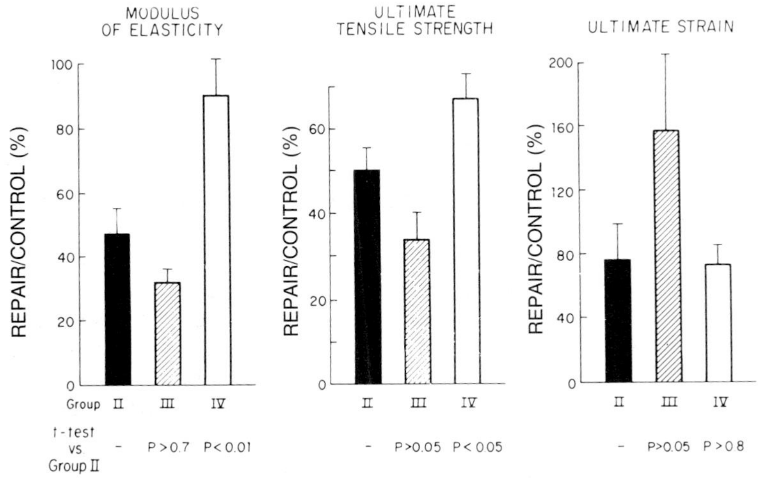

Figure 4.24

Material properties of bone strips from femora fixed with stainless steel plates (group II, 31% of intact bone stiffness), tubular stainless steel plates (group III, 20%), or titanium plates (group IV, 3%). Reducing the stiffness of the plate (group IV) increases the load sharing to bone and its resulting material properties. (From Ref 36 with permission.)

2 mm/day retarded osteogenesis. Also, bone could be formed parallel to the direction of the tensile strain, even when this was perpendicular to the long axis of the bone.[43] These observations indirectly confirm the concept of different tissues being formed with different interfragmentary strains.[15]

The difference between static and dynamic loading should be distinguished. Changing the magnitude of static compression has not been noted to alter the rate of bone remodelling.[44] In an interesting experiment, osteotomies of the femur on one side were treated by static compression alone, and on the contralateral by cyclic compression superimposed on the static load. No differences were found in any of the mechanical properties tested at any time period.[45]

Kenwright and Goodship[46] showed that controlled micromotion, consisting of an axial displacement at a fracture gap 3 mm wide, increased the bone mineral content within the fracture gap, if the maximum motion was 0.5 mm. This corresponds to an average interfragmentary strain of about 16%, although the true local strain may be much more complex. However, decreased bone mineral content was noted if the displacement was increased to 2.0 mm, as shown in Figures 4.25 and 4.26. Further, delaying the onset of this controlled micromotion treatment decreased bone mineral and fracture gap stiffness.[47] In view of the fact that increasing the compressive load in a rigidly fixed fracture does not stimulate healing, but controlled strain, whether compressive or tensile, does increase the rate of mineralization, strain and not load should be considered as the influencing factor.

Biodegradation of the implant

Using an implant that biodegrades over a period of time is an attractive approach to changing the properties of the implant as the fracture heals. A further benefit to the patient is that degradation

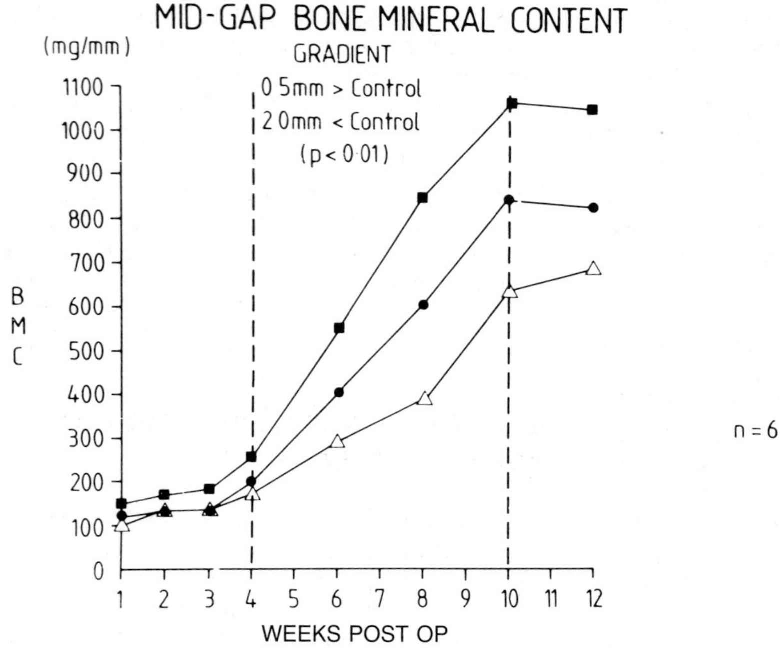

Figure 4.25

Bone mineral content in a fracture subjected to either rigid external fixation (control, ●), a controlled axial displacement of 0.5 mm applied as a total of 500 loading cycles over a period of 17 min daily (■), or a displacement of 2.0 mm at the same loading rate (△) (n = 6). (From Ref 46 with permission.)

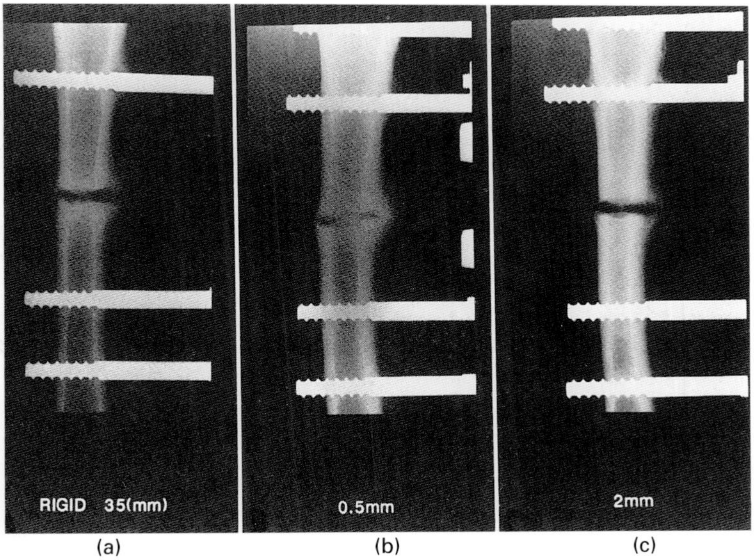

Figure 4.26

Radiographic comparisons of the appearance of a healing fracture at six weeks post surgery: (a) with rigid fixation; (b) with 0.5 mm displacement; (c) with 2.0 mm displacement. (From Ref 46 with permission.)

would potentially make removal of the hardware unnecessary. Poly(glycolides) and poly(lactides) are polymers frequently proposed as candidates for degradable implants based on a long history of use as degradable surgical sutures.[48] (Their properties are discussed in more detail in Chapter 5.) The shape, structure, composition, and purity of these devices along with their rate of degradation determine the inflammatory response.[49] The process of degradation involves absorption by giant cells (Figure 4.27),[50] and their degradation products, lactic acid and glycine (after conversion from glycolic acid), are incorporated into the tricarboxylic acid cycle.[51]

The rate of degradation is influenced by factors such as the molecular weight, degree of crystallinity, polymer/copolymer ratio (Figure 4.28),[50,52] local pH,[53] shape (surface area/volume ratio), and the magnitude of mechanical stress experienced.[54] The elastic modulus and tensile strength of these materials are much lower than those of commonly used metals such as titanium or stainless steel.[49] Therefore attempts have been made to fabricate plates that are composites of polymer and either nondegradable fibers such as carbon[55] or, preferably, degradable fibers of the same polymer but in a highly crystalline form.[56] Another ingenious reinforcement that has been proposed is calcium metaphosphate fiber, which would be biodegradable.[57] The decrease in bending strengths with implantation time of various diameters of self reinforced poly(glycolic acid) rods is shown in Figure 4.29.[56] Recent reports have described the clinical use of biodegradable rods and screws for the fixation of bimalleolar fractures of the ankle,[58,59] intra-articular fractures of the elbow joint,[60] and for bony avulsions.[61]

4.5 The effect of implants on bone vascularity

In the evaluation and selection of implants for fracture fixation, the effect of the implant on the vascular supply of the healing fracture must be considered. Chidgey et al[10] demonstrated a direct relationship between vascular structure and stiff-

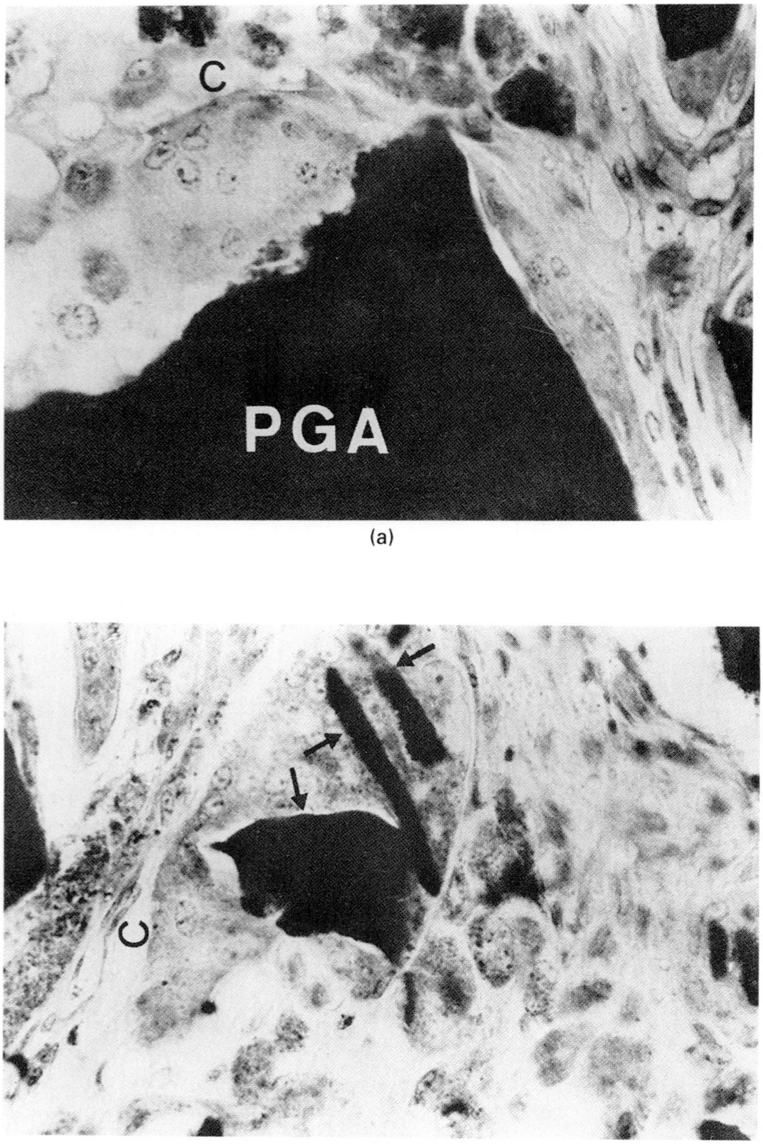

Figure 4.27

Histologic sections demonstrating the process of resorption of a poly(glycolide) implant. (a) Implant being absorbed by a giant cell (labelled C in the figure). (b) PGA debris (arrows) within the giant cell. (From Ref 50 with permission.)

ness of the healing osteotomized radius in the canine. They classified fracture vascularity into three definable patterns: (i) an avascular gap, (ii) vessels bridging the medullary canal and the cortex with medullary circulation supplying the callus, and (iii) return to a normal vascular pattern, examples of which are shown in Figure 4.30. These patterns were shown to be related to mean values of 10%, 30%, and 104% of the bending rigidity of the normal contralateral radius (Figure 4.9). A recent study has shown that blood flow at a healing osteotomy site is affected by the inter-

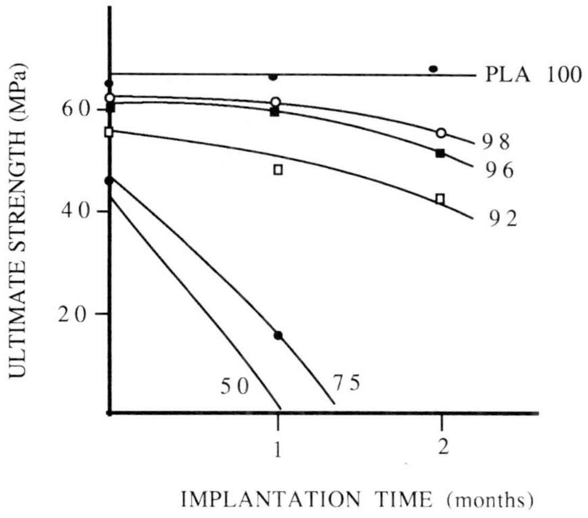

Figure 4.28

Change in the tensile strength of biodegradable polymers with time of implantation for implants with various poly(lactic)/poly(glycolic) stereocopolymer ratios (PLA 100 = 100% PLA, 50 = 50% PLA, 50% PGA). (From Ref 50 with permission.)

fragmentary strain in the fracture gap. With larger strains, both cortical and medullary blood flow are significantly higher, possibly because a larger mass of callus is required to stabilize this lower stiffness fracture.[62]

The effects of several standard orthopedic procedures for fracture fixation on the disruption of bone blood supply have been investigated. Daum et al[63] compared the changes in blood flow in five regions of the canine femur six months after either drilling a hole, drilling and applying screws, or drilling and applying a plate and screws. As shown in Figure 4.31, significant increases in blood flow occurred in the midshaft and metaphyseal/diaphyseal regions due to drilling and applying screws (without plates) and with plates applied. These procedures disrupt the local blood supply; however, only plating resulted in significant cortical thinning and porosity.

The disruption of the blood supply by plates has been considered by Perren et al[64] to be the cause of the late cortical thinning and porosity commonly seen after plate removal. Fixation of plates to bone impedes the radial blood supply from the medullary cavity to the periosteum[65] by clotting and accumulation of blood under the plate, as well as by impeding the access of external vessels to the periosteum.[66] Loss of blood supply has been demonstrated to stimulate remodelling and result in bone porosis.[64] Plates with reduced direct contact area between plate and bone have been found to reduce the region of disturbed circulation in the bone underneath the plate, and the area in the bone undergoing remodelling (Figure 4.32).[64] However, Uhthoff et al[67] have shown that there are two independent mechanisms by which increased porosity in bones can result. The short term process is, as outlined above, the interference with blood supply to the cortex, causing necrosis and porosis. This effect decreases with time. Long term changes, discussed previously, involve remodelling of bone due to decreased bone stress with the plate applied.

The effects of intramedullary reaming have also been investigated. Open intramedullary reaming of canine tibiae produced five times greater blood flow at the fracture site, and plating three times, compared with controls.[68] Intramedullary reaming has been demonstrated to interrupt the medullary vasculature and occlude vessels with fat emboli and bone particles.[69,70] Unreamed nailing has been proposed to reduce trauma to the vascular circulation. With reaming, disturbed circulation was found in at least the outer two thirds of the cortex and regionally throughout the entire cortex. Insertion of a nail without reaming affected only the inner third of the cortex.[71]

4.6 Summary

This material has been presented in order to develop a basis for the discussion of biomechanical testing results to be presented in the third part of this volume. The mechanical environment for fracture healing appears to allow for some range in selecting the optimal rigidity of fracture fixation. Rigid fixation (about 60% of intact bone) with a small fracture gap produces primary healing with little callus formation, while more flexible fixation (about 20%) with a larger fracture gap produces more callus; however, the end result is similar in terms of mechanical properties of the healed bone. Load sharing in the late stages of healing

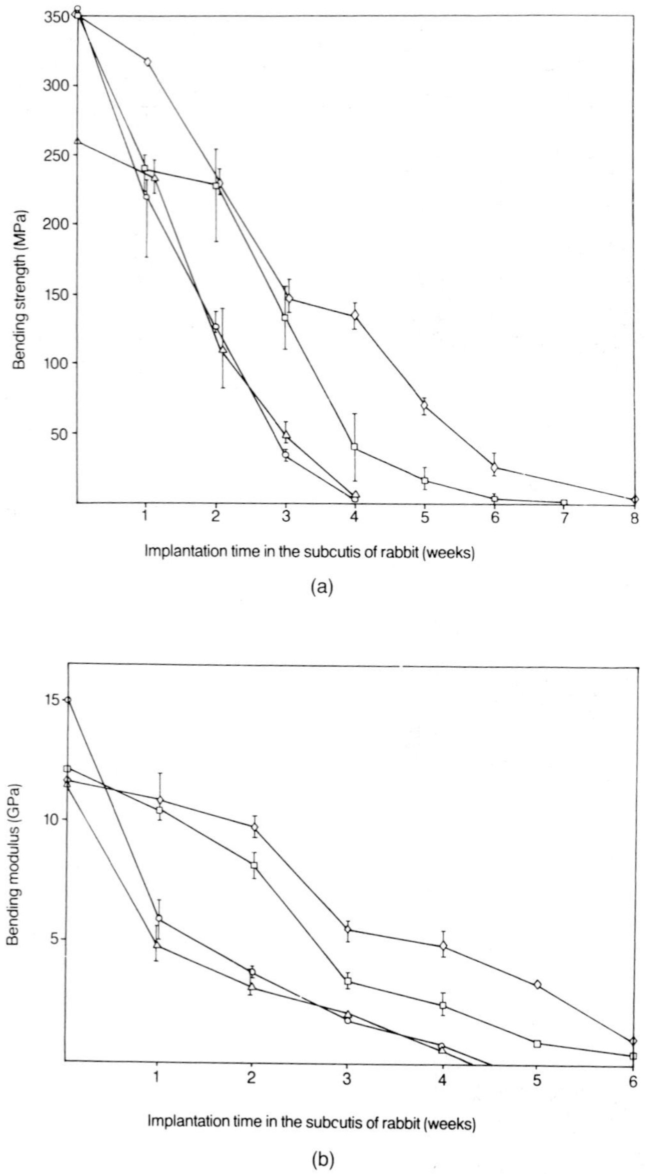

Figure 4.29

(a) Change in the bending strength of self reinforced poly(glycolic acid) rods of various diameters after different periods of implantation in the subcutis of the rabbit. (b) The rate of change in bending modulus varies with rod diameter. ○, 1.5 mm dia rod; △, 2.0 mm; □, 3.2 mm; ◇, 4.5 mm. (From Ref 55 with permission.)

is desirable, and can be produced by unlocking (dynamizing) intramedullary nails, partial disassembly of an external fixator, or early removal of plate hardware. Experiments in controlled loading of healing fracture demonstrate that repetitive loading is a key factor in stimulating new bone formation, as compared with static loading (i.e. static compression). This approach may be applicable to some classes of fractures. When choosing the type of fixation to use, the potential for minimizing damage to the vascular supply should be a key consideration.

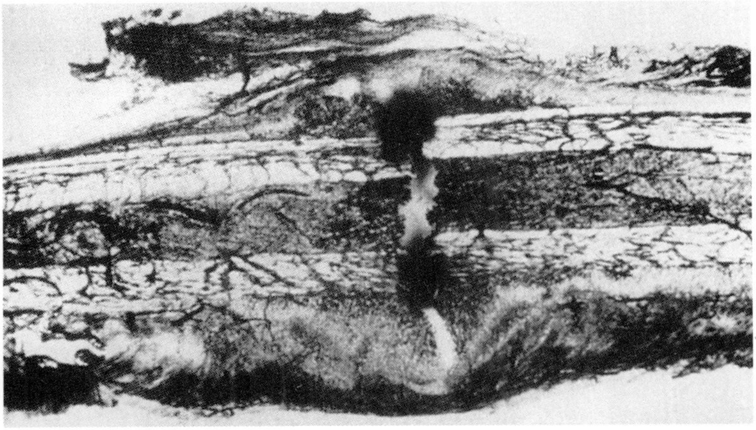

(a)

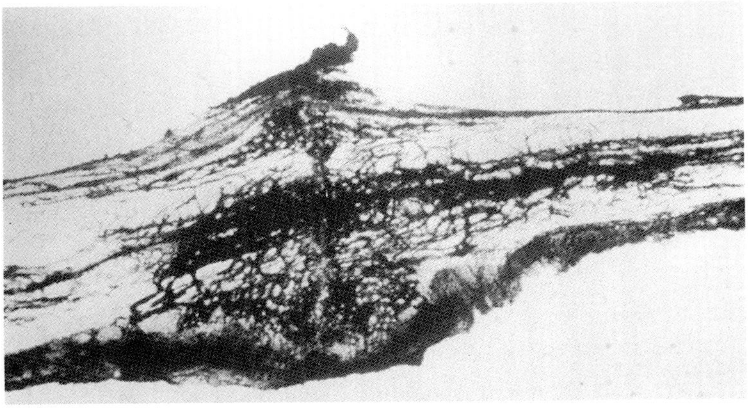

(b)

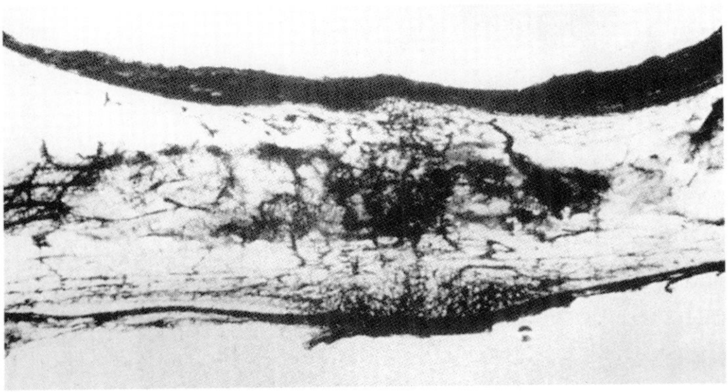

(c)

Figure 4.30

Differences in fracture vascularity. (a) An avascular gap. (b) Vessels bridging the medullary canal. (c) A normal vascular pattern. (From Ref 10 with permission.)

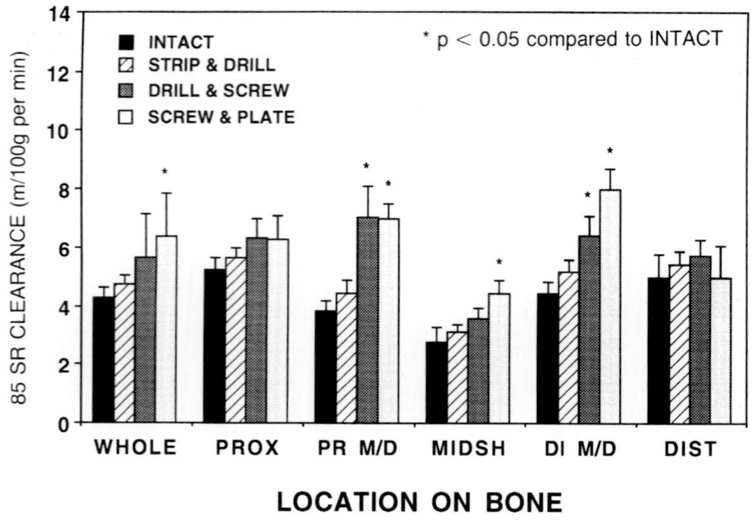

Figure 4.31

Disruption of the blood supply of the cortex of five regions of the canine femur at six months due to drilling alone, drilling and application of screws, and drilling and application of screws and a plate. WHOLE, whole bone; PROX, proximal end, PR M/D, proximal part of the middiaphysis, MIDSH, midshaft; DI M/D, distal part of the middiaphysis; DIST, distal. (Data adapted from Ref 63.)

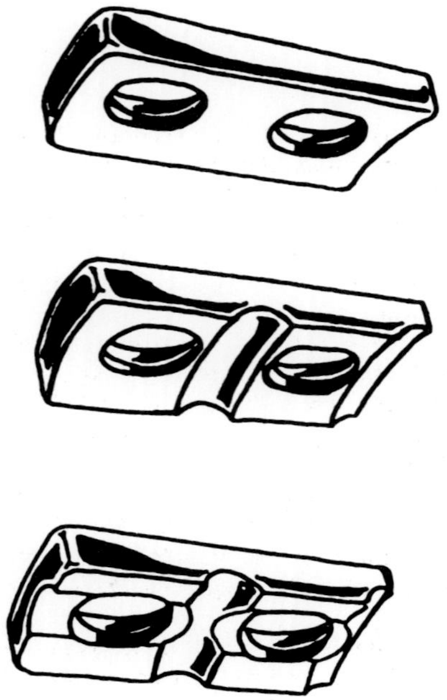

(a)

Figure 4.32

The effect of plate contact area on the vascularity in the bone below the plate. (a) Undersurface profiles of three different plates. (b) Measured area of disturbed circulation underneath the plate decreases with lower plate–bone contact. (From Ref 64 with permission.)

(*Continued next page*)

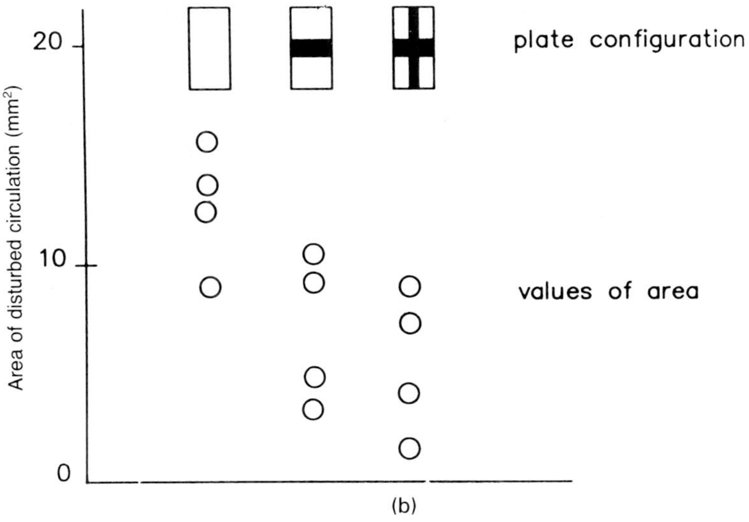

Figure 4.32

(*Continued*)

4.7 References

1. Cruess RL, Dumont J, Fracture healing, *Can J Surg* (1975) **18:** 403–13.
2. Ficat RP, Horvath E, Durroux R, Boussaton M, Senve JN, Bone circulation in fractures and pseudoarthroses. In: Arlet J, Ficat RP, Hungerford DS, eds, *Bone circulation* (Williams & Wilkins: Baltimore 1984) 126–34.
3. Henricson A, Hulth A, Johnell O, The cartilaginous fracture callus in rats, *Acta Orthop Scand* (1987) **58:** 244–8.
4. Dvonch VM, Murphy JM, Dawson PJ, Bunch WH, Grotendorst GR, Cellular and molecular biology of repair in a stable osseous defect, *Trans 38th Orthopedic Research Society Meeting* (1992) **17:** 584.
5. Joyce ME, Jinguishi S, Bolander ME, Transforming growth factor in the regulation of fracture repair, *Orthop Clin North Am* (1990) **21:** 199–209.
6. White III AA, Panjabi MM, Southwick WO, The four biomechanical stages of fracture repair, *J Bone Jt Surg* (1977) **59A:** 188–92.
7. Aro HT, Wippenman BW, Hodgson SF, Wahner HW, Lewallen DG, Chao EYS, Prediction of properties of fracture callus by measurement of mineral density using micro-bone densitometry, *J Bone Jt Surg* (1989) **71A:** 1020–30.
8. Perren SM, Physical and biological aspects of fracture healing with special reference to internal fixation, *Clin Orthop* (1975) **138:** 175–94.
9. Markel, MD, Wikenheiser MA, Chao EYS, A study of fracture callus material properties: relationship to the torsional strength of bone, *J Orthop Res* (1900) **8:** 843–50.
10. Chidgey L, Chakkalakal D, Blotchky A, Connolly JF, Vascular reorganization and return of rigidity in fracture healing, *J Orthop Res* (1986) **4:** 173–9.
11. Danis R, *Théorie et pratique de l'ostéosynthèse* (Masson: Paris 1949).
12. Venable CS, An impacting bone plate to attain closed coaption, *Ann Surg* (1951) **133:** 808–13.
13. Boreau J, Hermann P, Plaque d'ostéosynthèse permettant l'impaction des fragments, *Presse Méd* (1952) 60–356.
14. Bagby GW, James JM, The effect of compression on the rate of fracture healing using a special plate, *Am J Surg* (1958) **95:** 761–71.
15. Perren SM, Cordey J, The concept of interfragmentary strain. In Uhthoff HK, ed, *Current concepts of internal fixation of fractures* (Springer-Verlag: Berlin 1980) 63–77.
16. DiGioia III AM, Cheal EJ, Hayes WC, Three dimensional strain fields in a uniform osteotomy

gap, *J Biomech Eng* (1986) **108**: 273–80.
17. Rubin CT, Lanyon LE, Regulation of bone formation by applied dynamic loads, *J Bone Jt Surg* (1984) **66A**: 397–402.
18. Parsons JR, Alexander H, Corcoran SJ, Weiss AB, In vivo evaluation of fiber reinforced absorbable polymer bone plates. In: *Proceedings of the Second International Symposium on Internal Fixation of Fractures, Lyon, France, September 1982*, 355–62.
19. Kaplan SJ, Hayes WC, Mudan P, Lelli JL, White AA, Monitoring the healing of a tibial osteotomy in the rabbit treated with external fixation, *J Orthop Res* (1985) **3**: 325–30.
20. Benirschke SK, Mirels H, Jones D, Tencer A, The use of resonance frequency measurements for the noninvasive assessment of mechanical stiffness of the healing tibia, *J Orthop Trauma* (1993) **7**: 64–71.
21. Jernberger A, Measurement of stability of tibial fractures, *Acta Orthop Scand* (1970) Supp 135.
22. Tencer AF, Johnston WD, Gill K, Johnson KD, A biomechanical comparison of various methods of stabilization of subtrochanteric fractures of the femur, *J Orthop Res* (1984) **2**: 297–305.
23. Tencer AF, Claudi B, Pearce S, Bucholz RW, Johnson KD, Development of a variable stiffness fixation system for stabilization of segmental defects of the tibia, *J Orthop Res* (1984) **1**: 395–404.
24. Aro HT, Chao EYS, Biomechanics of external fixation: a dynamic approach to fracture union problems: Part II, *Surg Rounds for Orthop* (July 1990) 43–50.
25. Terjeson T, Apalset K, The influence of different degrees of stiffness of fixation plates on experimental bone healing, *J Orthop Res* (1988) **6**: 293–9.
26. Woodard PL, Self J, Calhoun JH, Tencer AF, Evans EB, The effect of implant axial and torsional stiffness on fracture healing, *J Orthop Trauma* (1987) **1**: 331–40.
27. Gilbert JA, Dahners LE, Atkinson MA, The effects of external fixation stiffness on early healing of transverse osteotomies, *J Orthop Res* (1989) **7**: 389–97.
28. Chao EYS, Aro HT, Lewallen DG, Kelly PJ, The effect of rigidity on fracture healing in external fixation, *Clin Orthop* (1989) **241**: 24–35.
29. Wu JJ, Shyr HS, Chao EYS, Kelly PJ, Comparison of osteotomy healing under external fixation devices with different stiffness characteristics, *J Bone Jt Surg* (1984) **66A**: 1258–64.
30. Dietschi C, Zenker H, Refrakturen und neue Frakturen der Tibia nach AO-Platten und Schrauben Osteosynthesen, *Arch f. Orthop Unfall-Chir* (1973) **76**: 54–65.
31. Richon A, Livio JJ, Saegesser F, Les refractures apres ostéosynthèse par plaque à compression, *Helv Chir Acta* (1967) **34**: 49–64.
32. Blaimont P, Considerations théoriques au sujet de la fragilisation osseuse par les implants métallique, *Acta Chir Belg* (1968) **67**: 118–26.
33. Slatis P, Karaharju E, Holmstrom T, Ahonen J, Paavolainen P, Structural changes in intact bone after application of rigid plates with and without compression, *J Bone Jt Surg* (1978) **60A**: 516–22.
34. Uhthoff HK, Dubuc FL, Bone structure changes in the dog under rigid internal fixation, *Clin Orthop* (1971) **81**: 166–70.
35. Strömberg L, Dalén N, Låftman P, Sigurdson F, Atrophy of cortical bone caused by rigid plates and its recovery. In Uhthoff HK, ed, *Current concepts of internal fixation of fractures* (Springer-Verlag: Berlin 1980) 289–90.
36. Woo SLY, Hothringer KS, Akeson WH, Coutts RD, Less rigid internal fixation plates: historical perspectives and new concepts, *J Orthop Res* (1984) **1**: 431–49.
37. Carter DR, Shimaoka EE, Harris WH, Gates EI, Caler WE, McCarthy JC, Changes in long bone structural properties during the first 8 weeks of plate implantation, *J Orthop Res* (1984) **2**: 80–9.
38. Uhthoff HK, Bardos DI, Hiskova-Kiar M, The effect of stainless steel and of titanium alloy plates on fracture healing. In Uhthoff HK, ed, *Current concepts of internal fixation of fractures* (Springer-Verlag: Berlin 1980) 398–403.
39. Brown SA, Merritt K, Mayor MF, Internal fixation with metal and thermoplastic plates. In Uhthoff HK, ed, *Current concepts of internal fixation of fractures* (Springer-Verlag: Berlin 1980) 334–41.
40. Tonino AJ, Klopper PJ, The use of plastic plates in the treatment of fracture. In Uhthoff HK, ed, *Current concepts of internal fixation of fractures* (Springer-Verlag: Berlin 1980) 342–8.
41. Cheal EJ, Hayes WC, White III AA, Perren SM, Stress analysis of compression plate fixation and its effects on long bone remodeling, *J Biomech* (1985) **18**: 141–50.
42. Ilizarov GA, The tension–stress effect on the genesis and growth of tissues: Part II. The influence of the rate and frequency of distraction, *Clin Orthop* (1989) **239**: 263–85.
43. Ilizarov GA, The tension–stress effect on the genesis and growth of tissues: Part I. The influence of stability of fixation and soft tissue preservation, *Clin Orthop* (1989) **238**: 249–81.
44. Matter P, Brennwald J, Perren SM, The effect of static compression and tension on internal remodelling of cortical bone, *Helv Chir Acta* (1975) Supp 12.
45. White III AA, Panjabi MM, Southwick WO, Effects of compression and cyclical loading on fracture healing – a quantitative biomechanical study, *J Biomech* (1977) **10**: 233–9.

46. Kenwright J, Goodship AE, Controlled mechanical stimulation in the treatment of tibial fractures, *Clin Orthop* (1989) **241**: 36–47.
47. Goodship AE, Adams MA, Kenwright J, The influence of mechanical stimulation on different stages of fracture healing, *Trans 35th Orthopedic Research Society Meeting* (1989) **14**: 592.
48. Frazza EJ, Schmitt EE, A new absorbable suture, *J Biomed Mat Res Symposium* (1971) **1**: 43–58.
49. Gogolewski S, Resorbable polymers for internal fixation. *AO/ASIF Dialogue* (1991) 3 (Issue 2) 6–8.
50. Vert M, Christel P, Chabot F, Leray J, Bioabsorbable plastic materials for bone surgery. In: Hastings GW, Ducheyene P, eds, *Macromolecular biomaterials* (CRC Press: Boca Raton, FL 1984) 119–41.
51. Hollinger JO, Battistone GC, Biodegradable bone repair materials (synthetic polymers and ceramics), *Clin Orthop* (1986) **207**: 290–305.
52. Cutright DE, Perez B, Beasley III JD, Larson WJ, Posey WR, Degradation rates of polymers and copolymers of polylactic and polyglycolic acids, *Oral Surg* (1974) **37**: 142–52.
53. Chu CC, Comparison of the effect of pH on the biodegradation of two synthetic absorbable sutures, *Ann Surg* (1982) **195**: 55–9.
54. Daniels AU, Smutz WP, Andriano KP, Chang MKO, Heller J, Dynamic environmental testing of biodegradable polymers, *Trans 15th Meeting of the Society for Biomaterials* (1989) **12**: 74.
55. Zimmerman M, Parsons JR, Alexander H, The design and analysis of a laminated partially degradable composite bone plate for fracture fixation, *J Biomed Mat Res* (1987) **21**: 345–61.
56. Tormala P, Vasenius J, Vainionpaa S, Laiho J, Pohjonen T, Rokkanen P, Ultra-high-strength absorbable self-reinforced polyglycolide (SR–PGA) composite rods for internal fixation of bone fractures: in vitro and in vivo study, *J Biomed Mat Res* (1991) **25**: 1–22.
57. Kelley BS, Casper RA, Dunn RL, Totally resorbable high-strength plate for internal fracture fixation. In: BW Sauer, ed, *Proceedings of the Fourth Southern Biomedical Engineering Conference, Jackson, MI 1985*, 26–31.
58. Bostman O, Hirvensalo E, Vainionpaa S, Vihtonen K, Tormala P, Rokkanen P, Degradable polyglycolide rods for the internal fixation of displaced bimalleolar fractures, *Internat Orthop* (1990) **14**: 1–8.
59. Bostman O, Vainionpaa S, Hirvensalo E, Makela A, Vihtonen K, Tormala P, Rokkanen P, Biodegradable internal fixation for malleolar fractures. A prospective randomized trial, *J Bone Jt Surg* (1987) **69B**: 615–19.
60. Hirvensalo E, Bostman O, Vainionpaa S, Tormala P, Rokkanen P, Biodegradable fixation in intraarticular fractures of the elbow joint, *Acta Orthop Scand* (1988) **59**: Supp 227.
61. Tunc DC, Rohovsky MW, Zadwadsky JP, Spieker JE, Strauss ED, Evaluation of body absorbable screw in avulsion type fractures. In: *Trans 12th Meeting of the Society for Biomaterials, Minneapolis, May 1986*, 168.
62. Wallace AL, Draper ERC, Strachan RK, Fleming RH, Wyatt BC, McCarthy ID, Hughes SPF, Inter-relationship of haemodynamics and interfragmentary strain in the osteotomized ovine tibia, *Trans 38th Orthopedic Research Society Meeting* (1992) **17**: 10.
63. Daum WJ, Simmons DJ, Calhoun JH, Blood flow and histomorphometric changes in long bone after six months of plate fixation, *Trans 34th Orthopedic Research Society Meeting* (1988) **13**: 510.
64. Perren SM, Cordey J, Rahn BA, Gauthier E, Schneider E, Early temporary porosis of bone induced by internal fixation implants, a reaction to necrosis, not to stress protection?, *Clin Orthop* (1988) **232**: 139–51.
65. Brookes M, *The blood supply of bone* (Butterworth: London 1971).
66. Gunst MA, Interference with blood supply through plating of intact bone. In: Uhthoff HK, ed, *Current concepts of internal fixation of fractures* (Springer-Verlag: Berlin 1980) 268–76.
67. Uhthoff HK, Foux A, Yeadon A, McAuley J, Black RC, Two processes of bone remodeling in plated intact femora: an experimental study in dogs, *J Orthop Res* (1993) **11**: 78–91.
68. Rand JA, An KA, Chao EYS, Kelly PJ, A comparison of the effect of open intramedullary nailing and compression-plate fixation on fracture-site blood flow and fracture union, *J Bone Jt Surg* (1981) **63A**: 427–42.
69. Danckwardt-Lilliestrom G, Lorenzi L, Olerud S, Intramedullary nailing after reaming, *Acta Orthop Scand* (1970) Supp 134: 1–78.
70. Kessler SB, Hallfeldt K, Perren SM, Schweiberer L, The effects of reaming and intramedullary nailing on fracture healing, *Clin Orthop* (1986) **212**: 18–25.
71. Klein MPM, Rahn BA, Frigg R, Kessler S, Perren SM, Reaming versus non-reaming in medullary nailing: interference with cortical circulation of the canine tibia, *Arch Orthop Trauma Surg* (1990) **109**: 314–16.

CHAPTER 5

Biomaterials used in fracture fixation

In this chapter the properties of materials used in fracture fixation are discussed. These include metals, principally stainless steel and titanium alloys which are used for fracture hardware, adhesives such as cyanoacrylates and fibrin for repair of small nonload bearing fragments, biodegradable polymers, and allografts or ceramics, which can be used as alternatives to autogenous bone to fill bone defects.

5.1 Metals

Methods of fabrication

The characteristics of metals used for fracture implants have been well defined. Stainless steel (316L) and titanium (6AL–4V ELI), which are commonly used for screws and hardware, are governed by national standards for maximum content of alloys and impurities[1] and mechanical properties.[2] These standards are necessary to define the minimum compositional requirements of the material and the maximum allowable percentage of impurities.

The actual mechanical properties of the metal are a function partly of its composition and partly of its *grain structure*, shown in Figure 5.1. In general, a finer grain structured metal is both stronger and more ductile, useful attributes in fracture implants, which are frequently shaped in the operating room. Grain structure is affected by the method of fabrication of the metal into its finished shape. *Casting* consists of heating the metal to a molten state and pouring it into a mold. Few implant parts, if any, are currently fabricated in this manner, because the act of pouring the molten metal into a mold results in internal impurities, pores, and other defects that reduce fatigue life. In addition, the grains of the cast part are large, resulting in low strength and brittleness. An improvement to regular casting is *hot isostatic pressing*, forming the part under high pressure in an inert gas filled chamber, which reduces the sizes of defects in the casting. The part may then be machined or finished in various ways.

Mechanical forming techniques are currently in wide use for fabricating fracture implants. *Rolling* (between rollers) and *drawing* (through a hole in a hardened plate) are used to form bar and wire. The material is plastically deformed in the process and the grains become elongated in the direction of deformation. *Machining* is used on parts that require holes, grooves or other geometric features. Machining may work harden the surface of the material but does not change its grain structure. *Forging* consists of gradually shaping a metal by compressive impact between die pairs, in conjunction with controlled heating or cooling.

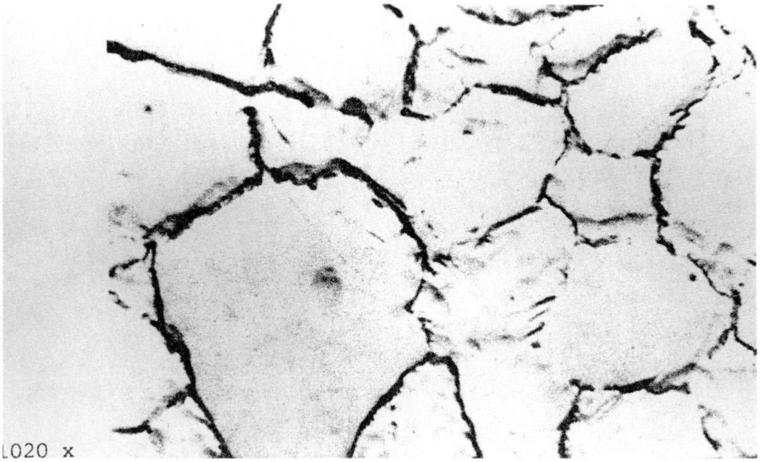

(a)

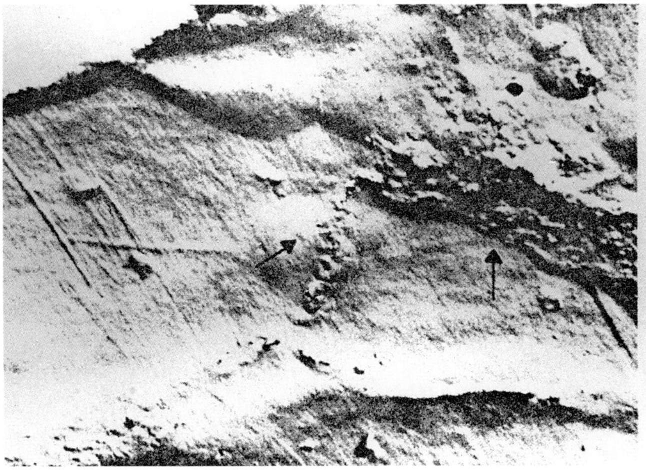

(b)

Figure 5.1

Microscopic views of the surface of a metallic implant show the interlocking metallic grains. This example shows carbide precipitations within the grain boundaries of the surface of a fixation plate: (a) × 1020; (b) × 5100. (From Ref 4 with permission.)

After forming, metal parts undergo heat treatment to alter structure and properties. In particular, *annealing* (heating to about half the melting point followed by controlled cooling) reverses the effects of work hardening and restores ductility and toughness to the metal. Finishing the surface by *polishing* removes scratches, which could act as local stress risers. Acid treatment is used to *passivate* the surface of stainless steels by creating an oxide layer on the surface, which protects against corrosion. *Nitriding,* or allowing the surface to react with ammonia or potassium cyanate, is used to harden the surface of titanium implants. The following discusses specifics of stainless steels and titanium alloys, the most common metals used in fracture implants.

Stainless steel

Stainless steel, an alloy primarily of iron, chromium, and nickel (Table 5.1) is protected from corrosion primarily by the addition of *chromium*. The chromium forms a passivating chromium oxide layer on the surface, which aids in preventing oxidation of the iron (corrosion).[3] The *carbon* component increases strength, but the implant may be subject to corrosion if carbon, which is diffused throughout the alloy, is allowed to precipitate at the grain boundaries, a result of improper heat treatment (Figure 5.1). Carbon can react with chromium to form carbides.[4]

When immersed in an electrolytic solution, the alloy will corrode anodically while the carbides at

Table 5.1 (a) Compositions and (b) mechanical properties of some stainless steels used in fracture fixation implants. (From Ref 3 with permission.)

(a)

Alloy				
ASTM	F 55[a], F 138[a]	F 745		
ISO	5832-1			
Other	AISI 316L		22-13-5	Ortron 90
Elements (w/o)				
C	<0.03	<0.06	<0.03	0.05
Cu	<0.5		<0.5	
Cr	17–20	17–19	22.5–23.5	21.5
Fe	← balance (>58%) →			
Mn	<2	<2	<2	4
Mo	2.25–3.5	2–3	2–3	2.6
N				0.39
Nb			0.1–0.3	0.3
Ni	13–16	11–14	11.5–13.5	9
P	<0.025	<0.045	<0.025	0.017
S	<0.01	<0.03	<0.01	0.005
Si	<0.75	<1	<0.75	0.25
V			0.1–0.3	

[a]Grade 2

(b)

Alloy				
ASTM	F 55, F 138	F 745		
ISO	5832-1			
Other	AISI 316L		22-13-5	Ortron 90
Mechanical properties				
Tensile modulus Y (GPa)	193	#	#	#
0.2% Yield strength $\sigma_{0.2\%}$, min (MPa)	170a	205c		479a
	250hf		785hf	
	310cw		1175cw	928cw
	1200cf[b]			
Ultimate strength σ_u, min (MPa)	480a	480c		834a
	550hf		930hf	
	655cw		1300cw	1035cw
	1300cf[b]			
Strain to failure ε_u, min (%)	40a	30c		72a
	55hf		37hf	
	28cw		15cw	64cw
	12cf[b]			
Hardness	85RBa			
	30RCcw			

a, Annealed; c, as cast; cw, 30% cold worked; cf, cold forged; hf, hot forged; RB, Rockwell B; RC, Rockwell C; #, not reported, close to F 55.
[b]F138.

the grain boundaries act as cathodes, a form of galvanic corrosion. (Galvanic corrosion requires the presence of two dissimilar materials immersed in an electrolyte, with one giving up ions and the other receiving them, as shown in Figure 5.2.) Also, the carbides degrade the mechanical properties of the material. The addition of small quantities of *titanium* or *niobium* reduces the formation of intergranular carbides by competing for carbon. Stainless steel is protected from corrosion by a protective surface chromium oxide layer, which is enhanced by the addition of small quantities of *molybdenum*. This can decrease the rate of slow passive dissolution by up to 1000-fold.[5] Molybdenum also hardens the alloy and makes it more difficult to work.[3] Surface treatment also reduces corrosion. Implants are surface finished by grinding and polishing to a specified roughness, which reduces the exposed surface area, and then cleaned with an alkaline cleaner. The oxide layer is then produced by immersion in 20–40% nitric acid by volume for a minimum of 30 min.[6]

Several stainless steels are currently in use. The commonly designated AISI (American Iron and Steel Institute) 316L (carbon content $<0.03\%$), has the composition shown in Table 5.1. Its strength can be greatly altered by the method of manufacture, and it can be extremely ductile (up to 55% strain to failure), as indicated in Table 5.1. The alloy designated F 745 is a high strength casting material, while 22-13-5 has much greater yield strength than 316L for the same treatment method (Table 5.1). Stainless steels are popular because the base materials are relatively inexpensive, they can be formed using common techniques, and their ranges of mechanical properties can be controlled over a wide range for strength and ductility.[3]

Titanium

Titanium derives its excellent resistance to corrosion from the formation of an oxide layer that binds tightly to its surface. *Impurities* such as oxygen, hydrogen, and nitrogen tend to make it brittle, which is why only minimal amounts are acceptable in titanium alloys used in surgical implants (Table 5.2). *Aluminium* stabilizes the alpha form of the material, while *vanadium* stabilizes the beta form. (Alpha and beta forms of a metal are commonly used to describe different phases of the alloy that have different properties.) The higher strength beta form exists at higher temperatures. Combinations of both components form a two phase alloy with good strength properties and one that can be heat treated.[2] In general, the mechanical properties of titanium and its alloys are in the range of half those of stainless steel alloys (Table 5.2). It is important to note that the ductility of titanium alloy is considerably lower than that of most stainless steels.[3] The alloy Ti–5Al–2.5Fe is more ductile than Ti–6Al–4V (Table 5.2), and the absence of vanadium may be of biological benefit.[3]

Corrosion of metals

Corrosion describes a chemical reaction in which material is removed from an object. *Passivation* describes a chemical reaction in which an oxide layer is formed on the surface and prevents corrosion. A number of corrosion processes can occur in fracture implants. In general, they require the components of a *galvanic cell*: two different electrically conducting solids, an electrically conductive path between them, and an electrolyte solution containing free ions (Figure 5.2). *Galvanic corrosion*, shown in Figure 5.3(a), may occur at the surface of an implant having an impurity. *Stress corrosion* involves both chemical and mechanical effects. Figure 5.3(b) demonstrates how a scratch or crack acts as both a stress concentrator and as a small corrosion cell. The implant is passivated by the oxygen layer formed over it. At the tip of an opening crack, there may be limited oxygen, so that an oxide layer is not present. In the area near the crack, there are effectively two dissimilar materials. The corrosion effect accentuates the progession of the crack through the material. *Crevice corrosion* occurs in a similar manner, but between components that may have some relative motion between them, such as a screw head within a plate (Figure 5.3c). Pitting corrosion occurs when abrasion creates a pit and allows the entrance of foreign materials through the oxide layer. The pit area is anodic with respect to the rest of the material (Figure 5.3d). The ability of a material to repassivate or regenerate its protective oxide film after scratching or abrasion is important in reducing its susceptability to corrosion. As shown in Figure 5.4, titanium and its alloys can repassivate considerably more quickly than can stainless steels.[5]

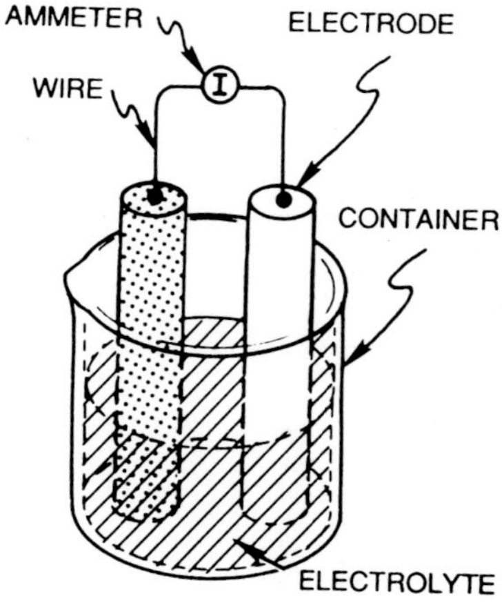

Figure 5.2

A basic galvanic cell, consisting of two different metals, an electrically conductive path between them, and an electrolyte containing free ions. (From Ref 3 with permission.)

Table 5.2 (a) Compositions and (b) mechanical properties of titanium and alloys used in fracture fixation implants. (From Ref 3 with permission.)

(a)

Alloy			
ASTM	F 67[a]	F 136	
ISO		5832-3	
Other	Pure Ti	Ti–6Al–4V	Ti–5Al–2.5Fe
Elements (w/o)			
Al	—	5.5–6.5	4.5–5.5
C	<0.1	<0.08	<0.08
Fe	<0.5	<0.25	2–3
H	<0.01	<0.015	<0.0125
N	<0.05	<0.05	<0.05
O	<0.4	<0.2	<0.2
Ti	>99	← Balance	→
V	—	3.4–4.5	—

[a]Grade 4.

(b)

Alloy			
ASTM	F 67[a]	F 136	
ISO		5832-3	
Other	Pure Ti	Ti–6Al–4V	Ti–5Al–2.5Fe
Mechanical properties			
Tensile modulus Y (GPa)	100	105	—[b]
0.2% Yield strength $\sigma_{0.2\%}$, min (MPa)	485ac	795a	818a 900f,a
Ultimate strength σ_u, min (MPa)	550af	860af	963a 985f,a
Strain to failure ε_u, min (%)	15af	10af	36a 33f,a

a, annealed; af, as fabricated; f, forged.
[a]Grade 4.
[b]Similar to F 138.

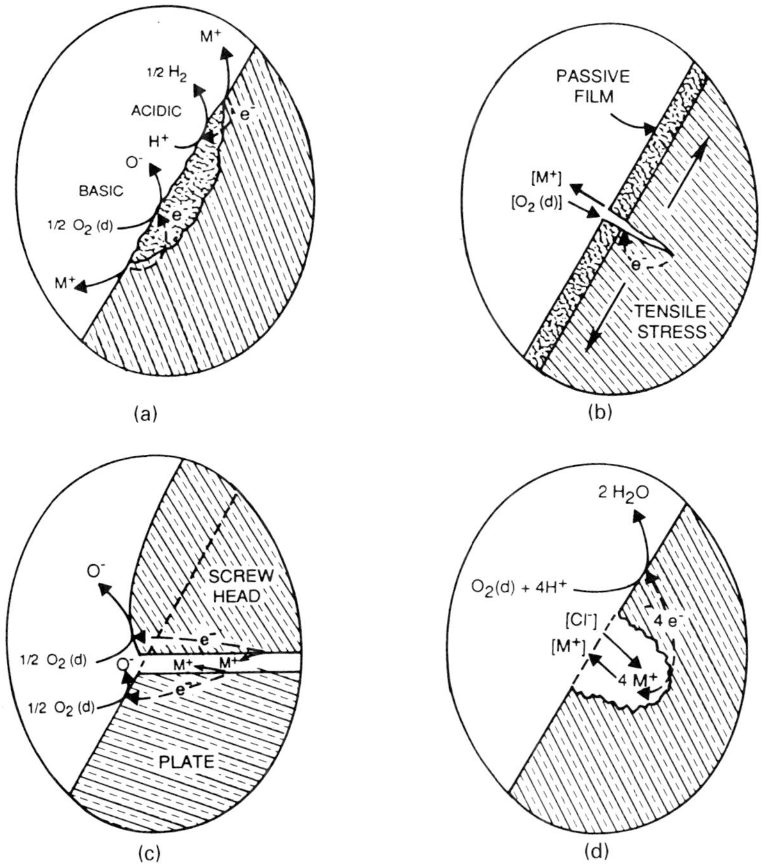

Figure 5.3

(a) Example of a galvanic cell formed by an impurity in the surface of an implant (M^+ = metal ions, different reactions depending on the pH of the electrolyte). (b) A surface scratch on a metal implant acts as both a stress riser, and as the crack opens, as a galvanic corrosion cell, causing stress corrosion. (c) Crevice corrosion results from relative movement between two surfaces, such as a screw head in a plate hole, which removes the passivating layer from the surface. (d) Pitting corrosion is a local form of crevice corrosion. (From Ref 3 with permission.)

Ion release

Another consideration in the use of metallic implants is the long term release of metal ions into surrounding tissues. Table 5.3 demonstrates that there can be a significant increase in the concentrations of metal ions compared with controls in tissues surrounding implants. In particular, the concentration of titanium increased from a mean of 11.4 parts per million (ppm) to 236.8 ppm, a 20-fold gain.[5] In vivo observations of the effects of ion release from implants is controversial. French et al[7] studied the reactions of tissues in patients undergoing hardware removal, and concluded that tissue reaction decreases with time, and that since tissue reaction is not a major clinical factor, internal fixation devices need not be removed routinely. In a study by Brunet et al,[8] the ultrastructure of tissues covering an implant were found to consist of a single layer of lining cells over fibroblasts and an outer layer of fibro-fatty tissue, with few inflammatory cells. McNamara and Williams[9] embedded discs of various materials in the paraspinal muscles of rats, and showed that cobalt produced an intense toxic reaction, while nickel induced polymorph activity in perivascular areas along with some cell necrosis.

As discussed by Black,[3] the literature reports the presence of implant site tumors associated with fracture fixation devices. However, many of the implants reported on were pre-1980 vintage or

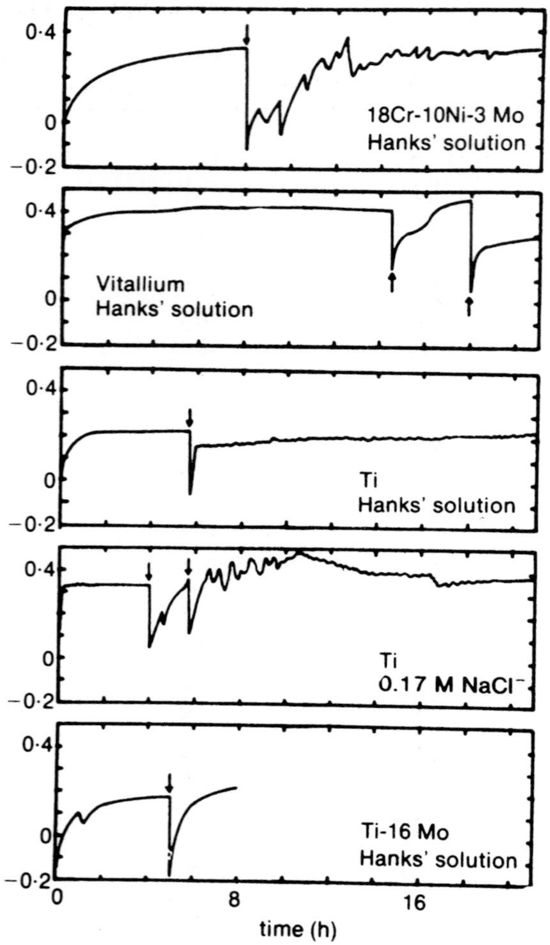

Figure 5.4

Electrical potential of various implant alloys in Hanks' solution or sodium chloride before and after scratching the surface (indicated by the arrow). (From Ref 5 with permission.)

even older. Patients may be sensitive to chromium or nickel found in stainless steel implants. Black reported on a study in which, of 32 patients presenting for internal fixation, 16 were found to be sensitive to implant metals. After removal, 3 more had become sensitive.[3] At this time, there are risks and benefits to implant retention and removal. The most obvious is the high cost and risk of a second operative procedure for removal. The procedure may be complex because bone remodelling around the implant makes removal difficult. On the other hand, the long term effects of retention of the implant are unclear. One solution may be the further use of titanium materials, which appear to be more biologically benign.

Comparison of stainless steel and titanium for fixation

Both materials have relative benefits and deficiencies. Stainless steels can be produced with higher elastic modulus and ductility than, and equivalent endurance limits (mean stress at which fatigue failure does not occur) to, titanium alloys. Ductility is an important property for implants such as wires or plates that have to be contoured during the operative procedure. The machinability and relative cost of the base metals allow stainless steel implants to potentially cost less. The significant advantage of titanium alloy is corrosion resistance and the lack of potentially toxic ions such as chromium and nickel, found in stainless steels.

5.2 Adhesives

Adhesives are not common in orthopedic fracture treatment; however they represent a potentially useful alternative method of fixation, particularly for small fragments that are difficult to hold in position by mechanical means. The two adhesives that have received most attention are cyanoacrylate and fibrin. Clinical results using these materials have been variable, which may be partly due to the (lack of) attention paid to surface preparation, a critical aspect in the use of any adhesive system, and the problem that some adhesives cannot tolerate a gap between the mating surfaces. Any bonding agent to be used surgically should[10]

- have sufficient bond strength
- be biocompatable

Table 5.3 Concentrations (in ppm) of elements found in tissues next to metallic implants of various types, in rabbits, compared with controls. (From Ref 5 with permission.)

Element	*Alloy*[a]	*No. of specimens*	*Mean concentration*[b]	*Standard deviation*
Fe	Control	97	37.9	34.6
	AISI 316	61	76.8	45.7
	A 286	16	46.1	19.0
	Inconel X	14	39.3	18.0
	Hastelloy C	18	17.2	6.6
Ni	Control	132	8.0	9.3
	AISI 316	66	40.5	41.2
	A 286	16	54.9	20.2
	Inconel X	14	41.5	19.4
	Hastelloy C	18	15.7	8.2
Cr	Control	75	3.7	4.9
	AISI 316	63	76.0	55.7
	A 286	16	26.9	24.9
	Inconel X	14	7.6	1.6
	Hastelloy C	18	7.3	3.8
	Co–Cr–Mo	37	67.0	43.6
	Co–Cr–Ni–W	9	74.9	99.8
Mo	Control	124	1.8	3.2
	AISI 316	65	8.4	9.2
	A 286	19	2.6	3.2
	Hastelloy C	18	3.2	1.8
	Co–Cr–Mo	46	11.5	8.9
Co	Control	280	2.9	6.4
	Hastelloy C	18	4.7	7.6
	Co–Cr–Mo	54	76.7	45.9
	Co–Cr–Ni–W	9	63.8	77.8
Ti	Control	225	11.4	17.4
	A 286	17	27.1	32.4
	Titanium	25	236.8	168.8

[a]AISI 316, stainless steel, surgical grade; A 286, stainless steel containing Ti, Inconel X, Ni 80%, Cr 14%, Fe 6%; Hastelloy C, Mo 17%, Fe 5%, Cr 14%, W 5%, Ni bal; Co–Cr–Mo, cast cobalt–chromium alloy; Co–Cr–Ni–W, wrought cobalt–chromium alloy.
[b]The figures give the concentration of metallic dissolution products in parts per million dry ash of the various elements found in the tissues surrounding implants of selected alloys in rabbits.

- be able to adhere to moist surfaces
- permit healing across the bond line
- be sterilizable

Methylmethacrylate, though commonly termed "bone cement," does not meet enough of the criteria given above to be defined as a true adhesive.

Cyanoacrylates

Isobutyl cyanoacrylates have been widely used in general surgery, ophthalmology, gynecology, and dentistry.[11–13] However, their use in bone fractures has been controversial. Cyanoacrylates have fallen out of favor because of concerns of tissue toxicity leading to high rates of nonunion and infection, and problems with displacement of bonded fracture fragments.[14–16] Hampel et al[17] reported that in oblique cortical fractures at the tibiofibular junction in rabbits, periosteal healing took place around the glue line but no healing occurred across the bonded fracture (Figure 5.5). Bond strengths achieved, even in carefully prepared in vitro bone specimens, have been highly variable,[18] which may be due to sensitivity in surface preparation and the requirement for intimate contact between bonded surfaces without gaps. These observations may help to explain some of the problems encountered clinically.

In an extensive study by Weber and Chapman,[10] the bonding strengths of various cyanoacrylates applied to bovine cortical and cancellous bone specimens were determined. Figure 5.6 shows the results of bonding strength tests in cortical bone specimens. The longer alkyl chain cyanoacrylates did not cure within the 10 min time period considered by the authors as the maximum acceptable in surgical use, and therefore had very low bonding strengths. They also noted large standard deviations in their results, although most of the adhesives surpassed bonding strengths that they defined to be clinically the minimum acceptable. Surface treatments using chloroform and acetone increased bond

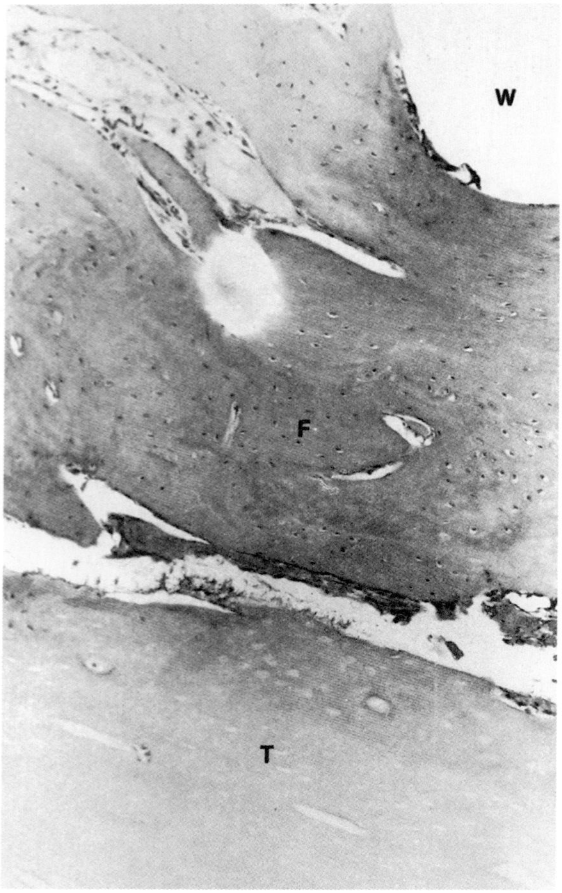

Figure 5.5

Histological appearance of an osteotomy of the tibiofibular junction in the rabbit that was bonded using isobutyl 2-cyanoacrylate. The fracture gap is occupied by glue, with no healing across it. The periosteal callus heals normally. (From Ref 17 with permission.)

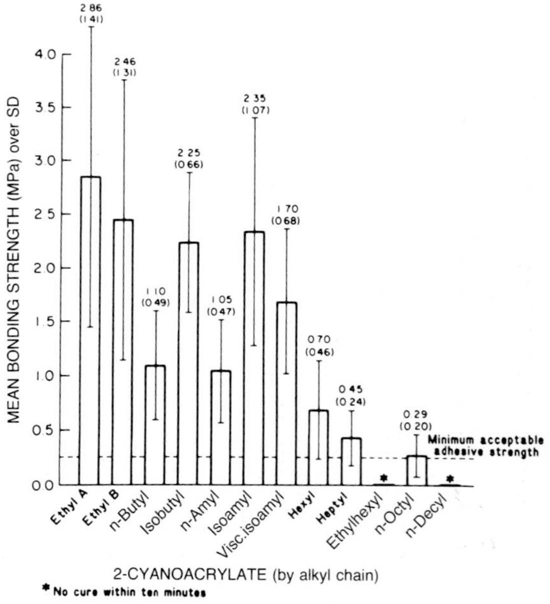

Figure 5.6

Bond strengths achieved in cortical bone tested in tension using various cyanoacrylates. (From Ref 10 with permission.)

strengths, although not sufficiently to establish statistical significance, while Tween 50 reduced bond strength. The bond strengths of cancellous specimens, shown in Figure 5.7, were much lower than those of cortical bone, with only four of the cyanoacrylates achieving minimum acceptable strengths. Again, the longer chain adhesives demonstrated poorer performance, and the scatter in the data was large. Considering the sensitivity of the bond strength to both surface preparation and intimate contact of the bone surfaces, these adhesives were not considered practical for fracture surgery use in their present forms.

Recently Harper[19] described the use of a viscous adhesive, isoamyl 2-cyanoacrylate, which allows bonding across surface gaps. In an experimental model, an oseotomized section of the femoral condyle in the rabbit was bonded using adhesive limited to the perimeter regions, to allow healing across the central part of the defect. In 23 of the 24 animals, reduction was maintained and healing proceeded with no abnormal histologic appearance. The author attributed the success of this experiment to the ability of the viscous adhesive to act as a gap filler and possibly produce mechanical interlock as well as true adhesion. Also, the concept of applying the bonding agent in limited regions is important, since it has been shown that bone will appose but not grow through the adhesive, as Figure 5.5 shows. Since more adhesive area will improve the immediate strength of fixation but will inhibit long term bone healing, the decision of how much

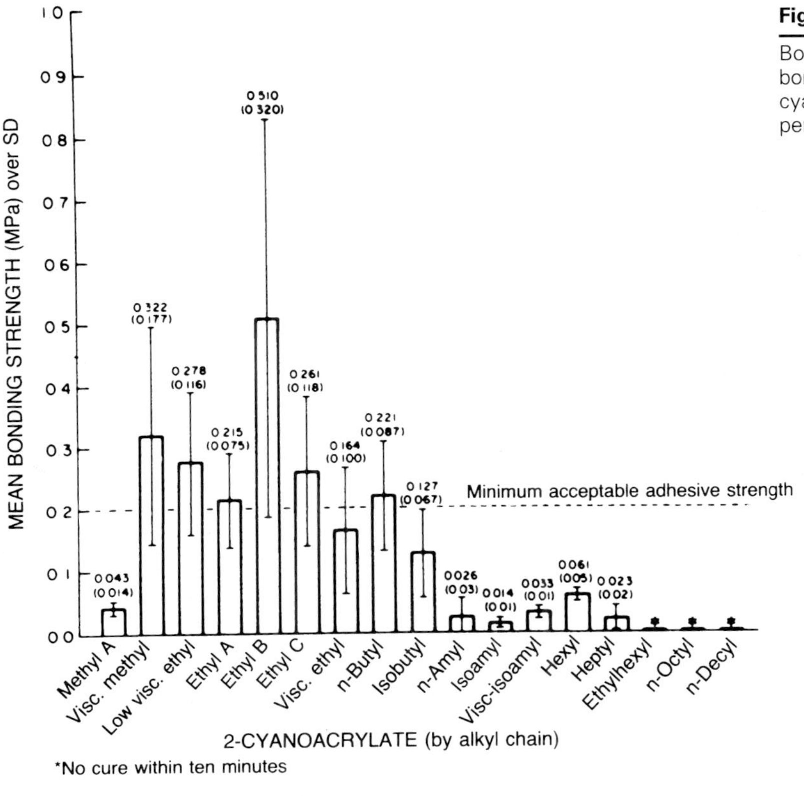

Figure 5.7

Bond strengths achieved in cancellous bone tested in tension using various cyanoacrylates. (From Ref 10 with permission.)

adhesive to apply in fragment fixation is important. The long term fate of the adhesive has not been addressed.

Fibrin

A second adhesive that has been extensively investigated for fracture fixation is fibrin, which plays an important role in the natural coagulation of blood and in wound healing. Fibrin has found use in the sealing of defects in visceral organs[20] and in cardiac surgery.[21] Fibrin glue simulates the last step in the process of coagulation.[22] As discussed by Lerner and Binur,[23] fibrinogen and factor XIII are activated by thrombin in the presence of calcium ions. The fibrinogen converts to fibrin, which polymerizes to form a stable clot. Factor XIII stimulates fibroblast proliferation, which is assisted also by fibronectin. Cold insoluble globulin encourages the adhesion of fibroblasts to the clot. Bosch[24] demonstrated that optimal clotting occurred with a 5:1 ratio of fibrinocryoprecipitate with 600 NIH units of thrombin in a 250 mM calcium chloride solution.

Fibrin adhesive has been described in the repair of osteochondral defects,[25] and in bone grafting.[26,27] Faster revascularization of a cancellous bone graft was found if a thin layer of fibrin was used for adhesion of the graft (Figure 5.8). However, a thicker layer of fibrin, similar to a clot, must be fragmented before revascularization can proceed.[28] Results from an experimental study of osteotomy healing have also demonstrated better callus bridging, faster reconstruction of the osteotomy site, and greater bending strength with the use of fibrin adhesive (Figure 5.9).[29]

Weber and Chapman,[10] in their extensive testing of osteoadhesives, also reported on the tensile strengths of bone bonds using fibrin adhesives after clamping the bonded pieces for

Table 5.4 Tensile bonding strength of fibrin adhesive compared with equivalent samples bonded using isobutyl cyanoacrylate or polymethylmethacrylate, and the tensile strength of intact bone. (From Ref 10 with permission.)

Adhesive	*Bonding Strength Mean (MPa) (S.D.)*
Bovine fibrinogen in solution[a]	
Thrombin (in Ringer's[b])	
Factor XIII[c]	0.016 (0.005)[d]
Bovine fibrinogen (dry)	
Thrombin (in Ringer's)	
Factor XIII	0.017 (0.005)
Bovine fibrinogen in solution	
Thrombin (in calcium sol.)	
Factor XIII	0.016 (0.007)
Human cryoprecipitate	
Thrombin (in calcium sol.)	
No factor XIII	0.005 (0.002)
Human cryoprecipitate	
Thrombin (in calcium sol.)	
Factor XIII	0.006 (0.003)
Isobutyl cyanoacrylate	0.127 (0.067)[e]
Polymethylmethacrylate	1.01 (0.51)[d,e]
Intact bone	5.77 (2.19)

[a]Fibrinogen made up 90 mg/ml.
[b]Thrombin made up 600 NIH U/ml in either CaCl or Ringer's lactate.
[c]Factor XIII made up 65 U/ml.
[d]$t = 6.14$: $p < 0.001$.
[e]$t = 5.52$: $p < 0.001$.

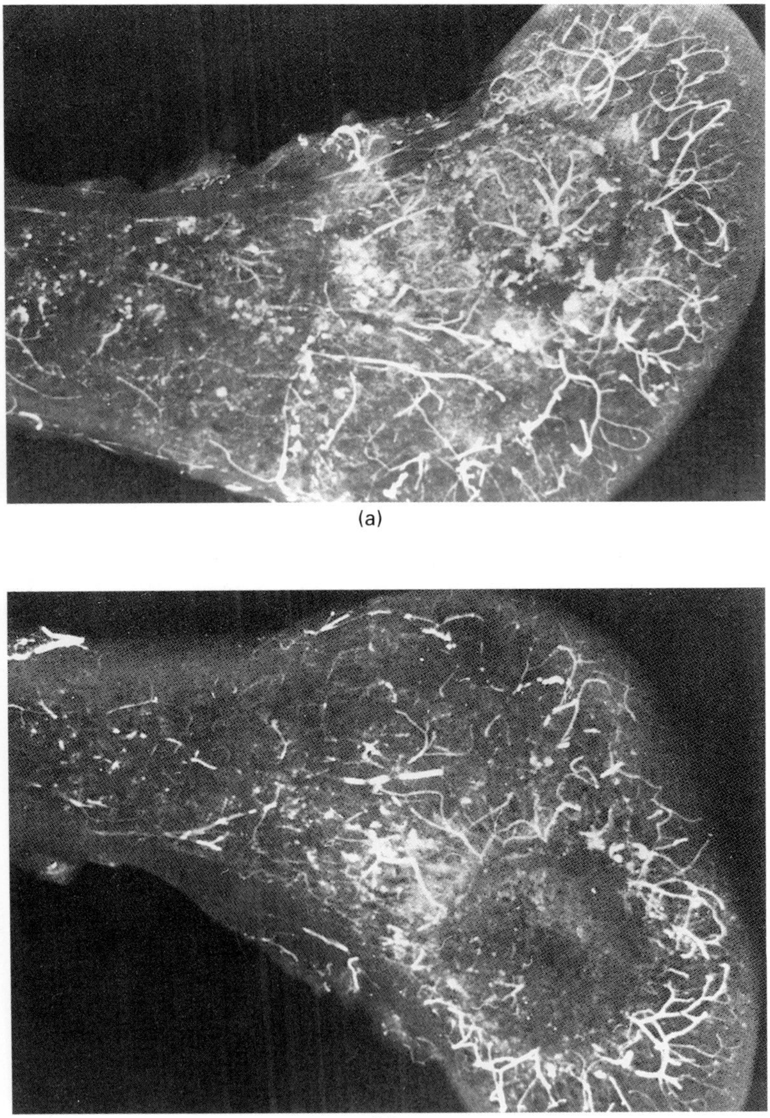

(a)

(b)

Figure 5.8

In experimental cancellous bone grafting of the femoral condyle of the dog, the graft with fibrin adhesive (a) demonstrates more vascularity than the contralateral without adhesive (b) three days postoperatively. (From Ref 28 with permission.)

10 min. The results, shown in Table 5.4, indicate that the bond strength formed by fibrin was significantly lower than that produced by cyanoacrylate. They concluded that fibrin adhesives should find use only for fracture fragments either having considerable inherent stability or being nonload bearing.

5.3 Biodegradable polymers

Degradable polymers represent an area of increasing interest in orthopedic fracture fixation. Their attractiveness lies in the potential that implants made from these materials will hydrolyze in situ and therefore make hardware removal unnecessary. This would present a significant advantage in many clinical situations, since no secondary procedure with its associated trauma, potential morbidity, and additional cost would be necessary.

While a large number of degradable polymers have been identified,[30] the polyesters, poly(lactic acid) (PLA), poly(glycolic acid) (PGA), and their copolymers have received the most study. These materials were initially proposed for use as degradable sutures,[31] and are commonly used today under tradenames such as Vicryl and Dexon. In order to find use in fracture fixation, a fixation implant made of a biodegradable material should exhibit the following properties:

- adequate mechanical strength for the application
- sufficient strength over an appropriate time period to maintain stability of the fracture components during healing and prevent loss of reduction
- degradability into products that do not encourage an adverse biological reaction, and that can be easily eliminated from the body

Poly(alpha-hydroxyacids) form a class of polyesters with repeating units [O–CO–CH–R], derived from glycolic (R = H) and lactic (R = CH_3) acids as shown in Figure 5.10. Lactic acid has two enantiomeric forms, L and D, which have opposite configurational structures. The structures of PGA, PLA, and their copolymers are shown in Figure 5.11.[32] Degradation of polyhydroxyacids occurs in aqueous media via bulk hydrolysis of the ester bonds in the polymer chain. Chu[33] proposed that PGA sutures consist of alternate regions of crystalline and amorphous structures with polymer tie chains passing between regions. He observed that degradation did not proceed at the same rate throughout the whole material, and considered that the process began in the amorphous regions, which were more permeable to water, and specifically in the backbone ester linkages of the polymer tie chains. This process dominated the initial degradation procedure.

(a)
(b)

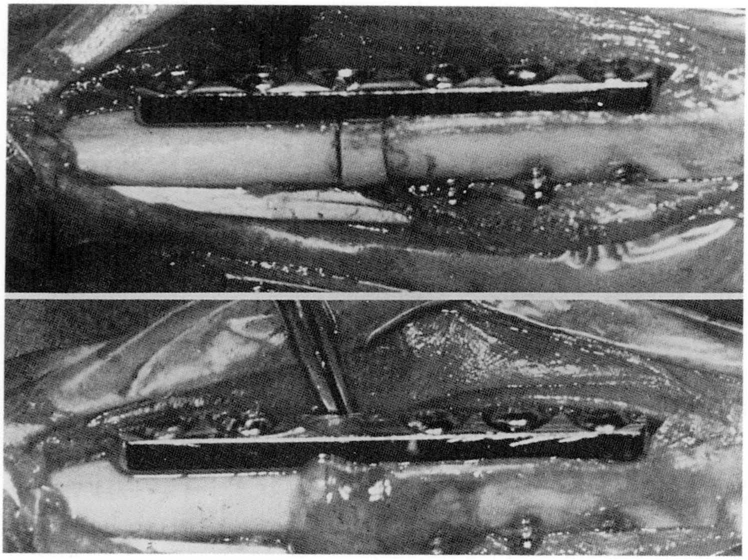

Figure 5.9

Response of an osteotomized segment of bone in the rabbit. (a) Control bone. (b) Bone with fibrin adhesive. (From Ref 29 with permission.)

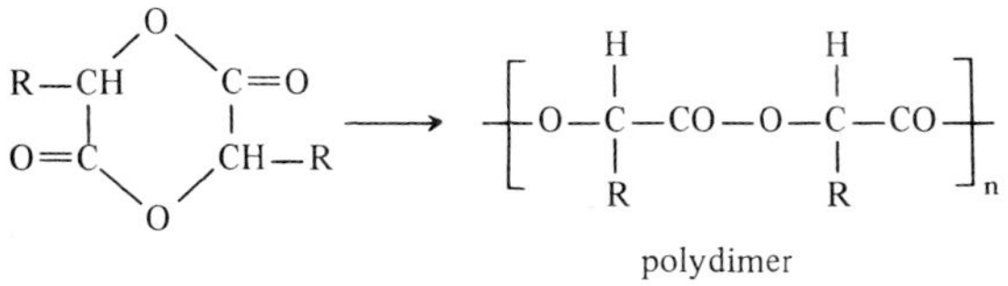

Figure 5.10

Basic molecular structure of glycolide and lactide and the polydimer. (From Ref 32 with permission.)

In vivo degradation proceeds in a similar fashion; however, enzymatic action may also be involved.[34] The degradation process converts PLA to lactic acid and glycine, which are incorporated into the tricarboxylic acid cycle. Brady et al[35] showed that implants in rats were ultimately eliminated primarily in respiration, and secondarily in the feces and urine (Figure 5.12). The biocompatability of polyhydroxyacids and the intensity of the tissue response to their degradation depends on their purity, shape, and size, and on their rate of degradation.[36] In general, inflammatory reactions have been reported as mild in experimental investigations.[32,37,38] In contrast, using PGA or PLA-CO-PGA rods for fracture or osteotomy fixation, Bostman[39] reported a total of 7.9% clinically manifest foreign body reactions, which produced a fluctuant swelling at the implant site after 12 weeks (41/516 patients). Daniels et al[40] explained the toxicity of rapidly degrading PGA as being due to the production of significant quantities of acid, when maintained in a confined space. In their experiments, the pH of the water bath around rapidly degrading PGA specimens decreased to below 3, while the pH of fluid around more slowly degrading PLA samples stayed between 7 and 5 at 12 weeks.

Both the degradation rate and mechanical properties of polyhydroxyacids are affected by a number of parameters. Degradation is dependent on the polymer–copolymer ratio of PLA to PGA. As

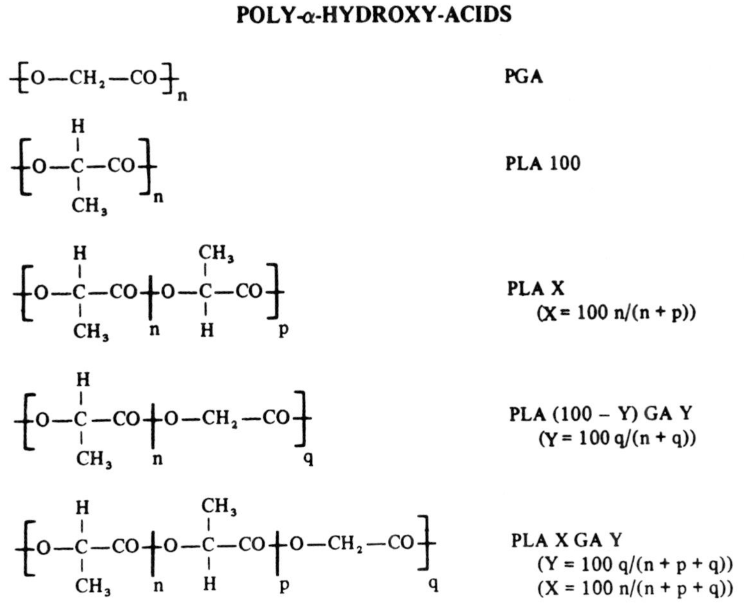

Figure 5.11

Structure of the polymers, poly(lactic acid), poly(glycolic acid), and copolymers, PLA (100 – Y) GA Y, and PLA X GA Y (GA = PGA; X = fraction PLA; Y = fraction PGA) (From Ref 32 with permission.)

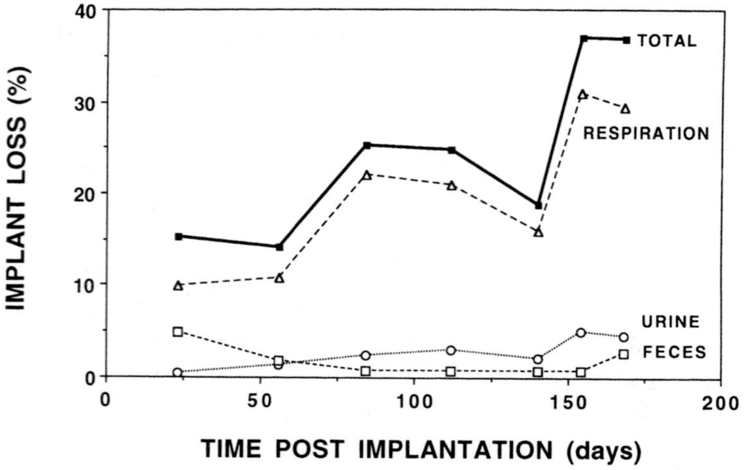

Figure 5.12

Proportion of PLA implants eliminated by various routes during in vivo degradation in the rat. (Adapted from data of Ref 35.)

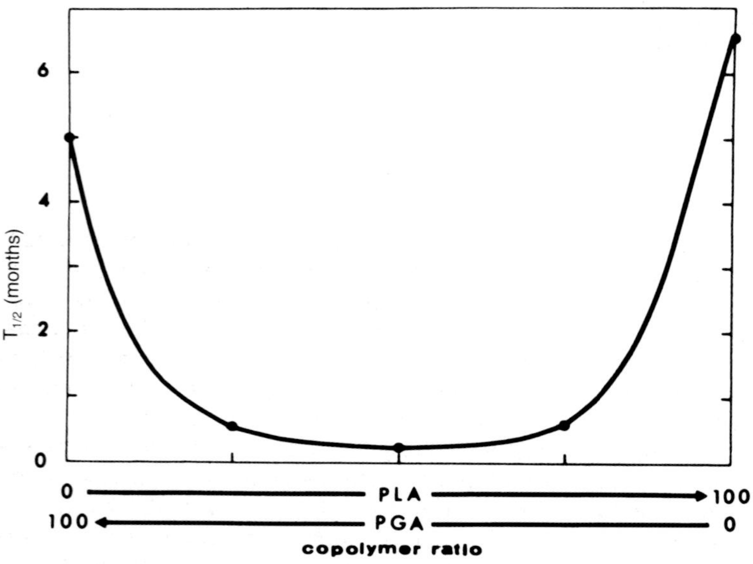

Figure 5.13

Half life of implants formed from various ratios of PLA and PGA. (From Ref 41 with permission.)

shown in Figure 5.13, a 50/50 PLA/PGA copolymer produces implants with the lowest half life, while implants of pure PLA exhibit the greatest half life.[41] Similarly, the ultimate tensile stress of 100% PLA samples is greater than any stereopolymer (PLA/PGA) of less than 100% PLA content (Figure 5.14).[32] The pH of the solution in which the implant is immersed affects degradation properties, with the slowest loss of mass and mechanical properties occurring at a solution pH of 7.5.[42] As discussed

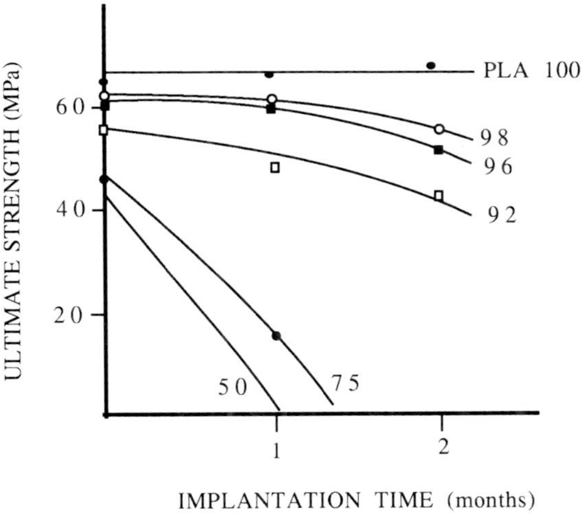

Figure 5.14

Ultimate tensile stress of samples of various stereocopolymers after in vivo implantation for varying periods of time. (From Ref 32 with permission.)

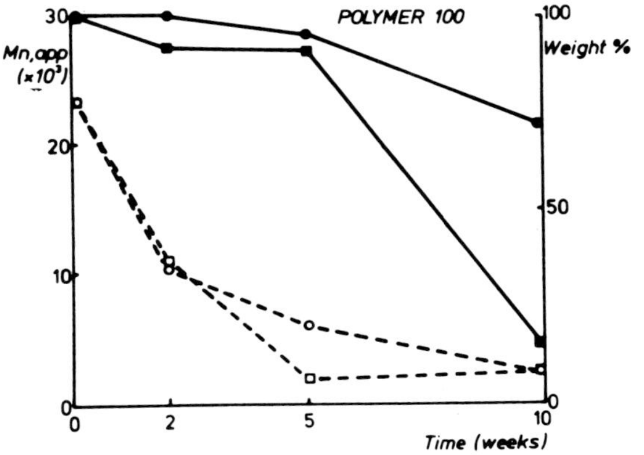

Figure 5.15

In vivo (○,●) and in vitro (□,■) degradation profiles of polyhydroxyacid copolymers of different molecular weights. The solid line shows % weight change, and the dashed line the molecular weight. (From Ref 43 with permission.)

above, slower degradation rates may be beneficial in terms of reducing the potential for tissue reaction to the implant.

Lower molecular weight samples also degrade more rapidly (Figure 5.15). It is also noteworthy that the rate of degradation for the same samples was found to be similar at most time points tested both in vivo and in vitro.[43] However, as Figure 5.16 shows, the in vitro decrease in mechanical properties of dynamically loaded degradable polymers is much more rapid than specimens immersed in solution but not exposed to mechanical loads.[44] This is an important consideration in designing implants for load bearing situations in orthopedic surgery, and has not been fully explored. Sterilization can also alter the properties of degradable polymers due to depolymerization and the breaking of crosslinks.[45,46] Rozema et al[46] compared seven different protocols for steam sterilization, and found that all reduce the mechanical strength of PLA to some extent; however, the minimum effect was produced using a sterilization cycle with lower temperature and smaller exposure time.

Given the concern that biodegradable materials have initially poorer material properties than metals commonly used for load bearing orthopedic fracture applications (Table 5.5), and that these properties are affected by factors such as sterilization, loading, pH, and time of implantation, practical biodegradable implants have been designed using the methods of composite materials to improve strengths. In this approach, stiffer fibers are incorporated in a more flexible matrix. The fibers improve strength properties while the matrix provides the structure with flexibility and fracture toughness. An early attempt to build composite fixation plates utilized carbon fibers preimpregnated with PLA, which were then cut and placed in a mold at specific orientations between 45° and 0° (parallel to the long axis of the plate), and molded under pressure and elevated temperatures.[47] Plates made in this way had significantly improved mechanical properties, which were further enhanced by molding instead of machining the screw holes, since machining the holes exposes the internal matrix. However, concern for the fate of nonresorbable carbon

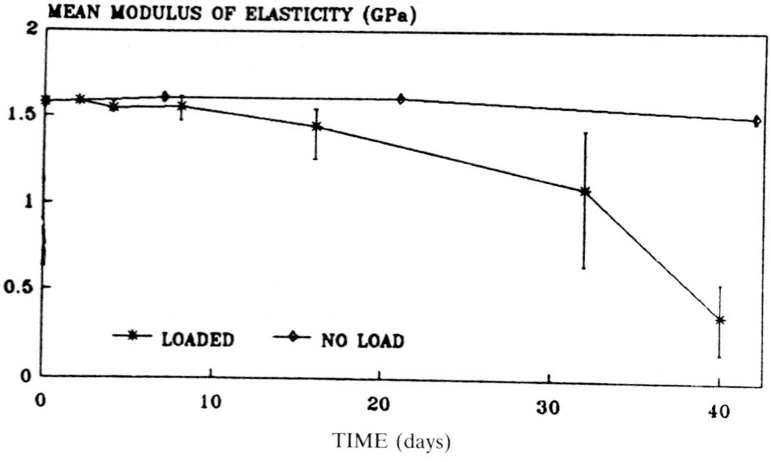

(a)

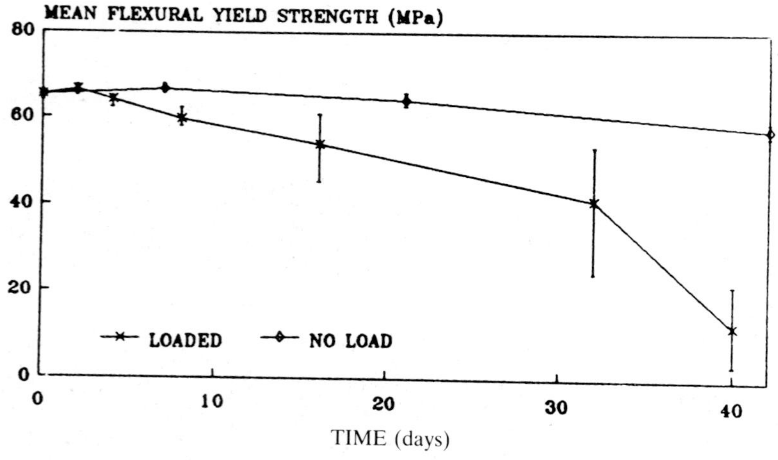

(b)

Figure 5.16

Mechanical properties of samples of the degradable polymer poly(orthoester), immersed and loaded in three point bending at 10% of flexural yield load for 630 cycles at 1 Hz: (a) modulus of elasticity and (b) flexural yield strength, both plotted as functions of time (◆, no load; *, loaded). (From Ref 44 with permission.)

fibers has led others to explore different methods for increasing the strength of implants fabricated from these materials.

Several groups have developed biodegradable implants with increased strength compared with the basic material. One approach is to produce a material with extremely high molecular weight, up to 10^6, with careful control of polymerization using low catalyst concentration and formation temperature.[48,49] Polymers with tensile strengths of up to 83 MPa have been fabricated using these techniques. The self reinforcement approach utilizes a composite material in which the reinforcing fibers are the same base material as the matrix, but of higher molecular weight. As shown schematically in Figure 5.17 and by scanning electron micrography in Figure 5.18, this technique consists of laying PGA sutures in a mold,

Table 5.5 Comparison of the mechanical properties of metals and resorbable polymers used in orthopedic surgery. (From Ref 36 with permission.)

Material	*Young's modulus (GPa)*	*Tensile strength (GPa)*
Bone	7–40	0.09–0.12
Steel 316L	200	0.80
Titanium (0% porosity)	100	0.70
Ti–Al–V (0% porosity)	124	0.90
Polylactides	3–5	0.06
Polylactides (oriented)	6–14	0.3–2.5
Polylactides/resorbable glass fiber	8–30	0.20

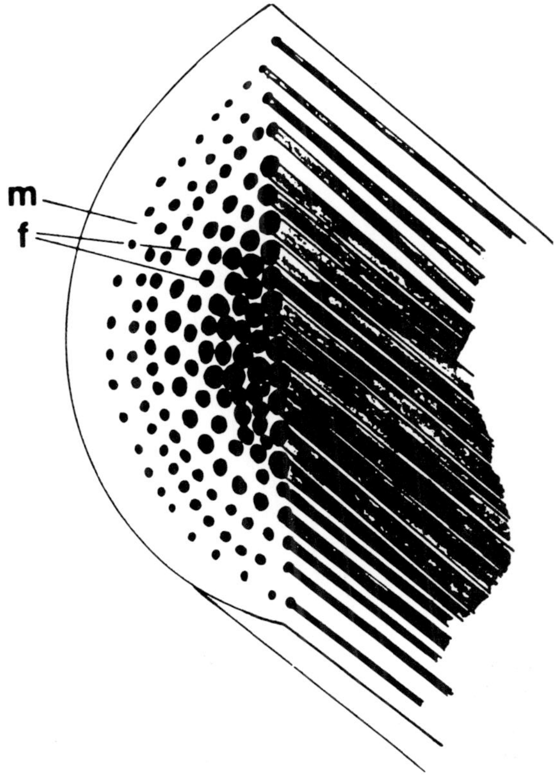

Figure 5.17

A schematic diagram of the construction of a self reinforced PGA rod formed from axially aligned PGA sutures (f) fused into an amorphous PGA matrix (m). (From Ref 50 with permission.)

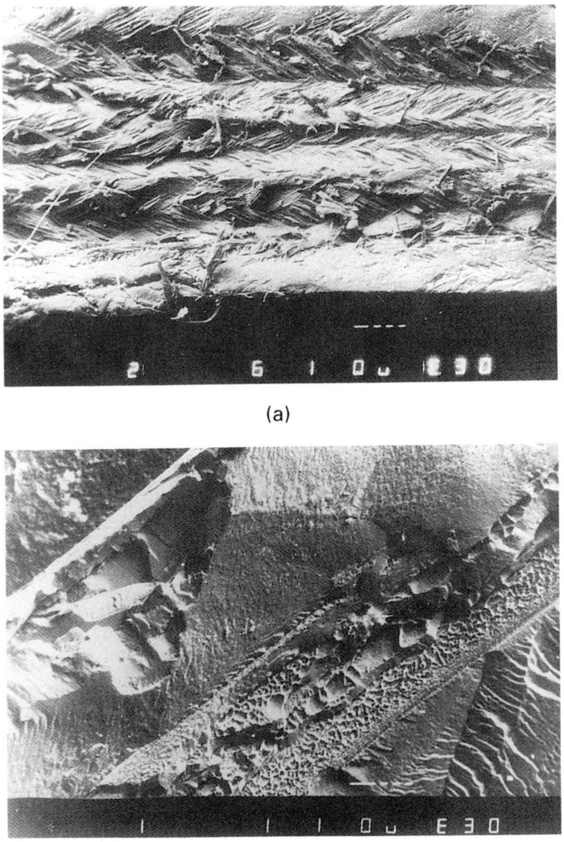

(a)

(b)

Figure 5.18

Scanning electron micrographs of sections of (a) a self reinforced PGA rod and (b) an injection molded PGA rod. (From Ref 50 with permission.)

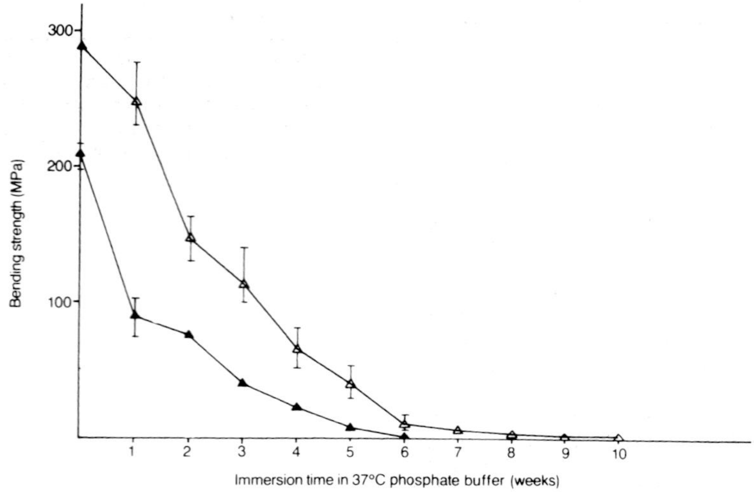

Figure 5.19

Comparison of the initial bending strengths and the change in bending strength with time for (upper curve) 3.2 mm diameter self reinforced and (lower curve) injection molded PGA rods. (From Ref 50 with permission.)

after which the exterior surface is melted and internally the sutures are fused together. The molecular chains of the sutures are highly oriented axially. This construction has been demonstrated to significantly increase bending strengths, shown in Figure 5.19, in comparison to injection molded rod of the same materials.[50] The modulus of elasticity of this material is 10–15 GPa, compared with 6.5 GPa for pure PGA,[50] 100 GPa for titanium, and 200 GPa for stainless steel used in conventional K wires. The fact that the modulus, and hence (for the same size and shape of implant) the bending stiffness, of implants of stainless steel is 20 times those of self reinforced PGA indicates that these devices should be considered for low load applications, or that larger diameter implants need to be used.

Apart from eliminating metal toxicity, and the requirement for hardware removal, degradable polymer implants may have another potential advantage in fracture fixation. Polyhydroxyacids have been described extensively for use in the controlled delivery of drugs. Recent experiments have described the use of controlled release agents for bone formation delivered from a biodegradable IM rod placed in the femur in rabbits.[51–53] Ultimately, these devices may, apart from providing fixation stability, be used to deliver antibiotic agents or stimuli to bone healing.

5.4 Bone graft substitutes

While ceramics and allograft bone are not used as materials in fracture implants, they have found use as defect fillers and buttressing devices in fracture fixation situations. Therefore they can constitute a significant mechanical component of the fracture construct. Their properties are reviewed here briefly. Autogenous bone remains the graft material of choice because of its inherent biocompatability and demonstrated osteogenic capacity, yet complications can occur with the harvest of bone from the iliac crest. These can include additional blood loss,[54,55] sepsis and pain,[54,56] pelvic instability,[54,56] fatigue fracture,[54,57] iliac hernia,[56,58,59] ureteral injury,[60] or heterotopic bone formation.[54] Younger and Chapman[61] noted an overall major complication rate of 8.6% with an additional minor rate of 20.6% for iliac crest bone grafting.

Damien and Parsons[62] presented a comprehensive review of bone graft substitutes. Allogeneic bone presents one alternative bone substitute. Freeze drying of harvested grafts is commonly used for preservation and storage; however, this alters mechanical properties, increasing stiffness by 175% and decreasing torsional strength to 80% of that of fresh fibular bone.[63–65] Drying, in effect, makes bone more brittle. Rehydration either in vacuo for 1 h or ex vacuo for 24 h returned the

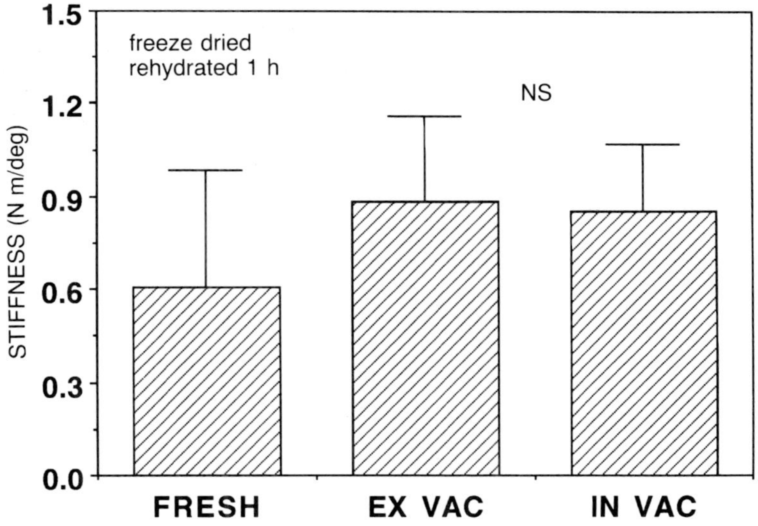

(a)

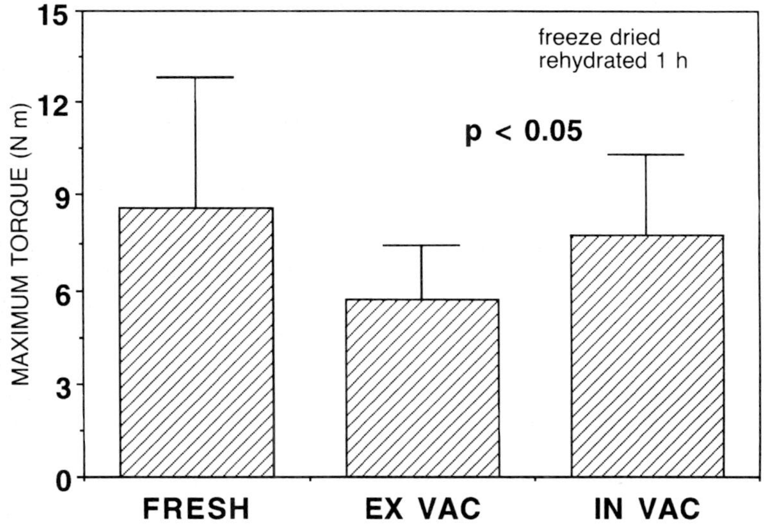

(b)

Figure 5.20

Comparison of the torsional properties of allograft bone, fresh or freeze dried followed by rehydration either ex vacuo or in vacuo for 1 h: (a) stiffness; (b) maximum torque.[65]

torsional strength of fibular grafts to that of fresh bone (Figure 5.20); however, the stiffness remained 135% greater compared with fresh bone.[65] In vacuo rehydration can be accomplished by injecting saline into the storage container in which the graft is packaged before surgery. Cancellous allograft mechanical properties in compression are similarly affected by freeze drying.[66] Apart from the differences in mechanical properties, bone formation occurs at a slower rate in allogeneic bone grafts compared with autografts,[67–69] and there is a potential for the transmission of viral infection from the donor to the recipient.[70]

Historically, plaster of Paris was the first ceramic proposed and extensively studied as a bone substitute.[71–73] As early as 1892, Dreesman reported its use in nine bone defect sites with healing occuring in six.[71] This material is the beta-hemihydrate form of calcium sulfate $[(CaSO_4)_2.H_2O]$. The addition of water results in setting of the material, with the generation of heat.[62] However, plaster is brittle, and has poor strength and abrasion resistance,[74] as well as being resorbed rapidly,[75] and therefore may be better suited as a method for the short term delivery of antibiotics[72,76] or bone morphogenic protein[77] than as a structural defect filling material.

Ceramics can be classified by material or structure. Typical materials used as bone defect fillers are tricalcium phosphates, hydroxyapatites, and composites containing a polymer component. Structurally, these materials come in block or particulate forms, in varying degrees of porosity. Porosity is probably the most important property, since greater porosity increases the potential for bone ingrowth and the rate of dissolution, while at the same time it decreases mechanical strength. In general, ceramics can be classified as being very brittle with little tensile strength and a susceptability to rapid crack propagation and fatigue. They have been found to be highly biocompatible,[78] but function mainly as a scaffold for new bone growth across a void (termed osteoconductive) as opposed to actually stimulating bone formation (osteoinductive).

Tricalcium phosphate (TCP) is one of the two most widely used ceramic materials. Its chemical composition is $Ca_3(PO_4)_2$, with a calcium to phosphorus ratio of 1:5. The more stable form is beta-TCP which has been reported to be highly biocompatable.[79] Klein et al[80] reported that, of implants of hydroxyapatite (HA) and TCP in dense, microporous, and macroporous form, only the porous TCP degraded, with disintegration occurring by breaking into smaller particles, which were transported to neighboring tissues as well as being digested by phagocytes. The pores of TCP implants were filled with new bone, in direct apposition to the implants, and had the morphologic appearance of osteons with haversian canals. By 12 months post implantation, only fragments of the TCP implants remained (Figure 5.21).

Synthetically formed hydroxyapatite is similar to the naturally occuring mineral component of bone, although in bone the crystals are usually smaller, being 100 μm or less in dimension.[78] Hydroxyapatite (HA) has a nominal composition $Ca_{10}(PO_4)_6(OH)_2$, with a calcium to phosphorus ratio of 1.67. It is an attractive material because of its similarity to bone mineral, and several reports have demonstrated direct apposition and bonding of bone to hydroxyapatite implants,[81–83] as shown in Figures 5.22 and 5.23. The biological reaction to implantation of HA has been described as initial roughening of the surface of the implant by

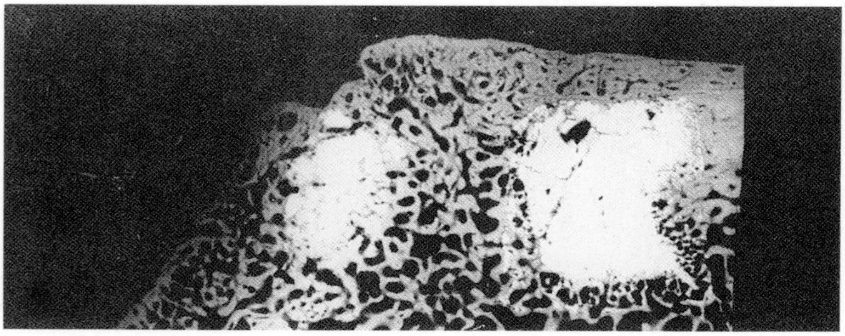

Figure 5.21

Microradiograph of a porous tricalcium phosphate implant one year after implantation into the middiaphyseal cortex of the dog femur, showing fragmentation and bone ingrowth. (From Ref 80 with permission.)

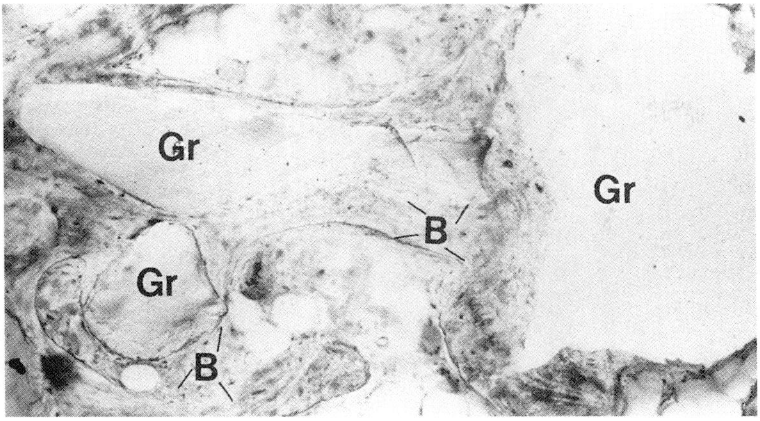

Figure 5.22

Histological appearance of hydroxyapatite granules (Gr) placed within cancellous bone (B). Bone connects the granules, and there is an absence of inflammatory cells (human specimen, ×5). (From Ref 82 with permission.)

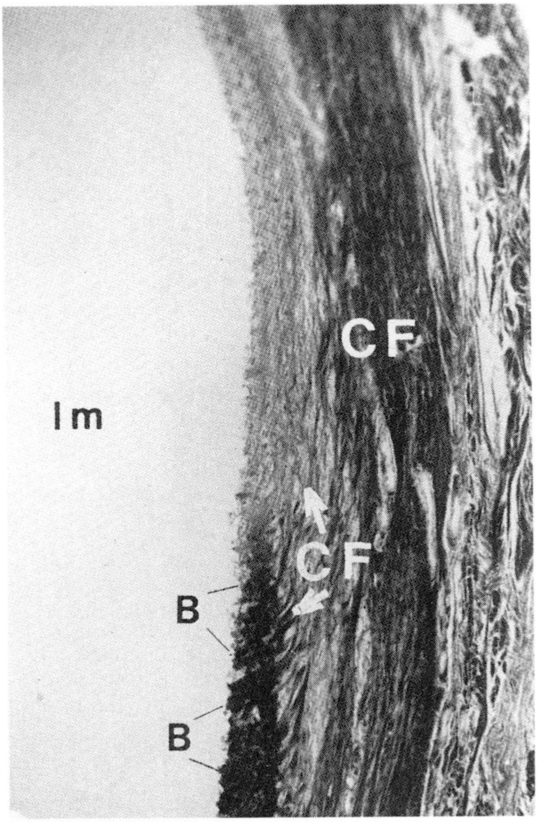

Figure 5.23

Detailed light micrograph of a hydroxyapatite/tissue interface, showing bone (B) deposited directly against the implant (Im), and collagen fibers (CF) within the bone tissue. (From Ref 82 with permission.)

macrophages, followed by migration of osteoblasts to the surface, where osteoid is laid down and progressively mineralized.[83] The response of osteoblasts to various orthopedic materials, including Ti–6Al–4V alloy, 316L stainless steel, and hydroxyapatite has been compared. Cell growth was found to be significantly lower on HA than any other material in the first four day period, indicating some initial hesitation by osteoblasts to respond to implanted HA.

Porosity is a key property of both HA and TCP implants. One method of fabrication of porous HA is sintering of granules, which form a pore between them as they fuse. The granule size and sintering temperature control the size of the pore produced.[78] The internal pore structure produced by this method is random, however, and is not similar to the oriented porosity of bone. A process of hydrothermal exchange has been described that converts calcium carbonate to pure hydroxyapatite.[84] This technique has been applied to the exoskeletons of several corals, which were selected based on pore size. The implant material demonstrates oriented porosity with longitudinal channels and crossfenestrations (Figure 5.24). As shown by Holmes,[85] in addition to the direct apposition of bone to the interstices of the implant, the crossfenestrations permit vascular channel formation (Figure 5.25). Morphometric studies have demonstrated that the microstructure of the coral, genus *Goniopora*, is very similar to that of cancellous bone derived from the iliac crest, as shown in Table 5.6.[86]

Three properties affected by pore size are bone ingrowth, mechanical strength, and possibly biodegradation. Bone ingrowth was found to be more rapid in porous coralline implants having a void fraction averaging 70% (pore size 260–600 μm) than those with a void fraction of 60% (pore size 190–230 μm) (Figure 5.26).[87] In implants with random instead of oriented porosity, the relation of pore size to the quantity of bone ingrowth has been found to be similar.[88] The degradation of HA implants is thought to be dependent on pore size;[89] however, up to 48 months post implantation in vivo, significant degradation of HA implants has not been demonstrated.[90]

Defining the mechanical properties of ceramic bone substitutes is complex, because the

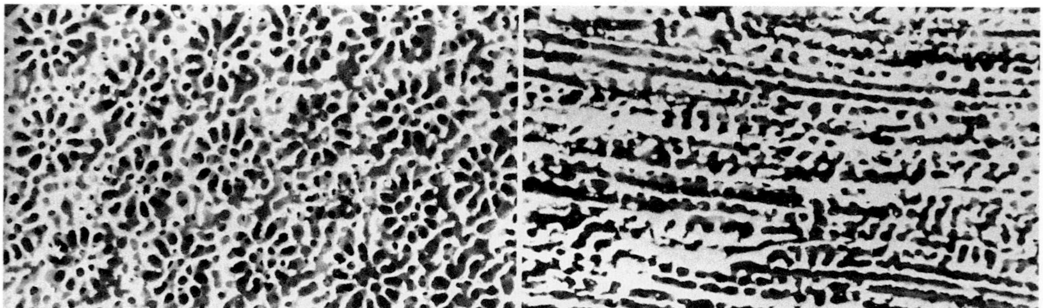

Figure 5.24

Oriented porosity of the coral, genus *Porities*, showing haversian-like voids in cross section and oriented channels with crossfenestrations in longitudinal section. (From Ref 85 with permission.)

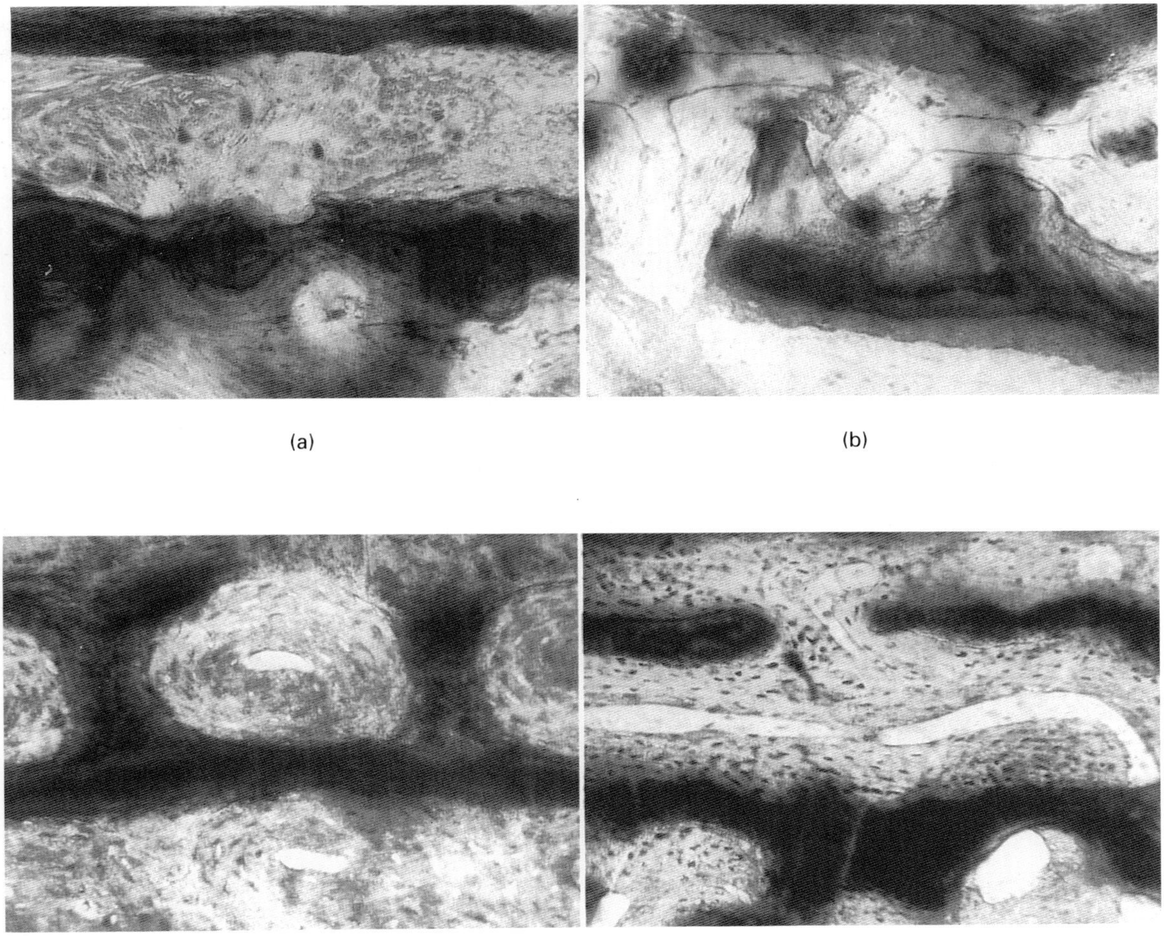

(a) (b)

(c) (d)

Figure 5.25

Bone formation within a porous hydroxyapatite implant with oriented porosity. (a) At four months, both woven and lamellar bone are present in the implant. (b) A vascular channel can be seen bridging a crossfenestration. (c) At six months, haversian osteons occupy the implant pores, with (d) interchannel communication. (From Ref 85 with permission.)

ingrowth of bone effectively decreases the porosity and increases the strength of the implant, while degradation, if it occurs, has the opposite effect. Thus, like a healing fracture, the properties of a bone substitute in vivo change with time. The lowest strength can be anticipated to occur at the time of implantation before ingrowth occurs. de Putter et al[91] described a relationship between the ultimate compressive stress (CS) and the total volume occupied by pores in the implant (VP) as follows:

$$CS = 700 \exp(-5VP) \quad \text{(with CS in MPa)}.$$

Table 5.6 Morphometric comparison (mean and standard error) of the microstructure of the hydroxyapatite bone substitute derived from the coral, genus *Goniopora* (IP500), and human iliac crest cancellous bone. (From Ref 86 with permission.)

	IP500	*Iliac bone*	*Iliac bone*
Volume fraction (%)	35.1 ± 1.5	20.5 ± 0.4	20.3 ± 0.4
Surface area (mm^2/mm^3)	5.3 ± 0.2	3.0 ± 0.1	3.4 ± 0.1
Ratio of surface area to volume fraction	15.3 ± 0.6	14.6 ± 0.6	17.3 ± 0.2
Mean trabecular width (μm)	131.9 ± 4.4	136.6 ± 4.5	120.3 ± 1.6
Mean pore width (μm)	245.0 ± 9.0	529.6 ± 22.9	468.2 ± 27.2

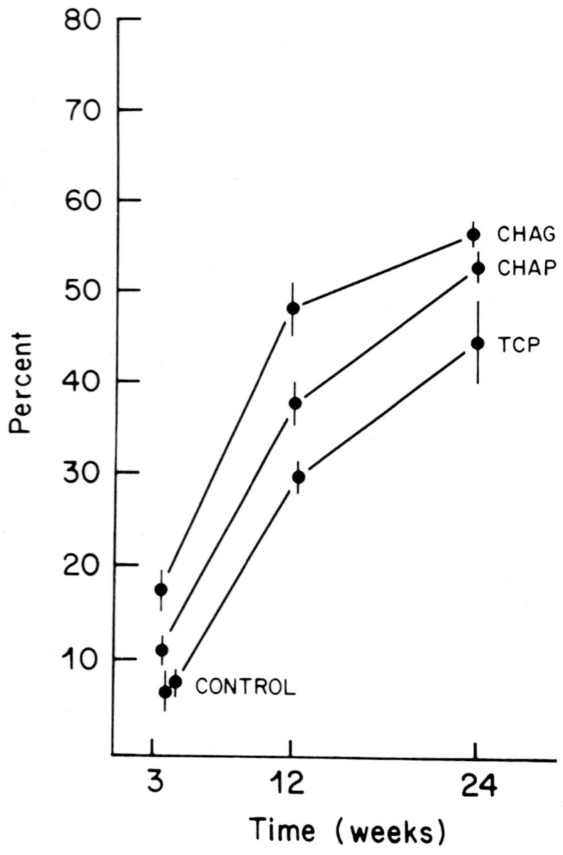

Figure 5.26

Bone ingrowth (percent of total volume) into porous coralline implants with different pore size ranges as a function of time post implantation: CHAG, hydroxyapatite, pore size 260–600 μm; CHAP, hydroxyapatite, pore size 190-230 μm; TCP, tricalcium phosphate, pore size 100-300 μm. (From Ref 87 with permission.)

This relationship demonstrates a strong dependence between pore volume and strength. Table 5.7 shows mechanical property data for hydroxyapatite implants of varying porosity. The compressive and tensile strengths of ceramics encompass those of bone; however, their moduli range from about three to eight times as great as that of bone.[92] For implants with oriented porosity, the orientation of the longitudinal channels significantly affects properties, as shown in Figure 5.27, with a more than 50% decrease in strength for only a 20° difference between channel and load axis.[93]

As discussed above, the properties of the implant can be expected to increase as bone invades it. The incorporation of the implant into the metaphyseal bone in the dog tibia, shown in Figure 5.28, can be well appreciated. Detailed scanning electron microscopy clearly distinguishes how new bone directly apposes the internal surfaces of the implant (Figure 5.29).[94] As shown in Table 5.8, six months post implantation, the ultimate strength of a cancellous autograft is about twice that of normal cancellous bone, while an incorporated hydroxyapatite implant (ingrown with bone) increases by about six times from its preimplantation compressive strength, from 60% of that of cancellous bone to more than 300%.[95]

Although the compressive strength of solid ceramics has shown to be in the range of that of bone, the use of materials of greater porosity to enhance ingrowth also reduces strength. Also, the modulus of ceramics is considerably greater than that of bone (Table 5.7). Reduced brittleness and

Table 5.7 Mechanical properties of hydroxyapatite materials compared with cancellous and cortical bone. (From Ref 62 with permission.)

Material	*Compressive strength (MPa)*	*Tensile strength (MPa)*	*Modulus (GPa)*
Bone			
Cortical	137.8	68.9	13.8
Cancellous	41.4	3.5	—
Calcium phosphates			
Porous	6.9–68.9	2.48	
Dense	206.7–895.7	68.9–192.9	34.5–103.4

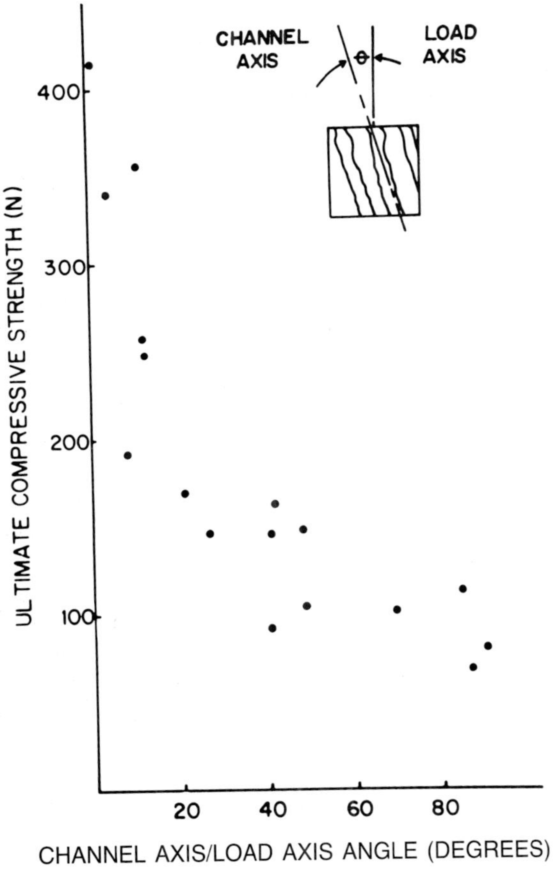

Figure 5.27

Relationship between longitudinal channel axis and ultimate compressive strength in a hydroxyapatite implant with oriented porosity. (From Ref 93 with permission.)

the ability to absorb greater energy of impact in bone is due to its two phase collagen/mineral structure. Therefore composites of hydroxyapatite and some other more flexible material, typically a polymer or collagen, have been explored. One example of a composite filler is hydroxyapatite granules bound with atelocollagen (calf skin collagen treated with pepsin).[96] This material does not have structural properties suitable for load bearing, nor does it maintain a pore structure; thus the collagen must be degraded before bone invasion can begin.

Alternatively, degradable polymers have been used either as binders for HA granules[97] or as coatings on implants.[98] Poly(lactic acid) coating of a porous implant of oriented porosity, similar to that shown in Figure 5.24, has been found to increase compressive strength, stiffness, and energy absorbed to failure, while still maintaining the internal pore structure of the implant. Bone ingrowth into this material was found to be slightly inhibited compared with implants without coatings, because the coating partly occludes the pores of the implant. Bone grows to the coating, as shown in Figure 5.30, but the coating must degrade before direct apposition between bone and the hydroxyapatite surfaces of the implant can take place.[98]

5.5 Summary

Various materials are available for use in orthopedic fracture surgery. Stainless steel will continue to be used, especially for implants requiring strength and ductility such as wires and screws,

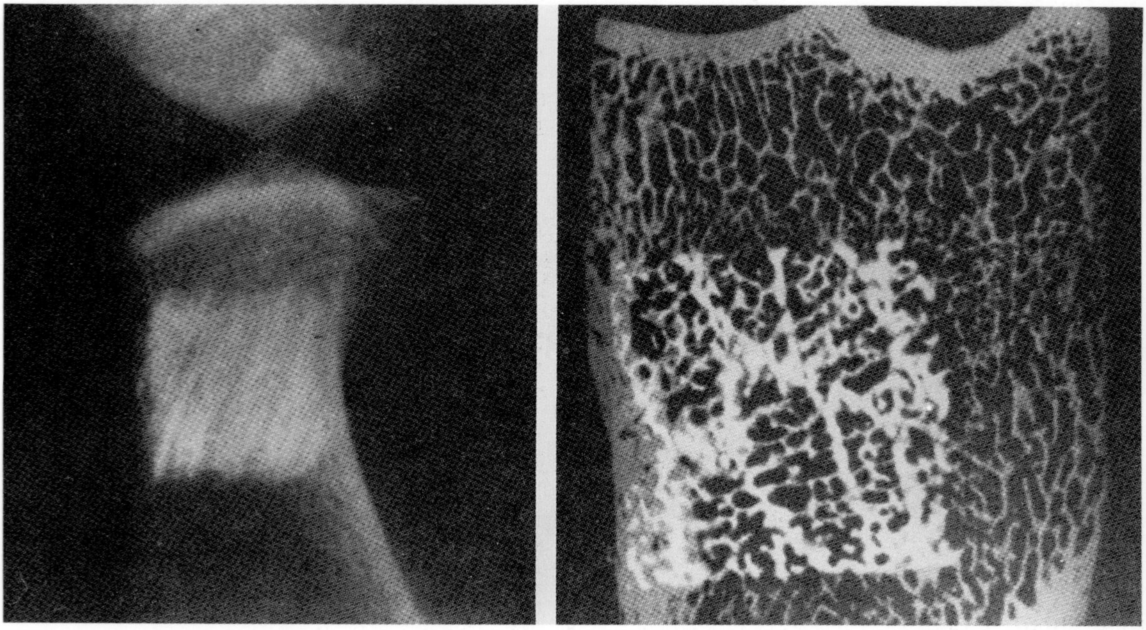

Figure 5.28

Incorporation of a coralline implant into the metaphysis of the tibia of the dog after six months. (From Ref 86 with permission.)

Table 5.8 Compressive properties of cancellous bone compared with cancellous autograft and corraline hydroxyapatite implant (CHAG) six months after implantation. (From Ref 95 with permission.)

	Average properties				*Ranges*		
Materials	*Stiffness (N/cm)*	*Ultimate strength (N/cm^2)*	*Energy absorbed (N cm)*	*No. of specimens tested*	*Stiffness (N/cm)*	*Ultimate strength (N/cm^2)*	*Energy absorbed (N cm)*
Cancellous bone	7950	754	93	6	14 760–3750	1150–485	166.7–25.5
CHAG (load parallel to channel axis)	6020	412	15.5	5	6560–5200	500–230	21.6–6.7
CHAG (load perpendicular to channel axis)	2360	84	2.1	4	3940–1280	175–50	5.6–0.3
Cancellous graft at 6 months under dog tibial plateau	24 110	1519	232.4	6	36 301–7160	2700–1000	609.6–93.6
CHAG graft at 6 months under dog tibial plateau	16 190	2488	389.7	6	6960–15 750	3500–1730	514.4–160.5

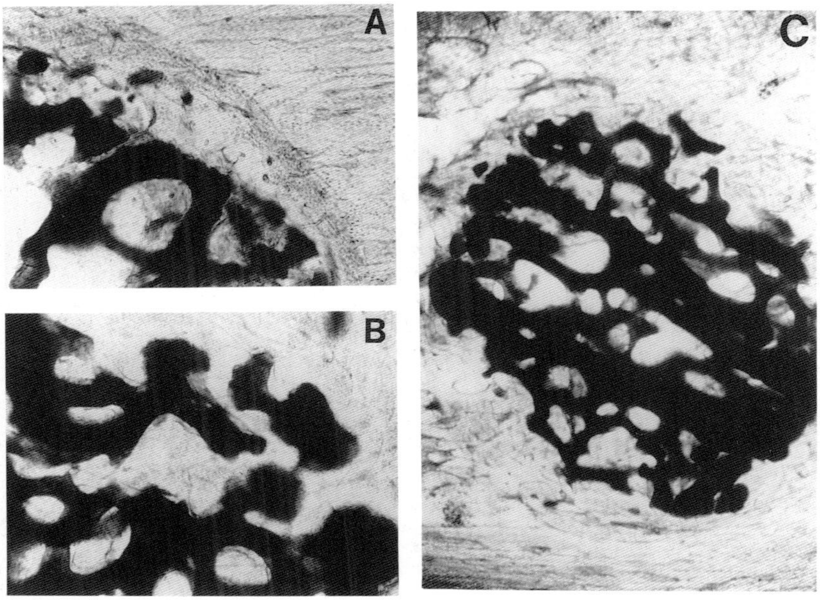

Figure 5.29

Sections at different magnifications from ingrowth through porous hydroxyapatite plugs placed transversely in the tibial cortex in the rabbit, simulating the filling of a bone defect. (A) Detail of approximation of the surface of the implant by new bone (original × 78); (B) bone invasion of the implant at 12 weeks (original × 78); (C) low-power view of the complete implant. (From Ref 98 with permission.)

(a) (b)

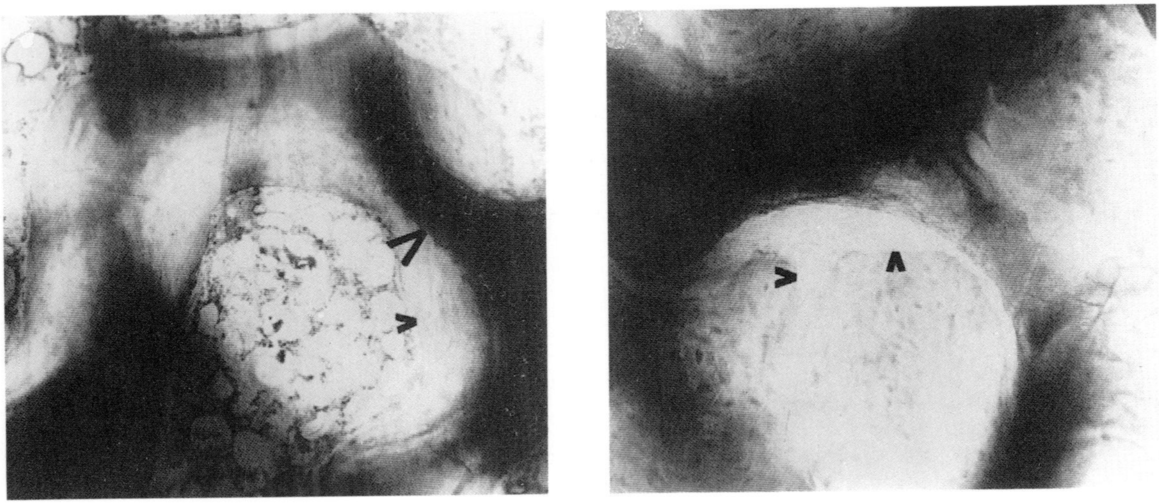

Figure 5.30

Bone ingrowth into porous coralline hydroxyapatite placed in the tibia of the rabbit at 24 weeks. (a) Uncoated implant. (b) Implant microcoated with poly(lactic acid) polymer. Black areas = hydroxyapatite; grey = new bone; arrowheads on (b) indicate polymer coating. (From Ref 98 with permission.)

although titanium alloys have significant advantages in terms of biocompatibility and resistance to corrosion. Adhesives have a potentially important role in repositioning of small, nonload bearing fracture fragments, which are difficult to handle using conventional hardware; however, to be practical, an adhesive must be viscous enough to fill gaps and be able to bond to wet surfaces. Fibrin and viscous cyanoacrylate are two promising adhesive materials.

Degradable polymers are finding use in fracture fixation, with their main advantage being that no hardware removal is necessary at a later date. However, these materials have elastic moduli that are only about 10% of those of conventional metals; therefore they should be considered mainly for low load bearing applications. Ceramics are used as bone fracture defect fillers. An appropriate pore size is required for adequate bone ingrowth, which decreases the strength of this very brittle material. However, bone ingrowth effectively reinforces the implant, improving its mechanical properties over time. Many of these materials, while not ideal in terms of meeting the requirements of the in vivo environment, offer important advantages, and will find their place in fracture surgery.

5.6 References

1. *Annual Book of Standards*, Section 13, Vol 13.01 (American Society for Testing and Materials: Philadelphia 1986) 3–9.
2. Fraker AC, Corrosion of metallic implants and prosthetic devices. In: *Metals handbook*, 9th edn, Vol 13, *Corrosion* (ASM International: 1987).
3. Black J, *Orthopaedic biomaterials in research and practice* (Churchill Livingstone: New York 1988).
4. Pohler O, Straumann F, Characteristics of the stainless steel ASIF/AO implants. In: *ASIF/AO basic course manual* (The Association for the Study of Internal Fixation: Davos, Switzerland 1975).
5. Mears DC, *Materials and orthopedic surgery* (Williams & Wilkins: Baltimore 1979).
6. *Annual Book of Standards*, Section 13, vol 13.01 (American Society for Testing and Materials: 1986) 15–17.
7. French HG, Cook SD, Haddad RJ, Correlation of tissue reaction to corrosion in osteosynthetic devices, *J Biomed Mat Res* (1984) **18**: 817.
8. Brunet J, Sarkar K, Uhthoff HK, Ultrastructure of the fibrous tissue surrounding internal fixation devices, *Clin Orthop* (1986) **208**: 84–94.
9. McNamara A, Williams DF, Enzyme histochemistry of the tissue response to pure metal implants, *J Biomed Mat Res* (1984) **18**: 185–97.
10. Weber SC, Chapman MW, Adhesives in orthopedic surgery. A review of the literature and in vitro bonding strengths of bone-bonding agents, *Clin Orthop* (1984) **191**: 249–61.
11. Markoff G, Quagliarello J, Rosen RJ, Beckman EM, Uterine arteriovenous malformation successfully embolized with a liquid polymer, isobutyl 2-cyanoacrylate, *Am J Obstet Gynecol* (1986) **155**: 659–60.
12. Barthelemy C, Audigier JC, Fraisse H, A nontumoral esophagobronchial fistula managed by isobutyl-2-cyanoacrylate, *Endoscopy* (1983) **15**: 357–8.
13. Lobene RR, Sharawy AM, The response of alveolar bone to cyanoacrylate tissue adhesives, *J Periodontol* (1968) **39**: 150–6.
14. Bonette GH, Experimental fractures of the mandible, *J Oral Surg* (1969) **27**: 568–74.
15. Corn RC, Corn O, Matsumoto T, Osteosynthesis employing isobutyl-cyanoacrylate monomer, *Int Surg* (1972) **57**: 483–7.
16. Hunter KM, Cyanoacrylate tissue adhesives in osseous repair, *Br J Oral Surg* (1976) **14**: 80–6.
17. Hampel NL, Pijanowski GJ, Johnson RG, Effects of isobutyl-2-cyanoacrylate on bone healing, *Am J Vet Res* (1986) **47**: 1605–9.
18. Brauer GM, Kumpula JW, Termini DJ, Davidson KM, Durability of the bond between bone and various 2-cyanoacrylates in an aqueous environment, *J Biomed Mat Res* (1979) **13**: 593–606.
19. Harper MC, Stabilization of osteochondral fragments using limited placement of cyanoacrylate in rabbits, *Clin Orthop* (1988) **231**: 272–6.
20. Spängler HP, Holle J, Braun F, Kovac W, Spängler H, Die Verklebung experimenteller Leberverletzungen mittels hochkonzentriertem Fibrin, *Acta Chir Aust* (1975) **7**: 89–93.
21. Spängler HP, Braun F, Holle J, Die lokale Anwendung von Fibrinogen und Kollagen zur Blutstillung der Herzchirurgie, *Wien Med Wochenschr* (1976) **126**: 86–9.
22. Stemberger A, Blumel G, Fibrinogen–fibrin conversion and inhibition of fibrolysis, *Thorac Cardiovasc Surg* (1982) **30**: 209–14.
23. Lerner R, Binur N, Current research review, current status of surgical adhesives, *J Surg Res* (1990) **48**: 165–81.
24. Bosch P, Die Fibrinspongiosaplastik. Experimentalle Untersuchungen und Klinische Erfahrung, *Wien Klin Wochenschr (Supp)* (1981) **93**: 1.
25. Zilch H, Animal experiments on cementing small

osteochondral fragments, *Handchirurgie* (1980) **12:** 71–75.
26. Arbes H, Bosch P, Lintner F, Salzer M, First clinical experience with heterologous cancellous bone grafting combined with fibrin adhesive system, *Arch Orthop Trauma Surg* (1981) **98:** 183–8.
27. Bosch P, Braun F, Spängler HP, Die Technik der Fibrinspongiosaplastik, *Arch Orthop Unfall-Chir* (1977) **90:** 63–75.
28. Zilch H, Der Einfluss des Fibrinklebers auf die Revaskularisierung des Knochentransplantates. In: Cotta H, Braun A, eds, *Fibrinkleber in Orthopädie und Traumatologie* (Georg Thieme Verlag: Stuttgart 1982) 62–4.
29. Bohler N, Bosch P, Sandbach G, Eschberger J, Schmid L, Experimentelle Erfahrungen, mit der Einklebung von Kortikaliszylindern. In: Cotta H, Braun A, eds, *Fibrinkleber in Orthopädie und Traumatologie* (Georg Thieme Verlag: Stuttgart 1982) 68–70.
30. Rosen HB, Kohn J, Leong K, Langer R, Bioerodible polymers for controlled release systems. In: Hsieh, DST, ed, *Controlled release systems: fabrication technology*, Vol II, Chapter 5 (CRC Press: Boca Raton, FL 1988) 83–110.
31. Kulkarni RK, Moore EG, Hegyeli AF, Leonard F, Biodegradable poly(lactic acid) polymers, *J Biomed Mat Res* (1971) **5:** 169–81.
32. Vert M, Christel P, Chabot F, Leray J, Bioabsorbable plastic materials for bone surgery. In: Hastings GW, Ducheyne P, eds, *Macromolecular biomaterials* (CRC Press: Boca Raton, FL 1984) Chapter 6.
33. Chu CC, An in vitro study of the effect of buffer on the degradation of poly(glycolic acid) sutures, *J Biomed Mat Res* (1981) **15:** 19–27.
34. Smith R, Oliver C, Williams DF, The enzymatic degradation of polymer in vitro, *J Biomed Mat Res* (1987) **21:** 991–1003.
35. Brady JM, Cutright DE, Miller RA, Battistone GC, Hunsuck EE, Resorption rate, route of elimination, and ultrastructure of the implant site of polylactic acid in the abdominal wall of the rat, *J Biomed Mat Res* (1973) **7:** 155–66.
36. Gogolewski S, Resorbable polymers for internal fixation, *AO/ASIF Dialogue* (1990) **3**(2): 6–8.
37. Wade CWR, Hegyeli AF, Kulkarni RK, Standards for in-vitro and in-vivo comparison and qualification of bioabsorbable polymers *J Testing and Evaluation* (1977) **5:** 397–400.
38. Cutright DE, Hunsuck EE, The repair of fractures of the orbital floor using biodegradable polylactic acid, *Oral Surg* (1972) **33:** 28–34.
39. Bostman O, Hirvensalo E, Makinen J, Rokkanen P, Foreign-body reactions to fracture fixation implants of biodegradable synthetic polymers, *J Bone Jt Surg* (1990) **72B:** 592–6.
40. Daniels AU, Taylor MS, Andriano KP, Heller J, Toxicity of absorbable polymers proposed for fracture fixation devices, *Trans 38th Orthopedic Research Society Meeting* (1992) **17:** 88.
41. Miller RA, Brady JM, Cutright DE, Degradation rates of oral resorbable implants (polylactates and polyglycolates): rate modification with changes in PLA/PGA copolymer ratio, *J Biomed Mat Res* (1977) **11:** 711–19.
42. Chu CC, A comparison of the effect of pH on the biodegradation of two synthetic absorbable sutures, *Ann Surg* (1982) **195:** 51–9.
43. Schakenraad JM, Nieuwenhuis P, Molenaar I, Helder J, Dijkstra PJ, Feijen J, In vivo and in vitro degradation of glycine/DL–lactic acid copolymers, *J Biomed Mat Res* (1989) **23:** 1271–88.
44. Daniels AU, Smutz WP, Andriano KP, Chang MKO, Heller J, Dynamic environmental exposure testing of biodegradable polymers, *Trans 15th Meeting of the Society for Biomaterials* (1989) **12:** 74.
45. Heponen V-P, Pohjonen T, Vainionpaa S, Tormala P, The effect of gamma-radiation on mechanical properties of biodegradable poly-*l*-lactide fibers. In: *Trans 3rd World Biomaterials Congress, Kyoto, April 1988* (Tokyo 1988) 281.
46. Rozema FR, Bos RRM, Boering G, van Asten JAAM, Nijenhuis AJ, Pennings AJ, The effects of different steam-sterilization programs on material properties of poly(L-lactide), *J Appl Biomaterials* (1991) **2:** 23–8.
47. Zimmerman M, Parsons JR, Alexander H, The design and analysis of a laminated partially degradable composite bone plate for fracture fixation, *J Biomed Mat Res* (1987) **21:** 345–61.
48. Leenslag JW, Gogolewski S, Pennings AJ, Resorbable materials of poly(L-lactide) fibers produced by a dry spinning method, *J Appl Polym Sci* (1984) **29:** 2829–42.
49. Leenslag JW, Pennings AJ, Bos RRM, Rozema FR, Boering G, Resorbable materials of poly(L-lactide). VI, Plates and screws for internal fracture fixation, *Biomaterials* (1987) **8:** 70–3.
50. Tormalla P, Vasneius J, Vainionpaa S, Laiho J, Pohjonen T, Rokkanen P, Ultra high strength absorbable self reinforced polyglycolide (SR–PGA) composite rods for internal fixation of bone fractures, *J Biomed Mat Res* (1991) **25:** 1–22.
51. Anderson PA, Copenhaver JC, Tencer AF, Clark JM, Response of cortical bone to controlled release of sodium fluoride: the effect of implant insertion site, *J Orthop Res* (1991) **9:** 890–901.
52. Guise JM, McCormack A, Anderson PA, Tencer AF, Effect of controlled release of sodium fluoride on trabecular bone, *J Orthop Res* (1992) **10:** 588–95.
53. Arm DM, Tencer AF, Controlled release of platelet derived growth factor. In: *Proc 4th World Congress of Biomaterials, Berlin, 1992.*

54. Prolo DJ, Rodrigo JJ, Contemporary bone graft physiology and surgery, *Clin Orthop* (1985) **200:** 322–42.
55. Friedlander GE, Current concepts review: bone banking, *J Bone Jt Surg* (1982) **64A:** 307–11.
56. Cowley SP, Anderson LD, Hernias through donor sites for iliac-bone grafts, *J Bone Jt Surg* (1983) **65A:** 1023–5.
57. Blakemore ME, Fractures at cancellous bone graft donor sites, *Injury* (1983) **14:** 519–22.
58. Challis JH, Lyttle JA, Stuart AE, Strangulated lumbar hernia and volvulus following removal of iliac crest bone graft, *Acta Orthop Scand* (1975) **46:** 230–3.
59. Lotem M, Maor P, Haimoff H, Woloch Y , Lumbar hernia at an iliac bone graft donor site, *Clin Orthop* (1971) **80:** 130–2.
60. Escalas F, Dewald RL, Combined traumatic arterio-venous fistula and ureteral injury: a complication of iliac bone grafting, *J Bone Jt Surg.* (1977) **59A:** 270–1.
61. Younger EM, Chapman MW, Morbidity at bone graft donor sites. *J Orthop Trauma* (1989) **3:** 192–5.
62. Damien CJ, Parsons JR, Bone graft and bone graft substitutes: a review of current technology and applications, *J Appl Biomaterials* (1991) **2:** 187–208.
63. Bright RW, Burchardt H, The biomechanical properties of preserved bone grafts. In: Friedlander GE, Mankin HJ, Sell, KW, eds, *Osteochondral allografts: biology, banking and clinical applications.* (Little, Brown: Boston 1983) 241–7.
64. Kmender A, Influence of preservation on some mechanical properties of human haversian bone, *Mater Med Pol* (1976) **8:** 13–17.
65. Miller E, Conrad III EU, Tencer AF, Mackenzie AP, Strong DM, The biomechanical effects of freeze-drying and rehydration on human cortical allograft bone, *Clin Orthop* (in press).
66. Conrad III EU, Ericksen DP, Tencer AF, Strong DM, Mackenzie AP, The effects of freeze drying and rehydration on cancellous bone, *Clin Orthop* (1993) **290:** 279–84.
67. Mellonig JT, Bowers GM, Cotton WR, Comparison of bone graft materials: Part II. New bone formation with autografts and allografts: a histological evaluation, *J Periodontol* (1981) **52:** 297–302.
68. Oklund SA, Prolo DJ, Gutierrez RV, King SE, Quantitative comparisons of healing in cranial fresh autografts, frozen autografts, processed autografts, and allografts in canine skull defects, *Clin Orthop* (1986) **205:** 269–291.
69. Burchardt H, Jones H, Glowczewskie F, Rudner C, Enneking WF, Freeze-dried allograft segmental cortical-bone grafts in dogs, *J Bone Jt Surg* (1978) **60A:** 1082–90.
70. Buck BE, Malinin TI, Bone transplantation and human immunodeficiency virus. An estimate of risk of acquired immunodeficiency syndrome (AIDS), *Clin Orthop* (1989) **240:** 129–36.
71. Peltier LF, The use of plaster of Paris to fill defects in bone. *Clin Orthop* (1961) **21:** 1–31.
72. Mackey D, Varlet A, Debeaumont D, Antibiotic loaded plaster of Paris pellets: an in vitro study of a possible method of load antibiotic therapy in bone infection, *Clin Orthop* (1982) **167:** 263–8.
73. Bahn SL, Plaster: a bone substitute, *Oral Surg, Oral Med, Oral Path* (1966) **21:** 672–81.
74. Sanad MEE, Combe EC, Grant AA, The use of additives to improve the mechanical properties of gypsum products, *J Dent Res* (1982) **61:** 808–10.
75. Calhoun NR, Neiders ME, Greene Jr GW, Effects of plaster-of-Paris implants in surgical defects of mandibular alveolar processes of dogs, *J Oral Surg* (1967) **25:** 122–8.
76. Dahners LE, Funderburk CH, Gentamicin-loaded plaster of Paris as a treatment of experimental osteomyelitis in rabbits, *Clin Orthop* (1987) **219:** 278–82.
77. Yamazaki Y, Oida S, Akimoto Y, Shioda S, Response of the mouse femoral muscle to an implant of bone morphogenic protein and plaster of Paris, *Clin Orthop* (1988) **234:** 240–9,
78. deGroot K, Klein CPAT, Wolke JGC, de Blieck-Hogervorst JMA, Chemistry of calcium phosphate bioceramics. In: Yamamuro T, Hench LL, Wilson J, eds, *Handbook of bioactive ceramics*, Vol II (CRC Press: Boca Raton, FL 1990) 3–16.
79. Cameron HU, Macnab I, Pilliar RM, Evaluation of a biodegradable ceramic, *J Biomed Mat Res* (1977) **11:** 179–86.
80. Klein CAPT, Patka P, den Hollander W, A comparison between hydroxylapatite and B-Whitlockite macroporous ceramics implanted in dog femurs, In: Yamamuro T, Hench LL, Wilson J, eds, *Handbook of bioactive ceramics*, Vol II (CRC Press: Boca Raton, FL 1990) 53–60.
81. Tracy BM, Doremus RH, Direct electron microscopy studies of the bone–hydroxyapatite interface, *J Biomed Mat Res* (1984) **18:** 719–26.
82. de Lange GL, The bone–hydroxyapatite interface, In: Yamamuro T, Hench LL, Wilson J, eds, *Handbook of bioactive ceramics*, Vol II, (CRC Press: Boca Raton, FL 1990) 61–75.
83. Kitsugi T, Yamamuro T, Nakamura T, Kokubo T, Takagi M, Shibuya T, Takeuchi H, Ono M, Bonding behavior between two bioactive ceramics in vivo, *J Biomed Mat Res* (1987) **21:** 1109–23.
84. Roy DM, Linnehan SK, Hydroxyapatite formed from coral skeletal carbonate by hydrothermal exchange, *Nature* (1974) **247:** 220.
85. Holmes RE, Bone regeneration within a coralline hydroxyapatite implant, *Plast Recon Surg* (1979)

63: 626–33.

86. Holmes RE, Bucholz RW, Mooney V, Porous hydroxyapatite as a bone graft substitute in metaphyseal defects, *J Bone Jt Surg* (1986) **68A**: 904–11.
87. Shimazaki K, Mooney V, Comparative study of porous hydroxyapatite and tricalcium phosphate as bone substitute, *J Orthop Res* (1985) **3**: 301–10.
88. Ito K, Ooi Y, Osteogenic activity of synthetic hydroxyapatite with controlled texture—On the relationship of osteogenic quantity with sintering temperature and pore size. In: Yamamuro T, Hench LL, Wilson J, eds, *Handbook of bioactive ceramics*, Vol II (CRC Press: Boca Raton, FL 1990) 39–44.
89. Legros RZ, Parsons JR, Daculsi G, Driessens F, Lee D, Liu ST, Metsger S, Peterson D, Walker M, Significance of the porosity and physical chemistry of calcium phosphate ceramics, biodegradation–bioresorption, *Ann NY Acad Sci* (1988) **523**: 268–71.
90. Holmes RE, Bucholz RW, Mooney V, Porous hydroxyapatite as a bone graft substitute in diaphyseal defects: a histometric study, *J Orthop Res* (1987) **5**: 114–21.
91. de Putter C, de Groot K, Sillevis Smitt PAE, Transmucosal application of implants of dense hydroxyapatite in prosthetic dentistry. In: Vincenzini P, ed, *Ceramics in surgery* (Elsevier: Amsterdam 1983).
92. Jarcho M, Calcium phosphate ceramics as hard tissue prosthetics, *Clin Orthop* (1981) **157**: 259–78.
93. Tencer AF, Mooney V, Brown KL, Silva PA, Compressive properties of polymer coated hydroxyapatite for bone grafting, *J Biomed Mat Res* (1985) **19**: 957–69.
94. Holmes RE, Wardrop RW, Wolford LM, Hydroxyapatite as a bone graft substitute in orthognathic surgery: histologic and histometric findings, *J Oral Maxillofac Surg* (1988) **46**: 661–71.
95. Holmes RE, Mooney V, Bucholz RW, Tencer AF, A corraline hydroxyapatite bone graft substitute, *Clin Orthop* (1984) **188**: 282–92.
96. Watanabe M, Harada K, Asahina I, Enomoto S, Implantation of hydroxyapatite granules mixed with atelocollagen and bone inductive protein in rat skull defects. In: Yamamuro T, Hench LL, Wilson J, eds, *Handbook of bioactive ceramics*, Vol II (CRC Press: Boca Raton, FL 1990) 223–8.
97. Higashi S, Yamamuro T, Nakamura T, Ikada Y, Hyon S-H, Jamshidi K, Polymer–hydroxyapatite composites for biodegradable bone fillers, *Biomaterials* (1986) **7**: 183–7.
98. Tencer AF, Woodward PL, Swenson J, Brown KL, Bone ingrowth into polymer coated porous synthetic coralline hydroxyapatite, *J Orthop Res* (1987) **5**: 275–82.

PART III
BIOMECHANICS OF FRACTURE FIXATION

In the following chapters the biomechanics of fracture fixation applied to specific anatomical areas is discussed in detail. Biomechanics is one of the important considerations in the application of fracture devices. Mechanically speaking, the fixation device must restore anatomical alignment of the fracture components and maintain this alignment under functional loading.

Fixation constructs (the composite structure of the implant and the bone fragments that it connects) are usually compared biomechanically in terms of stiffness, that is, their ability to minimize motion between fracture components under an applied load. In general, the loading of bones in the skeleton is complex, so a fixation system should be capable of withstanding forces and moments in multiple planes. However complex the actual loading situation may be, it can typically be broken into fundamental forces and moments. These include compression and tension along the long axis of the bone, torsion about the long axis, and bending in two perpendicular planes. Most physiological loading situations are superpositions of vector sums of these fundamental forces and moments. Therefore the comparative data to be presented are usually given in terms of these fundamental loads.

The implication of comparative biomechanical stiffness testing of fixation is that the most rigid construct is the "best." Certainly the desire to achieve rigid fixation is important; however, excessively rigid fixation can transfer too much load to the implant and not enough to the healing fracture. This has the combined negative effects of overstressing the implant while stress shielding the underlying bone. Considering the success of fixations of widely varying stiffnesses (for example a cast as compared with a plate), it is clear that the healing fracture can tolerate a range of mechanical conditions, and though responding differently to them, can achieve union.

If fixation is relatively flexible, greater callus formation can be expected, as shown in Figure 4.21 for the case of slotted or unslotted intramedullary rods. Using still quite incomplete data (see Figure 4.20), the optimal rigidity of a fixation construct can be estimated to be between 20% and 60% of the rigidity of the intact bone in bending. Other data (see Figure 4.25) suggest that 0.5 mm of micromotion in an axial direction stimulates fracture healing in a 3 mm wide gap, but that 2.0 mm is excessive. Therefore the additional complicating factor of the direction of the applied load must be considered. It appears that a fixation construct that controls bending (and probably torsion) but allows some movement along the axis of the bone provides a reasonable compromise. Where possible in the data presented, the rigidity of the construct is compared to percent of intact bone as a guide.

It should also be pointed out that fixation construct stiffness is directly affected by whether or not cortical contact can be achieved between the fracture components. Also, biomechanical tests of construct stiffness ignore the contribution of the fracture callus, in order to test worst case conditions. In reality, the construct stiffness increases as the callus matures, which is why achieving construct stiffnesses of about 50% of the intact bone initially (without any contribution from the fracture) is a better overall compromise that trying to achieve a rigidity approaching 100% of intact stiffness. Another aspect that must be considered is that applying hardware in an effort to increase fixation construct rigidity may result in excessive periosteal stripping or placement of a large number of holes in the bone, compromising its blood supply and creating avascular necrosis.

CHAPTER 6

General biomechanical principles of some common fracture fixation devices

This chapter provides some basic concepts related to the biomechanics of fracture fixation in general, before moving to specific anatomical areas and types of constructs. In this section the effects of drilling and the design of bone drills is discussed, as is the biomechanical effect of a hole in bone, the properties of screws and surgical wire, and the mechanics of the compression plate and lag screw.

6.1 Drilling holes in bone

Drilling is probably the most common single procedure performed in orthopedic surgery. The drill consists of a dead center (the point) and has two cutting edges or lips inclined away from the center (Figure 6.1). The cutting edges act as wedges that shear material from the surface being cut. As shown in Figure 6.2, in bone this shear cutting can occur transverse, across, or parallel to the predominant osteon direction. The cutting force increases considerably when cutting transverse to the osteon orientation,[1] as would be expected. Drilling is commonly performed perpendicular to the osteon axis, i.e. cutting either parallel or across osteons.

Factors affecting heat production

The process of drilling results in deformation of bone. Elastic deformation occurs as the tool indents the bone surface, and plastic deformation to failure in shear results as the material is cut away and forms a chip. The energy input to the cutting tool is converted partly to heat as a result of friction between the cutting edge of the drill and bone. About two thirds of the energy is absorbed by the action of cutting material, which disrupts atomic bonds. The rest is lost as heat, and a small fraction is converted to mechanical vibration and sound energy.[2] Heat generation is a very important consideration in drilling in bone, since exposure to elevated temperatures of 55°C for one minute in bone can result in osteocyte necrosis.[3] Among the effects of temperature elevation are the deactivation of alkaline phosphatase[4] and the degradation of the collagen–hydroxyapatite bond, resulting in irreversible alterations in material properties.[5] Therefore the consideration of heat production during drilling, both in terms of the maximum temperature produced and the time duration of the elevated temperatures, is important.

Matthews and Hirsch[4] demonstrated that a number of factors control heat production during drilling, and that peak temperature and time duration of temperature elevation in their 5 mm thick specimens of bone, drilled with standard surgical bits, could easily exceed levels known to

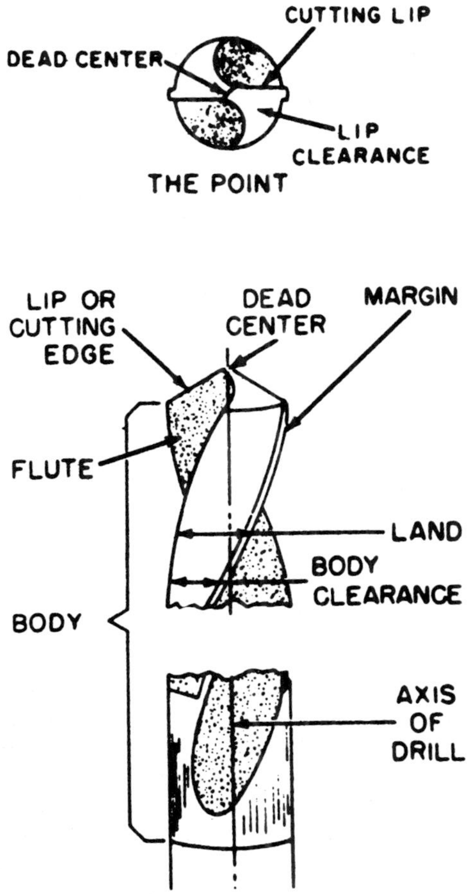

Figure 6.1

Nomenclature of a bone drill bit. (From Ref 2 with permission.)

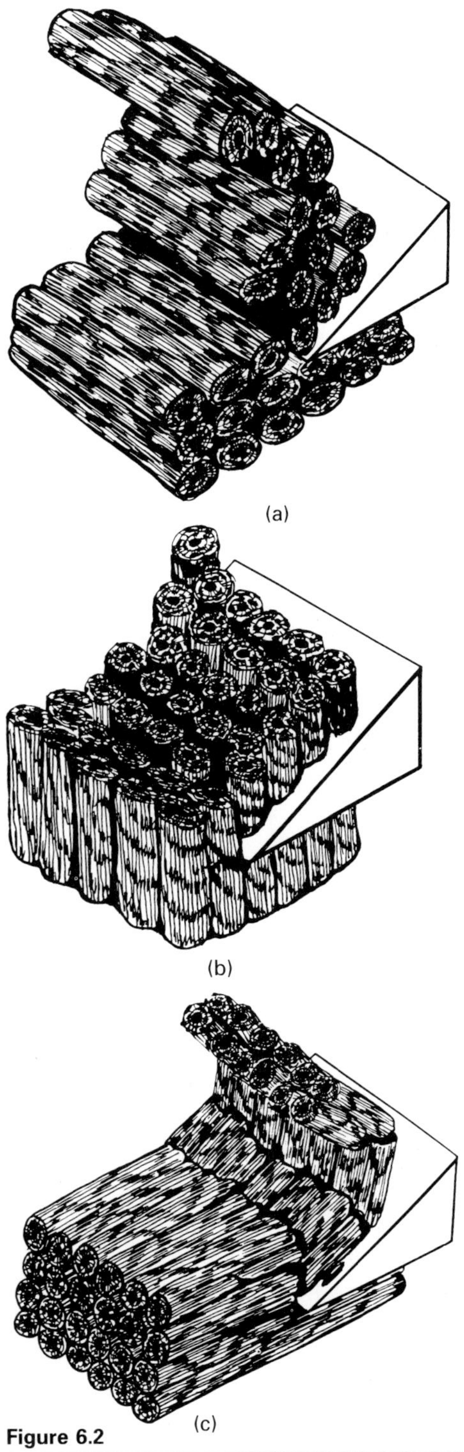

Figure 6.2

Schematic diagrams of the method by which a cutting tool shears osteons in cutting bone: (a) transverse; (b) across; (c) parallel. (From Ref 1 with permission.)

cause tissue necrosis. Using a lower force to drive the drill (2 kg instead of 12 kg) increased temperatures at the cutting surface significantly (Figure 6.3), since, with a smaller axial force acting on the drill, there is more friction as the cutting edges rub over the surface instead of engaging and cutting through it. Drill rotational speed does not affect the peak temperature of the sample; however, slower drill rotation produces a greater time over which the bone temperature remains elevated (Figure 6.4). An increase in the time of elevated temperature without a

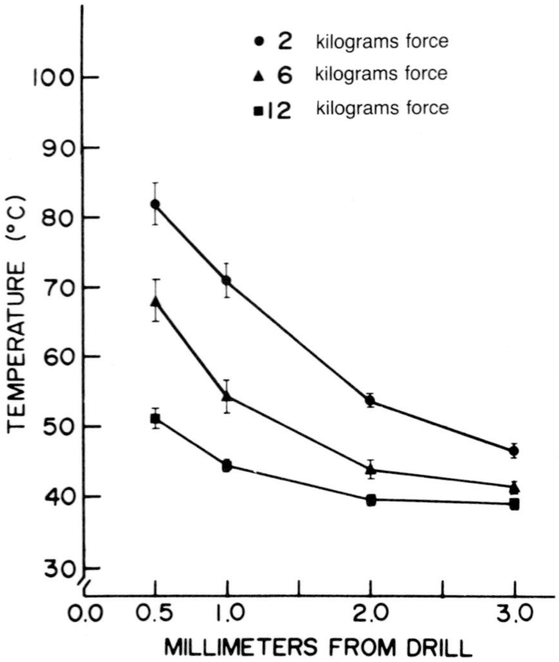

Figure 6.3

Elevation in temperature in bone samples due to drilling a hole with different axial forces applied to the drill bit. (From Ref 4 with permission.)

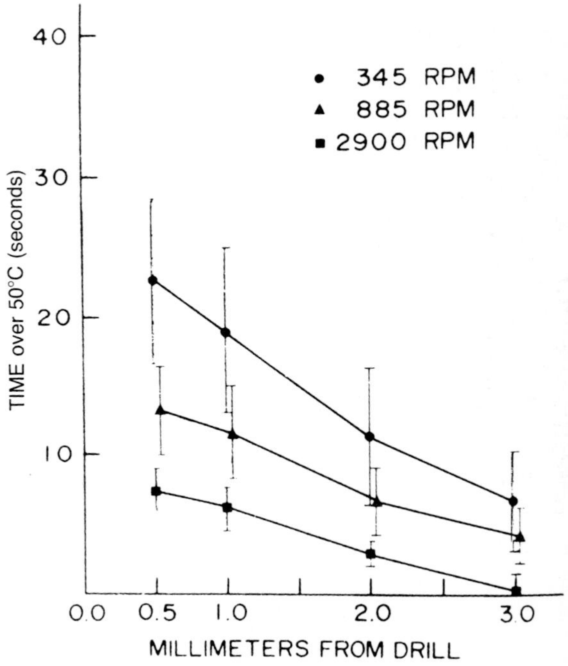

Figure 6.4

Time over which the sample temperature remained over 50°C for different drill rates of rotation. (From Ref 4 with permission.)

corresponding rise in the peak temperature implies a storage mechanism that converts heat, such as boiling of tissue fluid. Worn cutting edges on drills elevate bone temperature, as might be expected, since sharp cutting edges produce more shearing and less friction at the cutting surface. Predrilling (i.e. drilling a smaller hole first) significantly reduces bone temperature (Figure 6.5), as does irrigation while cutting, up to 500 ml/min (Figure 6.6). Manual tapping has no effect on temperature. Therefore rapid drilling of holes with adequate driving force, higher speed of rotation of the bit, the use of sharp bits, irrigation and use of a pilot hole will reduce temperature elevation in bone.

Bone drill design

The shape of the drill is another important factor in drilling effectively. The three specific geometric properties of the drill are, as shown in Figure 6.7, the cutting edge angle, the clearance angle, and the helix angle. The *cutting edge angle* determines the angle of the cutting surface with respect to the bone surface, while the *clearance angle* defines how much of the cutting surface of the drill is actually engaged in bone. With no clearance angle, the whole cutting surface of the drill, behind the cutting edge, engages the bone surface, increasing its temperature. Too high a clearance angle encourages chipping. The *helix angle* affects the speed at which material is removed from the hole and at the same time the speed at which the drill advances through bone. Typically, drills for relatively soft materials such as wood have smaller cutting edges and larger helix angles (cutting edge angle 86°, helix angle 17.2°) than those for harder materials such as metal (cutting edge angle 113°, helix angle 13.5°).[6] Since bone is softer than metal, but relatively brittle, a drill geometry is usually chosen that reduces the potential for chipping bone, yet

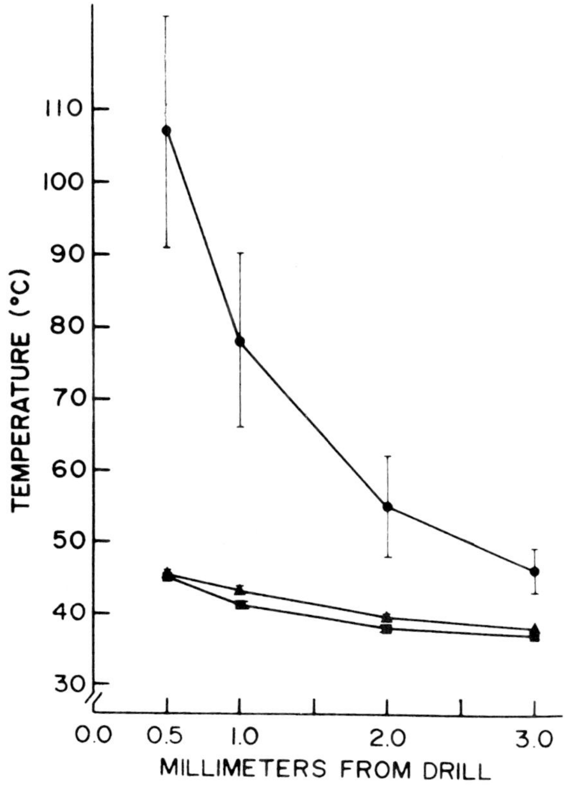

Figure 6.5

Maximum temperature in bone during drilling a 3.2 mm diameter hole with and without drilling a 2.2 mm diameter pilot hole first: ●, 3.2 mm hole without predrilling; ▲ 2.2 mm pilot hole; ■, pilot hole enlarged to 3.2 mm. (From Ref 4 with permission.)

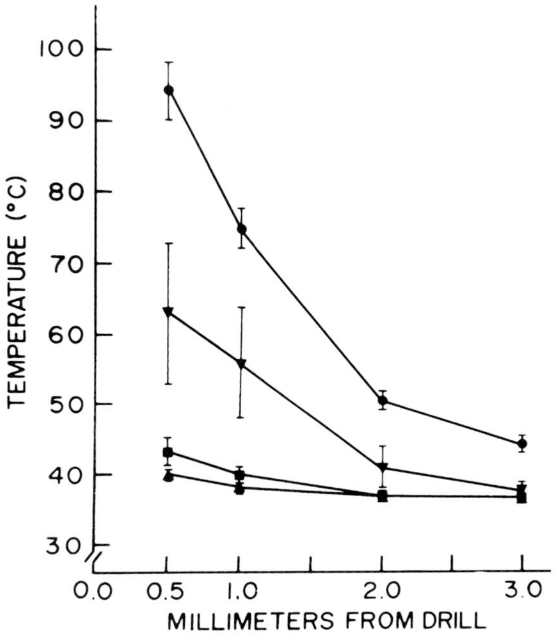

Figure 6.6

Effect of irrigation volume flow rate on maximum temperature generated in bone, during drilling: ▼, irrigation rate 300 ml/min; ■, 500 ml/min; ▲, 1000 ml/min; ●, control. (From Ref 4 with permission.)

allows rapid advance of the drill, which minimizes heating. Jacobs et al[6] reported, from comparisons of various drill types in cutting bone, that the drill geometry that produced the least drill thrust force at a given rotational speed and feed rate had a cutting edge angle of 110° and a helix angle of 24°.

6.2 The mechanical effects of holes in bone

Stress concentrator (riser)

The mechanical effects of holes produced in bone by drilling were covered in Chapter 2 briefly; however, that discussion did not describe the biological effect of removal and filling of the defect left by removal of the screw on the strength recovery in bone. From torsional tests of femora with holes of different diameters, Edgerton et al[7] showed that there is a critical hole diameter between 10% and 20% of the diameter of the cross section at which a sharp drop in bone torsional strength and in energy absorbed to failure occurs (Figure 6.8). For illustrative purposes, if a 4.5 mm diameter hole is drilled in a

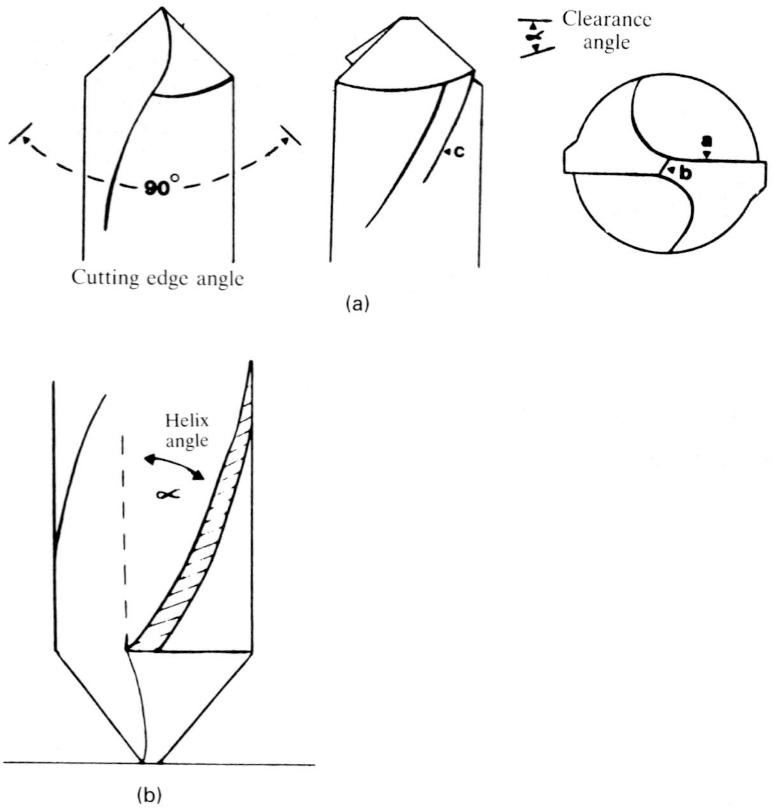

Figure 6.7

The three angles of the drill bit are (a) the cutting edge angle and the clearance angle or angle at which the cutting surface is raked away from the bone surface, and (b) the helix angle, which controls the rate of advance of the drill through bone. (From Ref 2 with permission.)

tibia of 22.5 mm diameter (hole diameter/cortex diameter = 20%) then the maximum torque and energy to failure are decreased to 64% of that of the intact bone. A study by Brooks et al[8] confirmed the reduction in bone energy absorption capacity due to drilling, and determined that the stress concentration factor (the ratio of stress around the hole to that in the bone away from the hole) was 1.6. Table 6.1 provides some data on the middiaphyseal (smallest) diameters of some long bones commonly fixed with screws, and the expected decreases in their properties due to drilling standard sized holes.

Leaving or removing screws in bone

The issue of the effect of the screw hole on bone strength is probably most important when hardware is removed after fracture healing, since refracture is a highly undesirable complication. It is tempting to consider leaving the screw in bone to reduce the stress concentration produced by the hole, since, as Schatzker et al[9] have shown, there is intimate contact between the screw and surrounding bone after 6–12 weeks. However, the modulus of the screw is significantly greater than that of the surrounding bone, so there will be a stress discontinuity at the hole (that is, the stresses will not be uniform within the screw and the surrounding bone) even if the screw completely fills the hole and is in intimate contact with the surrounding bone. While compressive stresses can be transmitted across the screw, the transmission of tensile stress depends on the bond between the screw and bone, if any, that occurs at the screw/bone interface.

Brooks et al[8] compared the torsional properties of rabbit femora with a hole drilled transversely and a self tapping screw inserted and either

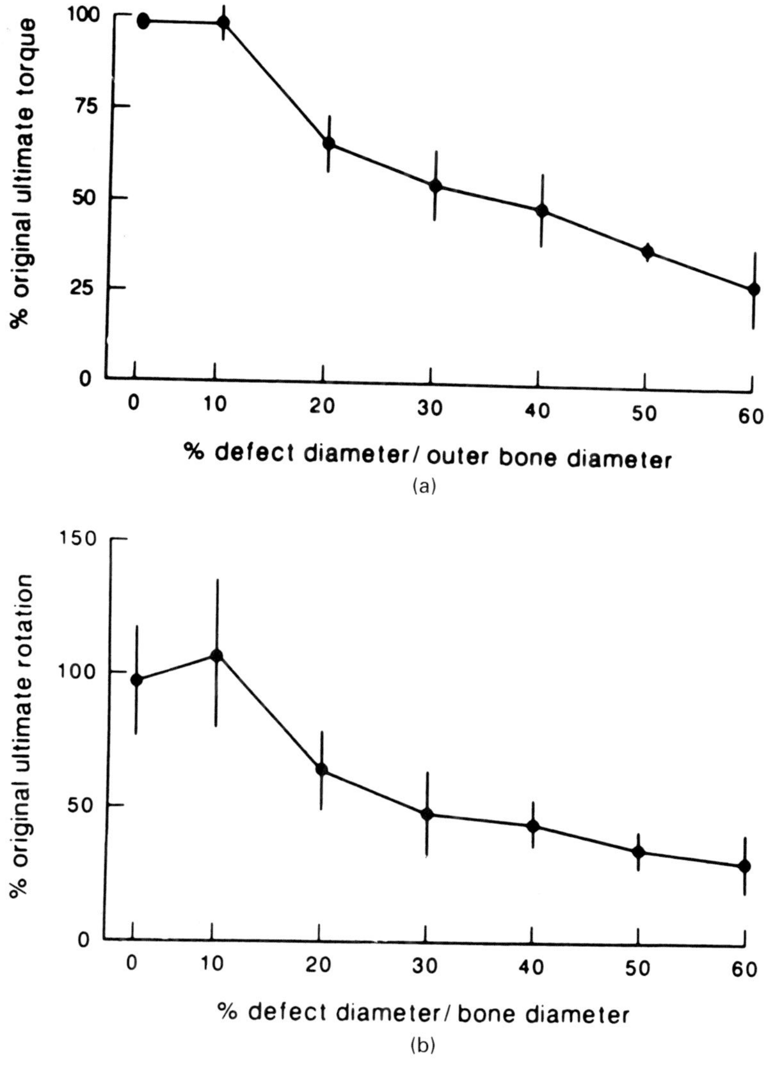

Figure 6.8

Changes in torsional properties of femora with holes of different diameters in percent of intact values. (a) Ultimate torque. (b) Ultimate deformation. (From Ref 7 with permission.)

removed immediately or left in place for up to eight weeks. The torsional properties were then tested at various periods post implantation. In some torsional tests, the screws were left in place, while in others, they were removed before testing to determine if the bone had remodelled to bypass the screw. As shown in Figure 6.9, initially having the screw in place does increase both the ultimate torsional strength and the energy absorbed to failure compared with bones with holes but without screws. However, this benefit (from about 48% of intact torsional strength for a bone with a hole to about 68% with a screw in place) is lost by two weeks, and in both cases, strength returns to about normal values at the same rate by eight weeks (in rabbits). If the screw is left in place for eight weeks and then removed, the torsional properties are similar to those of a bone that had a screw initially. Therefore leaving the screw in place provides an initial short term benefit in

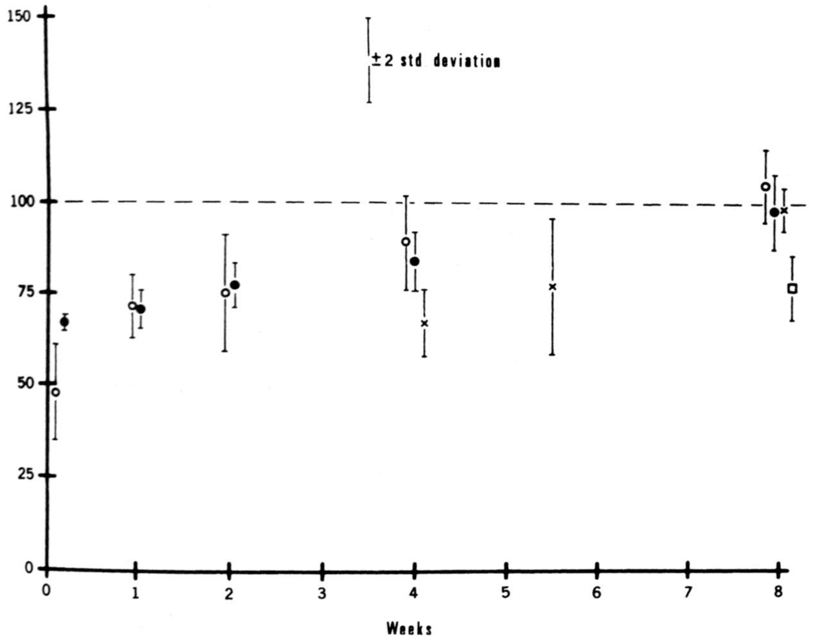

Figure 6.9

Torque ratio (ratio of experimental to intact bone) of rabbit femora as a function of time post implantation, for four conditions: ○, bones with a screw hole left to heal; ●, bones with the screws left in place after implantation and during testing; X, bones with a soft silastic plug in place of the screw; □, bones with screws left in place after implantation but removed before testing. (From Ref 8 with permission.)

Table 6.1 Estimates of the decreases in torsional properties of bones due to drilling a 3.2 mm diameter pilot hole for a 4.5 mm bone screw. (Based on the data of Ref 7.)

Screw (hole) dia (mm)	*Bone*	*Midshaft dia (mm)*	*d/D*	*Torsional strength (% of intact)*
4.5 (3.2)	Humerus	22.3	0.14	87
	Femur	30.5	0.10	100
	Tibia	27.9	0.11	96
	Radius	17.7	0.18	73

terms of improved torsional properties, compared with a bone with a hole; however, this is soon negated as the hole begins to fill with new bone. Brooks et al[8] also pointed out that although radiolucency at the screw holes was apparent, histologically, the hole was filled with lower density bone and not fibrous tissue. From the results of this study, one can conclude that there is no disadvantage to leaving a screw in place, since the torsional properties will return to normal, and that a small benefit results since the decrease in strength is not initially as great as with the screw removed.

6.3 Properties of surgical wire, cable, and pins

Wire

The material properties of stainless steel wire used for fixation have been specified by the American Society for Testing and Materials.[10] Material for pins and wire has a specified yield strength of 205 MPa and an ultimate strength of 515 MPa, at an elongation of 40%, if annealed (see Chapter 5). If the material is cold worked, these values change to 690 MPa, 860 MPa, and 12%

respectively. It is important to note that cold working material property changes can result simply from deforming the wire during surgery (for example by twisting), making it stiffer and less ductile.

The strength of surgical wire in tension increases directly with its diameter (Figure 6.10). A square knot decreases strength by about 30%.[11] Sharp bends, kinks, and damage from instruments affect strength to a variable degree depending on the amount of damage. Twisted wire is more flexible than single strand wire of equivalent maximum diameter, and, because of its irregular surface, less prone to slip. It is, however, less strong than a single wire of equivalent diameter. The tensile strength of twisted wire has been found to be maximized at between four and eight turns per inch, decreasing thereafter until it becomes less than that of untwisted wire when there are more than 13 turns per inch (Figure 6.11).[11] Wire supplied on spools is annealed, and so, as discussed above, it will have greater elongation but considerably lower strength than that which is cold worked and supplied in cut lengths. Although wire may have sufficient strength for fixation, failure may occur by fatigue. Notches as small as 1% of the diameter of the wire have been shown to reduce its fatigue life by 63% (Table 6.2).[12]

Cables

Recently, cables of various materials have been proposed for use in fixation because of the fatigue sensitivity of wires. Georgette et al[13] compared the fatigue properties of monofilament wire and cable of stainless steel to cables of commercially pure titanium, cobalt chrome, titanium alloy and MP35N (see Chapter 5). As shown in Figure 6.12, 1.2 mm outer diameter cable fabricated of 316L stainless steel had a fatigue resistance nearly 10 times that of stainless steel wire, while cables of Ti–6Al–4V and MP35N improved fatigue resistance more than 10-fold over stainless steel wire. They also noted that coating the wire could improve fatigue life by an additional factor of three. Also, it is interesting to note that though the fatigue properties varied greatly, the ultimate tensile strengths of all wire and cable tested (except Ti–6Al–4V) were nearly equivalent.

Cable systems require some method of tensioning and attaching the ends, since twisting them is

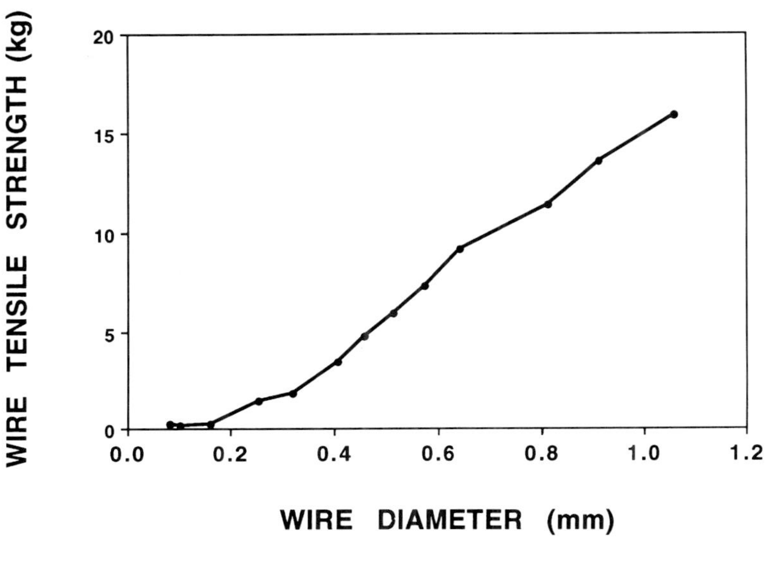

Figure 6.10

Relationship between surgical wire diameter and its tensile strength. (Adapted from data in Ref 10.)

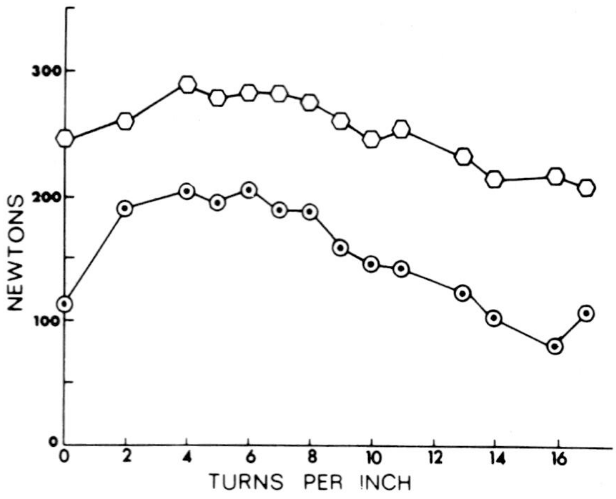

Figure 6.11

Effect on tensile yield (⊙) and ultimate strengths (O) of 0.5 mm stainless steel wire due to twisting. (From Ref 11 with permission.)

not practical. Methods for tensioning and crimping the ends have been provided by manufacturers. Luetzow et al[14] compared wire and cable techniques in reattaching the greater trochanter of the femur, and found smaller displacements for a load applied parallel to the osteotomy with wires as compared with cables. This may be related to differences in tension achievable with the different systems, or the crimp technique used.

Pins

Pins are commonly used in fixation, especially for small bones or fragments. The biomechanics of specific configurations of pins in metacarpal fixation is discussed in Chapter 7, and that for depressed tibial plateau fractures in Chapter 9. Threaded pins provide superior purchase in bone; however, the stiffness of a threaded pin is equivalent only to that of a smooth pin of diameter equal to the root diameter of the threaded pin (i.e. the diameter of the base of the thread).[2] The bending stiffness of a pin of circular cross section varies as the fourth power of its diameter (because of its moment of inertia), so threaded and smooth pins of equivalent outside diameter can be considerably different in stiffness. Applying axial tension to a pin creates a force that counteracts the applied bending moment (Figure 6.13), thereby reducing the deflection in the pin for a given load. As Figure 6.14 shows, tensioning smaller diameter pins is an effective way of stiffening them in bending.[2]

6.4 Bone screws

Screws are probably the most widely used of orthopedic implants. In considering screws, it is important to distinguish between their applications, either in cortical or in cancellous bone. The major difference is that in cancellous bone the properties of the material into which the screw is

Table 6.2 The tensile failure load and fatigue resistance, expressed as the number of cycles to failure, for orthopedic wire with notches of various depths (expressed as % of wire diameter). (Adapted from Ref 12.)

Notch size (% dia)	*Static tensile load (N)*	*Fatigue resistance (cycles to failure)*
0	622 ± 18	703 ± 43
1	665 ± 2	260 ± 21
5	663 ± 4	157 ± 19
10	663 ± 5	141 ± 19
15	661 ± 2	105 ± 15
20	667 ± 5	123 ± 12

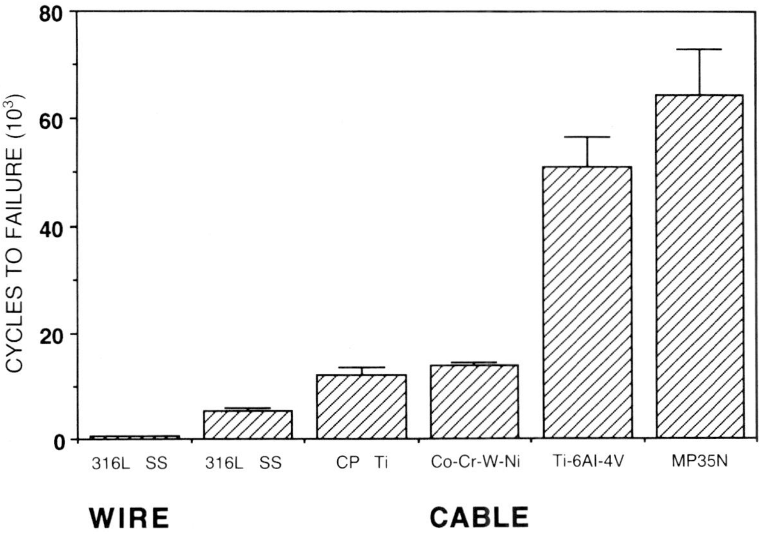

Figure 6.12

Comparison of the tensile strengths and fatigue resistance (number of cycles to failure at equivalent mean stress) of cables of 1.2 mm outer diameter, fabricated from various materials. (Adapted from data of Ref 13.)

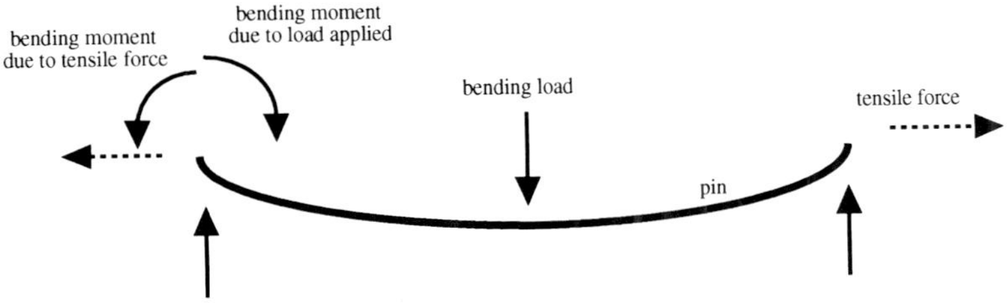

Figure 6.13

The effect of axial tension applied to a pin loaded in bending is to reduce the deflection due to bending by producing a countermoment, in effect stiffening the pin.

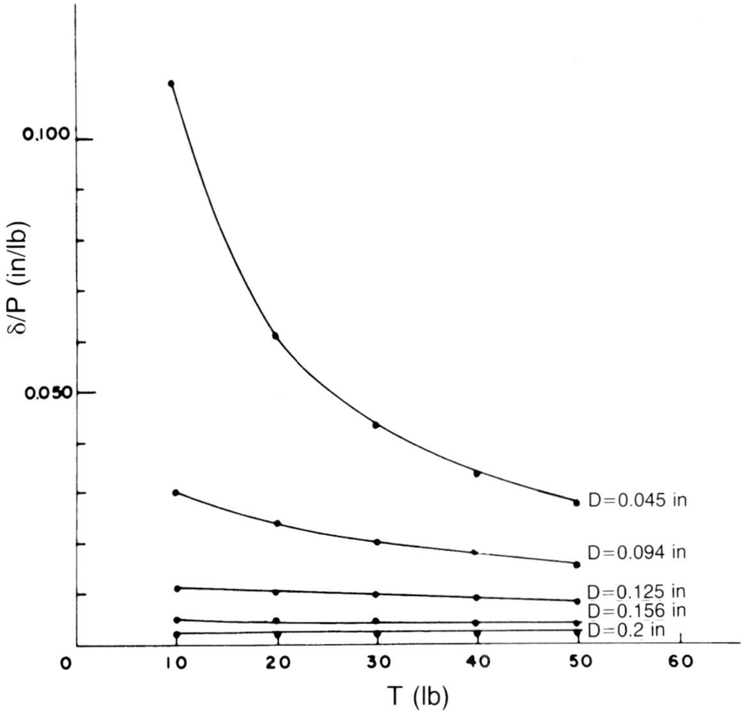

Figure 6.14

The compliance (the inverse of stiffness) (vertical axis) of pins of different diameters (curve labels) decreases with tension (horizontal axis) applied along the axis of the pin, especially for smaller diameter pins. (From Ref 2 with permission.)

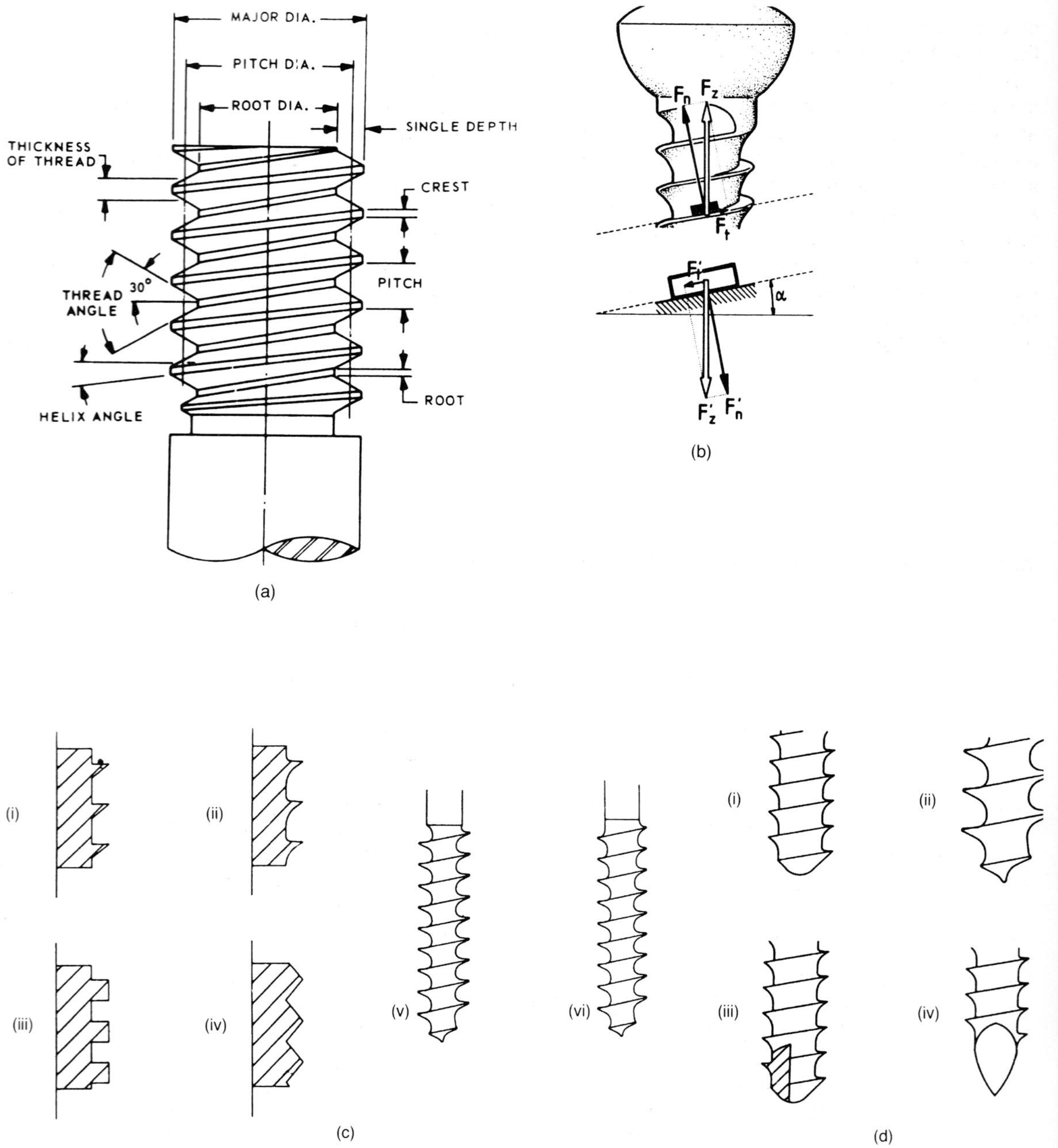

Figure 6.15

(a) Nomenclature related to screw threads (from Ref 2 with permission). (b) A screw thread can be thought of as an inclined plane with a block of material moving along its surface. It generates an upward force on the block, F_n, part of which lifts the block upwards, F_z, and part of which pushes the block along the surface, F_t, overcoming the friction between the surface of the block and the screw. F_t generates the tension in the screw and the compression that the screw applies. (c) Different thread profiles. The buttress thread profile (ii) allows transfer of force perpendicular to the axis of the screw, while the rounded base of the thread increases strength (v, vi). The transition between the threaded and smooth part of the screw should have as small and gradual a change in diameter as possible to avoid stress concentration effects. (d) Various tips: (i) blunt tip of non self tapping cortical screw; (ii) corkscrew tip of self tapping cancellous screw; (iii) flutes of self tapping screw; (iv) trochar of self drilling screw. (From Ref 16 with permission.)

placed become one of the dominant factors in their resulting pullout strengths.

A screw thread can be thought of as a long inclined plane or wedge that has been wrapped around a core (*root*) (Figure 6.15a). The wedge angle (*thread pitch*) determines the rate of advance of the screw (*lead*) through a material. A screw is essentially a machine that converts torque applied to it into internal tension along its axis as it produces compression between two surfaces. Screw threads may be of a "V" or buttress profile, with dimensions that are specified by ASTM standards (Table 6.3).[15]

Basic features

Perren et al[16] described some basic features of modern bone screw design. Most bone screws are formed with a hemispherical undersurface, which allows them to effectively contact the sides of the hole in a plate while permitting some inclination. Screws may be fully threaded, such as for holding a plate to bone, or may have a smooth shaft between the head and the thread, for lagging (screwing two components together; see Section 6.7), where gliding of the scew in one component must be allowed. Some screws have undersize

Table 6.3 Specified dimensions of cortical bone screws. (From Ref 15 with permission.)

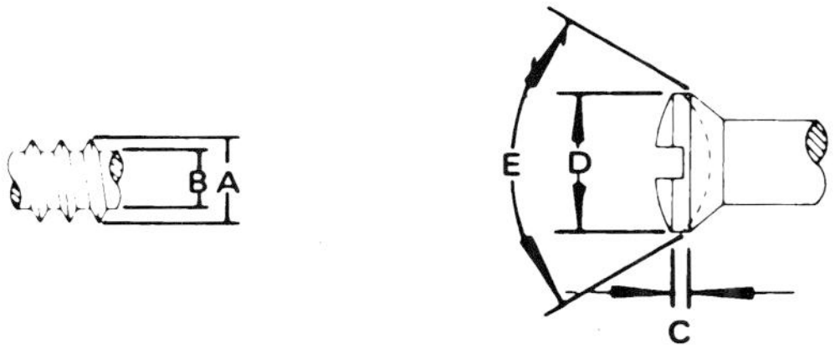

	Thread dimensions				*Standard head configuration*					
Size	*A*		*B*		*C*		*D*		*E*
	in	*mm*	*in*	*mm*	*in*	*mm*	*in*	*mm*	*deg*
Medical screws									
4M	0.112–	2.84–	0.082–	2.08–	0.040–	1.01–	0.187–	4.74–	82–
	0.110	2.79	0.080	2.03	0.035	0.89	0.182	4.62	78
6M	0.140–	3.56–	0.104–	2.64–	0.036–	0.91–	0.239–	6.07–	82–
	0.134	3.40	0.098	2.49	0.026	0.66	0.229	5.82	78
6.5M[a]	0.146–	3.71–	0.106–	2.69–	0.036–	0.91–	0.248–	6.30–	92–
	0.142	3.61	0.102	2.59	0.026	0.66	0.240	6.10	88
7M[a]	0.156–	3.96–	0.118–	3.00–	0.036–	0.91–	0.281–	7.14–	92–
	0.152	3.86	0.112	2.84	0.026	0.66	0.273	6.93	88
8M	0.166–	4.22–	0.127–	3.23–	0.036–	0.91–	0.239–	6.07–	82–
	0.160	4.06	0.121	3.07	0.026	0.66	0.229	5.82	78
Metric screws									
2.7mm	0.110–	2.80–	0.083–	2.10–	0.008	0.20	0.240–	6.10–	122–
	0.102	2.60	0.067	1.70	min	min	0.193	4.90	118
3.5mm	0.142–	3.60–	0.083–	2.10–	0.008	0.20	0.240–	6.10–	122–
	0.134	3.40	0.075	1.90	min	min	0.193	4.90	118
4.5mm	0.181–	4.60–	0.122–	3.10–	0.041–	1.05–	0.319–	8.10–	92–
	0.171	4.35	0.112	2.85	0.023	0.80	0.311	7.90	88

[a]These screws are produced by casting methods.

shafts, so that the pilot hole for the screw threads does not need to be overdrilled; however, this reduces the strength of the screw considerably. A buttress thread profile (Figure 6.15b) is used because it permits the transfer of force between bone and screw to occur at an interface that is perpendicular to the direction of the applied force. (The force generated in holding two objects together produces axial tension in the screw. The top of the buttress thread is perpendicular to the axis of the screw.) The transition between the thread and shaft can be the location of a significant stress concentrator (riser) if there are abrupt changes in diameter or sharp corners (Figure 6.15c). Screws with different functions have different types of tips (Figure 6.15d). Blunt tips are found on tapped screws that may protrude into tissues. The corkscrew tip is used in self tapping cancellous screws to open a threaded canal, since cutting a thread would break trabeculae. Self tapping screws may have flutes at their tips to cut threads, or a trochar (point) that allows for self drilling of the pilot hole as well.

Cortical screws

In cortical bone, both the strength of the screw itself and its holding power are important factors to consider. Typically, shearing of the screw during insertion occurs because the pilot hole is too small, the screw hole has not been tapped, or the screw is incorrectly aligned in the hole. Also, as the thickness of cortex through which the screw is inserted increases, the torque required to drive the screw goes up dramatically.[17] The stiffness of a cylinder increases with the fourth power of its diameter (polar moment of inertia; Chapter 1), and its ultimate torsional (shear) strength with the third power.[18] For a screw, its strength is dependent on its root diameter. As shown in Figure 6.16, doubling the root diameter of a screw increases the torque that it can withstand by a factor of 8.[19] Therefore large screws with deep threads may have good purchase, but this comes at the expense of inherent strength of the screw, because this type of screw has a relatively small root diameter.

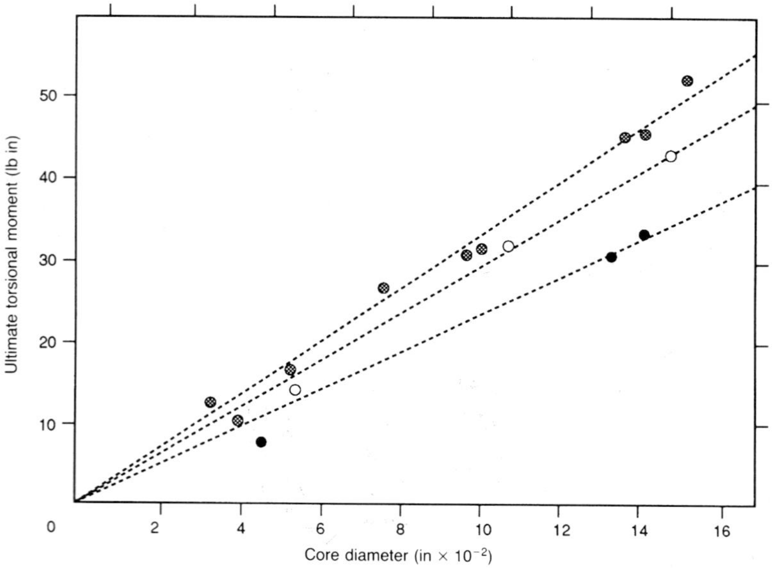

Figure 6.16

Relationship of ultimate torque that a screw can withstand and its core (root) diameter, for screws of different materials: Ti60 (●); Co–Cr–Mo (○); En 58j (◎). (From Ref 19 with permission.)

The pilot hole is an important factor, since if it is too small, screw breakage can occur, while if it is too large, screw purchase will be reduced. The root diameter of the screw and the material that it is made of limit the torque that can be applied. The useful component of the applied torque is that which is used to create tension in the screw (or compression of components such as a plate against bone). Hughes and Jordan[19] estimated that when applying a screw into an untapped hole with no lubrication, 35% of the torque is lost to cutting threads, 10% to friction at the screw/bone interface, and 50% at the countersink interface (i.e. between the bone or plate surface under the screw head and the base of the screw head), leaving only 5% that can be converted to tension in the screw (for compressing surfaces) (Figure 6.17). Increasing the pilot hole size or using a tap to prepare the hole increases the torque converted to tensile force in the screw itself to 65% of the torque applied. Hughes and Jordan[19] also showed that there is a critical pilot hole diameter beyond which pullout strength drops rapidly, as shown in Figure 6.18, and is independent of the number of threads engaged. Therefore the appropriate pilot hole size should be large enough to minimize the torque needed to drive the screw, but be below the critical diameter for pullout strength. Table 6.4 provides recommended pilot tap hole drill sizes for common bone screws.

The theoretical resistance of a screw to pullout depends, as shown in Figure 6.19, on its depth of insertion into bone, the shear strength of the bone into which it is embedded, and a geometrical factor which accounts for the volume of bone within the threads.[20] This geometric factor is complex and depends partly on volume and partly on thread profile. The pullout force is given by:

$$F = (L/P) \times (C \times S) \times G$$

where

F = pullout force per thread (N)
L = length of engagement of the screw (mm)
P = pitch (number of threads per mm)
C = outer circumference of the screw (mm)
S = shear strength of the bone into which the screw is placed (N/mm^2)
G = a geometric factor, which is less than 1 and accounts for the thread profile and the depth.

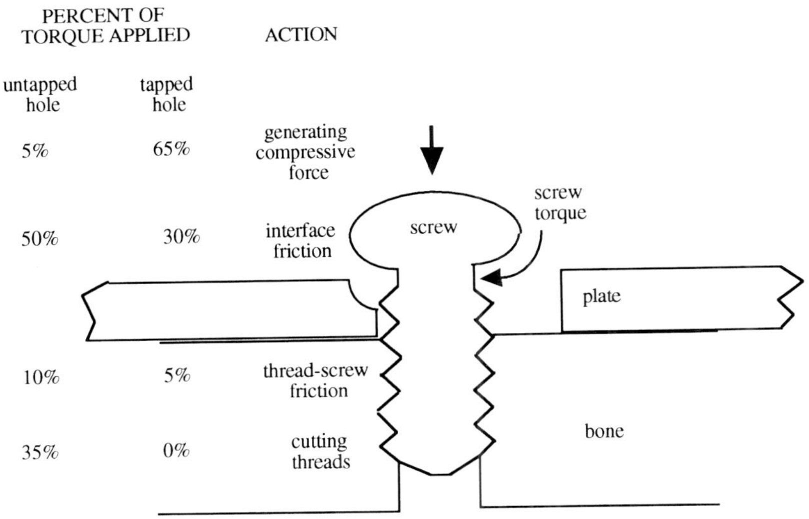

Figure 6.17

Schematic diagram showing the distribution of torque applied to the screw to different functions in an unthreaded or a threaded and lubricated screw hole. (Adapted from Ref 19.)

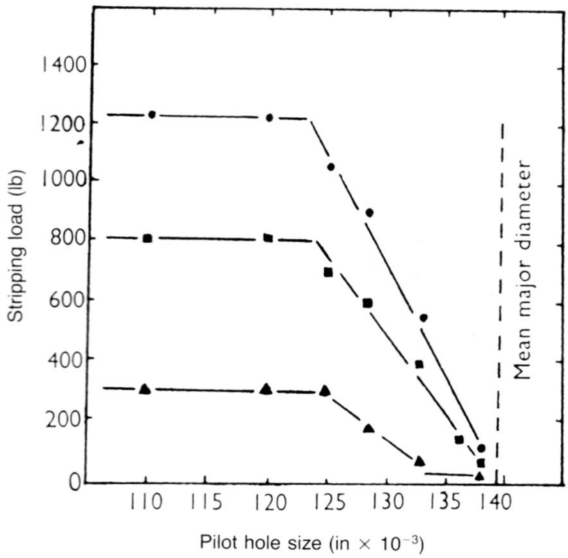

Figure 6.18

Pullout (stripping) load versus pilot hole diameter for a 3.5 mm diameter screw implanted in bone, at either of three different thread lengths. (From Ref 19 with permission.) (0.110 in = 0.279 mm; 0.140 in = 0.356 mm.)

The following relationship determining the geometric factor G accounts for the area of bone within the threads:[20]

$$G = 0.0197P + 0.0114(D_o - D_i)$$

Where D_o = outer diameter and
D_i = root diameter (both in mm).

In vivo, the pullout strength of screws implanted in bone increases with time, as shown in Figure 6.20. At the time of insertion, the screw is not in complete contact with bone in the hole, because the tap enlarges the hole and the threads (Figure 6.21).[21] Over the course of healing, the threads fill in with new bone, creating more intimate contact and increasing pullout strength (Figure 6.22).[9] Another important factor which controls the pullout strength of screws in cortical bone is the bone mineral content of the cortex, which, as shown by Trader et al[22] (Figure 6.23), correlates linearly with strength. It is also interesting to note that these authors reported no differences in pullout strength using either self tapping or non self tapping screws.

Table 6.4 Dimensions of recommended pilot hole drill diameters for common cortical bone screws. (From Ref 15 with permission.)

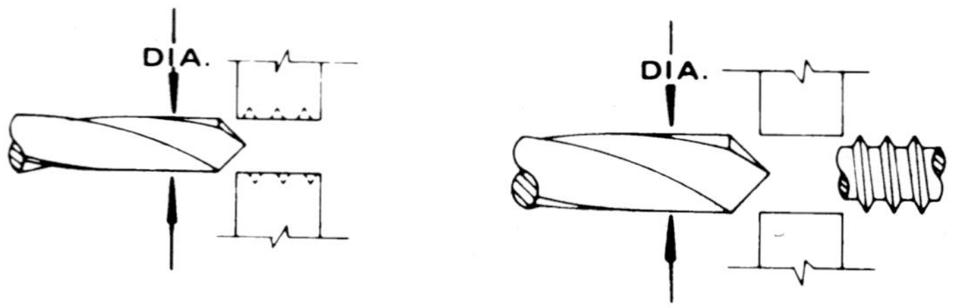

Screw size	*Drill size diameters*			
	Tap drill		*Clearance drill*	
	Fraction size (in)	*(mm)*	*Fraction size (in)*	*(mm)*
4M	3/32	2.3	7/64	2.9
6M	7/64	2.7	9/64	3.6
6.5M	7/64	2.7	9/64	3.8
7M	1/8	3.2	5/32	4.2
8M	9/64	3.6	11/64	4.2
2.7 mm	5/64	2.0	7/64	2.7
3.5 mm	5/64	2.0	9/64	3.6
4.5 mm	1/8	3.2	11/64	4.5

Note: The thread and drill dimensions shown are nominal.

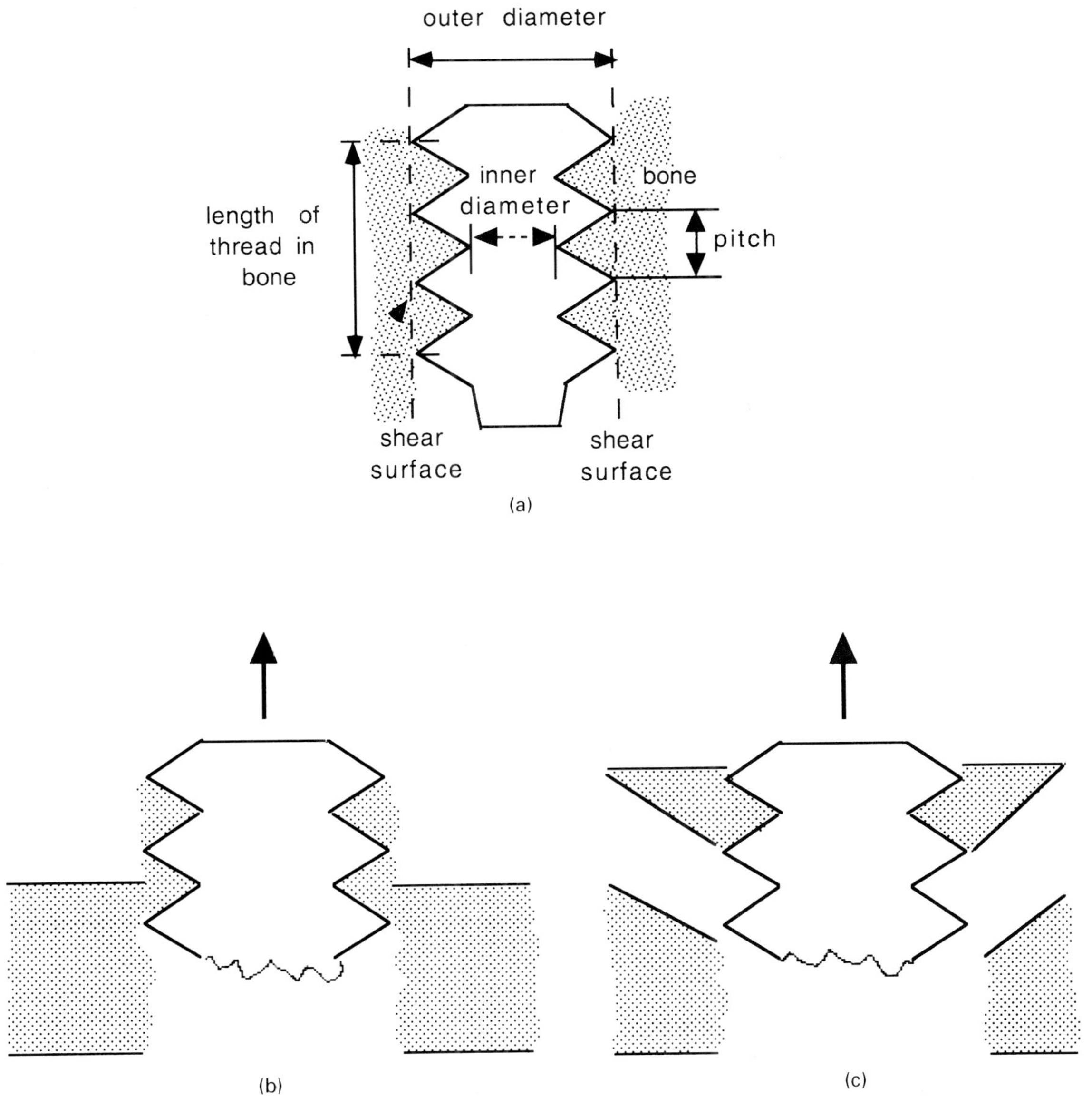

Figure 6.19

(a) The important parameters in determining screw pullout strength in cortical bone are the length of screw embedded into bone, the outside diameter, inside diameter, and pitch of the screw, and the shear strength of the bone. (b) Pullout failure may occur along a surface at the outer perimeter of the screw, where the screw thread cuts a cylinder of bone as it exits. This is a typical mechanism of failure in cancellous bone. (c) Alternatively, a wedge of bone may be pulled out, with failure along a shear (45°) plane. For a material of a given strength, the pullout strength will increase as this shear volume (the volume of material within the screw threads) increases.

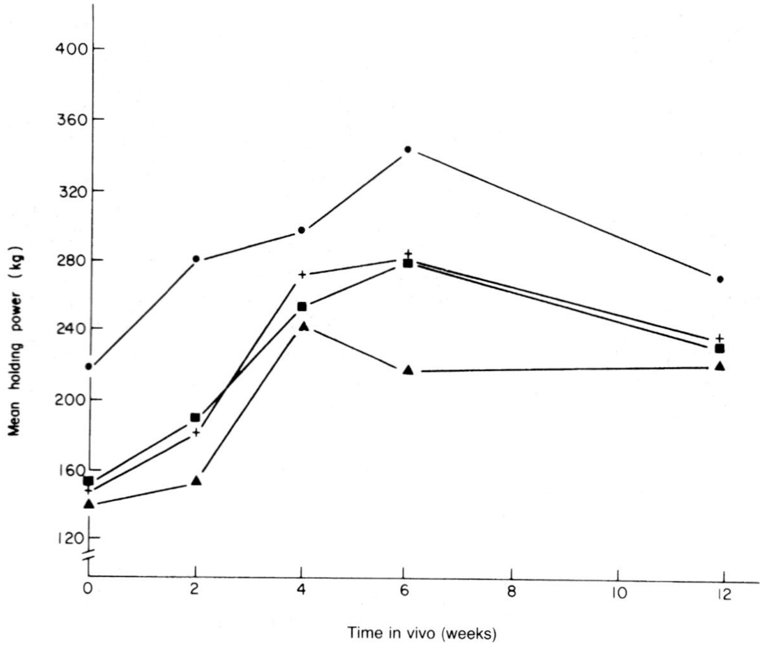

Figure 6.20

The increase in pullout strength with time in vivo due to bone growth to the screw threads. (From Ref 9 with permission.)

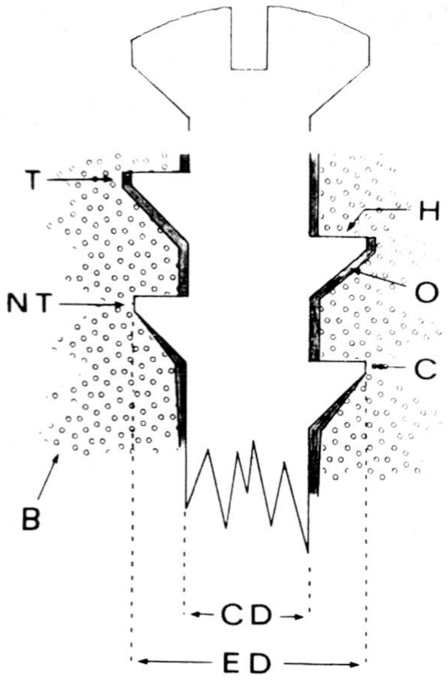

Figure 6.21

Schematic diagram of the fit of a screw into a hole in bone where the upper two threads show the fit after tapping (T), while the lower two are not tapped (NT). In the nontapped hole the crest of the thread is also in contact with bone. (From Ref 21 with permission.)

In summary, to increase the pullout strength of screws in cortical bone

- increase screw outside diameter
- decrease the root diameter
- increase the thickness of the cortex
- choose more dense cortex in which to implant the screw

In order to prevent breakage during insertion, increase the root diameter of the screw, and use a tapped pilot hole in cortical bone. The conflicting requirement is in the selection of an appropriate size of root diameter that does not compromise either pullout strength or screw torsional strength.

Cancellous screws

The parameters that affect the purchase of cortical screws also govern cancellous screw pullout strength; however, there are several differences

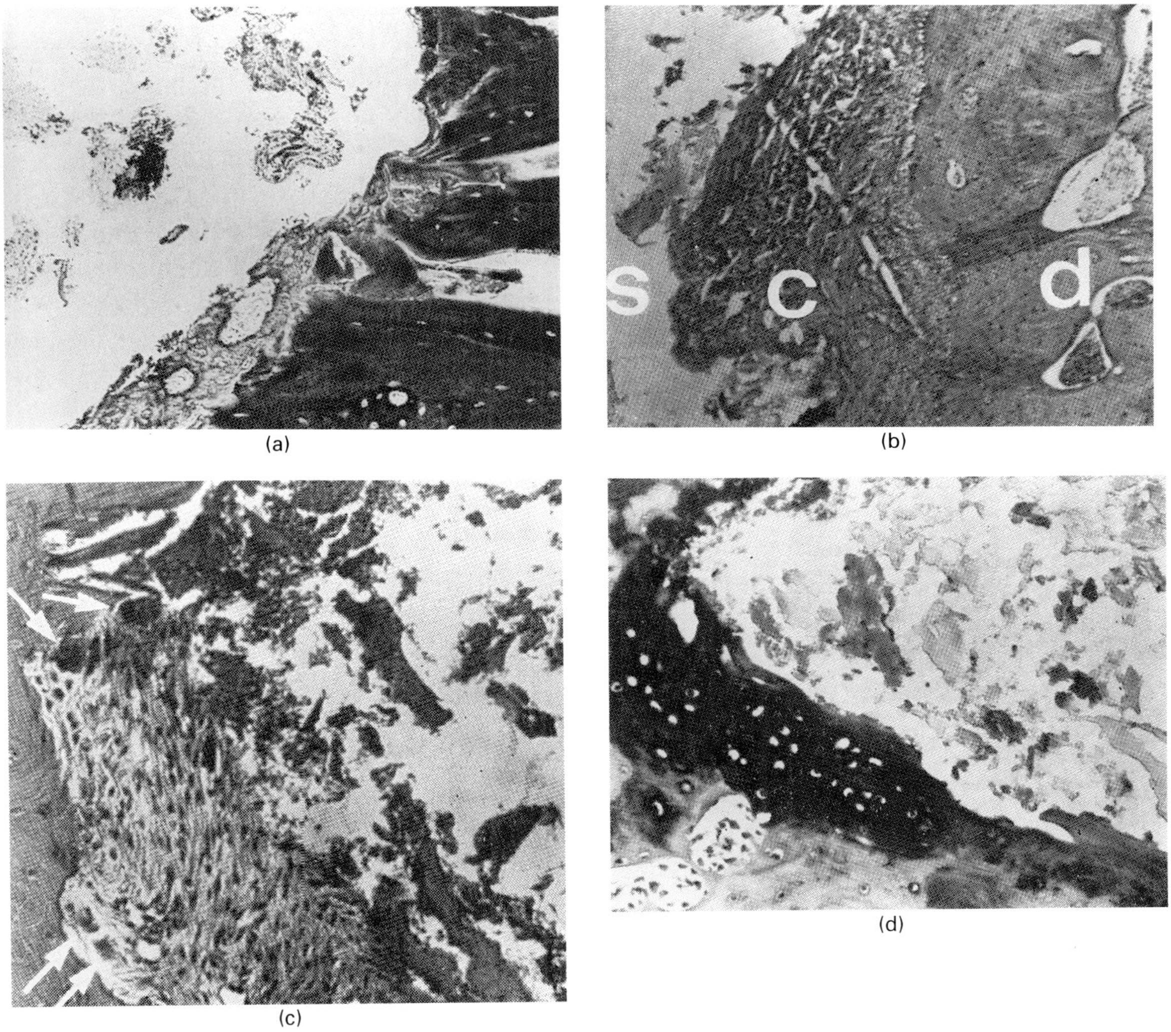

Figure 6.22

Histological sections showing new bone formation around the threads of a screw implanted in bone with (upper) sections from a stable screw and (lower) sections from an unstable screw. (a) At 8 weeks, haversian systems can be seen at right angles to the screw shaft. (b) At 8 months, the diaphysis (d) is being remodelled and the threads of the screw (s) are surrounded by collagenous tissue (c). (c) After unstable fixation, osteoclastic bone resorption and fibrous tissue formation are evident (arrows). (d) After 12 weeks, cartilage has formed around the threads. (From Ref 21 with permission.)

between screws implanted in cancellous and those in cortical bone. Screw breakage during insertion is less of a problem, and bone density – because it is so much more variable in trabecular bone than in cortical bone[23] – is much more of a factor in governing the strength of screw purchase.[24–27] Figure 6.24 shows examples of force–deformation plots of identical screws that have been inserted into and pulled out of polyurethane foams of different densities, all in the range of

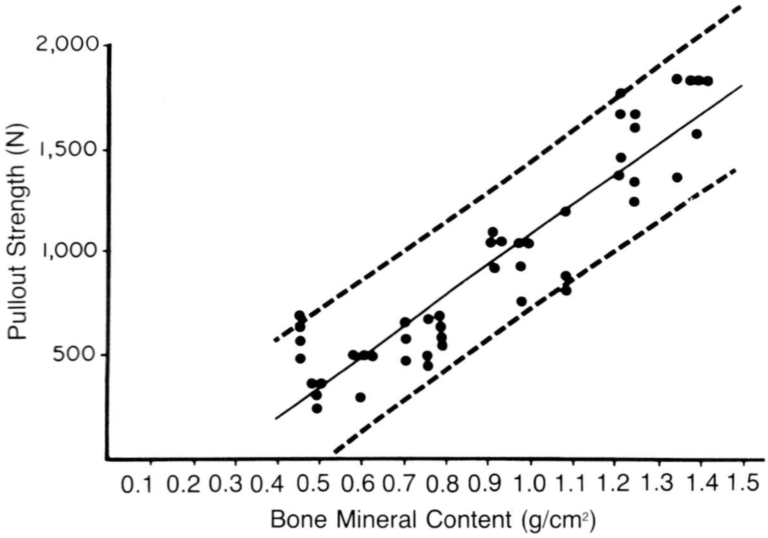

Figure 6.23

Pullout strength of screws in cortical bone as a function of bone mineral content. (From Ref 22 with permission.)

cancellous bone densities. The relationship between pullout strength and material shear strength is shown in Figure 6.25. The shear strength of cancellous bone has been found[28] to be proportional to its density to the power 1.65. Therefore doubling the density of cancellous bone into which a screw is placed will increase its pullout strength by a factor of 3.14.

Hole preparation is an important factor when dealing with cancellous bone. In cortical bone, as was shown in Figure 6.18, increasing the root diameter of the pilot hole has little effect on pullout strength of the screw until a critical size is reached, after which strength drops off considerably. In cancellous bone, the maximum pullout strength of large screws occurs when the pilot hole diameter is nearly equal to the root diameter, and drops off as diameter increases. For example, as shown in Figure 6.26, for a 6.5 mm screw in cancellous bone, pullout strength is greatest with a pilot hole of 3.2 mm diameter (screw root diameter 3.0 mm).[26]

A second aspect to consider in hole preparation for cancellous screws is whether or not to tap the hole. As discussed previously, tapping for cortical screw insertion reduces the tendency of the screw to fail during insertion and allows a greater percentage of the applied torque to be used to create compression between the surfaces across which the screw is placed. In porous materials, including cancellous bone, tapping before inserting the screw produces lower pullout strengths,

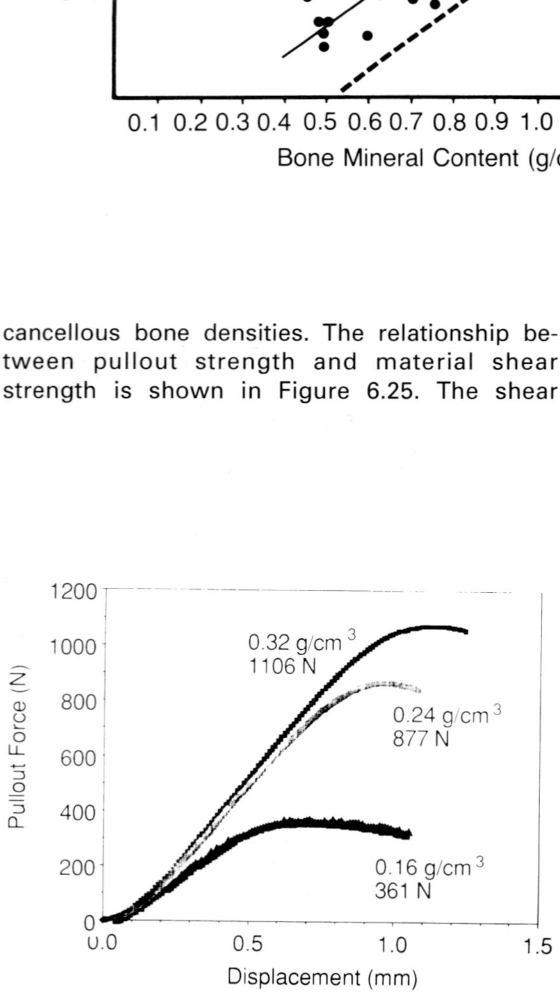

Figure 6.24

Sample force–deflection plots of identical scews (6.5 mm diameter × 16 mm length) that have been pulled out of polyurethane foams of three different densities, all within the range of the density of cancellous bone. (From Ref 25.)

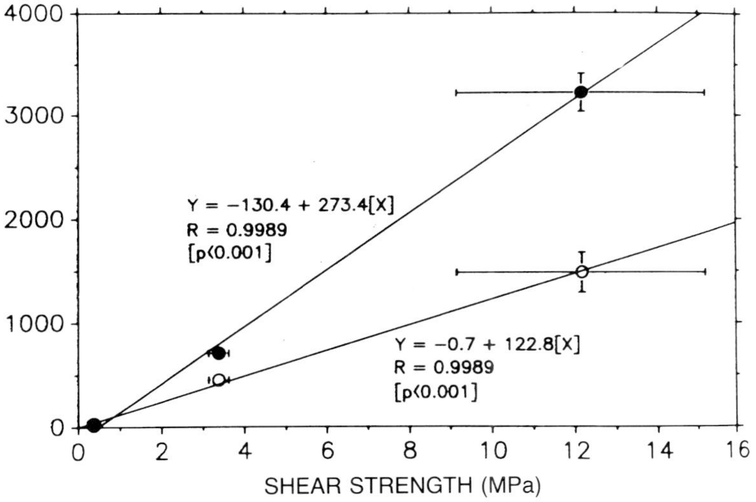

Figure 6.25

Relationship between screw pullout strength and shear strength of the material in which it is embedded: ○, screw diameter 3.8 mm; ●, 6.5 mm. (From Ref 26 with permission.)

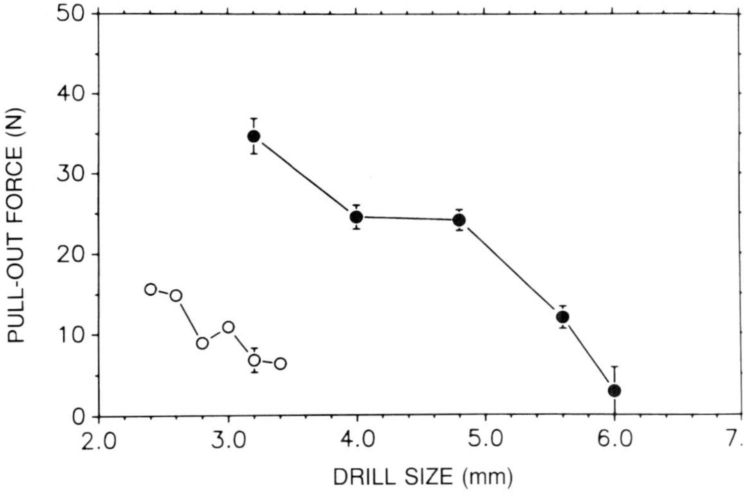

Figure 6.26

Pullout force of two sizes of screws (○, 3.8 mm diameter; ●, 6.5 mm) embedded into porous foam (mechanically representative of cancellous bone), as a function of the pilot hole size. (From Ref 26 with permission.)

for screws of equivalent length and diameter, as compared with not tapping (Figure 6.27).[25] Castings of the volumes of holes which had or had not been tapped demonstrate that the tap removes material from the hole, effectively enlarging it (Figure 6.28). The amount of material removed with tapping increases as the density of the material decreases. For bone, the mean volume increase is about 25%.[29]

Several design aspects of cancellous screws alter their achievable pullout strengths. Increasing the thread pitch (up to a point) significantly increases pullout strength (Figure 6.29).[25,27] This may be a result of the finite size of the trabeculae and the geometry of their fit between the threads of the screw. Cannulated screws are being used more frequently, since they allow initial placement of a guidewire to assess the orientation of the

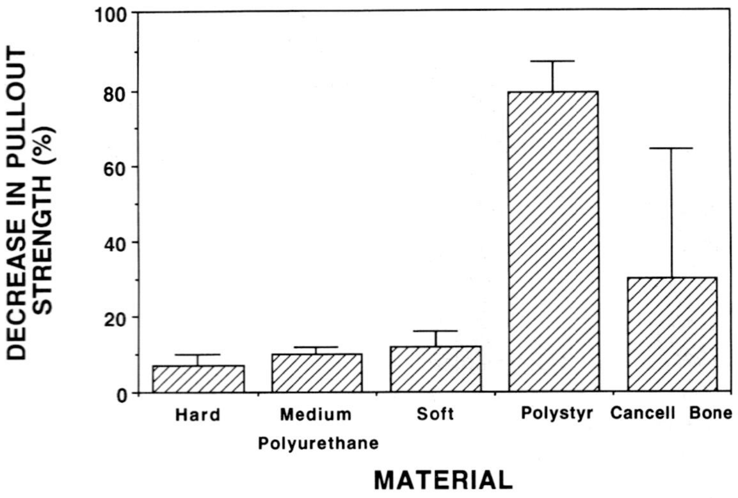

Figure 6.27

Tapping decreases screw holding power for similar screws in polyurethane foam in all density ranges (foam was used as a substitute for cancellous bone). (From Ref 25.)

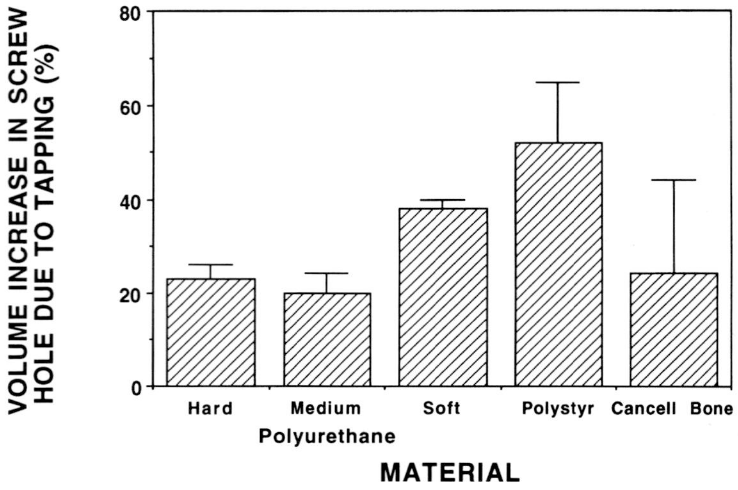

Figure 6.28

Percent increase in volume in tapped versus untapped holes for cancellous screws in various porous foam materials and in cancellous bone, demonstrating how tapping enlarges holes resulting in a decrease in screw pullout strength. (From Ref 29.)

screw before it is inserted. This reduces the problem of having to remove and reposition an incorrectly placed screw. However, as shown in Figure 6.30, cannulated screws of a size nearly equivalent to noncannulated screws have reduced pullout strength, because the larger root diameter needed to accomodate the central bore of the cannulated screw effectively decreases the volume of bone between the screw threads, compared with equivalent noncannulated screws.[25]

Additionally, an interesting observation was made about the effect of burying the threads of the screw below the surface of the material (for screws with smooth shafts between the thread and the head, such as lag screws). If the thread of the screw is buried 1 mm below the surface, only

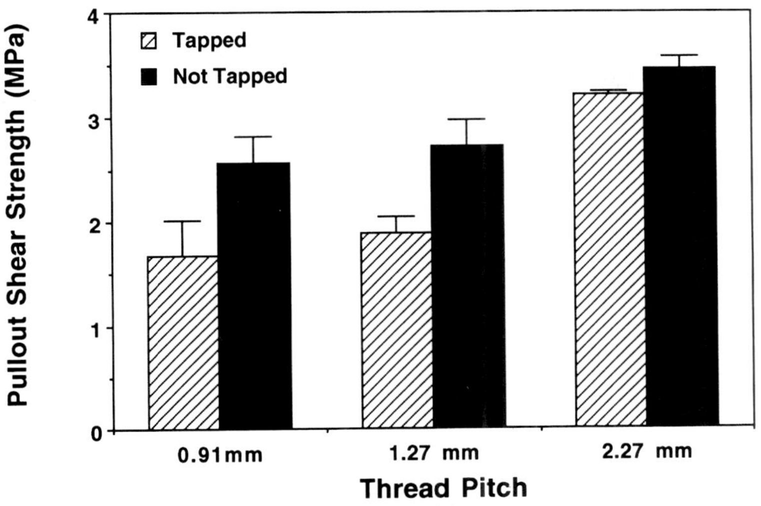

(a)

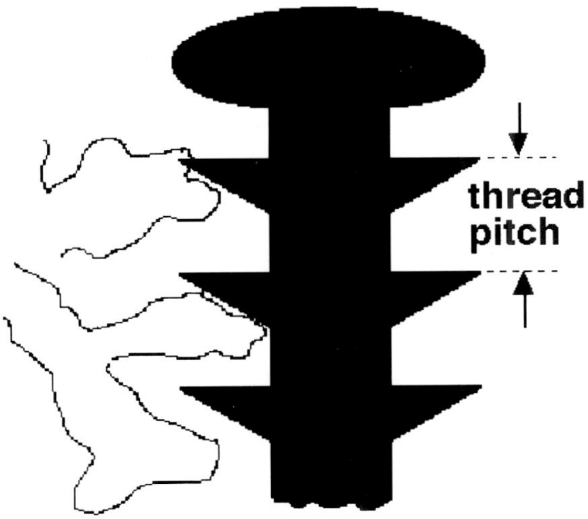

(b)

Figure 6.29

(a) Effect of increasing thread pitch (or reducing the number of threads per inch) on cancellous screw pullout strength in polyurethane foam. (b) Possible fit geometry of trabeculae within cancellous screw threads. (From Ref 25.)

60–70% of the theoretical maximum achievable pullout force has been measured. This increases to 90% of maximum when the threads are buried 5 mm below the surface (Figure 6.31).[25] Burying the threads in effect creates an additional volume of material above the screw threads that must be sheared in order for the screw to pull out (Figure 6.32). The practical implication of this result is that it provides an argument in favor of the cancellous lag screw with an undersized smooth shaft. The opposing argument is that the smaller shaft decreases screw strength.

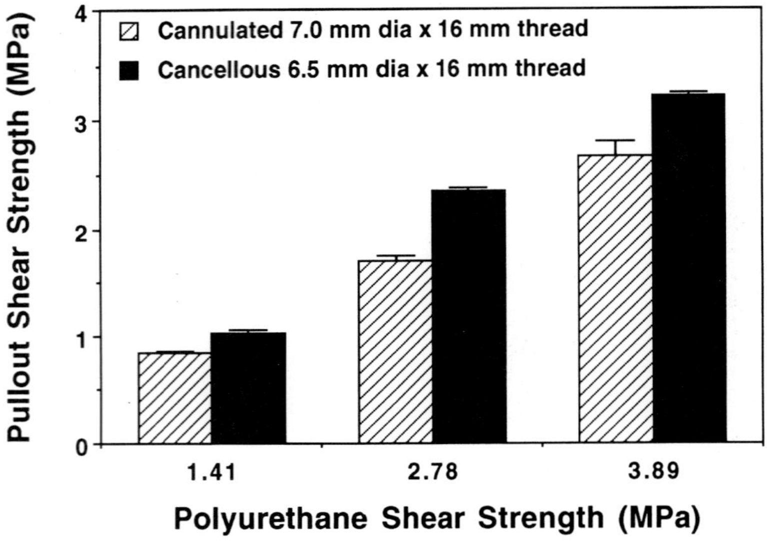

(a)

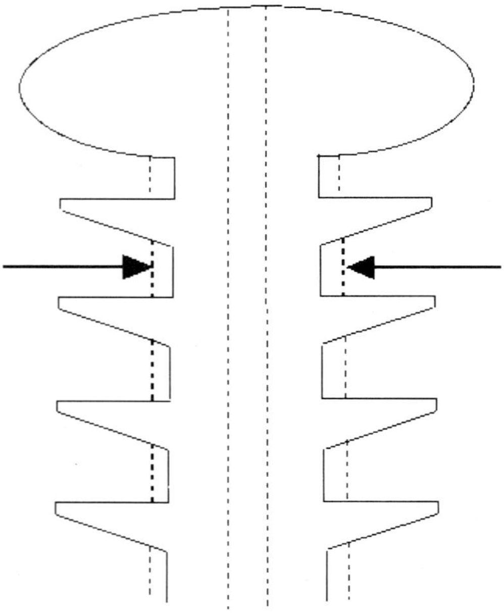

(b)

Figure 6.30

(a) Comparison of the pullout strengths (given as force divided by the product of screw outside diameter and length of insertion) of cannulated and noncannulated screws in polyurethane foams of different densities. (b) Difference in geometry between a cannulated and solid bore screw. Dotted outlines indicate central hole and enlarged root diameter of the cannulated screw. (From Ref 25.)

In summary, the best purchase of screws in cancellous bone can be achieved by

- using a screw of large pitch (small number of threads per inch)
- drilling a pilot hole equal to the root diameter of the screw
- not tapping except in very hard cancellous bone, and cortical bone where breakage of the screw might otherwise occur
- not using cannulated screws if possible
- using a screw of largest outside diameter and smallest root diameter
- achieving the longest length of purchase
- burying the threads at least 5 mm below the bone surface if a screw with an undersize smooth shaft is used
- placing the screw in the most dense cancellous bone possible

Screw loading and fatigue life

Assuming that a bone screw is inserted without damaging it, and that it has adequate purchase to allow the generation of compressive loads across the surfaces it spans (i.e. a plate against cortical bone, or one fracture component against the other), screw failure by fatigue has been found to occur in up to 6% of implanted fixation plates.[30]

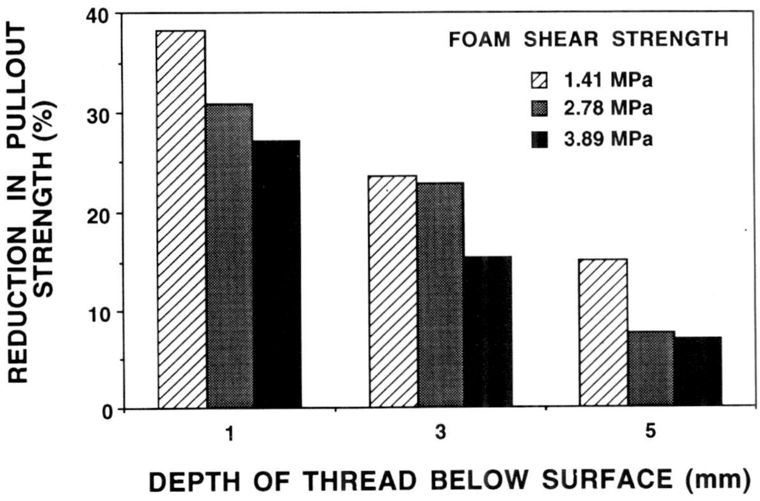

Figure 6.31

Relationship between the depth of the screw thread below the surface and the reduction from maximum theoretically achievable pullout force in polyurethane foams of three different densities. (From Ref 25.)

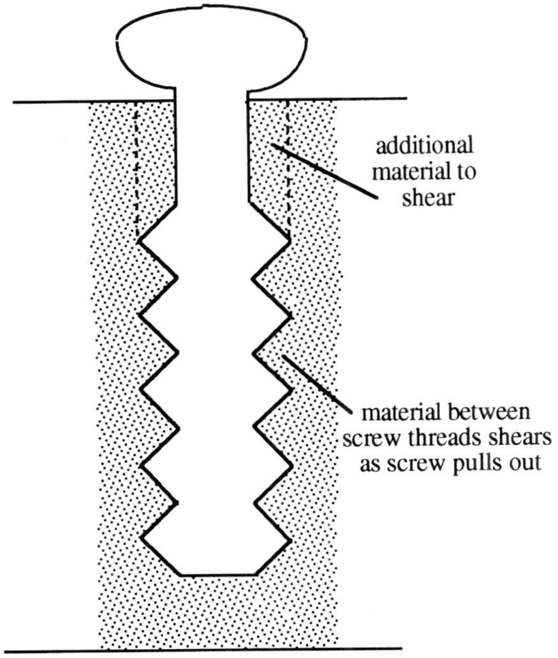

Figure 6.32

Schematic diagram showing how burying the threads of a cancellous screw can increase pullout strength by providing additional bone that must be sheared in order for the screw to be pulled out.

Taking the case of a screw implanted into bone cortex in order to secure a plate, applying a torque to the screw results in the screw driving the plate against the underlying bone surface. The torque applied to the head of the screw with a screwdriver is directly related to the axial compression achieved (Figure 6.33),[31] if the screw holes are prepared so that effort does not need to be expended in cutting threads (i.e. holes should be tapped in cortical and dense cancellous bone).

The frictional contact between the plate and bone (to be discussed in more detail in the next section) is governed by the force of the screw acting against the plate as well as the coefficient of friction between plate and bone. When a physiological load is applied to the plate, through bending of the bone or due to compression at the fracture site, this load is resisted partly by friction of the plate against bone, and partly by direct transfer of force to the screws as shown schematically in Figure 6.34, along with some load transfer across the fracture site. Zand et al[32] found that screws tightened to 488 N of compressive force sustained 2.5 million load cycles without fatigue, compared with screws loaded to

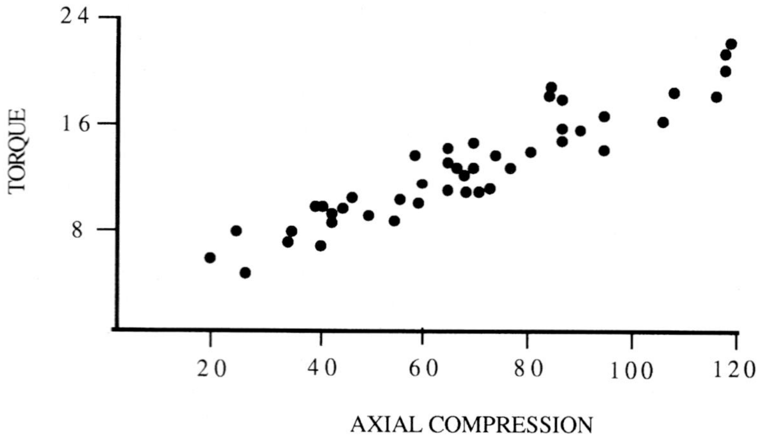

Figure 6.33

Relationship between torque applied to the head of a bone screw (4.5 mm diameter) and the compressive force achieved against the bone surface. (From Ref 31 with permission.)

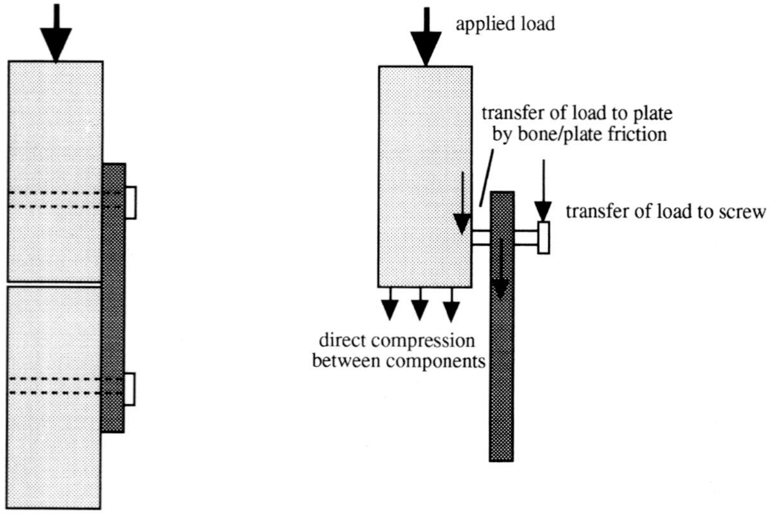

Figure 6.34

Force acting on a bone screw used to hold a plate against a bone surface. Part of the force applied to the bone is transferred across the fracture line. Part is transmitted to the plate by plate/bone friction, and part is supported by the screws. The bending load acting transverse to the long axis of the screw increases if the plate/bone friction decreases, which decreases the life of the screw.

between 400 and 418 N, which failed after as few as 1000 cycles. Therefore decreasing the potential for fatigue failure of the screws is critically dependent on generating sufficient compressive force so that the screw is released from significant bending loads. In practical terms, this is a strong argument for the use of tapped screws in cortical bone so that a greater part of the torque applied is converted to compressive force against the plate (Figure 6.17).

6.5 Plates for fracture fixation

Compression

A plate should be thought of as an internal splint holding together a structural defect (fracture in a bone), *but not as a load bearing member* itself. Its most important functions are to maintain alignment of the fracture components, and to create compression between the ends of a fracture so that load can be transferred across it. Achieving compression across the fracture components is important in protecting the plate from failure. (The effects of fixation rigidity on biological healing have been discussed in Chapter 4. There it was concluded that fixation rigidity should be in the range between 20% and 60% of the intact bone in bending.) For the three primary loads that a long bone must bear – axial compression, bending, and torsion – compression of the fracture ends is crucial in transmission of these forces through bone as opposed to through the plate. Considering Figure 6.35, which shows a plated fracture with a gap, a compressive load acting down the bone shaft produces bending in the plate, since this load is offset with respect to the plate. Bending may result in fatigue fracture of the plate, and/or pullout of the screws. Hayes and Perren[33] demonstrated significantly greater rigidity of fixation in bending when compression was applied across the fracture line (Figure 6.36). Compression also aids in resisting torsion applied to the bone about its long axis, by creating interdigitation and frictional contact of the fracture ends.

Compressive force can be generated across the fracture gap by two devices: a compressing plate and a lag screw (or both together). As previously discussed, the bone screw is a device that converts torque applied to it into compressive (clamping) force between two components, such as a plate and bone. Bone fragment compression with plating requires that the screw torque be converted to a force along the long axis of the bone, and can be accomplished by the wedge mechanism of the dynamic compression plate. As shown in Figure 6.37, in this system the head of the bone screw is spherical and fits into an oval hole with an inclined side in the plate. As the screw is tightened and its head moves towards the bone surface, the screw slides down the

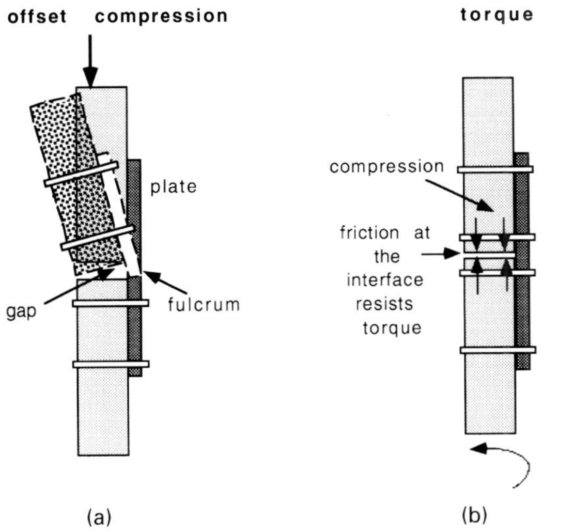

Figure 6.35

(a) A gap at the fracture surfaces, especially at the opposite cortex, allows bending of the plate, with the fulcrum at the upper edge of the distal fracture component. (b) Compression of the fracture surfaces creates friction and mechanical interlock at the interface, which helps to resist torsion, and transmits compressive loads through the bone.

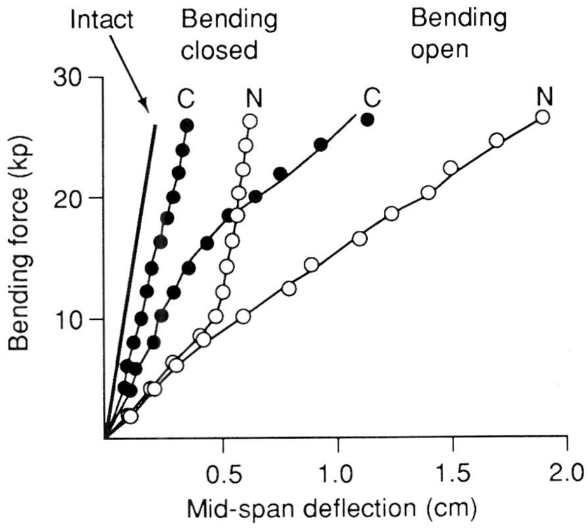

Figure 6.36

Comparison of the bending characteristics of a femur fixed with an eight hole dynamic compression plate. Bending closed (i.e. to close the fracture gap) produces less deflection than bending open because of the additional stability caused by contact of the cortices opposite the plate. With compression (C), both bending closed and bending open result in less deflection for the same applied force. (N = no compression.) (Adapted from Ref 33.)

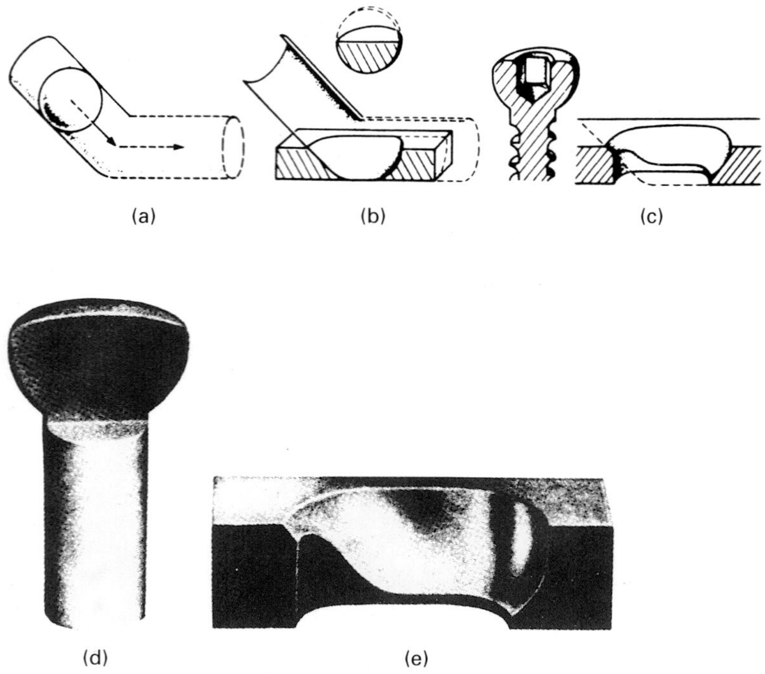

Figure 6.37

Schematic diagram of the operating principle of the dynamic compression plate. (a) A ball confined to a sloping path must move horizontally as it moves down. (b) If the ball is replaced by the spherical head of a bone screw (d) and the sloping path by the oval slot in the bone plate (e) then (c) as the screw is tightened and the screw head moves down (towards the bone surface), it must also move horizontally, carrying the bone fragment to which it is attached towards the other fragment, creating compression. (From Ref 34 with permission.)

inclined surface of the hole in the plate, causing the bone fragment to which the screw is attached to displace along the long axis of the plate. This can be used to produce apposition and compression of fracture components.[34]

Cordey et al[35] demonstrated the mechanics of the dynamic compression plate. The axial force (longitudinal force along the plate axis) that produces compression of bone fragments depends on the angle of the slope of the side of the hole, the thread pitch (which governs how far the screw descends for each turn; finer thread = more compressive force), and the coefficients of friction between the plate and bone and between the screw head and plate (Figure 6.38), reported to average 0.37.[36] They showed that there is a relationship between the torque applied to the screw and the compression ultimately achieved at the fracture site, as shown in Figure 6.39. The variability is partly dependent on variability in the bone/plate coefficient of friction.

It should be noted that friction developed between the plate and bone has counteracting effects on the mechanics of plating of fractures. If the bone/plate frictional force is large, there is less loading of the screws, enhancing their fatigue life. On the other hand, a smaller frictional force allows easier sliding of the plate, resulting in greater compression of the fracture site, important for mechanical stability of the fixation. Practically speaking, screws should be as tight as possible, since this protects them from fatigue as well as increasing the compressive force of the bone fragments. It should also be noted that the compressive force will decrease in vivo with time, although significant values have been recorded as late as 84 days after implantation of a compression plate.[37]

Application of plates

Taking the ideal case in which a straight plate is placed on a straight bone surface with a transverse fracture gap, uniform compression does not

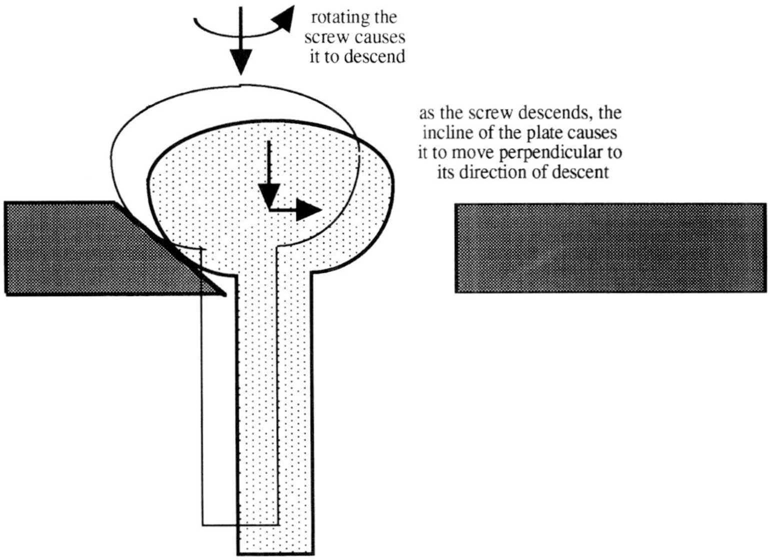

Figure 6.38

Schematic diagram showing the mechanics of conversion of torque on a bone screw to a longitudinal force capable of creating compression of bone fragments.

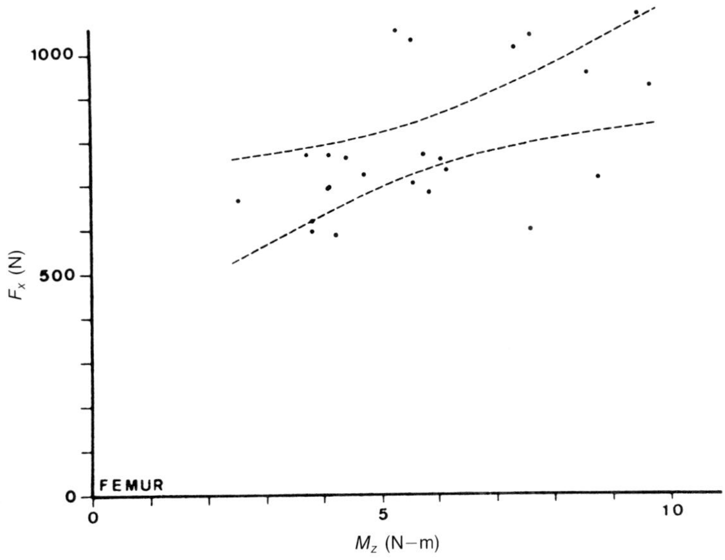

Figure 6.39

Relationship between the torque applied to a bone screw (M_z) and the compression achieved across the fracture line (F_x). (From Ref 35 with permission.)

result across the fracture gap. In fact, as shown in Figure 6.40, applying compression using a straight plate placed on one cortex causes compression just under the plate but gapping across the fracture line, with the fulcrum located at the fracture line just underneath the plate.[38] Prebending of plates has been advocated[39,40] to eliminate this problem. Figure 6.41 shows that bending the plate so that there is initially a slight gap between it and the surface to which it will be applied forces the bone fragments at the opposite cortex to contact and compress, thus distributing

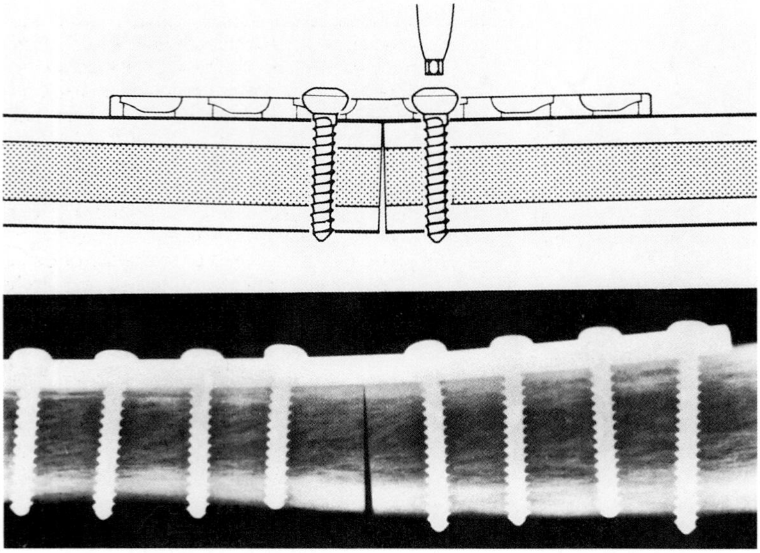

Figure 6.40

Example of gapping of the fracture with application and compression using a straight plate on a flat bone. (From Ref 35 with permission.)

the compressive force over the complete cortex. Similarly, when applying a plate to a convex curved surface, if the inner screws (the ones closest to the fracture line) are placed first, the fracture will tend to gap. On the other hand, if the outer screws are applied first, this in effect limits the length of fixed bone. Then bending the plate by tightening the inner screws effectively causes the distance between the outer screws to shorten, and thereby compresses the fracture (Figure 6.42).[40]

Stresses in plated bones and the tension band concept

In the simplest loading case, one can consider a compressive load acting on a long bone to produce bending as well as compression if either the load is not aligned with the long axis of the bone shaft or the bone is curved. In bending, the convex side of the bone will experience tension as it lengthens, and the concave side will experience compression. If the plate is located on the tension side of the bone in bending then the plate acts as a "tension band," and the fracture gap closes during loading (Figure 6.43). On the other hand, if the plate is applied on the compressive side of the bone then loading causes the fracture line to open, an undesirable event, since it could cause cyclic flexion and ultimately fatigue of the plate.

While this basic mechanical principle is correct, the difficulty may come in determining which are the tension and compression sides of a bone in vivo. In reality, the loading system of a plated weight bearing bone is complex. From in vivo implantation of strain gages in the canine femur, for example, Carter et al[41] showed that during a gait cycle, the femur experiences bending moments that produce predominantly tensile stresses on both the anterior and lateral cortices (Figure 6.44). Also, the plate itself alters the stress pattern in the bone/plate construct, so that part of the plate may be in tension and part in compression. This is best appreciated in Figure 6.45 by the position of the neutral axis (0- - - -0), the plane at which bending stresses change from tensile to compressive).

Further to the discussion of identifying the tensile and compressive sides of bones, Lanyon

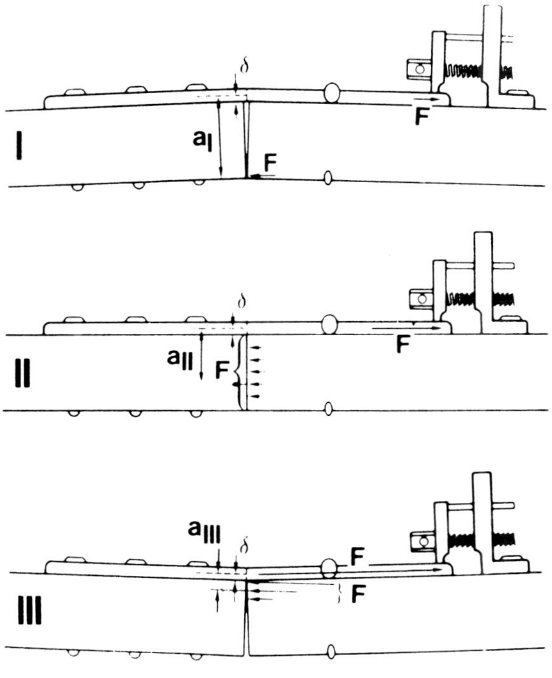

(a)

Figure 6.41

(a) Phases in tensioning of a prebent plate on the surface of a fractured bone (F, which causes fracture site compression): (I) with low tension applied, the opposite cortex is in contact because of the bend in the plate; (II) with greater tension, compression is more uniform across the fracture gap, and the center of compression moves from the opposite cortex towards the cortex under the plate; (III) with excessive tension, the advantage of prebending the plate is lost, and compression is limited to the cortex underneath the plate. (b) Relationship of the angle of bend of the plate and the tension applied to the plate (which creates fracture site compression) for the tibia and radius. The graph also indicates the location of the center of pressure at the fracture site (distance of the center of compression from the plate, %) and the three phases of tensioning, corresponding to (a). (From Gotzen L, Hatter J, Haas N, The prebending of AO plates in compression osteosynthesis. In: Uhthoff HK, ed, *Current concepts of internal fixation of fractures* (Springer-Verlag: Berlin 1980) 201–10, with permission.)

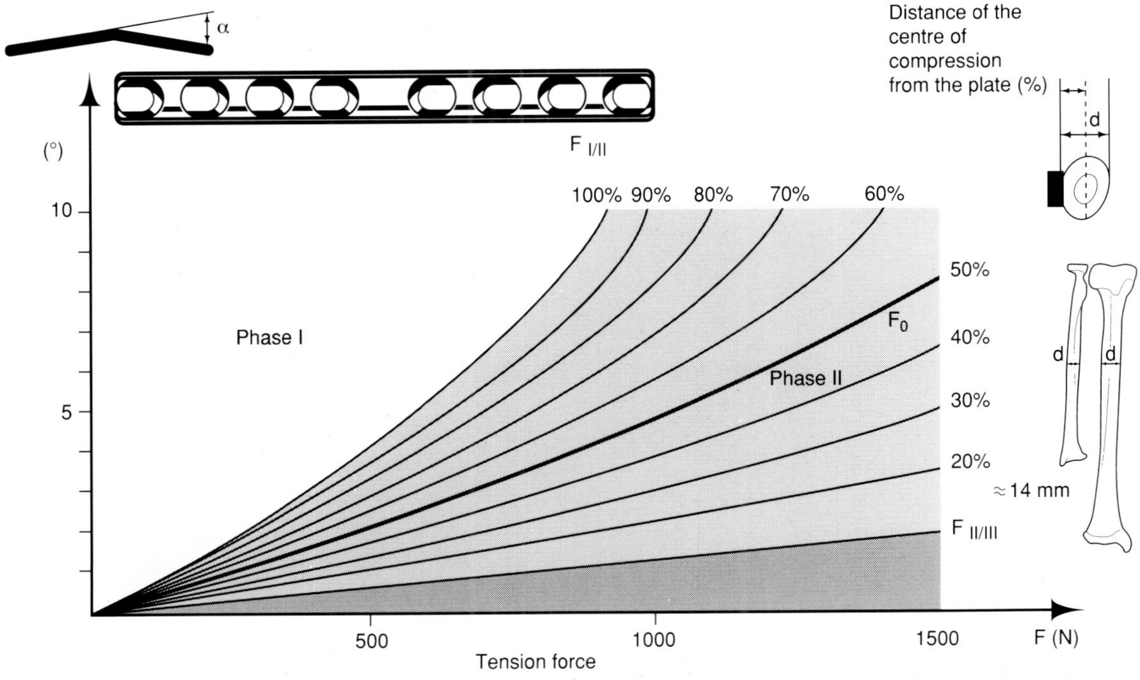

(b)

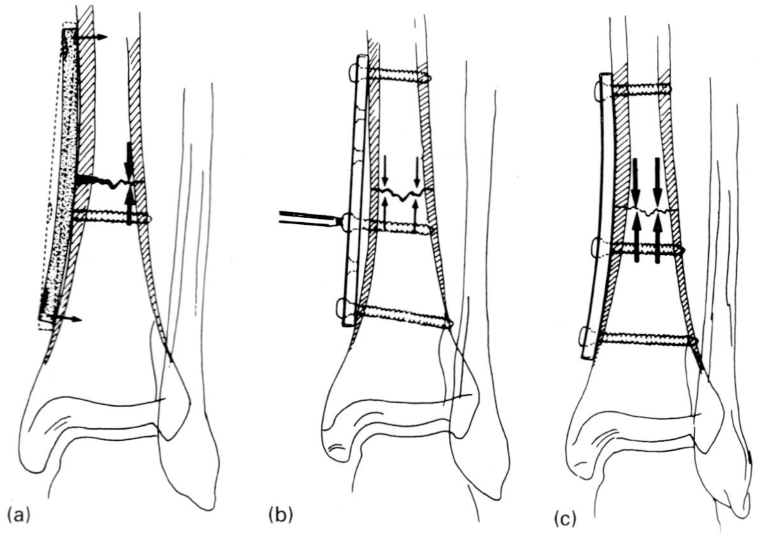

Figure 6.42

When applying a straight plate to a curved bone, (a) if the middle screws are applied first, the fracture gap near the plate will spread as the plate bends to approximate the bone; (b) if the screws are applied at the ends first and then near the fracture, curvature in the plate will effectively shorten it (c), creating compression across the fracture line. (From Ref 40 with permission.)

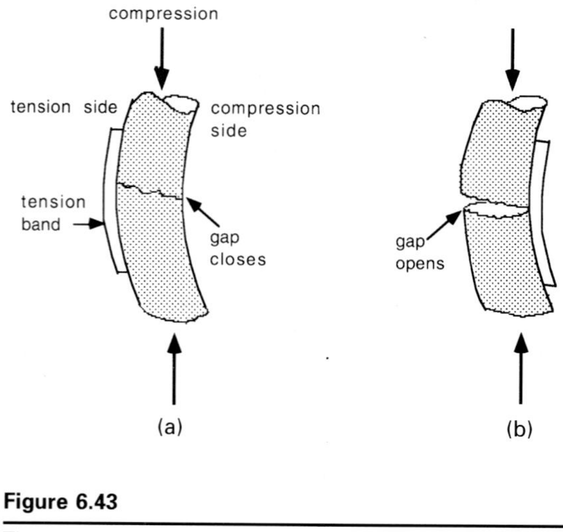

Figure 6.43

The application of a fixation plate as a tension band requires that it be placed on the tension side of the bone in bending. (a) When placed on the tension side, bending will cause the fracture gap to close. (b) When placed on the compression side, bending will cause the fracture gap to open.

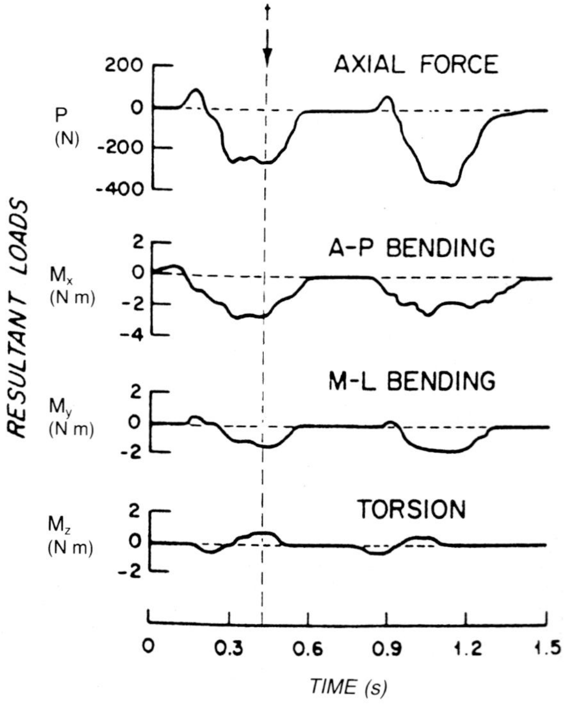

Figure 6.44

Resultant axial force, bending moments, and torsional moment acting on the femur of the dog in vivo during gait. The sign convention for the bending moments is such that a negative value indicates tensile stresses on the anterior and lateral aspects of the femur. (From Ref 41 with permission.)

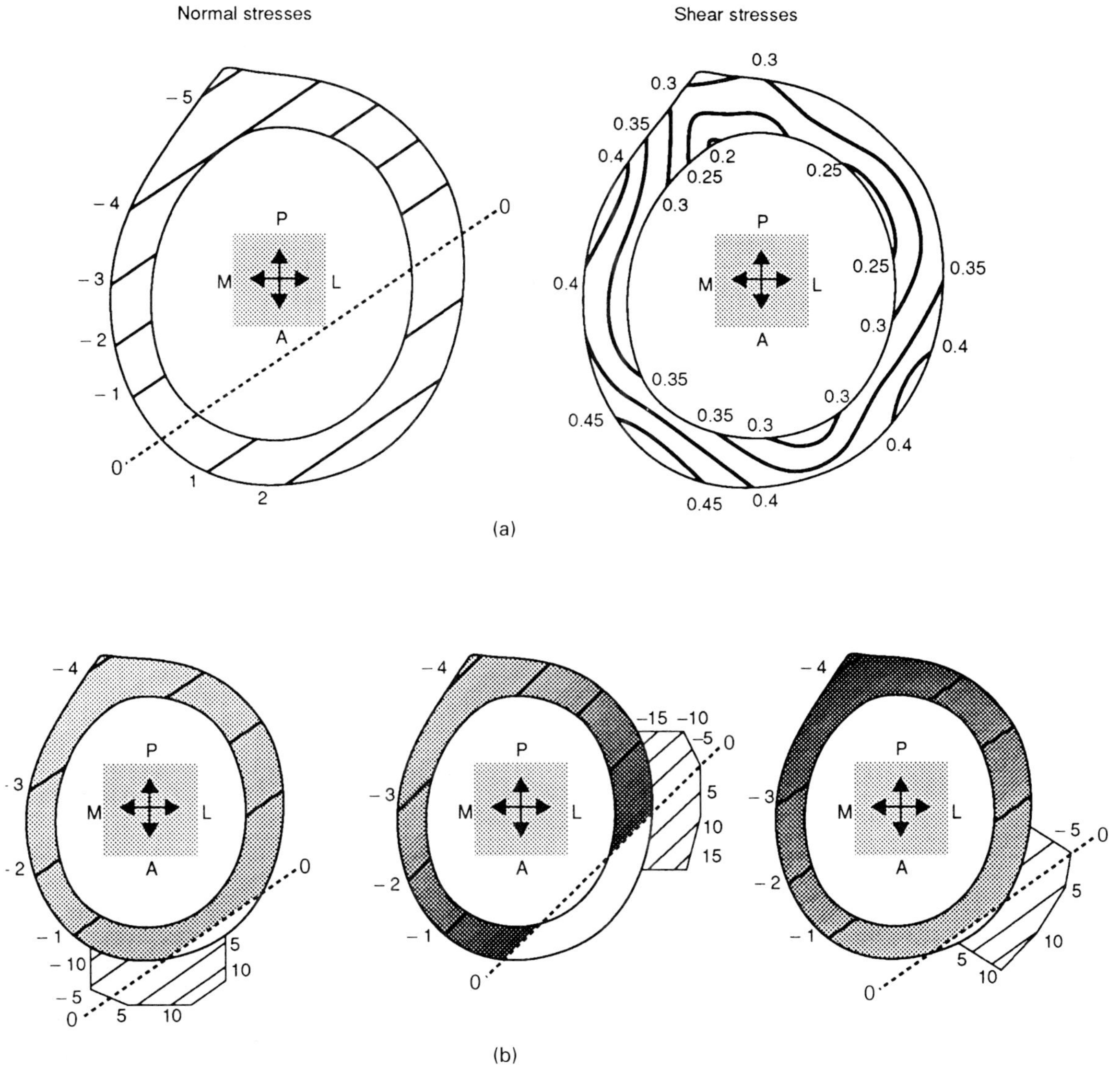

Figure 6.45

Bending (normal = tensile and compressive) stresses in the cross section of the canine femur: (a) intact; (b) with compression plates applied in anterior, lateral, or anterolateral locations. Anatomical orientation is indicated, as is the neutral axis (0- - - -0). Positive values indicate tensile and negative values compressive stresses during peak loading in the gait cycle in vivo.(From Ref 41 with permission.)

et al[42] showed that the tibia in humans is subjected to varying compressive and tensile strains during gait (Figure 6.46), which makes identification of a specific tensile side difficult. In particular, the angle of the bending strains changed considerably during gait, from being aligned with the tibial axis, to as much as 90° out of line. In the forearm, the dorsolateral aspect

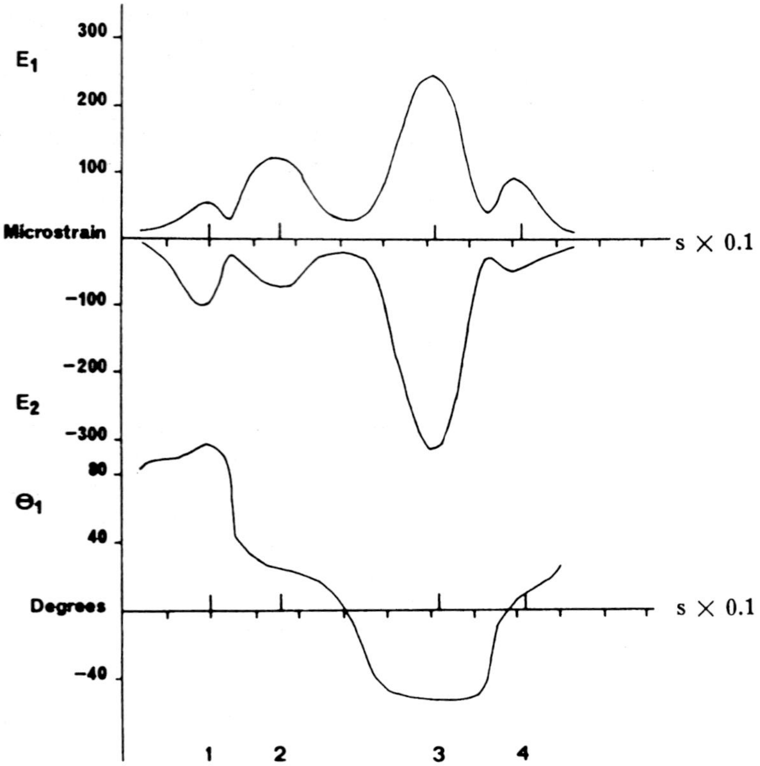

Figure 6.46

Strains in the human tibia during gait taken from in vivo recordings demonstrate changes in orientation of principal axes during different phases of motion: 1, toeoff; 2, swing phase; 3, heel strike; 4, stance phase. Θ_1 is the angle of principal tensile strain with respect to the long axis of the tibia, with 0° implying that the strains are aligned with the tibial axis, and 90°, perpendicular to the tibial axis. E_1 is the principal tensile strain, E_2 the principal compressive strain. S × 0.1 = time scale in 0.1 second intervals. (From Ref 42 with permission.)

of the radius and the flexor or extensor sides of the ulna have been proposed as the predominant tensile sides,[43] yet forearm loading is probably more complex than tibial loading. These examples have been given to demonstrate that loading of bone is complex and that application of the plate to the tensile side is not always obvious. The best way of ensuring survival of the plate is still to maintain compression across the fracture so there is minimal potential for the fracture gap to open regardless of the side that the plate is applied to.

Beaupre et al[44] also pointed out an interesting situation in which fixation of the plate to the compression side of a loaded bone may be desirable. If, as shown in Figure 6.47, there is no bony support across the fracture gap then the moment acting on the plate (which is the magnitude of the axial force times the perpendicular distance from the line of action of the force to the plate) may be smaller if the plate is on the compressive side of the bone.

Rigidity of plate fixation

Laurence et al[45] examined both the rigidity of fixation and the axial tension within the screws for the case of a plated fracture loaded in bending so as to open the fracture gap (so that all the load was carried by the plate and screws). They found that under load, the screws closest to the fracture on either side carried significantly greater axial loads than the other screws, and axial loads on the screws decreased towards the ends of the plate (Figure 6.48). The axial forces in the screws closest to the fracture were unaffected by either increasing the length of the plate or the distance between screws (Figure 6.49); however, as the distance between the innermost screws increased, the rigidity of the construct decreased. This is because the unsupported length of the plate in bending (the region of the plate between the innermost screws) increases as the screws are moved further apart. An empty screw hole

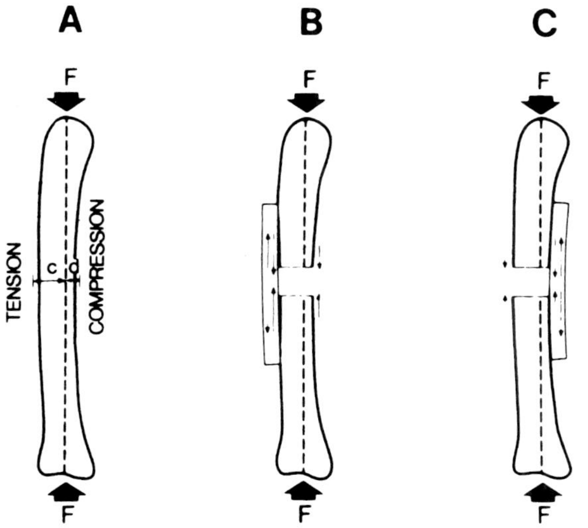

Figure 6.47

In a case of bone fixation with a gap, it may be advantageous to place the plate on the predominantly compressive side of the bone because the moment arm (distance from the line of action of the force to plate) may be smaller, resulting in a smaller bending moment acting on the plate. (From Ref 44 with permission.)

decreases rigidity, as well as creating a large stress riser. The rigidity of fixation can be increased by increasing the cross sectional moment of inertia, and the plate length.[46] Also, the orientation of the plate in relation to the direction of bending is important in determining the rigidity of the construct (Figure 6.50).[47]

6.6 Lag screws

Compression of fracture components can be produced by the action of a compression plate as described above; however, the amount of compression that can be achieved is limited by the bending stiffness of the screws, the plate/bone friction, and the torque that the screw can withstand.[48] Application of a lag screw can produce compression directly, and thereby considerably increase the stability of the construct.

Perrin et al[16] described some basic principles of lag screws. Lagging is a technique whereby a screw is placed directly across a fracture surface.

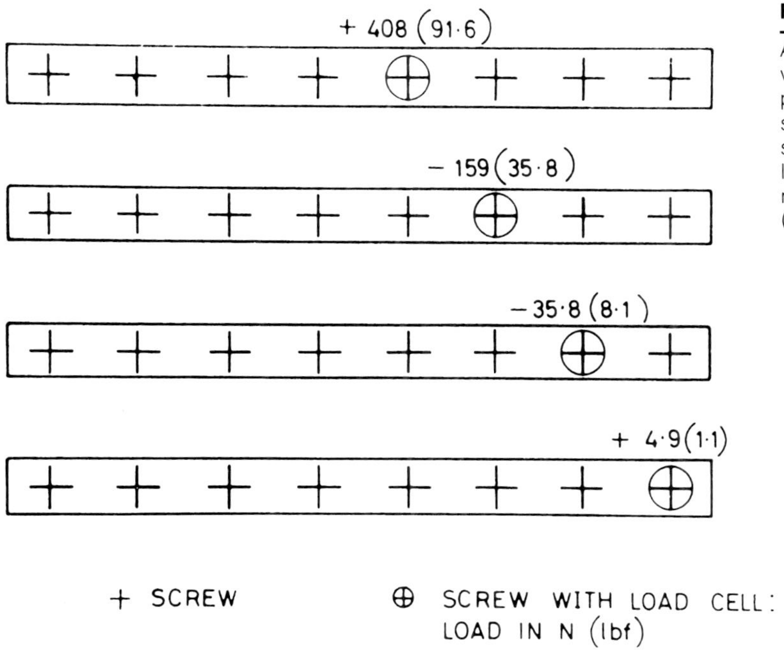

Figure 6.48

An eight hole plate mounted to a bone with a compressive load cell (whose position is indicated by ⊕) to measure screw axial force. The innermost screws carry considerably greater load, and the latter decreases on moving towards the end of the plate. (From Ref 45 with permission.)

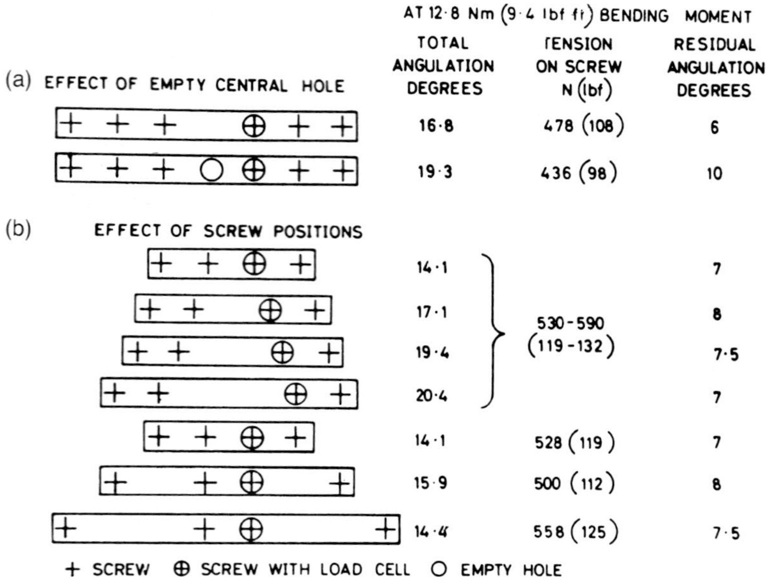

Figure 6.49

Angulation of a plate/bone construct in bending, axial tension in the screw, and residual angulation of the construct after load release due to (a) a central empty screw hole and (b) separating the screws or increasing the length of the plate. The tension in the innermost scews is unaffected by moving them farther apart. Lengthening the plate decreases its bending stiffness. (From Ref 45 with permission.)

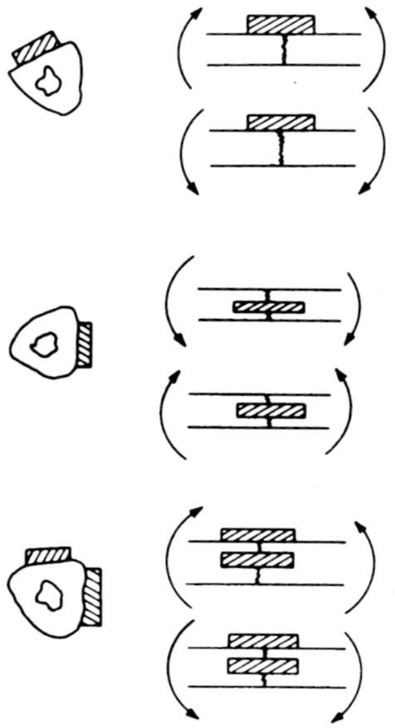

Configuration	Bending moment	Rigidity relative to (a)
(a)		1
(b)		200
(c)		60
(d)		35
(e)		218
(f)		235

Figure 6.50

Relative rigidity in bending (open and closed as indicated) of plates oriented in various configurations compared with configuration labeled (a). (From Ref 47 with permission.)

If the screw is allowed to slide in the hole of the upper component then as the screw is tightened in the lower component, the upper component is trapped by the screw head and is pulled against the lower component. In fact, the compression is not uniform across the fracture line, being greatest near the screw. A lag screw may produce up to five times the compressive force generated by a compression plate. A lag screw is subjected to tensile force during tightening, as well as a functional force when the bone is loaded, for example in bending, as shown in Figure 6.51. In this case, the fulcrum (the point around which the bone rotates when bending is applied) is located at the intersection of the bottom cortical surface and the fracture line. If the screw is nearer the upper surface, the moment arm is larger; therefore the additional force generated in the screw is smaller.

The inclination of the screw is a second important consideration. The optimum orientation of the screw is perpendicular to the fracture line. A small deviation in screw angle (greater than 20°) starts to displace the fracture components tangentially, because some of the screw force is acting parallel to the fracture line, and is sufficient to overcome bone-to-bone friction. In the case of a spiral fracture (Figure 6.52), the optimum orientation is perpendicular to the bisector of the angle between the fracture planes.[16]

In order to gain this compressive effect, the screw must be able to slide freely within one fragment while having its threads engaged in the other. When using a fully threaded screw, the threads of the lag screw may engage the cortices of both fragments, which can occur even if the hole is overdrilled in one of the bone fragments (to allow gliding of the screw) (Figure 6.53). In this case the lag compression effect can be reduced by up to 50%, as shown in Figure 6.54. Using a screw with a smooth shank just below the screw head eliminates this loss of compression.[48]

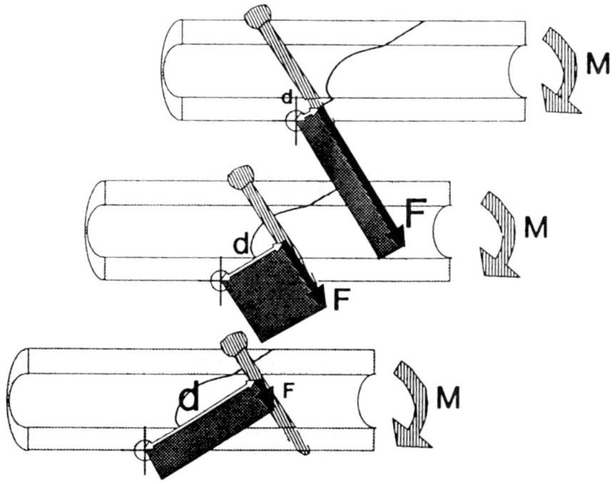

Figure 6.51

Effect of position of the screw on the force generated within it during bending. With the fulcrum at the bottom cortical surface/fracture line intersection point, the moment arm (distance from the screw to fulcrum) increases as the screw is positioned nearer the top surface. The resulting force in the screw decreases for the same applied moment. (Width of the shaded rectangle, d = moment arm; length along axis of screw, f = force in screw. In all cases F × d = M, the bending moment applied.) (From Ref 16 with permission.)

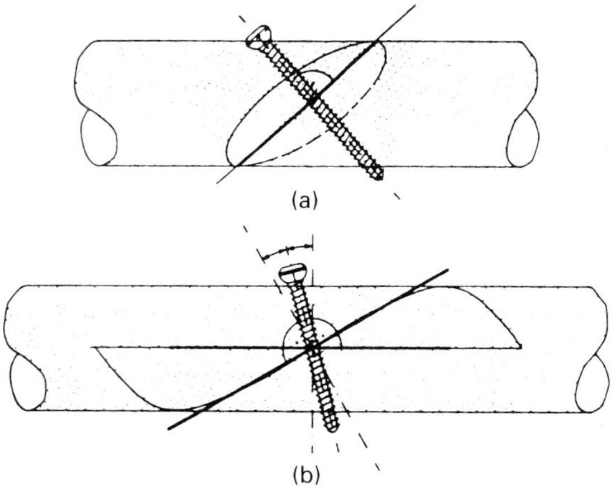

Figure 6.52

(a) The optimum inclination of a lag screw is perpendicular to the fracture plane. (b) In the case of a spiral fracture with a fracture plane that changes orientation, the optimum orientation is perpendicular to the bisector of the angle between the fracture planes. (From Ref 16 with permission.)

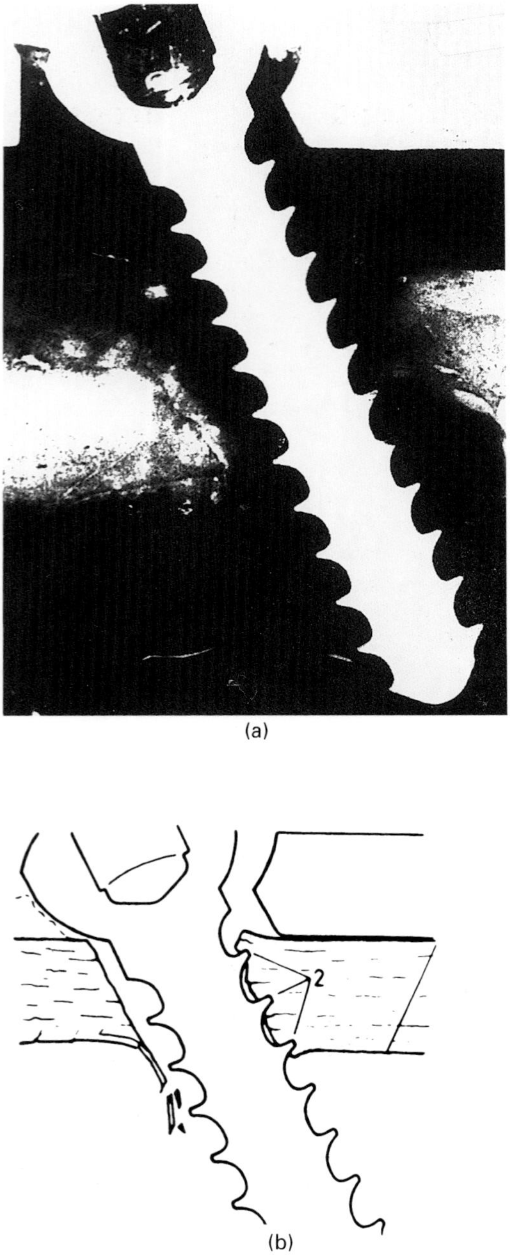

Figure 6.53

(a) Histological section and (b) schematic diagram of the way in which a fully threaded lag screw impinges on cortex, preventing complete compression of the fracture components. A screw with a smooth shank would allow gliding of the components together. (From Ref 48 with permission.)

6.7 Summary

Some basic biomechanical concepts related to commonly used devices for fracture fixation have been presented. Drilling holes in bone can cause heat related necrosis, so the use of drills of appropriate geometry with sharp cutting edges and copious irrigation while drilling is imperative. A hole of diameter equal to 20% of the diameter of the bone in which it is placed can act as a large stress riser, decreasing bone torsional strength by 64%. A screw left in place (e.g. during hardware removal) will result in higher torsional strength of the bone than if it is removed, and a hole left behind, until the screw hole fills with new bone or otherwise remodels.

Wire used for fracture fixation is prone to fatigue, with the fatigue life decreasing considerably, even with notches as small as 1% of the wire diameter. Cables of equivalent diameter can provide up to 10 times greater fatigue life than wires. When using pins, their bending stiffness can be significantly increased by applying axial tension to the pin, which counteracts the bending moment.

Screws placed in cortical bone can fail by shearing during insertion, by fatigue, or can be pulled out due to inadequate purchase in bone. Increasing the root diameter, providing a tapped pilot hole, and inserting the screw with lubrication can reduce the incidence of screw pullout by shearing, particularly in cortical bone. The purchase of a screw depends upon the shear strength of the material into which it is embedded, the length of engagement of the threads, and the volume of material between the threads. In low density cancellous bone, where failure of the screw during insertion is less likely, increased purchase can be gained by using a screw with a smaller root diameter, not tapping (which enlarges the screw hole), increasing the length of thread engagement, not using cannulated screws, and placing the screw in the most dense cancellous bone possible. The fatigue life of a screw used with a bone plate can be enhanced by applying maximum torque to it, which increases its axial load and plate/bone friction, and decreases the transverse load applied to the screw as a bending moment, since a greater part will be taken by the plate.

A dynamic compression plate is a device that converts the torque applied to a screw to a

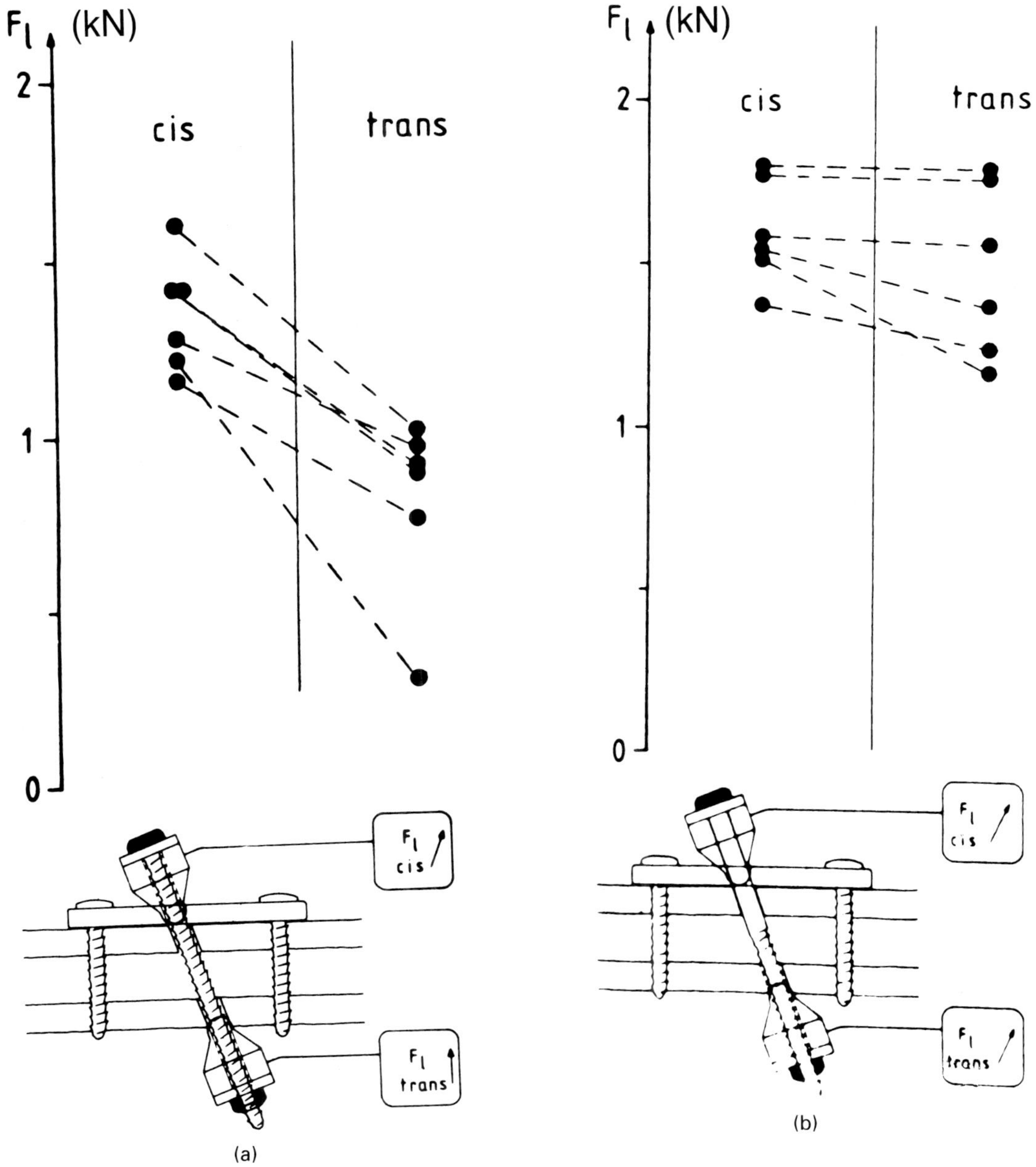

Figure 6.54

Comparison of the compression achieved by a lag screw at the cortex under the plate (cis) and on the opposite cortex (trans). (a) Using a fully threaded screw which permits binding of the screw in the cortex under the plate, the force at the screw on the opposite cortex is considerably lower than that of the cortex on which the plate rests. (b) Using a partially threaded screw with a smooth shank through the cortex under the plate results in similar forces in both ends of the screw. (From Ref 48 with permission.)

longitudinal force to compress bone fracture components. Prebending plates helps to create a more uniform compressive load across the fracture line, especially on the opposite cortex, which is important in ensuring the survival of the plate. Applying the plate to the tension side of a bone produces a situation where the fracture gap closes under load, thereby protecting the plate from excessive bending. However, the tension side of a bone may sometimes be difficult to identify, considering the complexity of physiological loading. The rigidity of plate constructs is decreased by increasing the separation between the innermost screws across the fracture or by leaving an empty screw hole at the fracture site. Lag screws are an effective way to increase the compressive force across the fracture site, necessary to ensure stability of the fixation and to protect the plate. A lag screw with a smooth shank whose threads only engage the opposite cortex is more effective in gaining compression than a fully threaded screw whose threads can bind in the cortex under the plate. Lag screws should be oriented within 20° of perpendicular to the fracture plane.

6.8 References

1. Jacobs CH, Pope MH, Berry JT, Hoaglund F, A study of the bone machining process—orthogonal cutting, *J Biomech* (1974) **7:** 131–6.
2. Albright JA, Johnson TR, Saha S, Principles of internal fixation, In: Ghista, DN Roaf, R, eds, *Orthopedic mechanics: procedures and devices* (Academic Press: New York 1978) 124–222.
3. Rouiller C, Majno G, Morphologische und Chemische Unterbuchungen an Koochen nach Hitzeeinwirkung, *Beitr Z Path Anat* (1953) **113:** 100–20.
4. Matthews LS, Hirsch C, Temperatures measured in human cortical bone during drilling, *J Bone Jt Surg* (1972) **54A:** 297–308.
5. Bonfield W, Li CH, The temperature dependence of the deformation of bone, *J Biomech* (1968) **1:** 323–9.
6. Jacobs CH, Berry JT, Pope MH, Hoaglund FT, A study of the bone machining process—drilling, *J Biomech* (1976) **9:** 343–9.
7. Edgarton BC, An K-A, Morrey BF, Torsional strength reduction due to cortical defects in bone, *J Orthop Res* (1990) **8:** 851–5.
8. Brooks DB, Burstein AH, Frankel VH, The biomechanics of torsional fractures. The stress concentration effect of a drill hole, *J Bone Jt Surg* (1970) **52A:** 507–14.
9. Schatzker J, Sanderson R, Murnaghan JP, The holding power of orthopedic screws in vivo, *Clin Orthop* (1975) **108:** 115–26.
10. *Annual Book of Standards*, Standard specification for stainless steel bar and wire for surgical implants, designation F138-82, Vol 13.01 (American Society for Testing and Materials: 1986) 31–4.
11. Taitsman J, Saha S, Tensile properties of reinforced bone cement, *J Bone Jt Surg* (1976) **59A:** 419–25.
12. Sander TW, Treharne RW, Baswell I, Oh I, Development of a new orthopedic wire tester, *J Biomed Mat Res* (1983) **17:** 587–96.
13. Georgette FS, Sander TW, Oh I, The fatigue resistance of orthopedic wire and cable systems. In: JM Anderson, ed, *Second World Congress on Biomaterials, Washington DC, 1984* (Society for Biomaterials: Birmingham, AL 1984) 146.
14. Leutzow WF, Markolf KL, Nasser S, Amstutz HC, Initial stability of the greater trochanter using newer methods of reattachment, *Trans 37th Orthopedic Research Society Meeting* (1991) **16:** 508.
15. *Annual Book of Standards*, Medical devices, Standard F 544, Vol 13.01 (American Society for Testing and Materials: 1986) 137–42.
16. Perren SM, Cordey J, Baumgart F, Rahn BA, Schatzker J, Technical and biomechanical aspects of screws used for bone surgery, *Int J Orthop Trauma* (1992) **2:** 31–48.
17. Ansell RH, Scales JT, A study of some factors which affect the strength of screws and their insertion and holding power in bone, *J Biomech* (1968) **1:** 279–302.
18. Dieter CE, *Mechanical metallurgy* (McGraw Hill: New York 1961) 273–5.
19. Hughes AN, Jordan BA, The mechanical properties of surgical bone screws and some aspects of insertion practise, *Injury* (1972) **4:** 25–38.
20. Oberg E, Jones FD, Horton HL, Bolts, nuts, screws, washers, pins, nails and spikes. In: Ryffel HH, ed, *Machinery handbook*, 22nd edn (Industrial Press: New York 1987) 1068–9.
21. Uhthoff HK, Mechanical factors influencing the holding power of screws in compact bone, *J Bone Jt Surg* (1973) **55B:** 633–9.
22. Trader JE, Johnson RP, Kalbfleisch JH, Bone mineral content, surface hardness, and mechanical fixation in the human radius, *J Bone Jt Surg* (1979) **61A:** 1217–20.
23. Hayes WC, Biomechanics of cortical and trabecular bone: implications for fracture risk. In: Mow VC, Hayes WC, eds, *Basic orthopedic biomechanics* (Raven Press: New York 1991) 93–142.
24. Wittenberg RH, Shea M, Swartz DE, Lee KS, White

III AA, Hayes WC, Importance of bone mineral density in instrumented spinal fusions, *Spine* (1991) **16**: 648–52.

25. Chapman JR, Harrington RM, Lee K, Forsyth E, Anderson PA, The influence of screw design and insertion technique on the pullout strength of screws in porous materials, *Trans 38th Orthopedic Research Society Meeting* (1992) **17**: 406.
26. Finlay JB, Jarada I, Boune RB, Rorabeck CH, Hardie R, Scott MA, Analysis of the pull-out strength of screws and pegs used to secure tibial components following total knee arthroplasty, *Clin Orthop* (1989) **247**: 220–31.
27. DeCoster TA, Heetderks DB, Downey DJ, Ferries JS, Jones W, Optimizing bone screw pullout force, *J Orthop Trauma* (1990) **4**: 169–74.
28. Stone JL, Beaupre GS, Hayes WC, Multiaxial strength characteristics of trabecular bone, *J Biomech* (1983) **16**: 743–52.
29. Lee KM, The effect of insertion technique on pull-out strength of cancellous bone screws in porous materials and cancellous bone, *Independent Study in Medical Science, University of Washington* (1992).
30. Scales JT, Perry P, Screw and plate devices in the fixation of fractures: a ten year survey, *Acta Orthop Belg* (1974) **40**: 836–45.
31. Nunamaker DM, Perren SM, Force measurements in screw fixation, *J Biomech* (1976) **9**: 669–75.
32. Zand MS, Goldstein SA, Matthews LS, Fatigue failure of cortical bone screws, *J Biomech* (1983) **16**: 305–11.
33. Hayes WC, Perren SM, Flexural rigidity of compression plate fixation of fractures. In: *Proceedings of the 2nd Nordic Meeting on Medical and Biological Engineering* (1971) 242.
34. Allgower M, Cinderella of surgery—fractures?, *Surg Clin NA* (1978) **58**: 1071–93.
35. Cordey J, Florin P, Klaue K, Perren SM, Compression achieved with the dynamic compression plate: effects of the inclined sloping cylinder and inclination of the screw. In: Uhthoff HK, ed, *Current concepts of internal fixation of fractures* (Springer-Verlag: Berlin 1980) 192–200.
36. Hayes WC, Perren SM, Plate–bone friction in the compression fixation of fractures, *Clin Orthop* (1972) **89**: 236–40.
37. Perren SM, Huggler A, Russenberger M, Straumann F, Muller ME, Allgower M, A method of measuring the change in compression applied to living cortical bone, *Acta Orthop Scand* (1969) Supp 125.
38. Askew MJ, Mow VC, Wirth CR, Cambell CJ, Analysis of the intraosseus stress field due to compression plating, *J Biomech* (1975) **8**: 203–12.
39. Nunamaker DM, Perren SM, A radiological and histological analysis of fracture healing using prebending of compression plates, *Clin Orthop* (1979) **138**: 167–74.
40. Schawecker F, *The practice of osteosynthesis. A manual of accident surgery* (Yearbook Medical Publishers: Chicago 1974).
41. Carter DR, Vasu R, Spengler DM, Dueland RT, Stress fields in the unplated and plated canine femur calculated from in vivo strain measurements. *J Biomech* (1981) **14**: 63–70.
42. Lanyon LE, Hampson WGJ, Goodship AE, Shah JS, Bone deformation recorded from in vivo strain gages attached to the human tibial shaft, *Acta Orthop Scand* (1975) **46**: 256–68.
43. Ruedi T, von Hochstetter AHC, Schlumpf R, *Surgical approaches for internal fixation* (Springer-Verlag: Berlin 1984).
44. Beaupre GS, Carter DR, Dueland RT, Caler WE, Spengler DM, A biomechanical assessment of plate fixation, with insufficient bony support, *J Orthop Res* (1988) **6**: 721–9.
45. Laurence M, Freeman MA, Swanson SA, Engineering considerations in the internal fixation of fractures of the tibial shaft, *J Bone Jt Surg* (1969) **51B**: 754–68.
46. Ray DR, Ledbetter WB, Bynum D, Boyd CL, A parametric analysis of bone fixation plates on fractured equine 3rd metacarpal, *J Biomech* (1971) **4**: 163–72.
47. Mears D, *Materials and orthopedic surgery* (Williams & Wilkins: Baltimore 1979) 298.
48. Klaue K, Perren SM, Kowalski M, Internal fixation with a self-compressing plate and screw: improvements of the plate hole and screw design, I. Mechanical investigation, *J Orthop Trauma* (1991) **5**: 280–8.

CHAPTER 7

Upper extremity fixation

In the following sections data and discussions are presented on fixation of fractures in the upper extremity. In general, there are two different locations for fixation: the diaphyseal regions of long bones, and the metaphyseal regions, including across articular surfaces. There are two major differences between these regions, related to fixation. First, diaphyseal cortical bone is denser and stronger than metaphyseal bone, which is primarily cancellous and requires a different strategy for gaining purchase for screws or pins. Secondly, the applied loads are different. The bone of the metaphysis is designed to support compressive forces across the joint, while the diaphysis is loaded in bending, torsion, and compression, by muscle forces and external loads.

This chapter is organized by region, moving distally to proximally in the upper extremity, where information on fixation technique is available. In each section, a biomechanical discussion of the loads that the anatomical region is likely to encounter is given, since without an understanding of the loading conditions, it is difficult to design an effective fixation system to stabilize the fracture. This is followed by a discussion and comparison of various techniques, ending with a short summary emphasizing basic principles, as opposed to specific fracture devices.

Table 7.1 Estimates of the forces occuring at each of the three joints of the finger, per unit of force applied due to a pinch or grasp. DIP, distal interphalangeal; PIP, proximal interphalangeal; MP, metacarpal phalangeal. (From Ref 1 with permission.)

	Prosthesis force and moment requirement (in units of applied force)				
Finger prosthetic joint	*Axial compressive force*	*Volar subluxation force*	*Radioulnar dislocation force*	*Radioulnar[a] bending moment*	*Axial[a] twisting moment*
DIP	6	4.5	1	4	4
PIP	10	6	1	7	8
MP	14	9	4	-	70

[a]Moment arm in mm.

7.1 Fixation of the interphalangeal joint

Loading conditions

Chao et al[1] define the finger as a beam, with a hinged joint at the base and passive and active tendons acting to counteract the external load (Figure 7.1). The moments generated by the tendons prevent excessive subluxation forces from acting on the joint and its capsule, while at the same time increasing the compressive force across the articular surfaces. For typical conditions such as pinch and grasp, which apply force perpendicular to the long axis of the phalange, the axial compressive force is 6–14 times the magnitude of the force applied, depending on the joint considered, as shown in Table 7.1. The volar subluxation force is considerably greater than that which produces radioulnar dislocation. Also the axial torque, especially at the metacarpal joint, can be large.

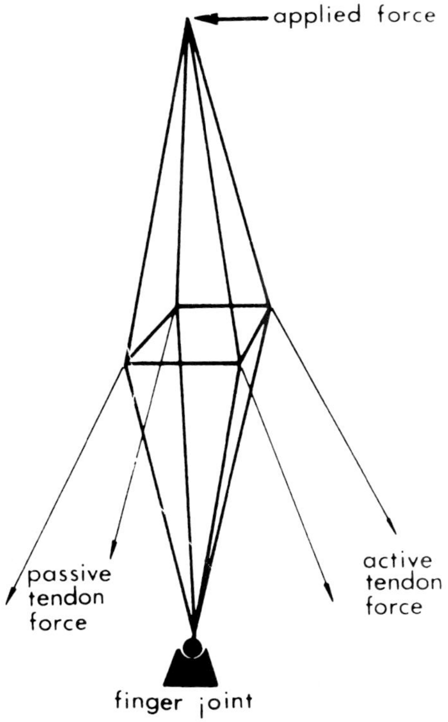

Figure 7.1

Schematic diagram of the finger as a beam supported by guy wires (active and passive tendon forces) rotating about a hinge at its base. (From Ref 1 with permission.)

Comparison of fixation techniques

Several alternative techniques have been proposed for fixation of the proximal interphalangeal joint.[2–8] Kovach et al[9] compared four techniques of fixation using K wires with different methods of cerclage wiring, as shown in Figure 7.2. As summarized in Figure 7.3, the double K wire with wire loop technique provided the greatest construct rigidity, supported the largest moments, and absorbed the most energy to failure in anterior–posterior three point bending and torsion. There were no statistical differences between fixation systems in lateral cantilever bending.

Summary

The mechanical superiority of the double K wire fixation technique with a figure of eight wire loop can be explained. In bending, the K wires are primarily responsible for construct stiffness. When a greater number are placed further from the neutral (central) axis and longitudinally, they will produce a construct that is stiffer in bending than fixations using only single K wires. In torsion, a single K wire acts as an axis about which the fixation components can rotate. This rotation is reduced using double K wires. The wire loop is important in producing compression of the bone surfaces, which further stabilizes the construct. This is why the double K wire with wire loop construct will be more rigid than a construct with K wires alone.

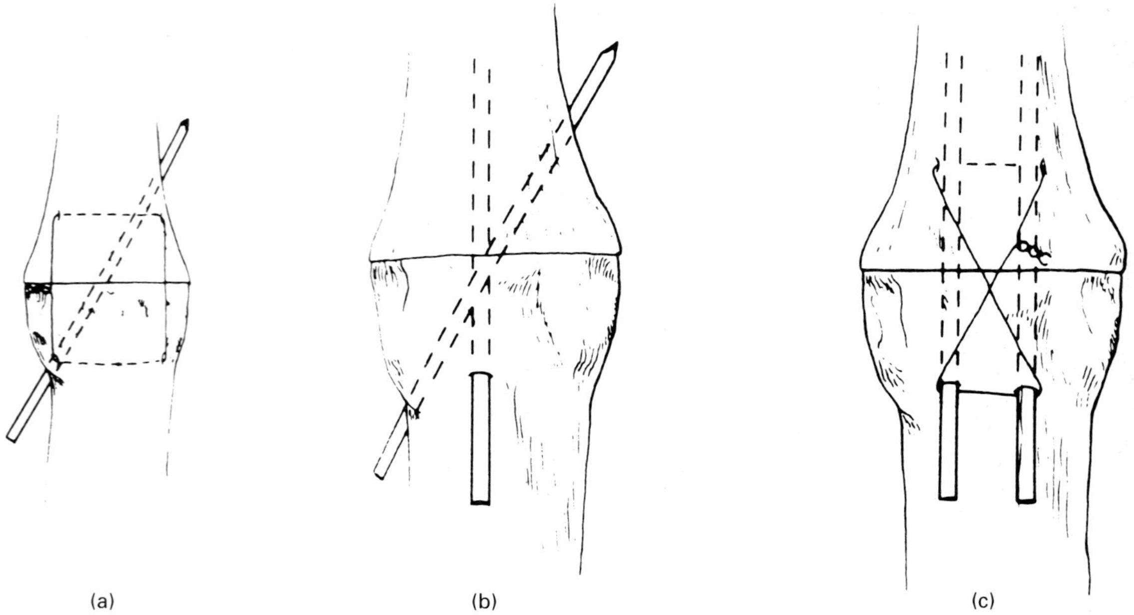

Figure 7.2

Techniques of fixation of interphalangeal joints. (a) Oblique K wire with cerclage wire placed either on the dorsal aspect (OKDW) (to act as a tension band) or through the midline of the joint (OKNW) (to apply compression). (b) One oblique and one longitudinal K wire (OKLK). (c) Two longitudinal K wires with a dorsal wire loop (LKDW). (From Ref 9 with permission.)

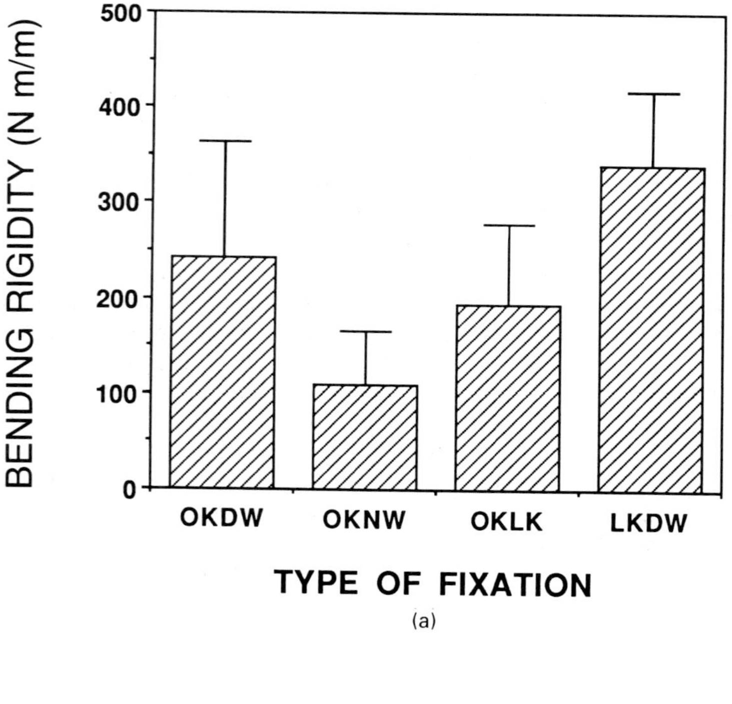

Figure 7.3

A comparison of (a) the anterior–posterior bending and (b) the maximum torsional and bending moments at failure of four methods of fixation of interphalangeal fusions: OKDW, oblique K wire and dorsal tension band; OKNW, oblique K wire and neutral tension band; OKLK, oblique and longitudinal K wires; LKDW; double longitudinal K wires and figure of eight dorsal wire loop (see Figure 7.2). (Data adapted from Ref 9.)

(*Continued next page*)

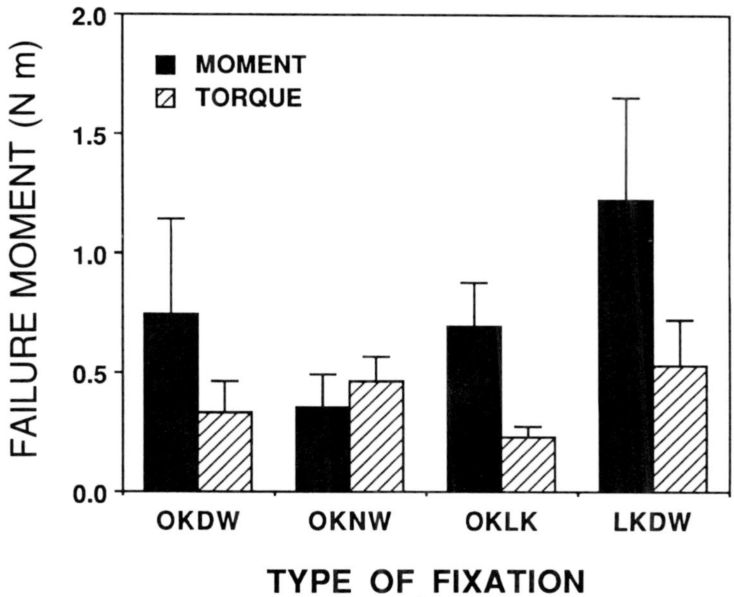

(b)

Figure 7.3

(Continued)

7.2 Fixation of metacarpal fractures

Loading conditions

The metacarpal is a load bearing bone during functional use of the hand, for example, in lifting. The metacarpals are attached distally by the transverse metacarpal ligaments, which prevent both tension along and torsion about the long axis of an individual bone. Therefore the predominant loads applied to the metacarpals will be in bending, due to the actions of the flexors and extensors of the fingers, as well as compression, applied both by external forces and internally by the dorsal and palmar interosseous muscles of the hand. An important consideration in fixation of metacarpal fractures is the prevention of angulatory deformity, particularly dorsally, by bending moments.

External fixation

Kato et al[10] compared the rigidity of various external fixation configurations for metacarpal fixation in apex dorsal bending. As shown in Figure 7.4, considering a four hole plate placed dorsally as the most rigid construct, a double half pin frame with Hoffman vice clamps mounted obliquely provides about 66% of the rigidity of the plate construct, followed by a double through pin configuration mounted in the plane of the applied bending moment (27.7%), a double half pin frame mounted dorsally and laterally (27%), single miniframes (17% and 9.6%), and crossed K wires (11.8%). As will be shown later, a dorsal plate construct is approximately equal to the bending stiffness of the intact metacarpal; therefore these values can be considered to reflect the approximate rigidity of the construct compared with the intact metacarpal.

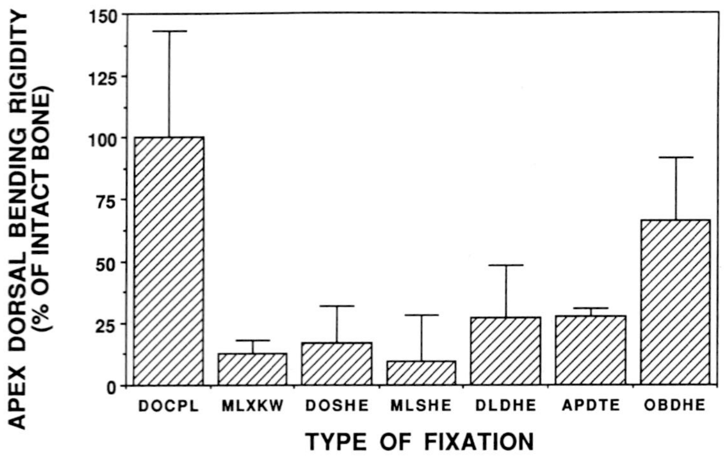

Figure 7.4

Rigidities of some methods of external fixation compared with a plate and crossed K wires, in apex dorsal bending: DOCPL, dorsal compression plate; MLXKW, medial–lateral crossed K wires; DOSHE, dorsal single half pin external fixator; MLSHE, medial–lateral single half pin external fixator; DLDHE, dorsal and lateral double half pin external fixator; APDTE, anterior–posterior double through pin external fixator; OBDHE, oblique double half pin external fixator. (Data adapted from Ref 10.)

Internal fixation

The use of various methods of internal fixation has been described in the literature.[11–16] In a study limited to internal fixation, Mann et al[17] compared plating and wiring techniques using human metacarpals and a transverse osteotomy model. In apex dorsal bending, a dorsally applied plate, with or without a lag screw, provides construct rigidity equal to that of the intact metacarpal. Crossed K wires (0.049 in diameter), with or without an intraosseous wire, produced equivalent construct rigidities, which were about 10% of that of the intact metacarpal (Figure 7.5). In apex palmar bending, which opens the fracture gap, the plate and lag screw maintained the same rigidity, while the rigidity of the dorsal plate construct was similar to that of metacarpal fractures fixed with K wires, as shown in Figure 7.6. In torsion, the dorsal plate with lag screw reached 66% of intact torsional stiffness, the dorsal plate alone 36%, and the wiring techniques 4–7.6%. In loading to failure in apex dorsal bending, plate fixed fractures failed by screw pullout, while K wire fixation failed by sliding and allowed the greatest angulation. Plate fixation absorbed the greatest amount of energy before failure.

Percutaneous fixation

Although K wire pinning of metacarpal fractures produces constructs with relatively low stiffness compared with plating, it may be desirable to apply this form of fixation for other reasons, such as ease of insertion, and avoidance of opening the wound and stripping the periosteum. Viegas et al[18] compared the rigidities of a number of alternative methods of percutaneous wiring as shown in Figure 7.7. It is important to consider the orientation of the fracture line, transverse or oblique, when considering percutaneous pin fixation alternatives. For transverse fractures, fixation using four crossed 0.028 in diameter wires produced the most rigid construct, followed by two crossed 0.028 or 0.035 in wires (Table 7.2). By estimation with the data of the previous study,[17] four crossed 0.028 in wire fixation produces a rigidity equal to about 37% of the intact metacarpal in apex dorsal bending, and 11% in torsion. For oblique fractures, Table 7.3 shows the most rigid construct to be three oblique 0.035 in K wires followed by two oblique K wires. In comparison to the intact metacarpal, three oblique 0.035 in K wires provide 31% and 13.8% of the rigidities of the intact metacarpal in apex dorsal bending and torsion respectively.

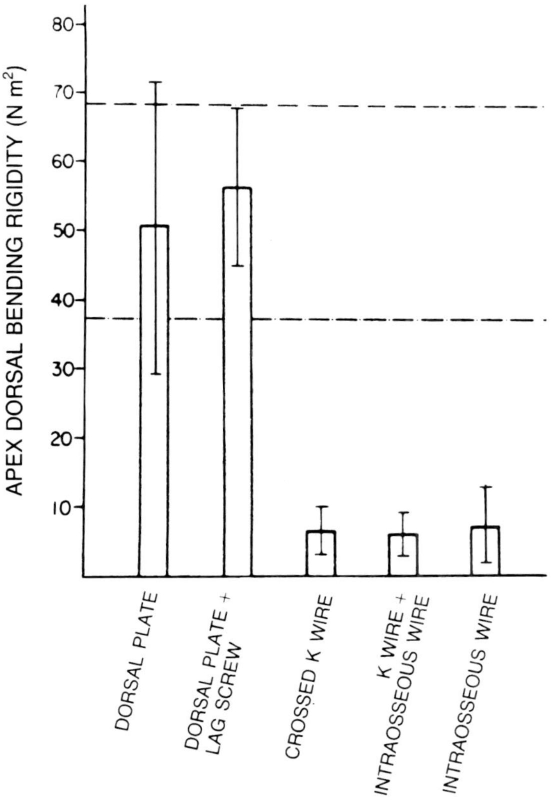

Figure 7.5

Apex dorsal three point bending rigidities of metacarpals with transverse osteotomies fixed using various techniques. (From Ref 17 with permission.)

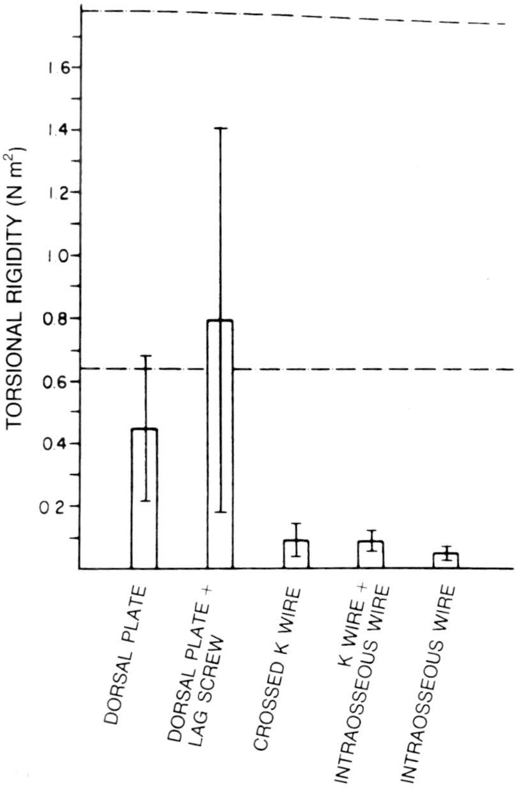

Figure 7.6

Apex palmar three point bending rigidities of metacarpals with transverse osteotomies fixed using various techniques. (From Ref 17 with permission.)

Summary

Considering previously discussed biomechanical guidelines for selecting a fixation method that will produce construct stiffness in the range of 20–60%, a double half pin external fixation frame or four crossed K wires provide the appropriate rigidity for fixation of a transverse fracture of a metacarpal. For oblique fractures, three oblique K wires provide adequate fixation stiffness.

It is important to consider the effects of bending when choosing the orientation of K wires. Bending, as shown in Figure 7.8, produces shearing across the fracture line, as does torsion. The appropriate direction of a fixation device in resisting shear is perpendicular to the fracture line.

This might imply using longitudinally oriented wires in a transverse fracture. However, the wires must be anchored in cortex in order to resist loads; therefore a crossed configuration is appropriate. Also, longitudinal pins are less effective in torsion, since they are nearly parallel to the torsional axis (i.e. the longitudinal axis of the bone). For an oblique fracture line, placing the pins parallel to each other and perpendicular to the fracture line is the appropriate orientation for fixation.

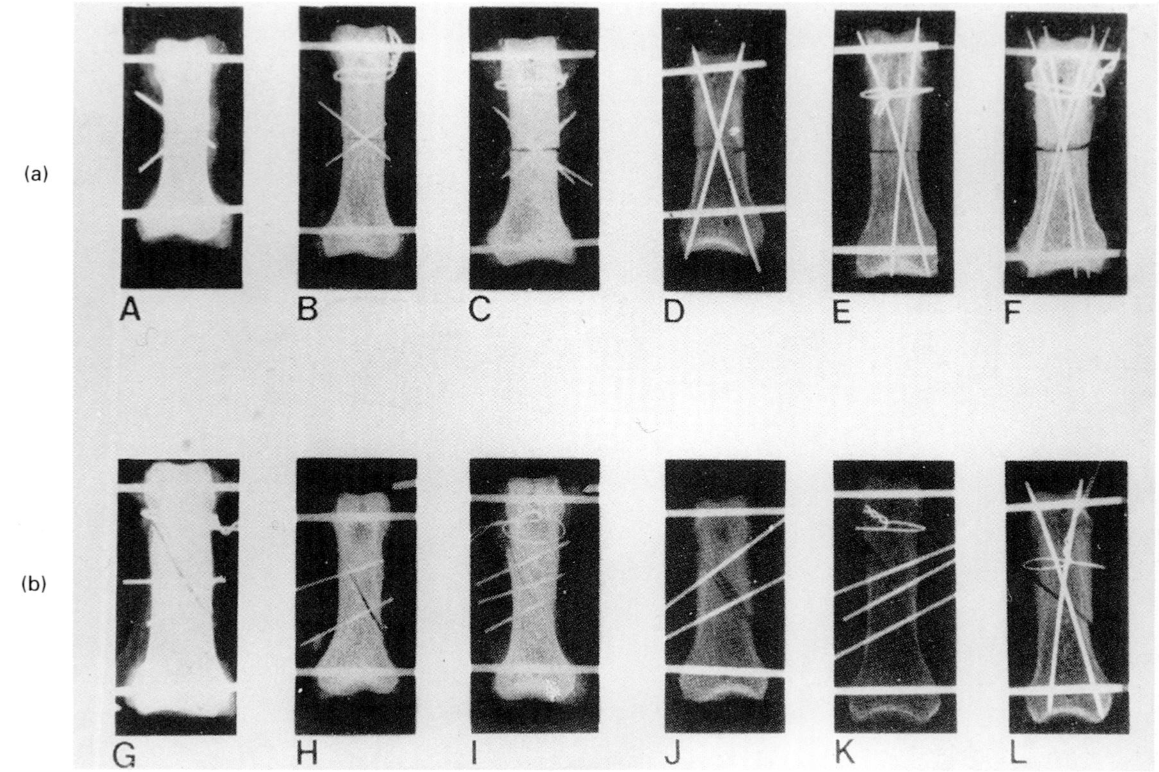

Figure 7.7

Alternative methods of percutaneous fixation of metacarpal fractures. (a) In transverse fractures: (A) two crossed 0.035 in diameter K wires; (B) two crossed 0.028 in K wires; (C) four crossed 0.028 in K wires; (D) two longitudinal 0.035 in K wires; (E) two longitudinal 0.028 in K wires; (F) four longitudinal K wires. (b) In oblique fractures: (G) two crossed 0.035 in K wires; (H) two oblique 0.028 in K wires; (I) three oblique 0.028 in K wires; (J) two oblique 0.035 in K wires; (K) three oblique 0.035 in K wires; (L) two longitudinal 0.035 in K wires. (From Ref 18 with permission.)

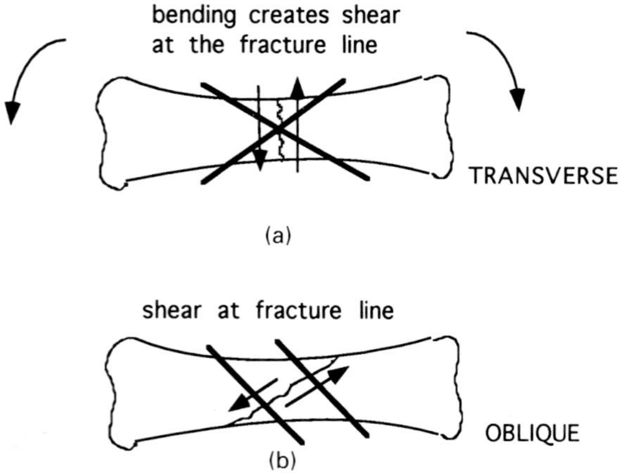

Figure 7.8

In bending, shear occurs at the fracture line therefore the fixation should be oriented so as to resist this motion. (a) For a transverse fracture pattern, pins crossed at 90° reduce shear at the fracture line, as well as resisting torque. (b) In an oblique fracture pattern, orienting the pins perpendicular to the fracture line resists shear and torsion.

Table 7.2 A relative comparison of the rigidities of constructs formed by each of six methods of percutaneous wire fixation of metacarpal fractures under various loading conditions with a transverse fracture line. (From Ref 18 with permission.)

	Fixation					
Loading mode	*2× −0.028*	*4× −0.028*	*2× −0.035*	*2L −0.035*	*2L −0.028*	*4L −0.028*
Apex palmar bend	1.5	1	1.5	2	1.5	1
Apex dorsal bend	1.5	1	2	2	1.5	2
Lateral bend	2	1	1.5	2	1.5	1
Torsion	1	1	1	2	2	2
Distraction	1.5	1	1.5	2	3	2
Overall	7.5	5	7.5	10	9.5	8

Key: 1, most rigid group; 1.5, intermediate rigidity between groups 1 and 2; 3, least rigid group.

Table 7.3 A relative comparison of the rigidities of constructs formed by each of six methods of percutaneous wire fixation of metacarpal fractures under various loading conditions with an oblique fracture line. (From Ref 18 with permission.)

	Fixation					
Loading mode	*2× −0.035*	*2O −0.028*	*3O −0.028*	*2O −0.035*	*3O −0.035*	*2L −0.035*
Apex palmar bend	2	2	2	1.5	1	2
Apex dorsal bend	1	2	2	1	1	2
Lateral bend	1.5	2	1	1	1	2
Torsion	2	2	2	1	1	2
Distraction	2	2	1.5	1.5	1	3
Overall	8.5	10	8.5	6	5	11

Key: 1, most rigid group; 1.5, intermediate rigidity between groups 1 and 2; 3, least rigid group.

7.3 Fixation of the scaphoid

Loading conditions

The load bearing role of the scaphoid has been demonstrated in biomechanical studies of the wrist by measurements of contact pressures between the scaphoid and radius with loads applied through the metacarpals.[19–21] Axial load applied to the metacarpals is transferred directly by the trapezium to the distal head of the scaphoid, as well as by the head of the capitate. This causes axial compression as well as cantilever bending, which tends to create a "humpback" deformity of the fractured scaphoid, where the proximal pole displaces palmarward (or volarward) (Figure 7.9).[22–24] Therefore resisting bending is an important consideration in fixation of these fractures,[25] and the orientation of the fracture line affects bending rigidity. Considering the forces applied (Figure 7.9), a more vertical (proximal–distal) fracture line will result in more shearing of the fracture components.

Comparison of fixation techniques

Carter et al[25] compared the rigidity of three methods of fixation of the scaphoid when subjected to bending, with failure defined as a 1 mm opening of the fracture site dorsally. In their model, the fracture line was transverse, and comparisons were made between the Herbert screw (Figure 7.10),[26] a cannulated screw, and parallel K wires. As shown in Figure 7.11, both the

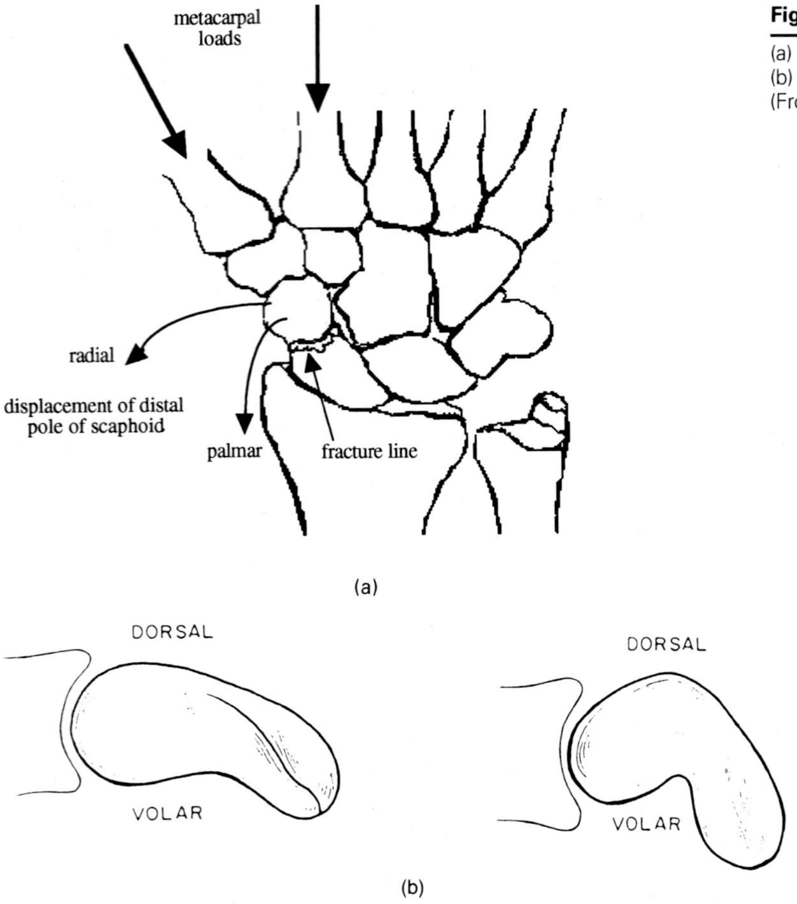

Figure 7.9

(a) Loads applied to a fractured scaphoid. (b) The resulting "humpback" deformity. (From Ref 24 with permission.)

Herbert screw and cannulated screw provide identical construct rigidity as well as supporting the same maximum bending moment, which are both approximately three times greater than for fractures fixed with crossed K wires.

Compression of the fracture site

Compression of the fracture site is important for gaining stability in scaphoid fractures, for the same reasons as discussed with reference to plate fixation. It is especially important in resisting torsion when using a single screw, which otherwise would allow rotation of the fracture components about its long axis. Shaw[27] showed that the interfragment compressive force generated by a 4.0 mm diameter cancellous screw was significantly greater than that produced by a Herbert screw (17.0 kg versus 4.4 kg) (Figure 7.12).

Summary

When fixing scaphoid fractures, consideration must be given to resisting bending, a major load applied to the construct. The rigidity of the fixed fracture will depend on the ability of the fixation to compress the fragments, the purchase of the screw, and the orientation of the fracture line.

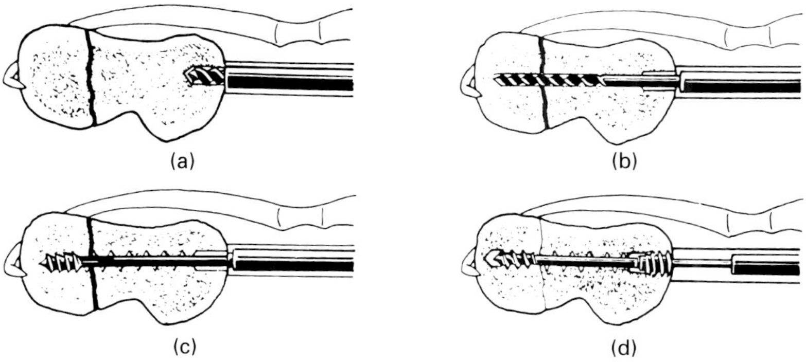

Figure 7.10

Schematic diagram of the method of insertion of the Herbert screw. (a) The pilot drill (for trailing end of screw). (b) Long drill (for leading edge of screw). (c) Tap (for leading thread). (d) The screw is inserted through the jig (the trailing thread is self tapping). The jig is used to align all instruments, and a built in stop ensures drilling to the exact length required. (From Ref 22 with permission.)

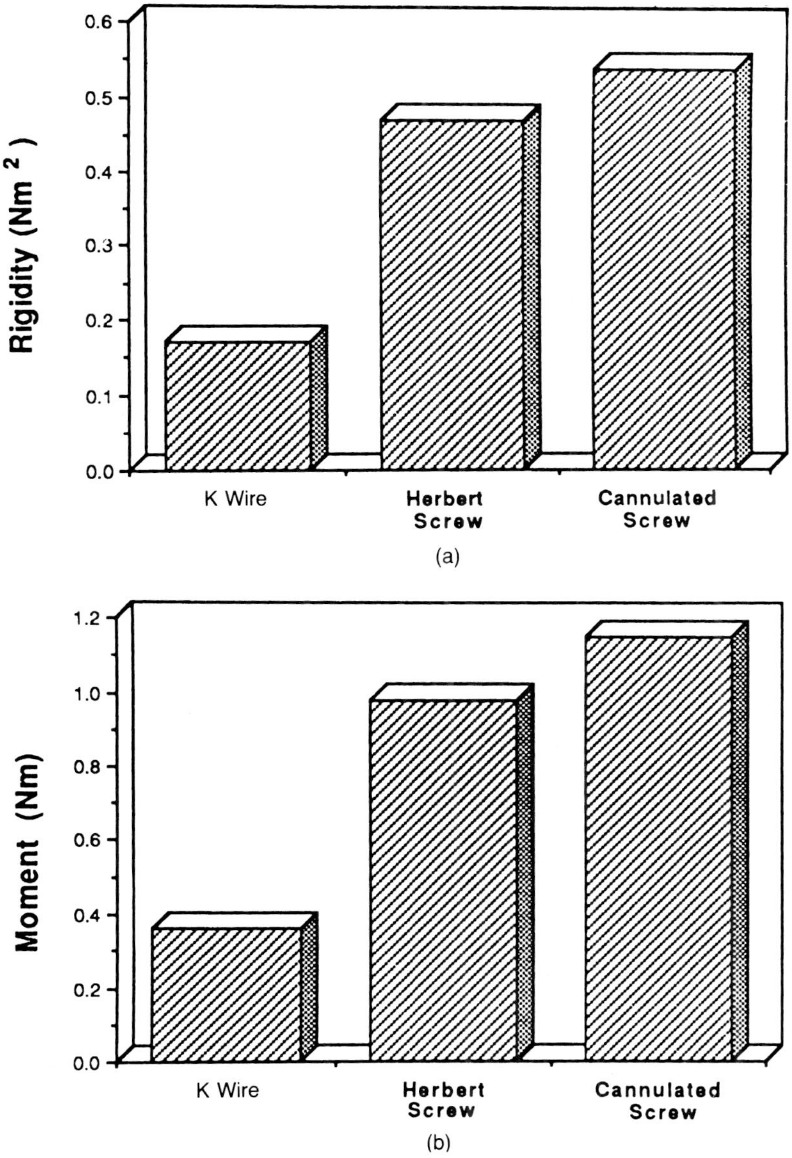

Figure 7.11

Biomechanical comparisons of scaphoid fixation constructs. (a) Construct rigidity in bending. (b) Maximum bending moment at failure. (From Ref 25 with permission.)

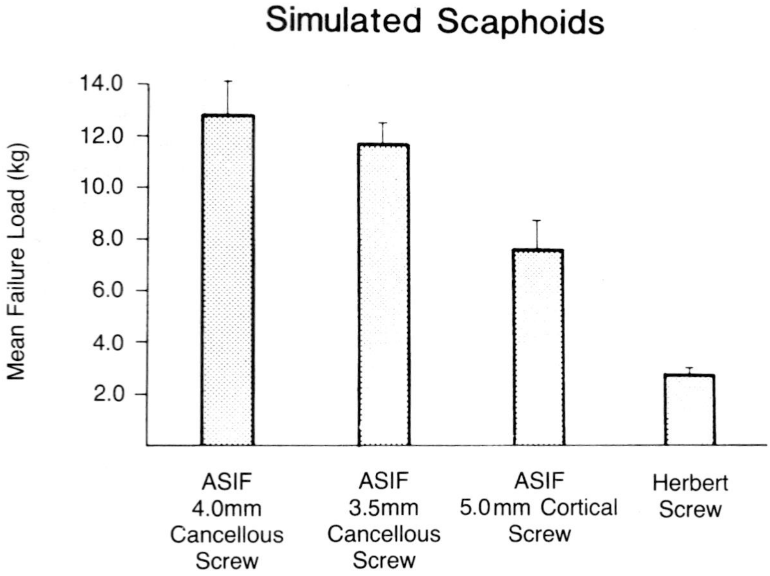

Figure 7.12

Comparison of the maximum interfragmentary compressive force generated by cancellous screws of different diameters and by the Herbert screw. (From Ref 27 with permission.)

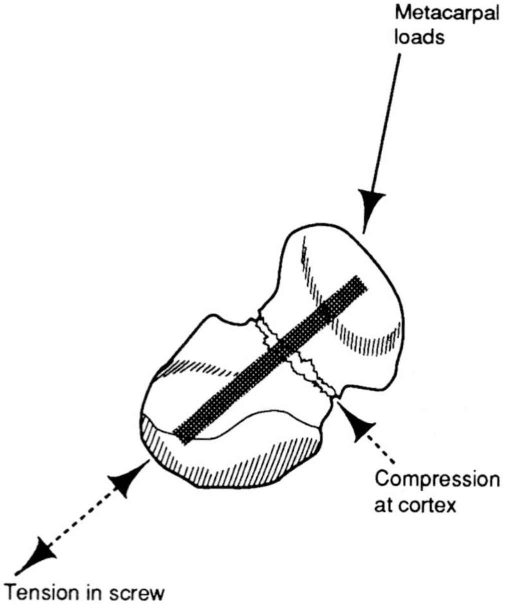

Figure 7.13

Schematic diagram demonstrating how a screw acts as a tension band to resist bending in the scaphoid.

The screw effectively acts as a tension band, while contact of the fracture components acts as a compressive buttress to resist bending (Figure 7.13).

7.4 Fixation of the trapezio-metacarpal joint

Loading conditions

Fixation across the trapeziometacarpal joint may be required due to trauma or other conditions such as joint surface degeneration. Unlike the fracture of a single bone, this joint is saddle shaped and allows a large range of flexion–extension and abduction–adduction motion.[28] Cooney and Chao[29] estimated that joint contact forces up to 164 kg, shear forces up to 21.5 kg, and axial rotation moments of up to 144 kg mm occurred in this joint during grasp. When fixed, bending moments, which the joint would not have been subjected to in its intact state are additionally applied across this articulation (Figure 7.14).

Comparison of fixation techniques

Stokel et al[30] compared four techniques of trapeziometacarpal fixation. As shown in Figure 7.15, these alternative constructs include the application of K wires, either single or crossed, or cerclage wire alone or in combination with a pin.[31–37] Both the stiffness and toggle of the fixed components were measured under various applied loads. Stiffness is defined as the applied load divided by the resulting deformation. Toggle is the looseness (movement without applying an appreciable load) that results after a complete loading cycle. This typically occurs due to cutting of wire through bone or slip of fixation pins.

The most significant differences in construct stiffness were found in axial and torsional loading. As shown in Figure 7.16, both methods of fixation using cerclage wiring produced constructs that were significantly stiffer than the other techniques in both axial tension and compression. In addition, the toggle of cerclage wire fixed constructs was lower. In torsion (Figure 7.17), results for both stiffness and toggle were similar to those of axial loading. There were few differences in fixation stiffness due to cantilever bending in any direction.

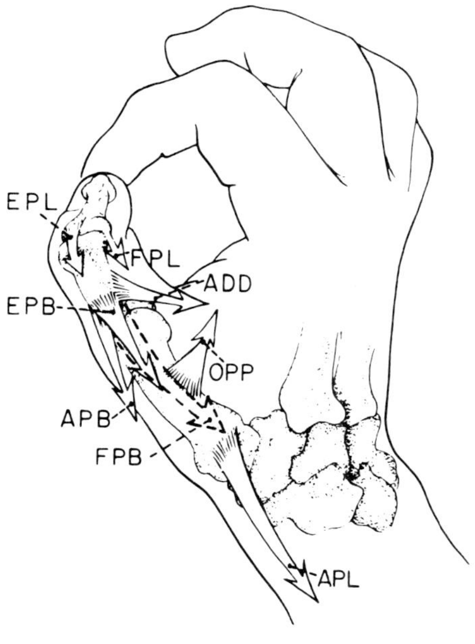

Figure 7.14

Schematic diagram demonstrating muscle loads acting on the trapeziometacarpal joint. These produce considerable bending as well as torsion about the joint. (From Ref 29 with permission.)

Summary

The differences in fixation stiffness can be attributed to the compression achieved by the wire applied in the cerclage and tension band techniques. Compression of the interfaces aids in resisting torsional moments and motion in axial loading, thereby increasing stiffness and decreasing toggle.

7.5 Fixation of fractures of the forearm

Loading conditions

Loading of the forearm is complex because of the many orientations it can assume, and the types of loads that can be applied. Three common loading modes are pure longitudinal tension, as when carrying an object with the arm at the side (elbow in 0° of flexion), torsion applied as when using the hand to twist an object, and bending with the elbow flexed and the hand either in a supinated or neutral position. Figure 7.18 illustrates a simple two dimensional free body diagram of the forearm with a load P applied near the wrist, which creates a bending moment that attempts to extend the elbow.[38] This is resisted by a combined muscle force M (biceps, brachialis, and brachioradialis), which produces a counteracting moment that flexes the elbow. A resulting joint force R must be present to maintain equilibrium. From

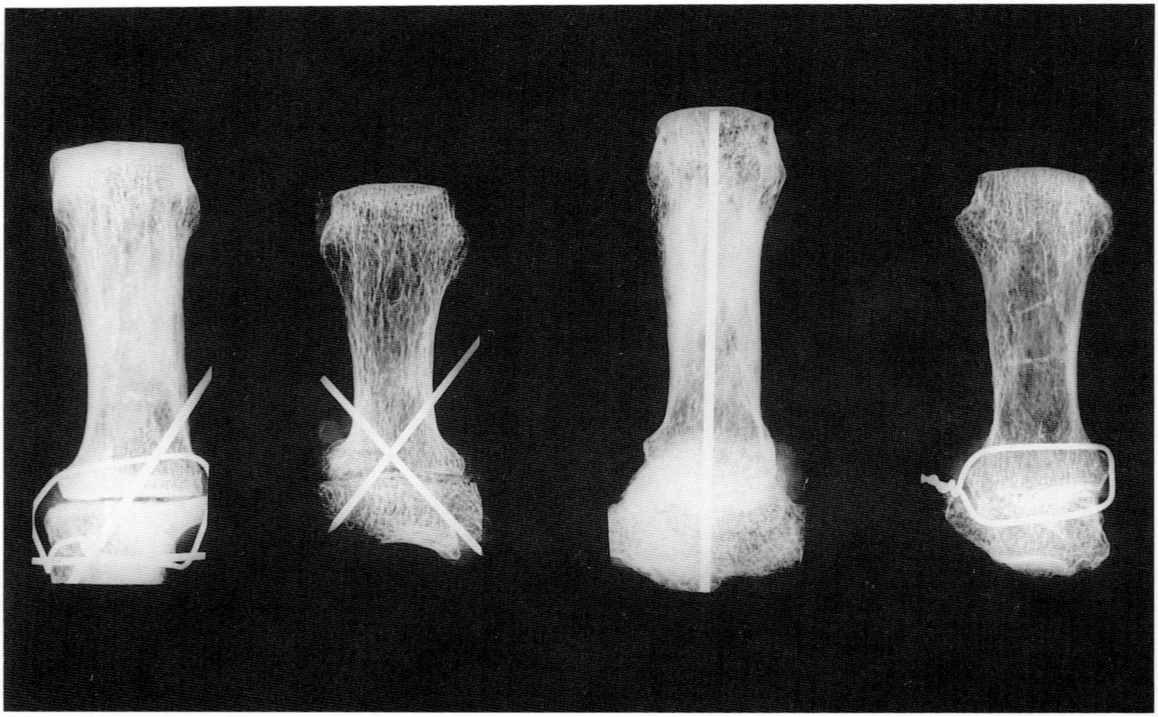

(a) (b) (c) (d)

Figure 7.15

Four alternative methods of fixation of the trapeziometacarpal joint: (a) tension band; (b) crossed K wires; (c) cup and cone; (d) cerclage wiring. (From Ref 30 with permission.)

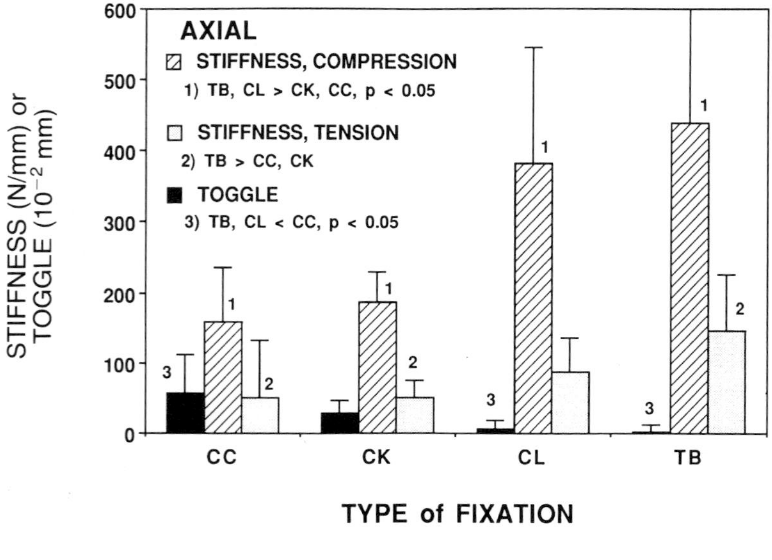

Figure 7.16

Comparison of the stiffness and toggle of trapeziometacarpal constructs fixed by four different methods loaded in axial compression and tension: CC, cup and cone; CK crossed K wires; CL cerclage wiring; TB, tension band (see Figure 7.15 for examples). (From Ref 30 with permission.)

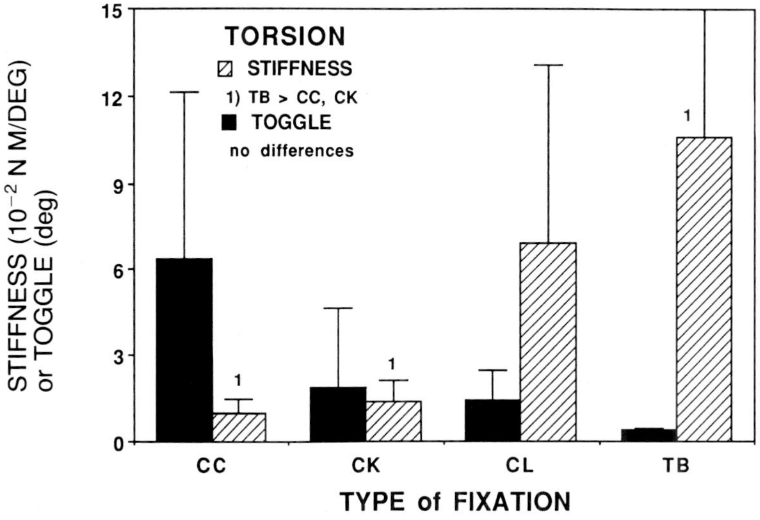

Figure 7.17

Comparison of the stiffness and toggle of trapeziometacarpal constructs fixed by four different methods loaded in torsion: CC, cup and cone; CK, crossed K wires; CL, cerclage wiring; TB, tension band (see Figure 7.15 for examples). (From Ref 30 with permission.)

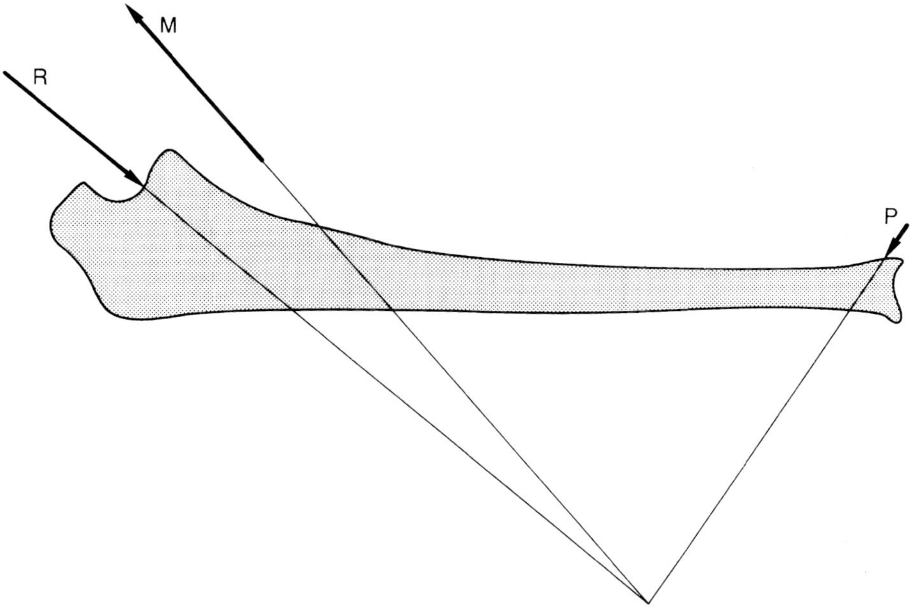

Figure 7.18

A two dimensional free body diagram of loads acting on the forearm. An external force *P* acting at the wrist produces a moment that tends to extend the elbow. It is counteracted by a combined muscle force *M* produced by the biceps, brachialis, and brachioradialis, acting across the joint. The joint reaction force *R* maintains equilibrium in the forearm. (After Ref 38.)

Table 7.4 Estimates of the maximum muscle force and elbow joint reaction force (as a percentage of body weight) due to a load applied at the wrist, based on a body weight of 670 N. BIC, biceps; BRA, brachialis; BRD, brachioradialis. (From Ref 38.)

Elbow flexion angle	*Maximum flexion strength at wrist (N)*	*Muscle force*			*Resultant joint force*
		BIC	*BRA*	*BRD*	
		(× body weight)[a]			
0°	90–150	0.79–1.19	1.2–1.81	0.29–0.39	2.15–3.2
30°	110–190	1.00–1.48	1.5–2.26	0.32–0.49	2.70–4.1
90°	220–383	0.90–1.33	1.3–2.02	0.29–0.43	2.10–3.1
120°	178–307	0.72–1.08	1.1–1.66	0.24–0.31	1.70–2.6

[a]Based on average body weight of 670 N.

analytical analyses, for maximum applied loads at the wrist at four different angles of elbow flexion, the forces in the three major flexors of the elbow as well as the magnitude of the resultant joint force have been determined as a percentage of body weight (Table 7.4). These data show that, for example, at 30° of flexion, with a 110–190 N (25–43 lb) load at the wrist, the biceps will generate 1.00–1.48 times body weight, and the joint reaction force can range from 2.7 to 4.1 times body weight. Clearly, forearm fixation must be able to resist surprisingly large moments, even though it is considered "non weight bearing".

Stability of forearm fixation

Jones et al[39] performed experiments to compare the stiffness of fixation provided by plates and intramedullary rods under several types of conditions. These included simulation of a single and double bone fracture, with or without cortical contact across the fracture gap. Examples of the fixation techniques are shown in Figure 7.19. As Figure 7.20, a comparison of the medial–lateral (ML) bending stiffnesses of the two constructs, shows, IM rodded radius fracture constructs are stiffer than the intact bone, while the plated radius is about 60% as stiff. Fixed ulnae are 70–80% as stiff as the intact bone, regardless of the fixation used. In torsion, plated fractures are significantly stiffer than rodded fractures in both the radius and the ulna (Figure 7.21).

Refracture after hardware removal

Because of the large functional loads applied to the forearm, the incidence of refracture after plate removal has been reported to range from 22 to 24%.[40,41] As shown in Table 6.1, a 3.2 mm pilot hole drilled for a 4.5 mm bone screw can reduce the torsional strength of the radius to 73% of its intact value. Naas et al[42] questioned whether a unicortical screw hole would reduce the loss of torsional strength in the forearm bones compared with a bicortical screw hole. They found no difference in the torsional strengths with either unicortical or bicortical screw holes, and concluded that removal of a forearm fracture plate should be carefully considered.

Summary

The forearm is subjected to a large and complex loading system. In particular, bending moments are produced by muscle forces that may exceed body weight in magnitude. Forearm plating produces constructs that are about 50% as stiff as intact bone in bending and 80–100% as stiff in torsion, while rodded bones are stiffer in bending and less stiff in torsion. The differences in bending stiffnesses produced by the different constructs is related to their shape (moment of inertia). In torsional loading, the difficulty in gaining purchase accounts partly for the low torsional stiffness of rodded bones. A 3.2 mm hole in the

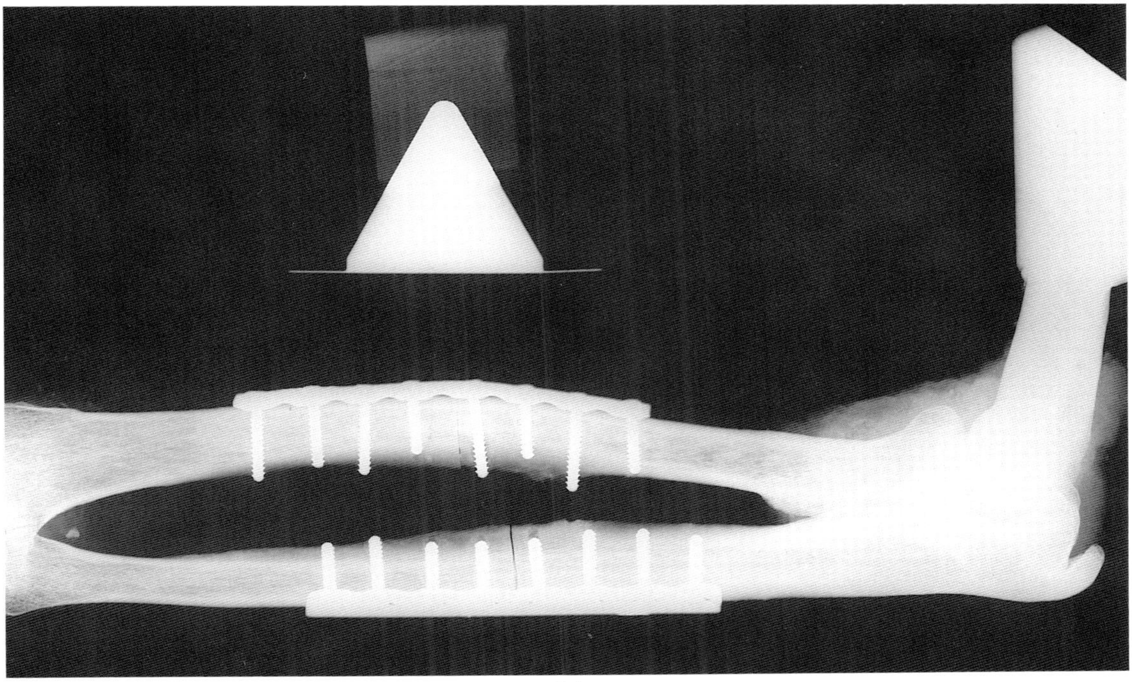

(a)

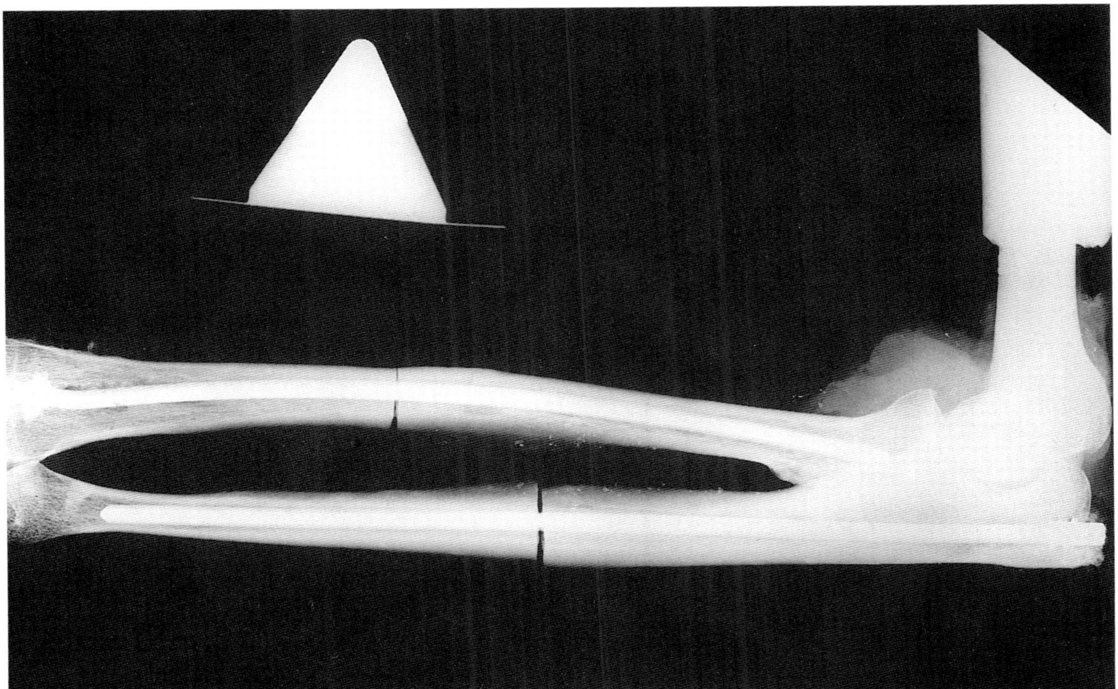

(b)

Figure 7.19

Examples of fixation of double forearm fractures with (a) plates or (b) intramedullary rods. (From Ref 39.)

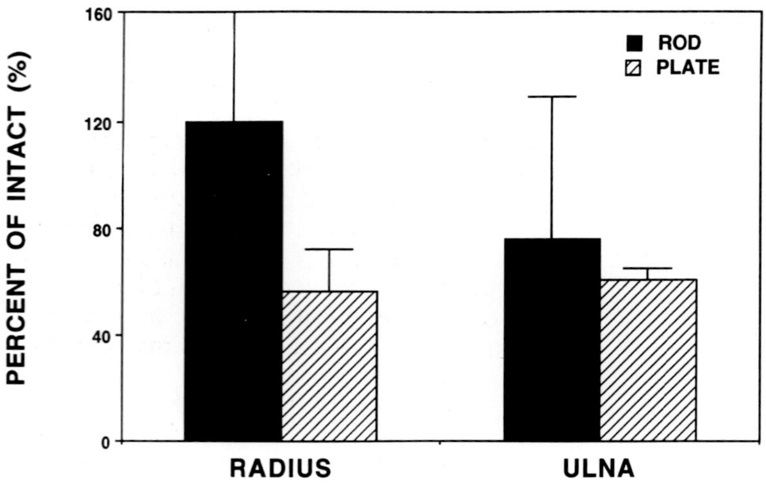

Figure 7.20

Stiffness of plated or intramedullary rodded fractures of the forearm in medial–lateral bending. (From Ref 39.)

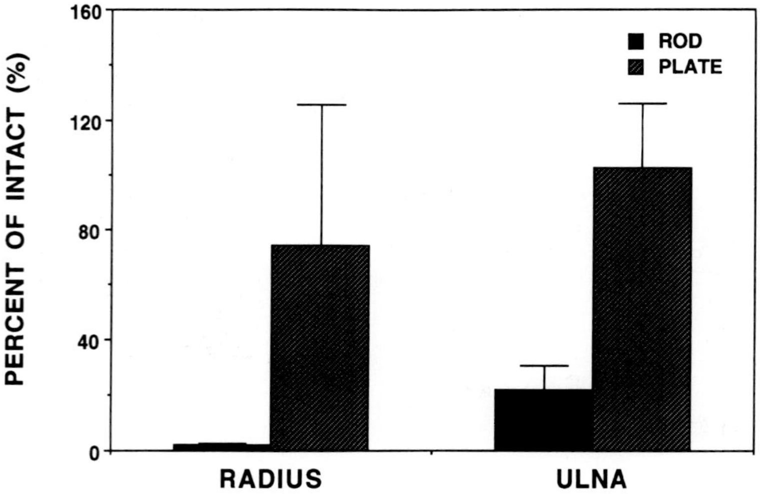

Figure 7.21

Stiffness of plated or intramedullary rodded fractures of the forearm in torsion. (From Ref 39.)

radius can reduce its torsional stiffness to 73% of intact. There is no benefit in terms of preventing refracture after hardware removal by using unicortical screws. Therefore careful consideration should be given to the decrease in strength that accompanies removal of a fracture plate from bones of the forearm.

7.6 Fixation of the distal humerus

Loading conditions

While the midshaft of a long bone is subjected to bending, the metaphysis is loaded primarily in compression. The compressive force arises from the joint reaction force that is required to maintain equilibrium between the external and muscle forces applied to the forearm (Figure 7.18). As shown in Figure 7.22 for the trochlea of the ulna, a contact pressure distribution will occur in the articular cartilage due to the joint reaction force. Its orientation and magnitude will change with both the orientation of the external load applied and the flexion angle of the elbow. The joint force magnitude may be as large as 4.1 times body weight (Table 7.4).[38]

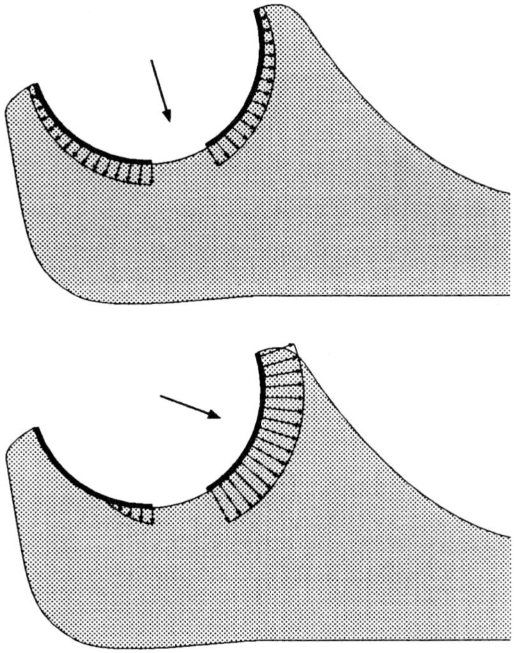

Figure 7.22

A schematic diagram of the trochlea of the ulna, showing how the joint reaction force is distributed over the articular cartilage for two different orientations of the joint reaction force. (After Ref 38.)

Fixation stability

Goulet et al[43] compared several currently used constructs[44–47] for the fixation of supra- and intercondylar fractures of the distal humerus when subjected to torsional loading, with and without cortical contact at the fracture site. Their results showed that reconstruction plates oriented at 90° (posteriorly on the lateral column and medially on the medial column of the distal humerus) were more effective in providing torsional stiffness to the construct than one third tubular plates or crossed K wires.

In a more comprehensive study that encompassed testing under axial compressive and tensile loads, torsion, and cantilever bending both in medial–lateral (ML) and anterior–posterior (AP) directions, Schemitsch et al[48] compared stiffnesses of fixation of five constructs, including reconstruction (R) plates, an anatomic (J) plate,[49] and combinations of the two, as shown in Figure 7.23. In axial loading, with no gap across the fracture, there was no difference in stiffness between the different constructs. However, with a gap (no cortical contact), the lateral J plate–medial R plate combination provided the greatest rigidity (Figure 7.24). In torsion with no fracture gap, the two plate fixations produced more rigid constructs than single plate constructs. With a gap, the J plate–R plate combination was again the most rigid construct. The results in both planes of bending were similar to those in torsion.

Summary

The distal metaphyseal region of the humerus is subjected mainly to axial compression and torsion. The most rigid fixation in a fracture with good cortical contact is provided by any two plate constructs, either an anatomic J plate or a reconstruction plate, applied on any aspect of the humerus. However, with little contact, the combination of a J plate applied laterally and an R plate applied medially produces the stiffest construct under any loading condition.

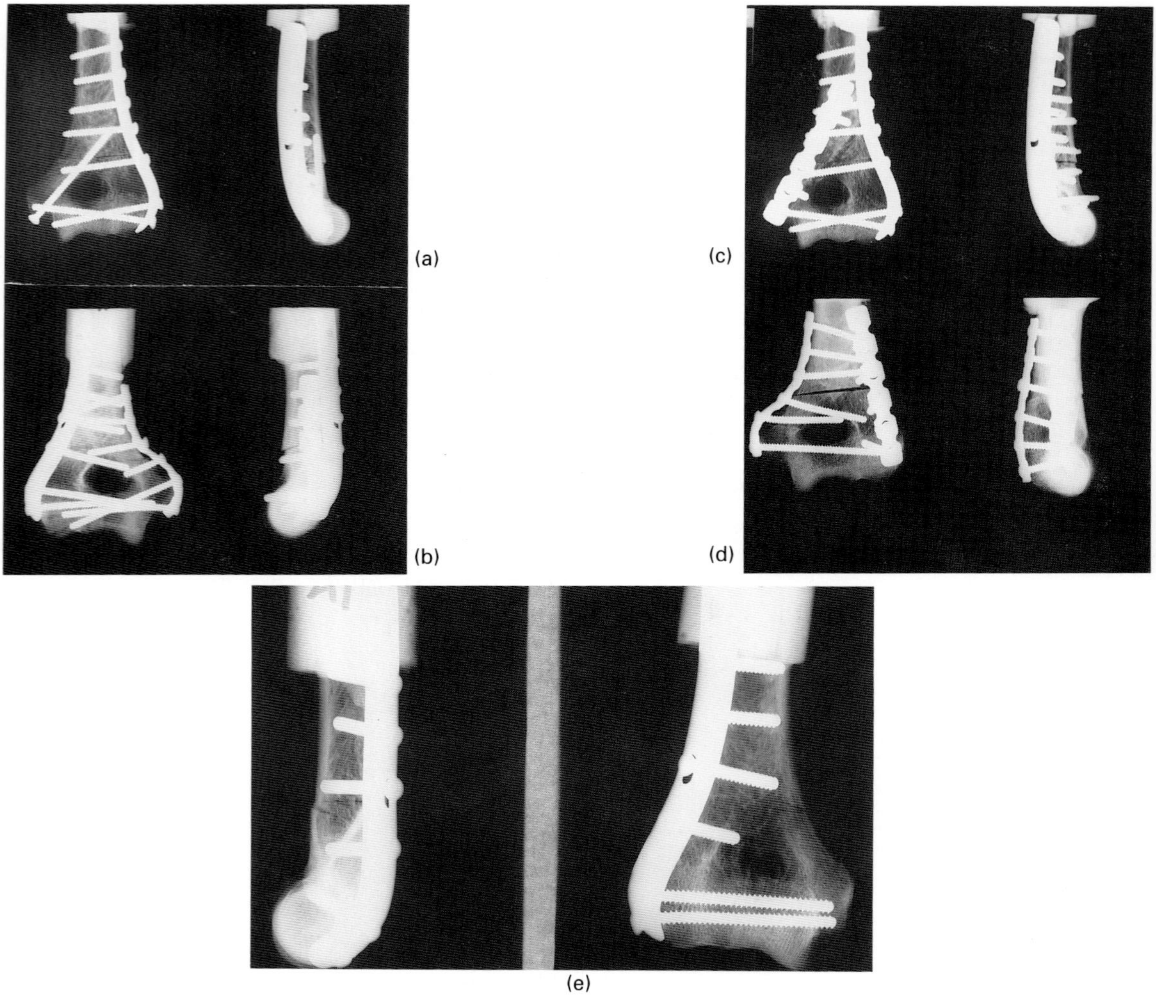

Figure 7.23

Five methods of internal fixation of a fracture of the distal humerus: (a) single J (anatomic) plate on lateral side with medial lag screw; (b) lateral J plate and medial R (reconstruction) plate; (c) lateral J plate and posteriomedial R plate; (d) posteriolateral and medial R plates; (e) single lateral J plate. (From Ref 48.)

7.7 Fixation of the humeral shaft

Loading conditions

The loads acting on the humerus are similar in many respects to those of the forearm. The arm is elevated by several muscle groups (deltoid, biceps, supraspinatus), which produce, along with external loads and the weight of the hand and forearm, bending moments along with joint compression. Inman et al,[50] as shown in Figure 7.25, estimated the force generated by the deltoid along with the joint reaction force at the glenoid for different positions of arm elevation. The peak deltoid force was determined to occur at 90° of arm elevation, and reached a magnitude of about 70% body weight (about 10 times the weight of the extremity), simply to lift the weight of the arm. These large forces occur because the distance of the center of gravity of the upper extremity from

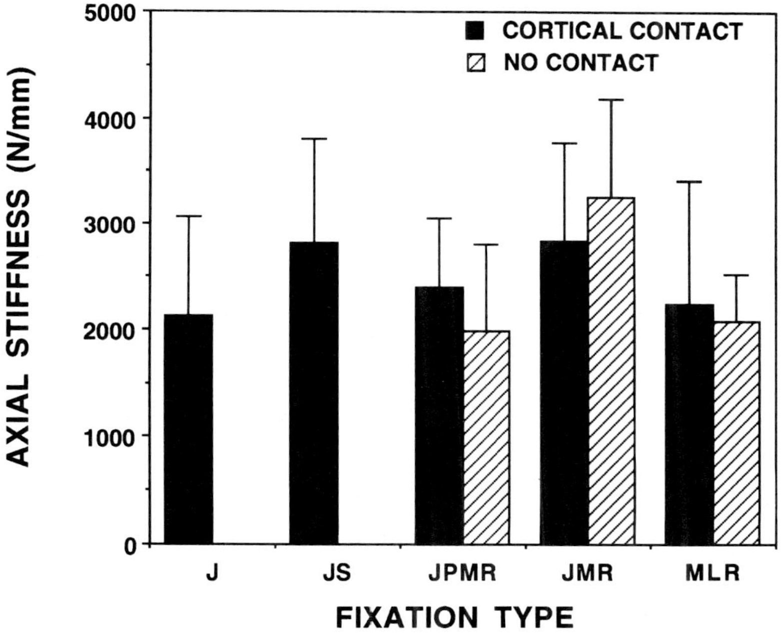

Figure 7.24

Comparison of the construct stiffnesses of five methods of fixation of distal fractures of the humerus in axial loading: J, lateral J plate; JS, lateral J plate and medial condylar screw; JPMR, lateral J plate and posteriomedial R (reconstruction) plate; JMR, lateral J plate and medial R plate; MLR, medial and posterolateral R plates. (From Ref 48.)

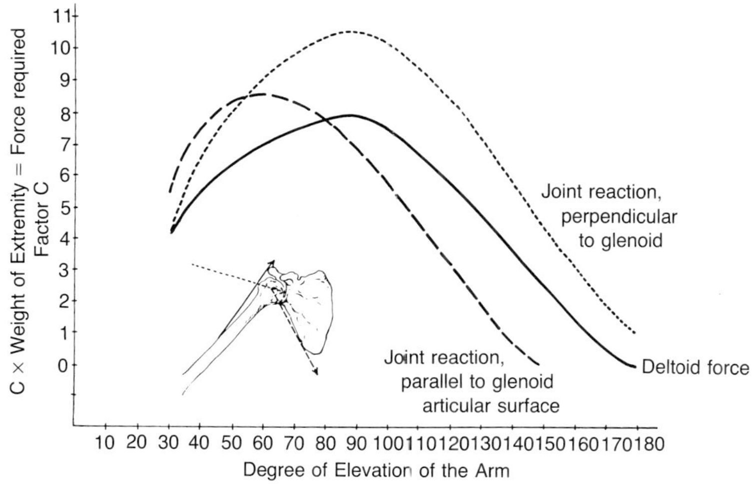

Figure 7.25

Estimated force in the deltoid and joint reaction force as a function of arm elevation angle. (From Ref 50 with permission.)

the center of the humeral head produces a large moment. In contrast, the moment arms of the muscles are small.

Comparison of fixation techniques

In a study by Henley et al,[51] the stiffness of several constructs that have been described for fixation of a fracture of the midshaft of the humerus[52–60] were compared. Alternatives for fixation included, as shown in Figure 7.26, two types of intramedullary flexible pins, a dynamic compression (DC) plate, and two tubular intramedullary nails (IM). In comparing the two types of flexible pins and also the two types of nails, constructs were not significantly different in stiffness from one another (Table 7.5). Nail constructs were stiffer than plate constructs in bending, but less stiff in torsion (a result similar to that found in forearm fixation). Relative to intact bone, in bending, the flexible pins produced constructs that ranged from 13% to 24%, the DC plate from 30% to 43%, and the IM nails from 64% to 104% (Figure 7.27). In

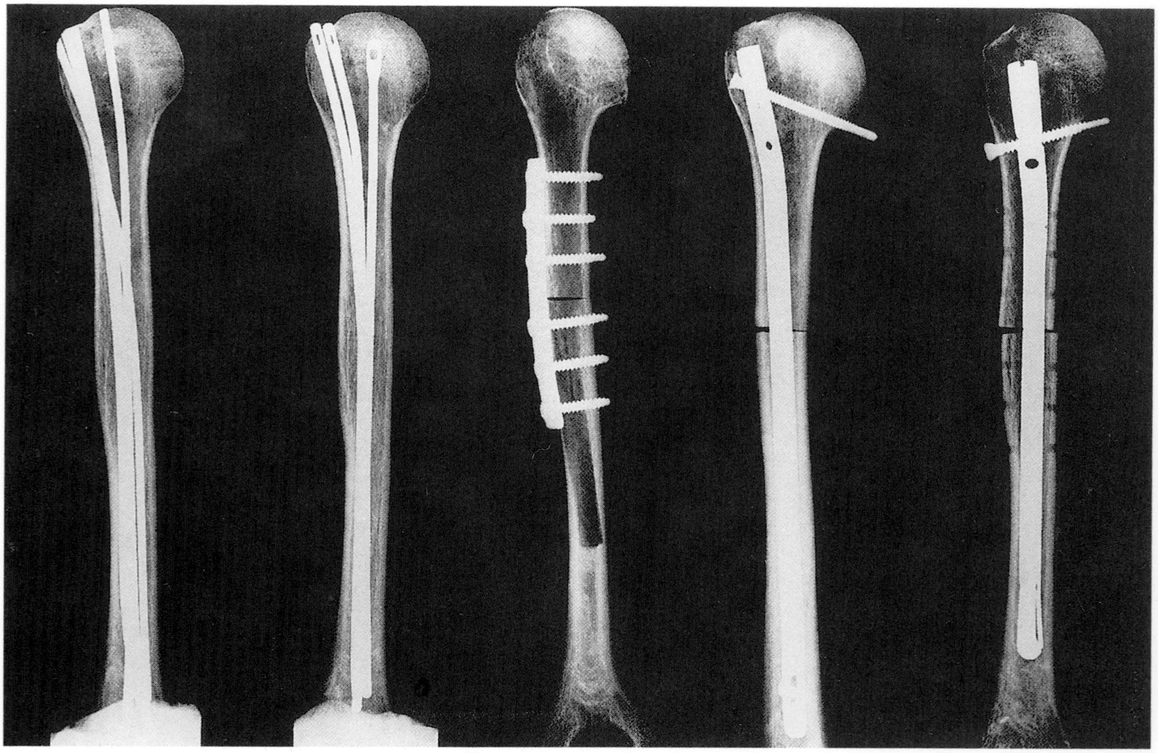

(a) (b) (c) (d) (e)

Figure 7.26

Alternatives for fixation of humeral shaft fractures: (a) Hackethal pins; (b) Enders pins; (c) dynamic compression plate; (d) Russell–Taylor 9 mm diameter nail; (e) Seidel 9 mm nail. (From Ref 51 with permission.)

Table 7.5 Paired comparison of the stiffness of humeral fracture constructs produced by various forms of fixation (units for bending are N/mm, for torsion, N m/deg (SD)). (From Ref 51 with permission.)

	Intact	*Flexible* IM *pins*			*Plate versus locking* IM *nail*			*Locking* IM *nails*		
		HP	*EP*	*Significance*	*DC*	*RN*	*Significance*	*RN*	*SN*	*Significance*
Posterior bending (N/mm)	7.52 (3.60)	1.82 (1.63)	1.69 (1.15)	NS	3.22 (0.93)	7.79 (2.90)	$p = 0.017$	7.79 (2.90)	5.50 (1.07)	NS
Lateral bending (N/mm)	13.81 (4.16)	2.70 (1.56)	1.85 (0.50)	NS	4.16 (0.49)	8.78 (2.66)	$p = 0.009$	8.78 (2.66)	10.19 (4.30)	NS
Torsion (N m/deg)	0.25 (0.09)	0.09 (0.05)	0.11 (0.07)	NS	1.37 (0.31)	0.43 (0.21)	$p = 0.001$	0.43 (0.21)	0.51 (0.37)	NS

Key: IM, intramedullary; HP, Hackethal IM pins; EP, Enders IM pins; DC, dynamic compression plates; RN, Russell–Taylor closed-section tubular interlocking IM nails; SN, 9 mm diameter interlocking Seidel IM nails; NS, not significant.

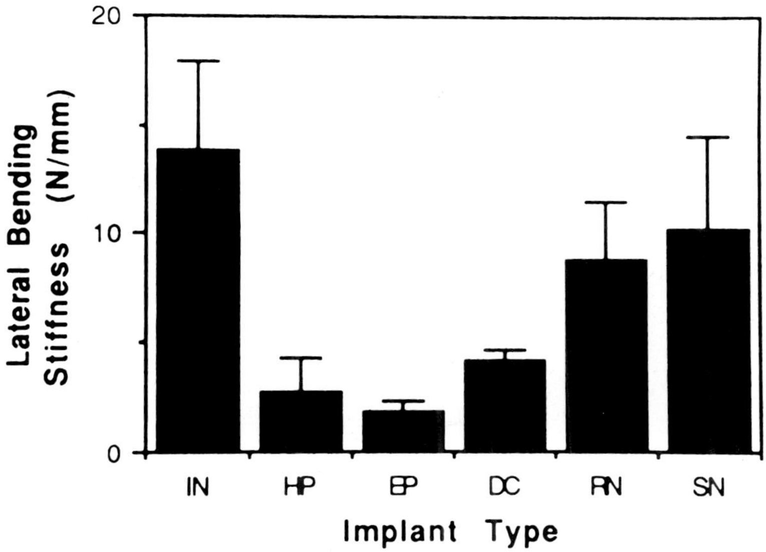

Figure 7.27

A comparison of the cantilever lateral bending stiffness of constructs formed by various implants: IN, intact; HP, Hackethal pins; EP, Enders pins; DC, dynamic compression plate; RN, Russell-Taylor 9 mm diameter IM nail; SN, Seidel 9 mm diameter IM nail. (From Ref 51 with permission.)

torsion, the stiffness values were 36–44% for pins, 548% for the plate, and 172–204% for IM nails. The maximum torque sustained by DC plate and IM rod constructs are not significantly different.[61]

Summary

The humerus is a bone that may be subjected to large loads, nearly equal to body weight, even when only lifting the arm against gravity. Therefore secure fixation is important for preventing fracture site motion. Comparatively, the IM nails produce constructs that, in bending, reach or exceed the desirable upper limit for fixation stiffness, discussed in Chapter 4. The IM rod is more rigid in bending because (disregarding load transfer through bone fracture surfaces) its area moment of inertia may be 6–8 times greater than that of a typical plate, depending on whether the rod is solid or tubular (Figure 7.28). In torsion, the plate fixed constructs are excessively rigid. There-

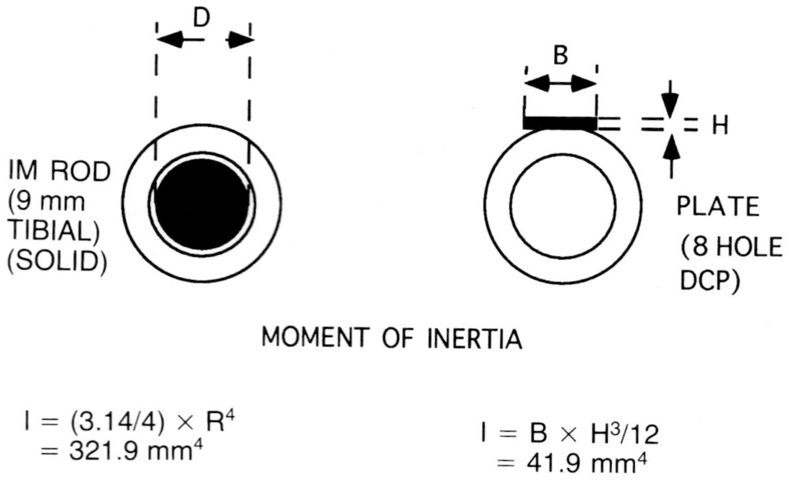

Figure 7.28

The moment of inertia of a typical IM rod for the humerus may be nearly 8 times greater than that of an eight hole DC plate, so for the same material, the rod will be considerably stiffer in bending.

fore the IM rod appears to be a better compromise, in terms of biomechanical performance, for fixation of midshaft humeral fractures.

7.8 References

1. Chao EY, Opgrande JD, Axmear FE, Three dimensional force analysis of finger joints in selected isometric hand functions, *J Biomech* (1976) **9**: 387–96.
2. Allende BT, Engelem JC, Tension band arthrodesis in the finger joints, *J Hand Surg* (1980) **5**: 269–71.
3. Carroll RE, Hill NA, Small joint arthrodesis in hand reconstruction, *J Bone Jt Surg* (1969) **51A**: 1219–21.
4. Harrison SH, Nicolle FV, A new intramedullary bone plug for digital arthrodesis, *Br J Plast Surg* (1974) **27**: 240–1.
5. Hogh J, Jensen PQ, Compression arthrodesis of finger joints using Kirschner wires and cerclage, *Hand* (1982) **14**: 149–52.
6. Watson HK, Schaffer SR, Concave–convex arthrodeses in joints of the hand, *Plast Reconstr Surg* (1970) **46**: 368–71.
7. Wexler MR, Rousso M, Weinberg H, Arthrodeses of finger joints by dynamic external compression, *Plast Reconstr Surg* (1977) **59**: 882–5.
8. Stern PJ, Drury WJ, Tension band arthrodesis of small joints, *Contemp Orthop* (1984) **8**: 59–62.
9. Kovach JC, Werner FW, Palmer AK, Greenkey S, Murphy DJ, Biomechanical analysis of internal fixation techniques for proximal interphalangeal joint arthrodesis, *J Hand Surg* (1986) **11A**: 562–6.
10. Kato S, Latta L, Burkhalter WE, Mechanical evaluation of external and internal fixation for metacarpal fractures, *Trans 32nd Orthopedic Research Society Meeting* (1986) **10**: 316.
11. Lister G, Intraosseous wiring of the digital skeleton, *J Hand Surg* (1978) **11**: 50–4.
12. Stern PJ, Wieser MJ, Reilly DG, Complications of plate fixation in the hand skeleton, *Clin Orthop* (1987) **214**: 59–65.
13. Green DP, Anderson JR, Closed reduction and percutaneous pin fixation of fractured phalanges, *J Bone Jt Surg* (1973) **55A**: 1651–4.
14. Joshi BB, Percutaneous internal fixation of fractures of the proximal phalanges, *Hand* (1976) **8**: 86–92.
15. Belsky MR, Eaton RG, Lane LB, Closed reduction and internal fixation of proximal phalangeal fractures, *J Hand Surg* (1984) **9A**: 725–9.
16. Clifford RH, Intramedullary wire fixation of hand fractures, *Plast Reconstr Surg* (1953) **11**: 366–71.
17. Mann RJ, Black D, Constine R, Daniels AU, A quantitative comparison of metacarpal fracture stability with five different methods of internal fixation, *J Hand Surg* (1985) **10A**: 1024–8.
18. Viegas SF, Ferren EL, Self J, Tencer AF, Comparative mechanical properties of various Kirschner wire configurations in transverse and oblique phalangeal fractures, *J Hand Surg* (1988) **13A**: 246–55.

19. Tencer AF, Viegas SF, Cantrell J, Chang M, Clegg P, Hicks C, O'Meara C, Williamson JB, Contact pressure measurements in the wrist, *J Orthop Res* (1988) **6**: 509–17.
20. Viegas SF, Patterson R, Peterson P, Roefs J, Tencer AF, Choi S, The effects of various load paths and different loads on the load transfer characteristics of the wrist, *J Hand Surg* (1989) **14A**: 458–465.
21. Augsburger S, Necking L, Horton J, Bach AW, Tencer AF, A comparison of scapho-trapezium–trapezoid fusion and four bone tendon weave for scapho-lunate dissociation, *J Hand Surg* (1992) **17**: 360–9.
22. Taleisnik J, Fractures of the carpal bones. In: Green DP, ed, *Operative hand surgery*, 2nd edn (Churchill Livingstone: New York 1988) 813–74.
23. Weber ER, Biomechanical implications of scaphoid wrist fractures, *Clin Orthop* (1980) **149**: 83–9.
24. Smith DK, An KN, Cooney III WP, Linscheid RL, Chao EYS, Effects of a scaphoid waist osteotomy on carpal kinematics, *J Orthop Res* (1989) **7**: 590–8.
25. Carter II FM, Mackessy RP, Dipaola DM, Zimmerman MC, Parsons JR, Biomechanical comparison of scaphoid fracture fixation devices, *Trans 37th Orthopedic Research Society Meeting* (1991) **16**: 179.
26. Herbert TJ, Fisher WE, Management of the fractured scaphoid using a new bone screw, *J Bone Jt Surg* (1984) **66B**: 114–23.
27. Shaw JA, A biomechanical comparison of scaphoid screws, *J Hand Surg* (1987) **12A**: 347–53.
28. Cooney III WP, Lucca MJ, Chao EYS, Linscheid RL, The kinesiology of the thumb trapeziometacarpal joint, *J Bone Jt Surg* (1981) **63A**: 1371–81.
29. Cooney III WP, Chao EYS, Biomechanical analysis of static forces in the thumb during hand function, *J Bone Jt Surg* (1977) **59A**: 27–36.
30. Stokel EA, Tencer AF, Driscoll HL, Trumble TE, A biomechanical comparison of four methods of fixation of the trapeziometacarpal joint, *J Hand Surg* (in press).
31. Carroll RE, Hill NA, Arthrodesis of the carpometacarpal joint of the thumb, *J Bone Jt Surg* (1973) **55B**: 292–4.
32. Dolye JR, Sliding bone graft technique for arthrodesis of the trapeziometacarpal joint of the thumb, *J Hand Surg* (1991) **16A**: 363–5.
33. Kvarnes L, Reikeras O, Osteoarthritis of the carpometacarpal joint of the thumb. An analysis of operative procedures, *J Hand Surg* (1985) **10B**: 117–20.
34. Leach RE, Bolton PE, Arthritis of the carpometacarpal joint of the thumb, *J Bone Jt Surg* (1968) **50A**: 1171–7.
35. Mattsson HS, Arthrodesis of the first carpometacarpal joint for osteoarthritis, *Acta Orthop Scand* (1969) **40**: 602–7.
36. Muller GM, Arthrodesis of the trapeziometacarpal joint for osteoarthritis, *J Bone Jt Surg* (1949) **31B**: 540–2.
37. Stark HH, Moore JF, Ashworth CR, Boyes JH, Fusion of the first metacarpotrapezial joint for degenerative arthritis, *J Bone Jt Surg* (1977) **29A**: 22–6.
38. An KA, Morrey BF, Biomechanics of the elbow. In: Morrey BF, ed, *The elbow and its disorders* (WB Saunders: Philadelphia 1985) 43–61.
39. Jones DJ, Schemitz E, Tencer AF, Henley MB, A comparison of the stability of forearm fractures fixed by plates or intramedullary rods (in preparation).
40. Anderson LD, Sisk TD, Tooms RE, Park III WI, Compression plate fixation in acute diaphyseal fractures of the radius and ulna, *J Bone Jt Surg* (1975) **57**: 287–97.
41. Hidaka S, Gustillo RB, Refracture of the bones of the forearm after plate removal, *J Bone Jt Surg* (1984) **66A**: 1241–2.
42. Nass PL, Hoeltzel DA, Gustilo RB, Biomechanical evaluation of unicortical vs. bicortical screw fixation for forearm fractures, *Trans 31st Orthopedic Research Society Meeting* (1985) **10**: 220.
43. Goulet J, Kirk P, Freiberg A, Goldstein S, A biomechanical evaluation of fixation methods for fractures of the distal humerus, *Orthop Trans* (1990) **14**: 674.
44. Helfet DL, Bicondylar intraarticular fracture of the distal humerus in adults: their assessment, classification, and operative management. *Adv Orthop Surg* (1985) **8**: 223–35.
45. Henley MB, Bone LB, Parker B, Operative management of intraarticular fractures of the distal humerus, *J Orthop Trauma* (1987) **1**: 24–35.
46. Müller ME, Allgöwer M, Schneider R, Fractures of the distal humerus. In: *Manual of internal fixation*, 3rd edn (Springer-Verlag: New York 1991) 446–51.
47. Waddell JP, Hatch J, Richards R, Supracondylar fractures of the humerus. Results of surgical treatment, *J Trauma* (1988) **28**: 1615–21.
48. Schemitsch E, Tencer AF, Henley MB, A biomechanical evaluation of methods of internal fixation of the distal humerus, *Trans 39th Orthopedic Research Society Meeting* (1993) **18**: 566.
49. Lecestre P, Dupont JY, Lortart JA, Les fractures complexes de l'extremité inférieure de l'humérus chez l'adult, *Revue de Chirurgie Orthopédique* (1979) **65**: 11–23.
50. Inman VT, Saunders JB, Abbot LC, Observations on the function of the shoulder joint, *J Bone Jt Surg* (1944) **26A**: 1–30.
51. Henley MB, Monroe M, Tencer AF, Biomechanical comparison of methods of fixation of a midshaft osteotomy of the humerus, *J Orthop Trauma* (1991) **5**: 14–20.

52. Chacha PB, Compression plating without bone grafts for delayed and nonunion of humeral shaft fractures, *Injury* (1974) **5:** 283–290.
53. Ruedi T, Moshlegh A, Pfieffer KM, Allgöwer M, Fresh fractures of the shaft of the humerus—conservative or operative treatment?, *Reconstr Surg Traumatol* (1974) **14:** 65–74.
54. Titze A, The operative treatment of fractures of the humerus, *Reconstr Surg Traumatol* (1974) **14:** 75–83.
55. Putz P, Treatment of humeral diaphysis fractures by Hackethal method, *Acta Orthop Belg* (1984) **50:** 521–38.
56. Dobozi WR, Hall Jr RF, Flexible intramedullary nailing of humeral shaft fractures. In: Browner BD, Edwards CC, eds, *The science and practise of intramedullary nailing* (Lea & Febiger: Philadelphia 1987) 305–18.
57. Hall Jr RF, Pankovich AM, Technique and results of closed intramedullary rodding of diaphyseal fractures of the humerus, *Orthop Trans* (1982) **6:** 359.
58. Hempel VD, Intramedullary nailing of the humerus, In: Browner BD, Edwards CC, eds, *The science and practise of intramedullary nailing* (Lea & Febiger: Philadelphia 1987) 319–23.
59. Rokkanen P, Slatis P, Vankka E, Closed or open intramedullary nailing of femoral shaft fractures? A comparison with conservatively treated cases, *J Bone Jt Surg* (1969) **51B:** 313–23.
60. War EF, White JL, Interlocking intramedullary nailing of the humerus, *Orthopedics* (1989) **12:** 135–41.
61. Waite AM, Zimmerman MC, Tovey JE, Oppenheim WC, Parsons JR, A biomechanical analysis of three humeral fracture fixation devices, *Trans 38th Orthopedic Research Society Meeting* (1992) **17:** 410.

CHAPTER 8

Spine and pelvis fixation

The goal of this chapter is to define the principles and performance characteristics of fixation techniques used in spine and pelvic fixation. Following a description of the biomechanics of the intact and injured spine, various forms of cervical spine fixation, both nonoperative and operative, are discussed. Thoracolumbar spine fixation is presented in relation to increasing severity and differing locations of injury. The biomechanical properties of lumbosacral junction and pelvic fracture fixation are then discussed.

8.1 Mechanics of the intact spine

Before selecting a fixation system to restore stability to the injured spine, it is important to understand the functions of the damaged structures and how the mechanics of the spine are changed by their loss. The complexity of the spine lies in its functional requirement both as a joint that provides mobility, and as a load bearing structure.

The vertebral motion segment can be considered mechanically as two vertebrae interconnected by three types of mechanical elements, the disc, the facet joints with their capsules, and the various spinal ligaments (Figure 8.1). The disc is composed of the annulus fibrosus, which contains bands of collagenous tissue of alternating fibers, with a semifluid nucleus in its center, and flexible end plates to prevent the nucleus material from escaping into the vertebral body. Under load, nucleus pressure increases,[1] creating vertical bulging in the vertebral endplates and radial bulging of the annulus.[2] Loss of nucleus material results in inward bulging of the inner layers of the annulus,[3] along with decreases in mechanical stiffness of the spine.[4] Because of its structure and wide attachment to the vertebral bodies, the annulus is the main load bearing member in the intervertebral joint. It contributes principally to resisting anterior/posterior and medial/lateral shearing movements of the inferior vertebra with respect to the superior one, axial compression and tension, flexion, torsion, and extension.[5] The relative contributions of the disc and facets to limiting motions in various loading directions are given in Table 8.1.

The lumbar facet joints, along with their capsules, play an important role in load sharing with the disc. The interference of the facet surfaces limits motion in anterior displacement of the superior vertebra, and in torsion about the long axis of the spine. The facet capsules play a significant role in limiting flexion and torsional rotations, along with the disc in the lumbar spine (Table 8.1).[5,6]

The spinal ligaments act as secondary stabilizers in comparison to the disc and facet joints, with their principal contributions being in flexion and extension.[5] Panjabi et al[7] found that the

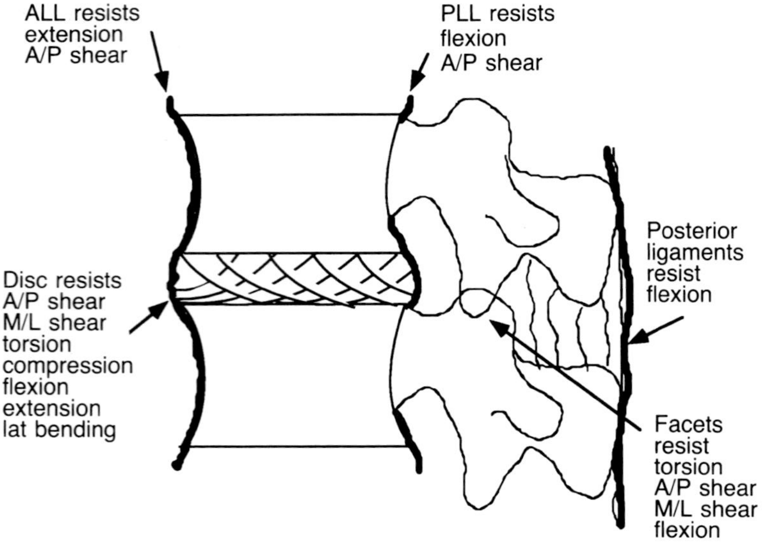

Figure 8.1

Mechanical function of the supporting and connecting structures of the intervertebral motion segment: ALL, anterior longitudinal ligament; PLL, posterior longitudinal ligament.

Table 8.1 Relative contributions of the disc and facets, including facet capsules, to limiting motion under various loading conditions in the lumbar spine. (Data adapted from Ref 5.)

Direction of motion	*Stiffness*	
	Facets injured (% of intact)	*Disc injured (% of intact)*
Right lateral shear	100	71.7
Anterior shear	100	84.6
Posterior shear	58.3	84.6
Axial compression	100	71.2
Flexion	81.5	87.7
Extension	86.8	88.3
Lateral bending	89.0	78.5
Axial torsion	49.8	55.9

maximum strain in the anterior longitudinal ligament (ALL) occurred during extension of the motion segment, while the posterior longitudinal (PLL), interspinous (ISL), supraspinous (SSL), and ligamentum flavum (LF) all had greatest strains in flexion. The greatest strains in the transverse ligament (TL) occurred on the side opposite the direction of lateral bending, and, for the facet capsules (CL), in the facet that opens when axial torque is applied (Table 8.2).

Table 8.2 Mean maximum strains for spinal ligaments: ALL, anterior longitudinal; PLL, posterior longitudinal; TL, transverse; LF, ligamentum flavum; CL, capsular ligament; ISL, interspinous ligament; SSL, supraspinous ligament. (From Ref 7 with permission.)

Ligament	*Strain (%)*	*Associated movement*
ALL	12.85	Extension
PLL	13.05	Flexion
TL	25.50	Lateral bending
LF	16.20	Flexion
CL	19.25	Rotation
ISL	27.90	Flexion
SSL	31.95	Flexion

Note: For each ligament, average maximum strain was computed as the sum of the maximum positive active strains during any of the three motions and half the corresponding neutral zone strain.

8.2 Cervical spine injury biomechanics

Loading conditions

The cervical spine is subjected to two types of external loads: the weight of the head due to gravity and the inertial forces that result when it is accelerated and decelerated, as well as forces and moments generated by the musculature acting about the neck. Figure 8.2 shows a cross section through the neck at the C4 level, indicating the various muscle groups that act on the cervical spine. With maximum voluntary lateral bending, axial twisting, flexion, and extension of the head and neck, Table 8.3 shows the expected forces and moments on the cervical spine.[8] The moments to which the cervical spine is subjected range to 25.9 N m in extension, and forces at the C4 level can be as large as 1164 N in compression and 135 N in shear. The large compressive forces, about 10 times the weight of the head, occur as a result of muscles that counteract the applied moments of other forces. Of importance from a fixation stability standpoint are the relatively large shear forces across the joint. Shear is particularly dangerous, since it tends to displace one vertebra horizontally with respect to another, and may reduce the cross section of the spinal canal, compressing the spinal cord.

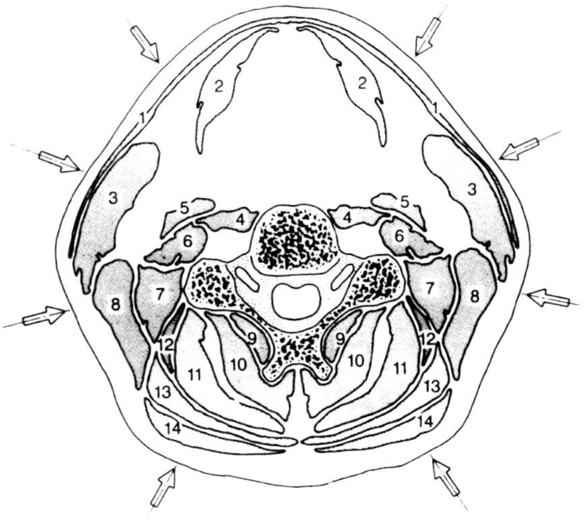

Figure 8.2

Schematic diagram of a cross section through the neck at the C4 level, showing the following muscle groups: (1) platysma; (2) infrahyoid; (3) sternocleidomastoid; (4) longus colli and cervicis; (5) scalene anterior; (6) scalene medius; (7) longissimus cervicis; (8) levator scapulae; (9) multifidus; (10) semispinalis cervicis; (11) semispinalis capitis; (12) spenius cervicis; (13) spenius capitis; (14) trapezius. (From Ref 8 with permission.)

Table 8.3 Estimated moments applied by neck musculature during maximum voluntary contractions in various directions, and the resulting shear and compressive forces acting at C4. (Data adapted from Ref 8.)

Direction of motion	*Bending moment (N m)*	*Lateral shear (N)*	*Ant/post shear (N)*	*Compression force (N)*
Relaxed	0	0 (0)	−2 (1)	122 (36)
Left twist	8.5 (3.1)	33 (8)	70 (24)	778 (36)
Extension	25.9 (13.4)	0 (0)	135 (69)	1164 (494)
Flexion	10.4 (6.3)	0 (0)	31 (63)	558 (375)
Lateral bend	12.8 (7.3)	125 (58)	93 (59)	758 (422)

Stability of the injured atlas

When applying a device for stabilization of the cervical spine, it is important to consider which structures have been injured and how this injury destabilizes the spine. Injuring certain structures may make the cervical spine unstable to specific loads but not to others. ("Unstable" as used in these discussions refers to the spine deforming to a greater extent than normal under load.) An example is fracture of the atlas. As shown by Panjabi et al,[9] who produced experimental fractures of C0–C2, the fracture pattern was predominantly failure of the anterior and/or posterior bony ring of C1, with occasional tearing of the transverse ligament (Figure 8.3). Testing range of motion and the neutral zone (the displacement of the joint in a certain direction without significant

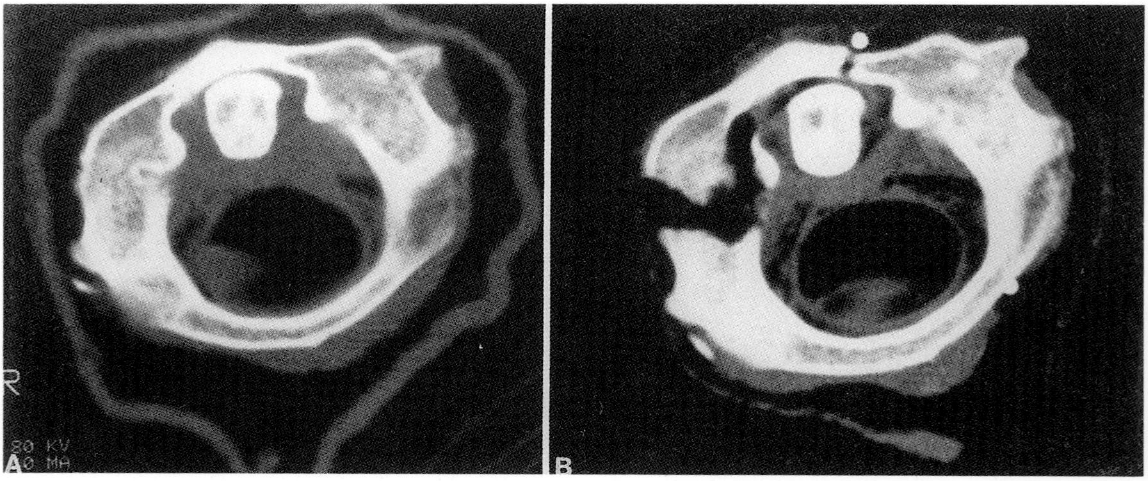

Figure 8.3

CT scan example of an experimentally produced fracture of the bony ring of C1. (From Ref 9 with permission.)

resistance under minimal load) demonstrated a large increase in motion in flexion–extension, but minimal change in axial rotation compared with the intact state (Figure 8.4). The residual stability in axial rotation between C1 and C2 after fracture is due to the intact facet joints which remain. Figure 8.5 shows that loss of the alar ligaments, but with the capsules remaining intact, produces only a 19% increase in axial rotation displacement at failure, compared with the intact joint.[10]

Injury to the cervical spine

Both ligamentous and bony injuries occur when the cervical spine is fractured. By progressively sectioning the ligamentous connections between cervical vertebrae, the effects of the extent of ligamentous injury on spinal stability can be determined. When an anterior ligamentous injury occurs and progresses posteriorly (Figure 8.6), the extension angulation at a specific load increases with the extent of injury. After disruption of the anterior longitudinal ligament (ALL), the disc, the posterior longitudinal ligament (PLL), and the transverse ligaments (TL), the motion segment cannot withstand an extension moment of 10.7 N m. This load is in the range of that

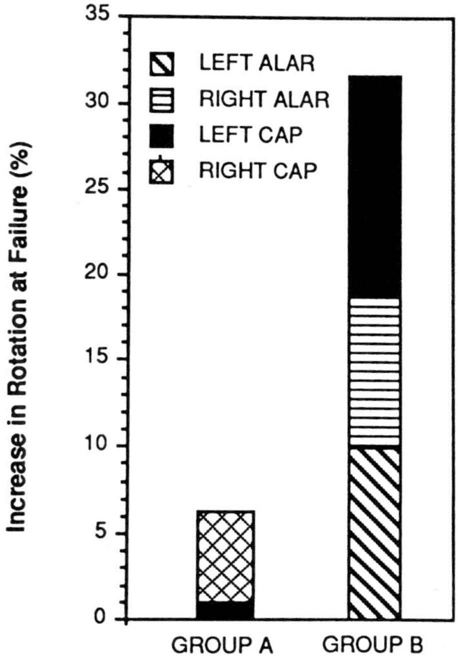

Figure 8.5

Percent increase in axial rotation angle of C1 with respect to C2, compared with intact, with progressive sectioning of the left and right alar and left and right capsular ligaments of C1–C2. Group A: capsular ligaments (CAP) only sectioned. Group B: alar and capsular ligaments sectioned. Stacked bars show progressive increase in displacement with progressive sectioning of structures. (From Ref 10 with permission.)

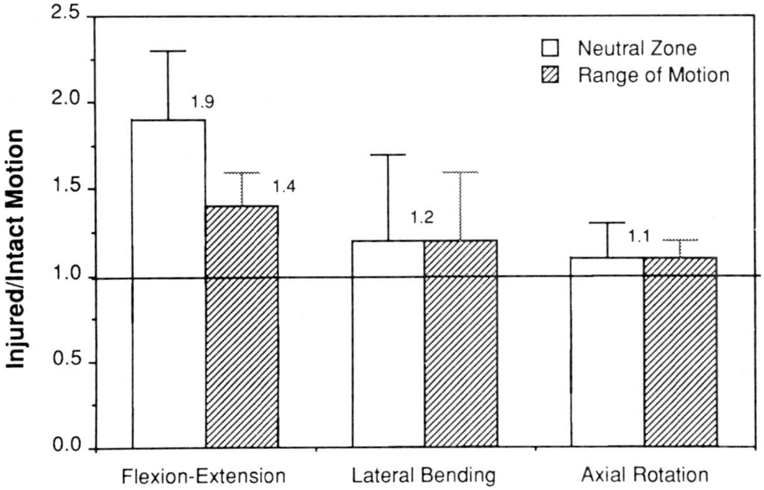

Figure 8.4

A comparison of the range of motion and neutral zone displacements of C1–C2 pre and post fracture of the bony ring of C1 in flexion–extension, lateral bending, and axial rotation. (From Ref 9 with permission.)

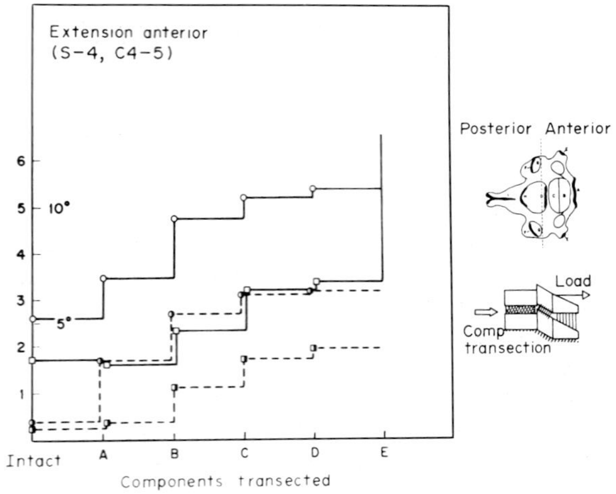

Figure 8.6

Extension–rotation of a cervical vertebra due to an extension moment of 10.7 N m, with progressive sectioning of ligamentous tissues from anterior: A, anterior longitudinal ligament sectioned; B, anterior half of disc; C, posterior half of disc; D, posterior longitudinal ligament; E, transverse ligaments; ○, angular displacement; □, horizontal displacement; ◑, residual angular displacement; ◨, residual horizontal displacement. (From Ref 11 with permission.)

produced by muscle forces, as shown in Table 8.3. Similarly, with the supraspinous, interspinous, ligamentum flavum, capsular ligaments, TL, and PLL cut, but with the disc and the other anterior structures intact, the spine is not able to support physiological flexion moments.[11]

Cervical spine injuries usually result in both bony and ligamentous disruptions, and are classified by the mechanism that is thought to create the injury. By creating cervical spine injuries through three different mechanisms, direct compression or compression combined with flexion or extension, and comparing pre and post injury motion of the spine, the effects of different injuries were determined. Panjabi et al[12] showed that flexion trauma creates significant spinal instability in flexion, extension, and torsional loading, but not in lateral bending (Figure 8.7). This is probably due to disruption of the disc

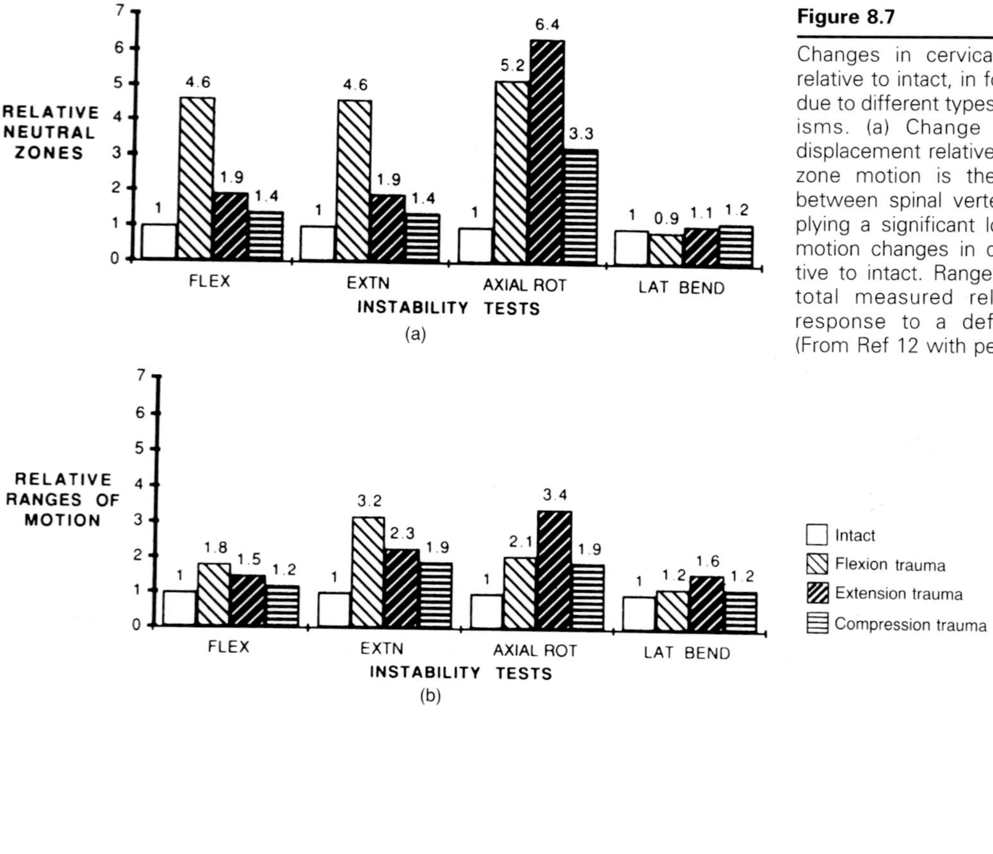

Figure 8.7

Changes in cervical spinal stability, relative to intact, in four loading planes due to different types of injury mechanisms. (a) Change in neutral zone displacement relative to intact. Neutral zone motion is the relative motion between spinal vertebrae without applying a significant load. (b) Range of motion changes in displacement relative to intact. Range of motion is the total measured relative motion in response to a defined load level. (From Ref 12 with permission.)

or vertebral body with a flexion type injury. Extension injuries cause the greatest instability in rotation and lateral bending, which may relate to disruption of the facet joints along with the disc, while direct compression creates significant instability mainly in axial rotation. This suggests that implants for fixation of the cervical spine should be chosen on the basis of their ability to regain lost stability in particular planes of motion, but that all devices must control axial rotation.

Summary

The cervical spine may be subjected to considerable loads. The type of injury (essentially the specific injuries to the interconnecting structures) governs the instability that results. For example, injury to the alar ligaments at the atlanto-axial joint does not significantly increase torsional instability. However, all cervical spine injuries, while creating various degrees of flexion–extension or lateral bending instability, do uniformly produce axial torsional instability.

8.3 Orthoses for the cervical spine

Comparisons of external cervical orthoses

During transport for hospital treatment of a cervical spine fracture, protection against spinal cord injury is accomplished by immobilization of the cervical spine. Comparison of various methods for immobilization demonstrates that supporting the cervical spine with sandbags and taping significantly reduces motion and is by far superior to the use of any type of cervical orthosis (Figure 8.8).[13]

The motion-restricting abilities of six commonly used orthoses for the management of cervical spine instability, some of which are shown in Figure 8.9, have been compared by Wolf and Johnson.[14] In comparison to the unstabilized cervical spine, the soft collar permitted 74.2–92.3% of normal motion. All other devices except for the halo vest allowed 12.8–28.9% of normal motion in flexion–extension, 45.9–66.4% in lateral bending, and 18.2–43.7% in axial rotation (Figure 8.10).

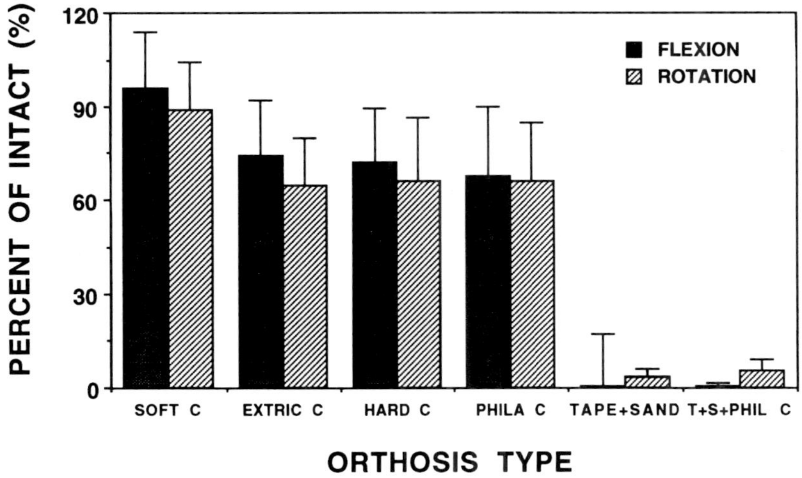

Figure 8.8

Comparison of the total cervical motion without immobilization, and with various methods of restricting motion in four directions of motion, expressed as percent of intact spinal motion: SOFT C, soft collar; EXTRIC C, extrication collar; HARD C, hard collar; PHILA C, Philadelphia collar; TAPE+SAND, tape and sandbags; T+S+PHIL C, tape and sandbags and Philadelphia collar. (Data adapted from Ref 13.)

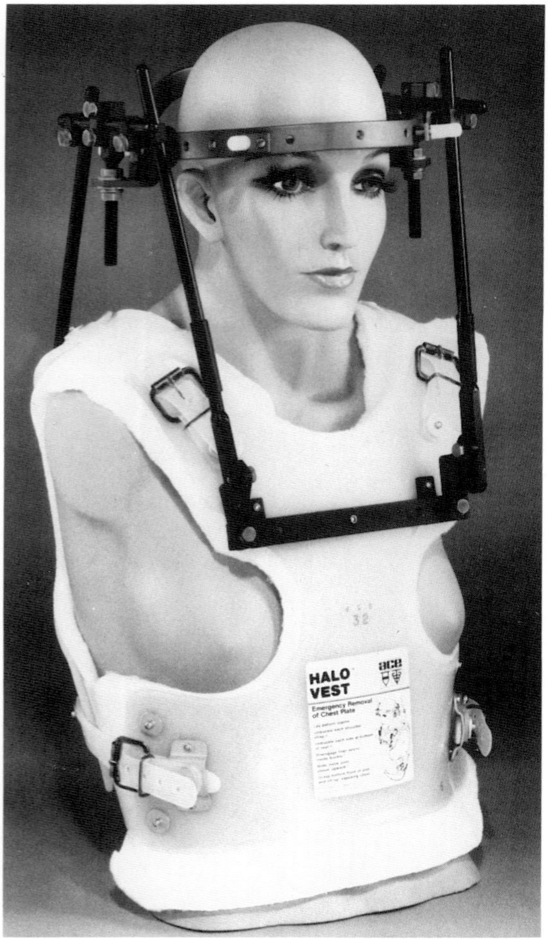

Figure 8.9

Halo orthosis for control of cervical spine motion in treatment of cervical spine fracture. The orthosis has a ring fastened to the skull by percutaneous pins; it is connected by braces to a jacket that fits about the chest.

Biomechanics of the halo orthosis

Controversy exists over the ability of the halo apparatus to stabilize the cervical spine. Cervical spine motion with the halo in place has been reported to be as low as 1–4% of normal;[14] however, other laboratory studies[15] and clinical observations[16,17] describe significant displacements occurring in the cervical spine stabilized with this device. The restriction of motion by the halo apparatus has been found to be least in the upper cervical spine and greatest in the lower spine in patients (Figure 8.11).[15]

Since the halo device is not rigidly attached to the thorax, and the latter can change shape depending upon activity, both the restriction of cervical motion and the distraction force applied to help maintain axial alignment of the spine can change with different activities.[15] Distraction forces on the spine were noted to be greatest when the patients studied were supine and least when sitting, which was partly attributed to the weight of the head counteracting the distractive force when seated (Figure 8.12). Shear forces on the skull pins[18] and cervical spine motions[15] were also found to be larger when seated than when standing or supine.

There are potentially three areas within the halo device that permit motion. First is the vest/throax interface, where motion is governed by (i) vest/thorax fit, (ii) vest/thorax interface friction, (iii) tightness of the vest straps, and (iv) changes in shape of the thorax (Figure 8.13). Even if no motion occurs at the vest/thorax interface, there can still be cervical spinal instability due to the flexibility of the vest itself. Finally, motion can also occur in the frame that connects the vest to the halo ring.[19,20] Using a model of the thorax and simulating a cervical spinal lesion, the relative contributions of these factors in standard halo devices were determined for loads causing flexion–extension and lateral bending of the head. As shown in Figure 8.14, the vest/thorax interface is the prime contributor to halo and cervical motion. Therefore halo device performance, in terms of limiting spinal motion, can be improved by either improving the fit, and/or increasing the coefficient of friction between the vest and the skin.

Krag and Beynnon[20] compared motion of different halo vests with respect to the thorax on normal volunteers. These experiments demonstrated the validity of increasing vest/thorax contact area in relatively rigid areas of the thorax such as the sternum anteriorly, the lateral aspects of the trunk, and the interscapular region posteriorly, while decreasing contact in mobile areas such as the upper aspect of the shoulder girdle, the pectoralis major muscles, the upper part of the

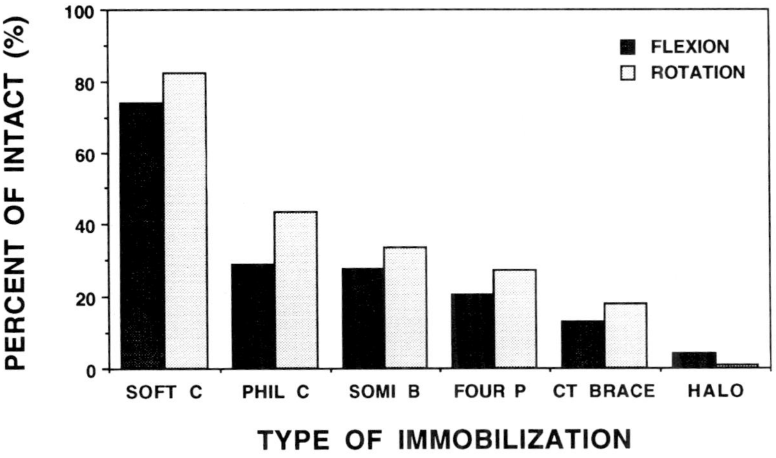

Figure 8.10

Cervical spine motions in flexion and axial rotation allowed with any of six external cervical orthoses in comparison with normal spine motion. (SOFT C = soft collar; PHIL C = Philadelphia collar; SOMI B = Somi brace; FOUR P = four poster brace.) (Data adapted from Ref 14.)

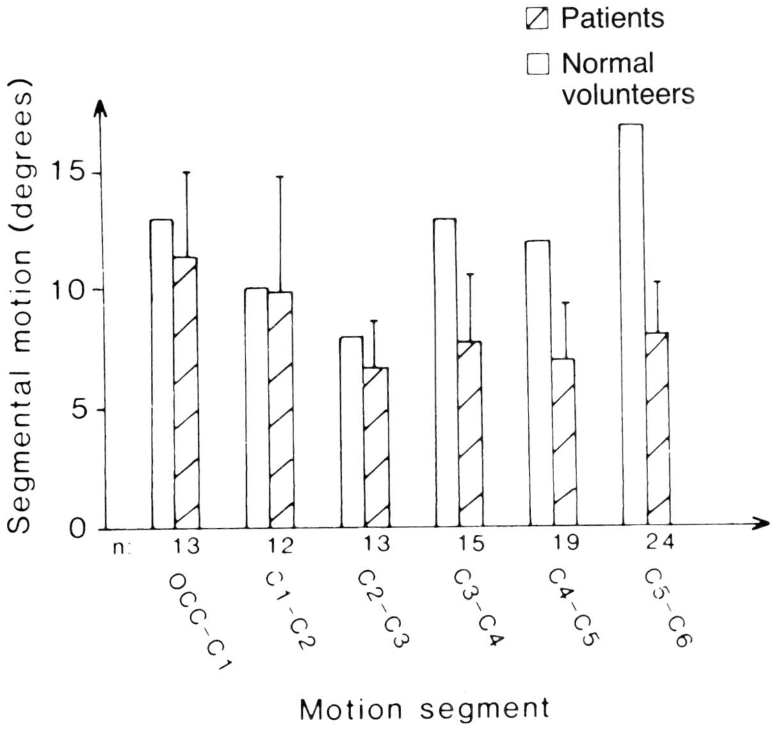

Figure 8.11

Segmental cervical spinal motion in normal volunteers and patients with a halo apparatus. (From Ref 15 with permission.)

abdomen, and the posterior aspects of the scapula. Further, permitting adjustability of the trunk contact pads and maintaining rigid connections between them enhances fit and decreases vest flexibility, thereby reducing vest/trunk motion. Lengthening the vest has been demon-

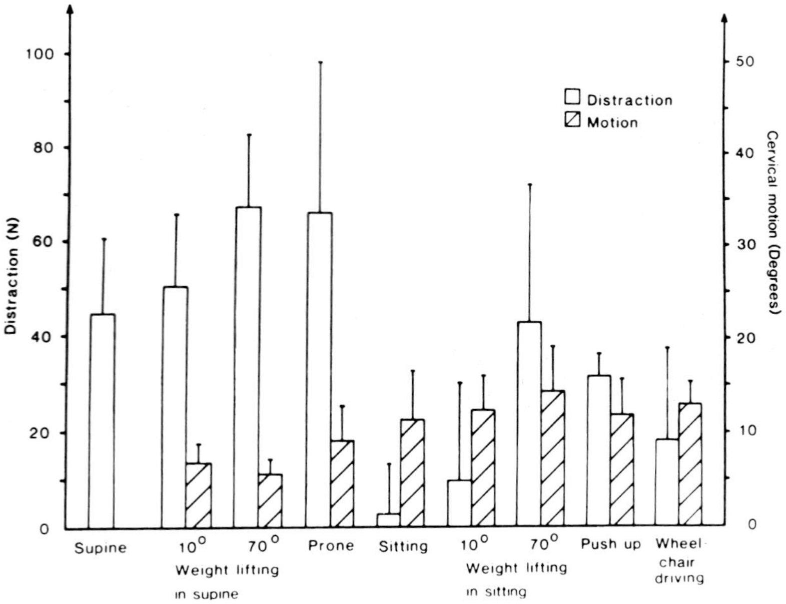

Figure 8.12

Distractive force acting on the cervical spine through the halo apparatus, and motion of the spine for various activities. (From Ref 15 with permission.)

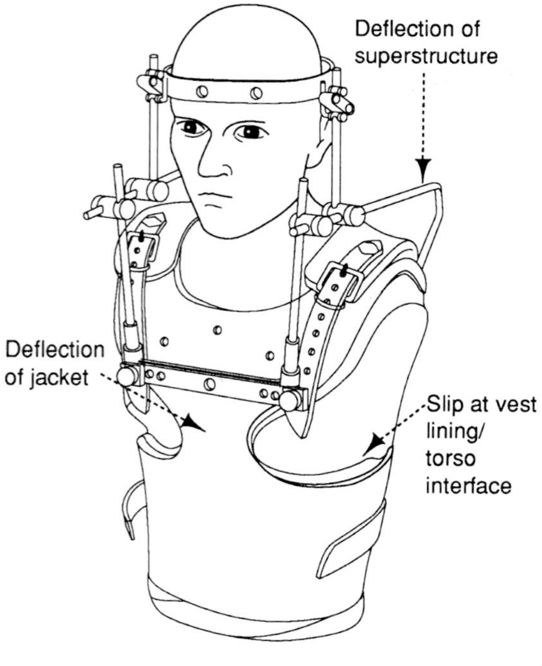

Figure 8.13

Potential sources of motion in the halo apparatus that can cause cervical spine motion. (Adapted from Refs 19,20.)

strated not to be effective in reducing cervical motion, because extending it over the abdomen does not provide an improved contact surface.[21]

Summary

The halo is the most effective method for fixation of cervical spine injuries without surgical intervention. However, spinal instability has been reported with halo fixation. Halo fixation rigidity is related principally to fit of the vest, including tightness and vest interface materials, which control the friction generated at the vest/thorax interface, as well as the stiffness of the surfaces that the vest is in contact with. Figure 8.15 compares the lateral bending stability of currently used vests.[19]

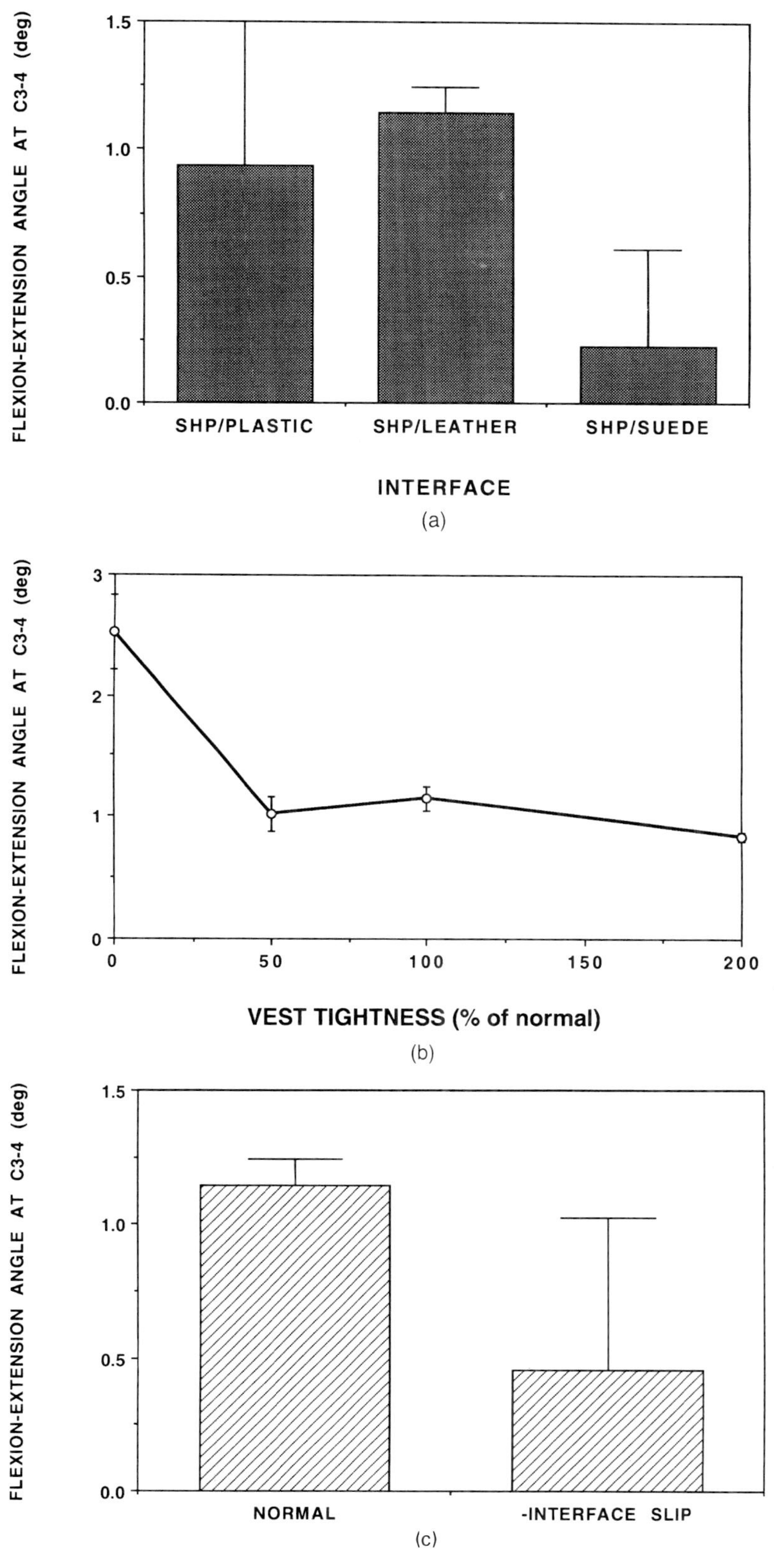

Figure 8.14

Relative motion at the C3–C4 level with complete transection, except for the anterior longitudinal ligament. (a) Effect of different frictional interfaces between the vest and halo (SHP/PLASTIC = sheepskin–plastic < skin frictional coefficient; SHP/LEATHER = sheepskin–leather = skin frictional coefficient; SHP/SUEDE = sheepskin – suede > skin frictional coefficient). (b) Effect of vest side strap tightness with a sheepskin–leather interface (100% = normal orthotist application tightness). (c) Contribution of vest slip to flexion–extension angulation of the vertebrae at the lesion. (Interface slip = vest bolted at base to eliminate slip on thorax.)[19]

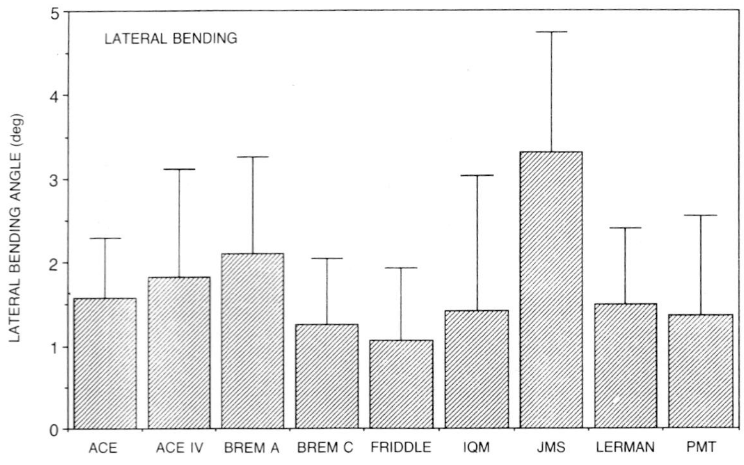

Figure 8.15

Lateral bending angle measured at cervical lesion site for vests tested. ACE: Ace mark III; ACE IV: Ace mark IV (Ace Medical, Los Angeles, CA); BREM A: Bremer Airflow; BREM C: Bremer Classic (Bremer Medical, Jacksonville, FL); FRIDDLE: Friddle MRI Model D (Friddle Mfg, Horea Path, SC); IQM (Innovative Quality Medical, Phoenix, AZ); JMS (Jerome Medical Systems, Mount Laurel, NJ); LERMAN: Lerman low profile (US Mfg Co, Pasadena, CA); PMT: PMT Model 1200 (PMT Corp, Chanhassen, MN). (From Ref 19 with permission.)

8.4 Internal fixation of atlanto-axial fractures

Comparison of fixation techniques

The atlanto-axial joint of C1–C2 provides a unique problem in spinal fixation because of the lack of a vertebral body at C1. Stability at this level is provided by ligamentous connections and the articular facets. Four methods have been commonly used for posterior fixation of fractures in this region. As shown in Figure 8.16, the Gallie type fixation[22] uses a single posterior bone graft between the arch of the atlas and the spinous process of C2, which is wired in place. The Brooks fixation[23] uses double wires placed over the posterior arch of C1 and the lamina of C2, which capture double bone grafts fitted between the arch and the lamina, as well as providing compression across the injury. In the Magerl transarticular screw technique,[24,25] the screws are placed from the junction of the lamina and articular mass of C2 into the mass of C1. Additionally, small grafts are placed posteriorly between the arch and lamina of C1–C2 and are wired in place. The Halifax method[26] uses clamps placed between the arch of C1 and the lamina of C2.

In a study by Grob et al,[27] these four methods were compared biomechanically in terms of their ability to limit angulation as well as anterior–posterior translation at C1–C2. In flexion, the Brooks, Magerl, and Halifax techniques reduced angulation to between 4.7% and 8.7% of normal motion, while the Gallie method allowed 26% of normal. Anterior–posterior (AP) translations were equivalent for all techniques, permitting 17.5–27% of normal values. In extension, the Gallie method allowed 27.6% of normal angulation, while with the other methods, angulation ranged from 5.7% to 10.4%. Again all techniques limited AP motion to between 10.3% and 24.3% of normal. For axial rotation, shown graphically in Figures 8.17 and 8.18, the Gallie method allowed 32.8% of normal rotation, while the other three techniques permitted 2.0–14.9% of normal motion. AP translations ranged from 5.6% to 19.3% of normal. In lateral bending, the Gallie technique permitted 52.9% of normal angulation, compared with between 5.9% and 6.7% with the other methods. In AP translation, allowable motions ranged from 25.3% to 10.2%.

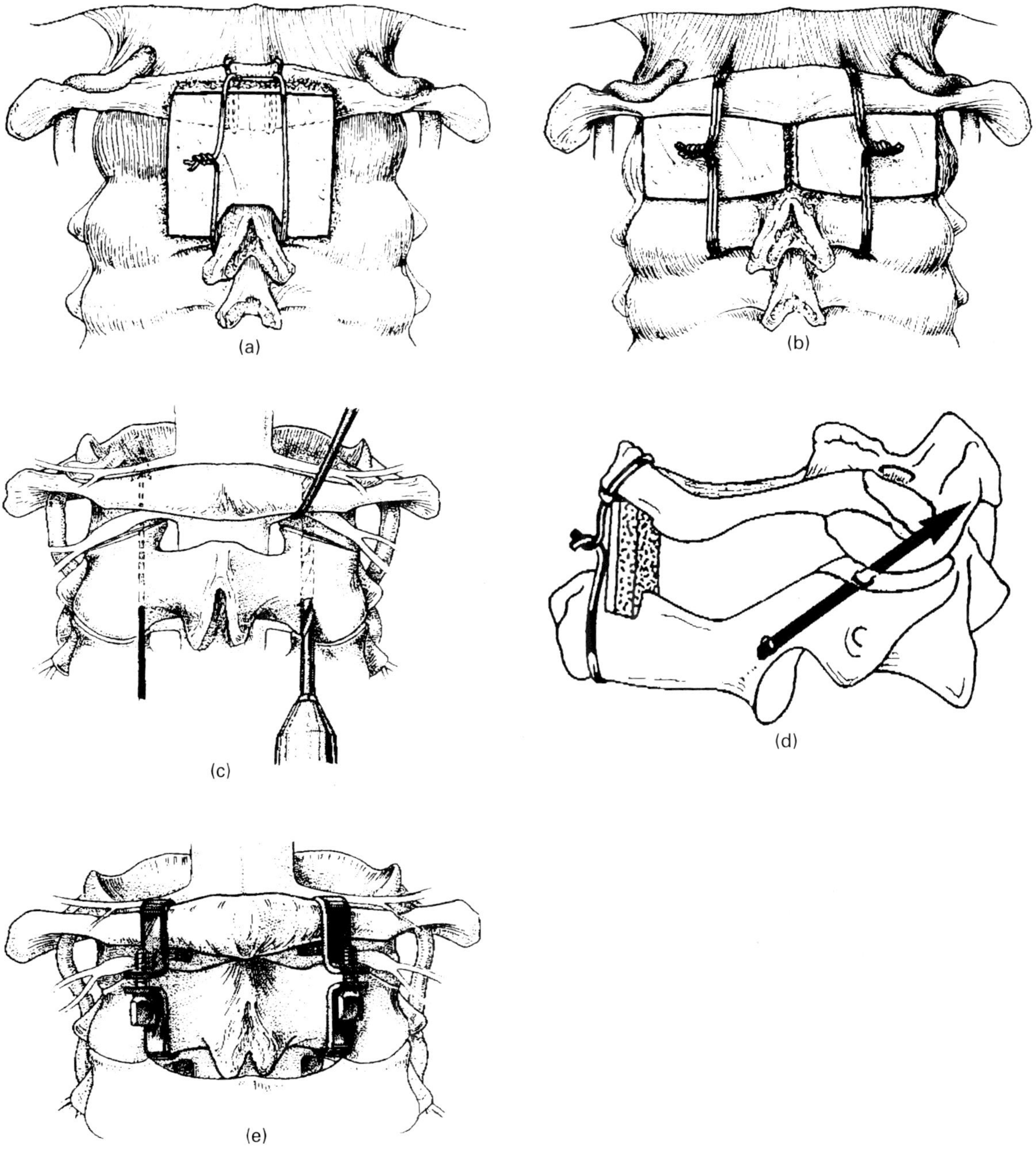

Figure 8.16

Four common methods of fixation of the atlanto-axial (C1–C2) articulation. (a) Gallie[22] posterior bone graft notched to fit the spinous process of C2 and wired in place. (b) Brooks' technique[23] has bone graft placed between the posterior arches of C1 and C2 with double wires compressing the graft. (c,d) Magerl[24,25] transarticular screws between C2 and C1, with posterior bone grafts secured by wire loops. (e) Halifax clamps[26] around the posterior arches of C1 and C2. (From Ref 27 with permission.)

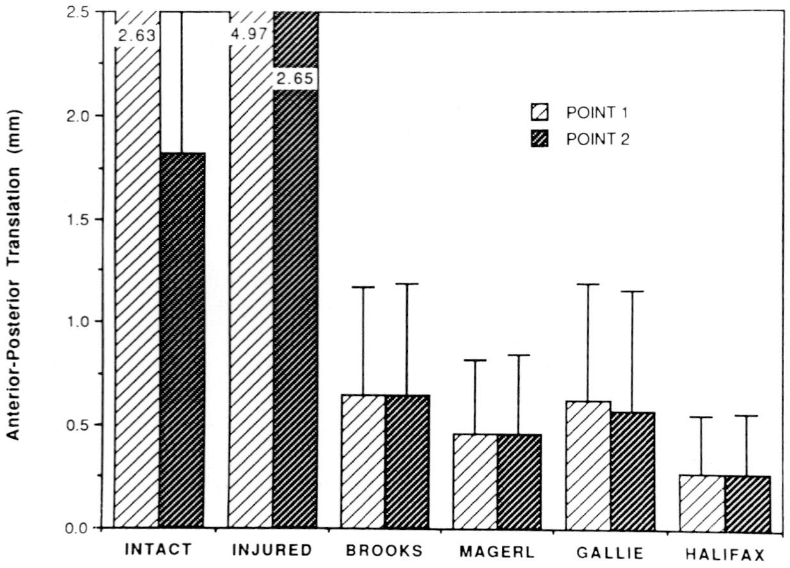

Figure 8.17

Mean anterior–posterior translation motion between reference points at the midline on the anterior aspect of C1 (point 1) and the posterior aspect of C1 (point 2) with respect to C2 for intact, injured, and posteriorly fixed atlanto-axial joints loaded in extension. (From Ref 27 with permission.)

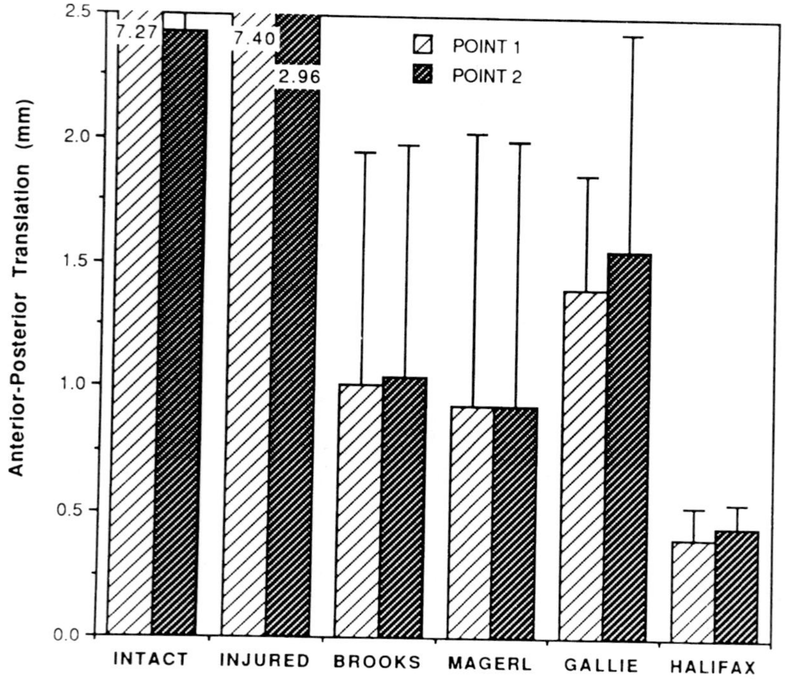

Figure 8.18

Mean anterior–posterior translation between points 1 and 2 on C1 with respect to C2 for intact, injured, and posteriorly fixed atlanto-axial joints loaded in axial torsion. (From Ref 27 with permission.)

Summary

In the experimental model described above there was major ligamentous disruption, but the bony structures remained intact. The central axes of motion of this joint lie through the articular facets for flexion–extension, and the dens for axial rotation. Therefore fixation applied posteriorly such as in the Halifax and Brooks techniques or locking the facets as in the Magerl method are effective in limiting motion at this joint. In the Gallie method, the wire acts only as a tension band. There is no provision for resisting an applied extension or lateral bending moment with the Gallie method, as opposed to the Brooks and Magerl methods, where the posterior bone graft serves this purpose. Similarly, the clamping action applied between the atlas and axis in the Magerl, Halifax, and Brooks techniques resists relative axial rotation between the fixed vertebrae.

8.5 Internal fixation of cervical spine injuries

Biomechanical principles

In fixation of cervical spine injuries, the magnitudes of the loads, primarily compression, and moments, flexion–extension, lateral bending, and axial rotation, must be appreciated. With a compromised vertebra (such as in a bursting or flexion compression injury), the fixation system should be able to withstand considerable compressive loading (see Table 8.3). Also, without the buttressing effect of the vertebra, the motion segment is less able to withstand flexion moments. As shown in Figure 8.19, appreciating the location of the center of rotation is important in improving the stability of fixation. The further from the center of rotation the fixator is located, the lower the forces on the implant and at the implant/bone interface, and the greater the moments it will be capable of resisting. Also, the degree of injury is a very important parameter, as has been discussed and will be shown again later.

Comparison of fixation techniques

A number of techniques have been used for fixation of cervical spine fractures. Pelker et al[29] compared the stabilizing potential of some common techniques, including spinous process wiring,[30] laminectomy with facet fusion,[31] H grafting,[32] and H grafting with facetectomy,[33] anterior plating[34] and posterior plating[35] (Figure 8.20). In addition, the effect of stiffening the structure by placing methylmethacrylate (PMMA) over the graft with wiring was investigated.

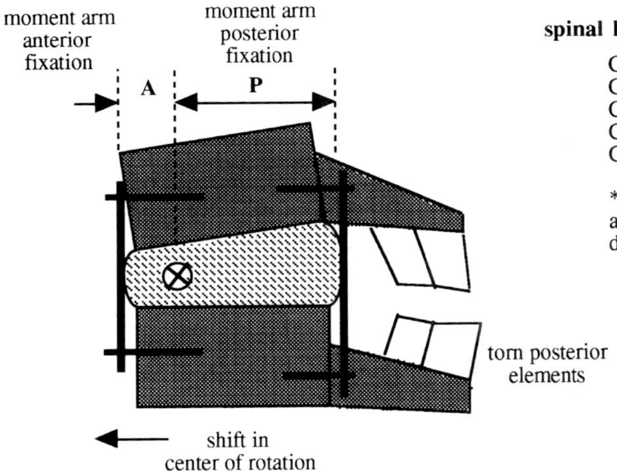

spinal level	A*	P*
C2-3	0.27	0.73
C3-4	0.32	0.68
C4-5	0.36	0.64
C5-6	0.39	0.61
C6-7	0.44	0.56

* in % of anterior-posterior diameter of verebra

Figure 8.19

Lateral view of a cervical motion segment with flexion–extension center of rotation location as described by Amevo et al.[28] In this example, a posterior fixation device would be more effective in limiting flexion–extension motions than one placed anteriorly, because of its longer moment arm (distance of the points of fixation to the center of rotation).

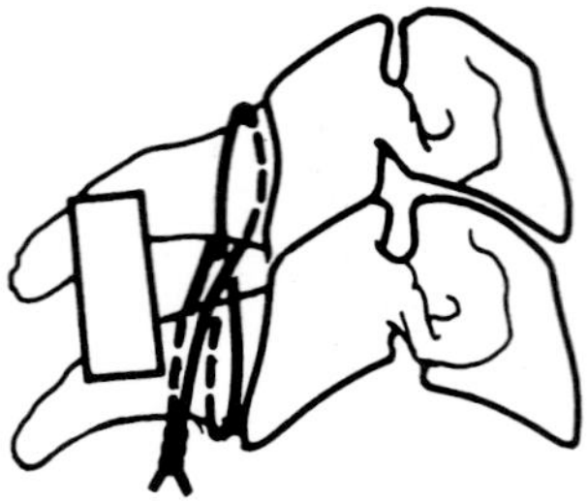

(a)

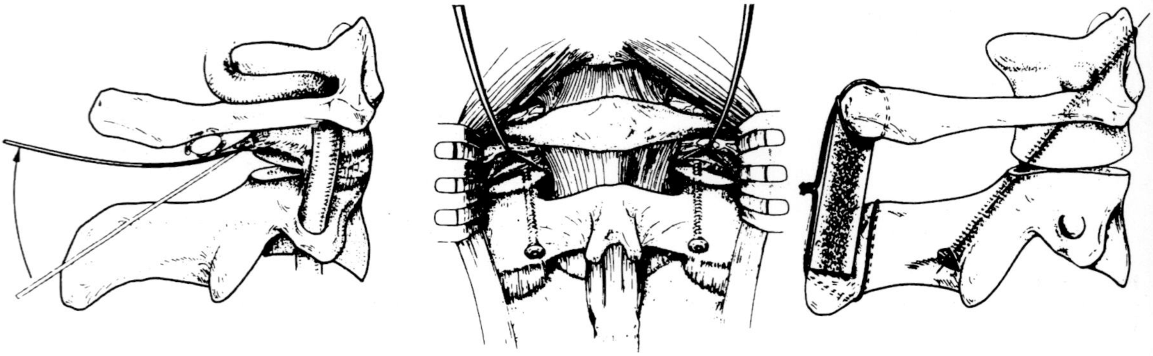

(b)

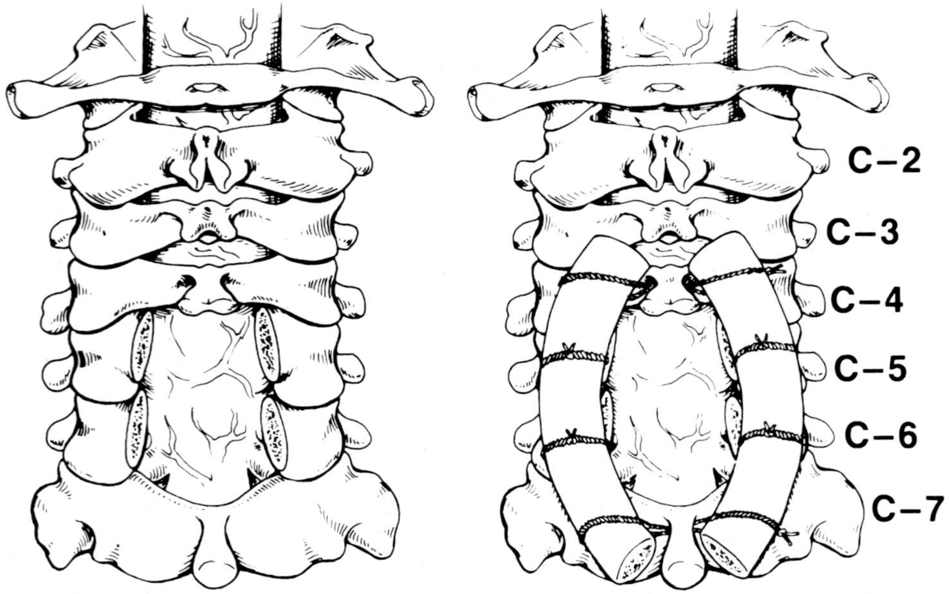

(c)

Figure 8.20

Methods for fixation of cervical spinal injury: (a) spinous process wiring;[30] (b) facet fusion;[31] (c) facet wiring;[33] (d) anterior plating;[34] (e) posterior plating.[35] (From Refs 29,31,33,35 with permission.)

(*Continued next page*)

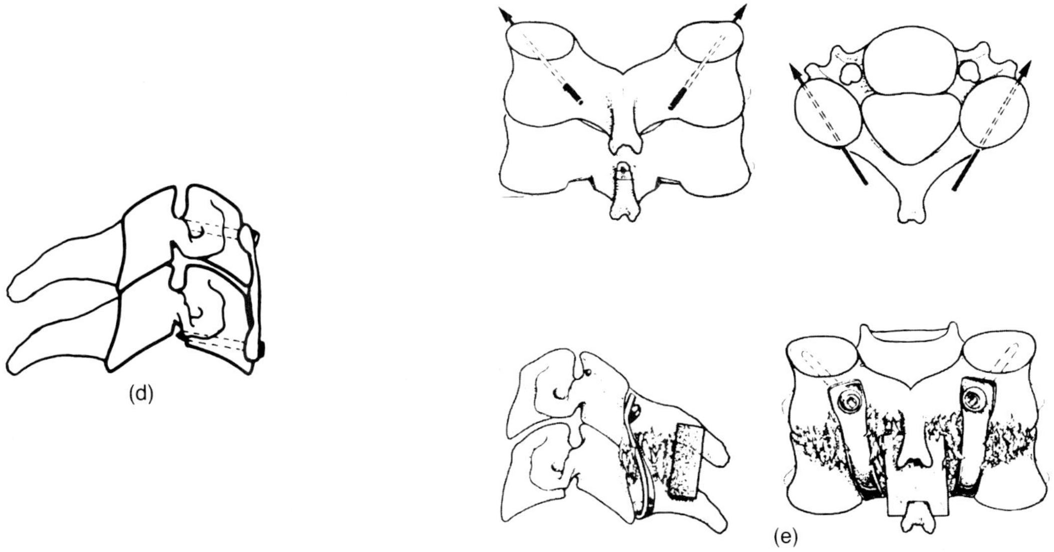

(d)

(e)

Figure 8.20

(Continued)

Comparisons of stiffness of some constructs are shown for extension (Figure 8.21) and axial rotation (Figure 8.22). Spinous process wiring of the injured joint limited motion to 75% of intact in flexion, but allowed motions considerably greater than intact in other planes. The addition of PMMA to the wire stiffened the construct and considerably reduced motion, especially in axial rotation (Figure 8.22) and lateral bending. Facet fusion using wired bone graft limited motion to 66% of intact in flexion and 40% in lateral bending, but allowed considerable movement in extension and axial rotation. H grafting was most successful in limiting axial rotation (to 68% of intact) and lateral bending (to 38% of intact), and its fixation to either the facets or the vertebrae did not change the stiffness of the fixation. Overall, the most effective method, an H graft wired to the vertebrae, with PMMA placed over the wires, graft, and spinous processes, limited motions to 35% of intact in flexion, 117% in extension, 46% in axial rotation, and 18% in lateral bending.

Recently, plates have been introduced as an alternative method of fixation. The anterior plate,[33] as shown in Figure 8.20, produces a construct in a flexion injury model (supraspinous, interspinous, ligamentum flavum, capsular ligaments disrupted), capable of limiting flexion angulation to 27.9% of intact. When the anterior H plate is combined with either a posterior hook plate[34] or spinous process wiring in a flexion injury model, flexion angulation is limited to 14.2% of intact, and AP translation to 17.7% of intact. With a complete lesion (disc removed) and a vertebral bone graft in place, combined fixation results in a limitation of flexion angulation to 12.5% of intact, compared with posterior wiring alone, at 57% of intact. The anterior plate alone was incapable of providing adequate stability in flexion (222% of intact) (Figure 8.23). In axial torsion with a flexion injury, the anterior H plate/posterior hook plate produced a construct with 48.4% of intact motion, and the hook plate alone 86.7% of intact. No other construct was able to limit motion to below intact levels (Figure 8.23).[35]

The most rigid constructs are produced by double posterior plates with screws through the lateral masses. With this fixation, constructs were found to have 8.5% of intact cervical motion in flexion, 12% in extension, 7.8% in lateral bending,

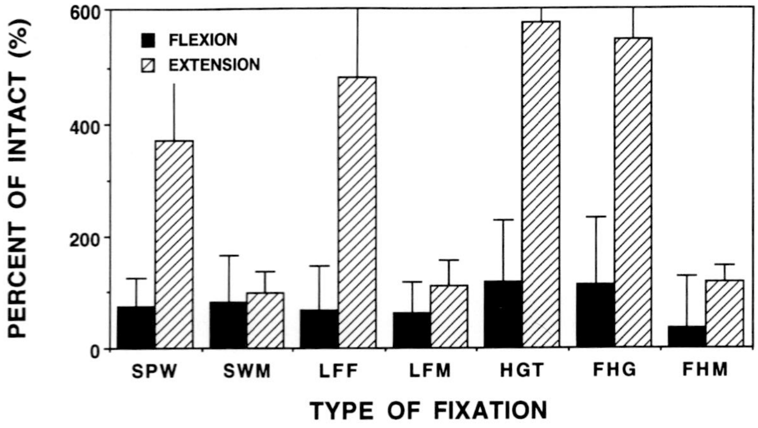

Figure 8.21

Motions of the superior vertebra with respect to the middle vertebra in extension for seven different repair techniques expressed as a percent of intact joint motion: SPW, spinous process wiring; SWM, spinous process wiring augmented with methylmethacrylate; LFF, laminectomy and facet fusion; LFM, laminectomy, facet fusion and methacrylate; HGT, H graft; FHG, facetectomy and H graft; FHM, facetectomy, H graft, and methacrylate. (Data adapted from Ref 29.)

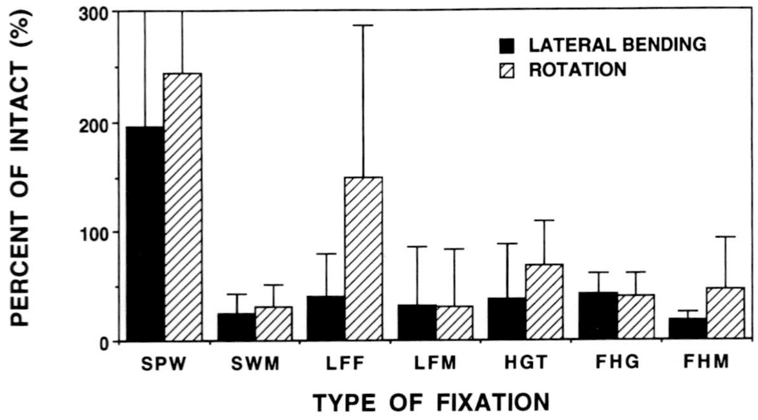

Figure 8.22

Motions of the superior vertebra with respect to the middle vertebra in axial rotation for seven different repair techniques expressed as a percent of intact joint motion. (Data adapted from Ref 29.)

and 11.3% in torsion.[36] Creating a more rigid construct transfers greater load to the implant and the implant bone interface; however, there was no change in fixation stiffness after 10 000 load cycles if the screws used to secure the plate were placed in ''adequate'' vertebral bone, and the facet joints were placed into apposition and compression.

Summary

As discussed in preceeding paragraphs, the most biomechanically rigid cervical spine fixation is obtained using a posteriorly mounted plate. This device acts as a tension band to flexion moments, and can resist extension moments as well since the moment is converted to compressive force within the plate (Figure 8.24). If the plates are widely separated, such as by attachment to the lateral masses, they are in the most effective location for resisting lateral bending moments. Resisting axial rotation requires that the plates not be permitted to pivot around the screw heads (Figure 8.24d). The anterior plate is not effective in stabilizing a flexion moment in a flexion injury pattern (i.e. posterior elements disrupted), because it cannot act as a tension band (being placed on the anterior surface of the vertebra) and

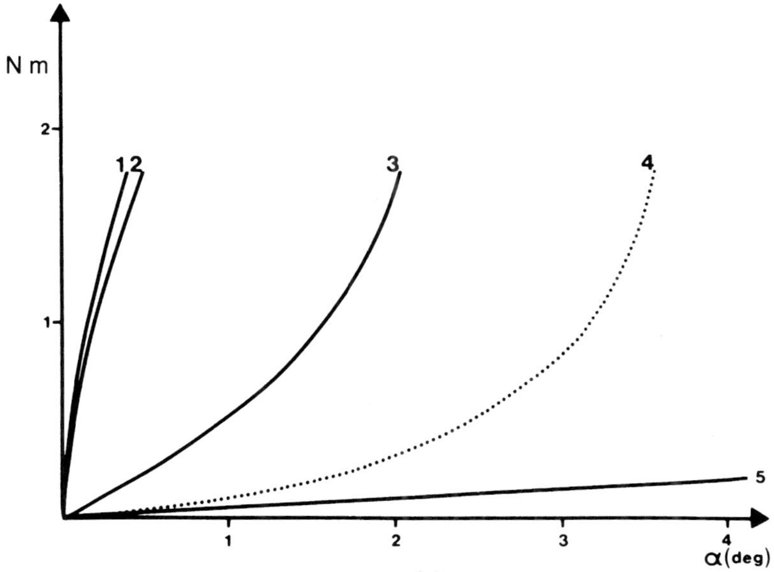

(a)

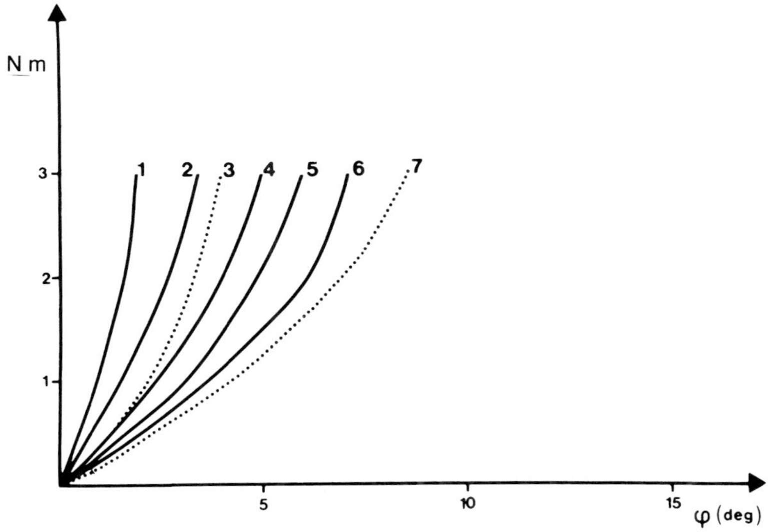

(b)

Figure 8.23

Comparison of stiffnesses of cervical spine constructs in a complete lesion. (a) Flexion angulation: (1) anterior H plate and posterior hook plate; (2) anterior H plate and posterior wiring; (3) posterior wiring alone; (4) intact spine; (5) anterior plate alone. (b) Axial torsion: (1) anterior H plate and posterior hook plate; (2) posterior hook plate alone; (3) intact spine; (4) anterior H plate and posterior wiring; (5) anterior H plate alone; (6) posterior wiring; (7) specimen with posterior injury. (From Ref 35 with permission.)

is too flexible to resist a flexion moment in this location. Additional posterior fixation should be used in this type of injury. The major biomechanical application of the anterior plate would be in an extension injury, where the posterior structures are intact and it can act as a tension band in resisting extension moments.

Wiring is not as effective at limiting spinal motion as plating. This is because load transfer in a wired joint occurs by friction between the graft and vertebral bone generated by tension in the wire. Shearing forces (which cause one surface to slip parallel to the other) are more effectively resisted by a screw, since shear causes

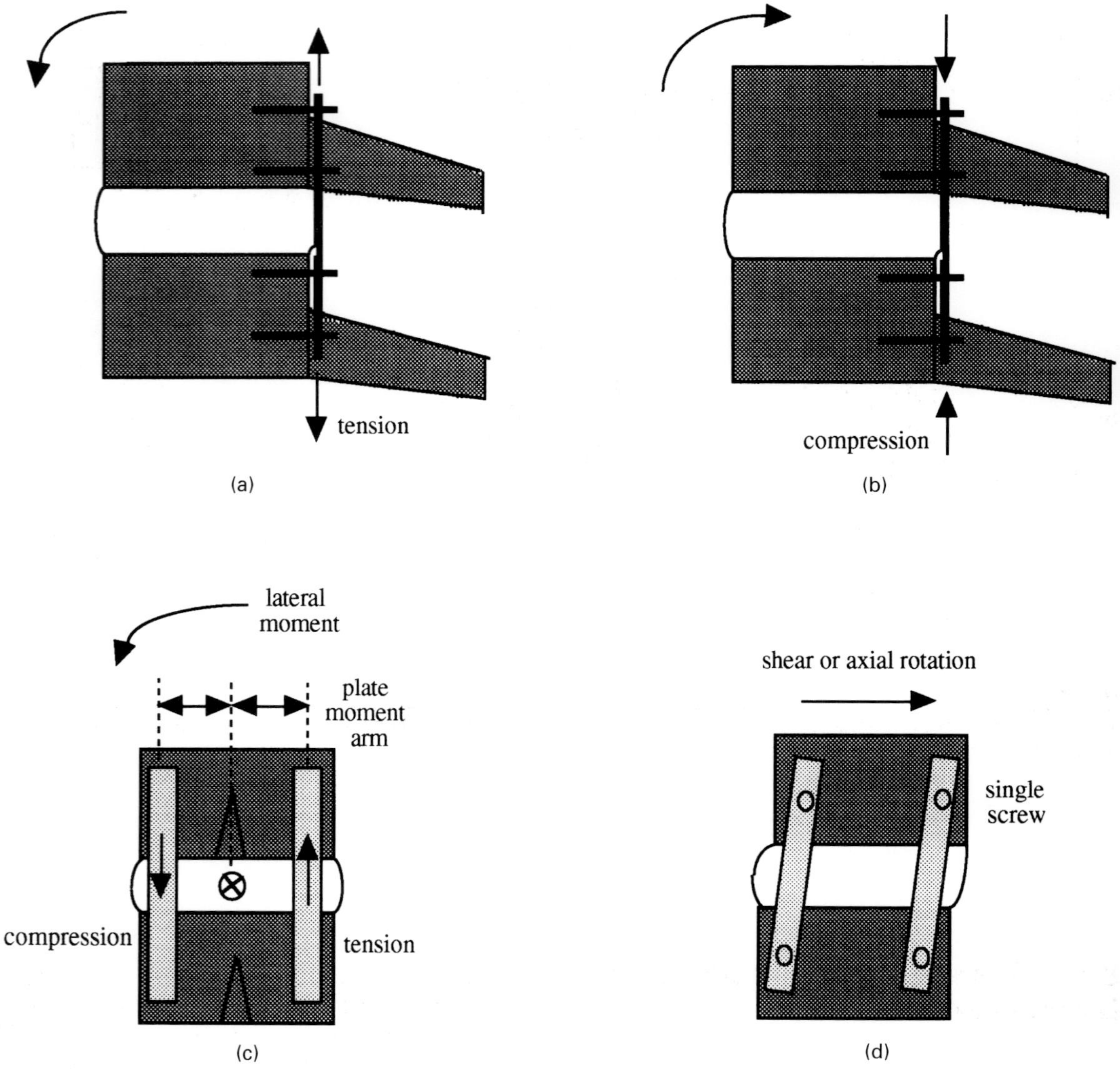

Figure 8.24

Effectiveness of posterior plating in resisting cervical spine loading. (a) a posterior fixation device acts as a tension band in flexion. (b) The device resists extension moments by loading the implant in compression. (c) In lateral bending, the fixation devices should be as far lateral as possible. One device will be in tension and the other in compression. (d) In axial torsion, the fixation device should not permit one lamina to shear laterally with respect to the other. Therefore the connection of the device to bone should not permit pivoting.

bending in the screw and slip between the surfaces is less likely (Figure 8.25). A hook, as used in the hook plate fixator,[34] effectively resists loads which are applied only against (as opposed to away from) the hook surface.

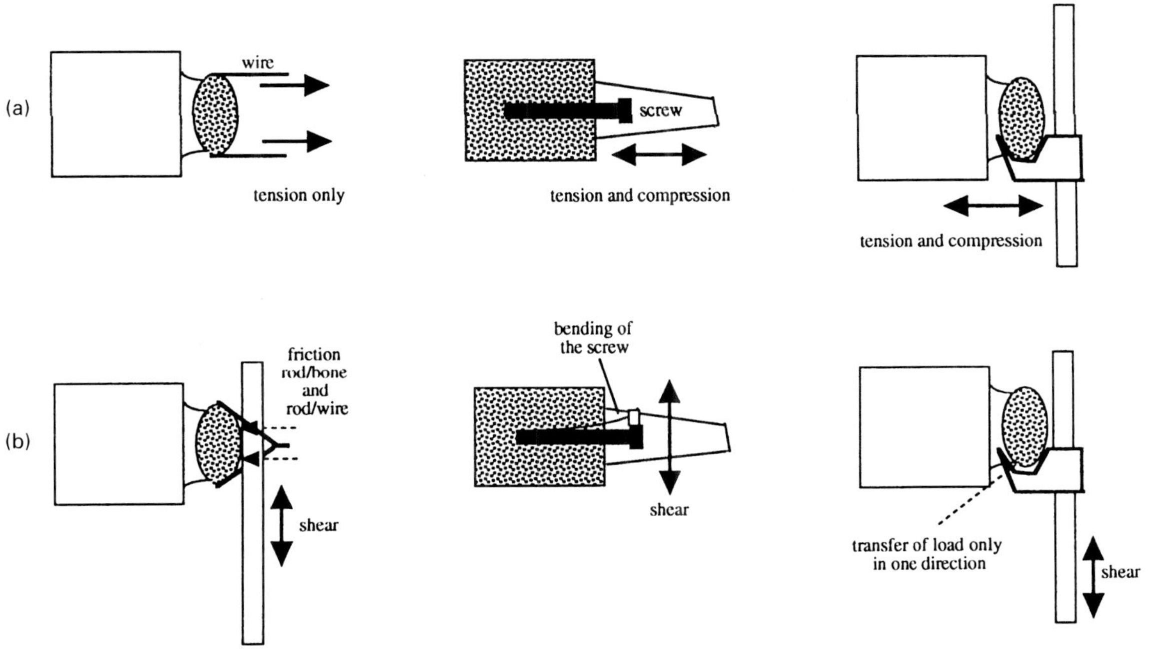

Figure 8.25

Methods of transferring load between two surfaces with wire, a screw, or a hook. (a) Tension and compression. (b) Shear parallel to the long axis of the spine.

8.6 Thoracolumbar spine injury biomechanics

Loading conditions

The lumbar spine is challenging to immobilize because of the multidirectional loads acting upon it, which are also large in magnitude. In its most simple form, there will be a large compressive load acting on the lower lumbar discs because the erector spinae muscles must counteract the flexion moments produced by the weight of the trunk and external loads anterior to the spine. Since the moment arms of the spinal muscles are small, the muscle forces must be large in order to produce an effective counteracting moment (Figure 8.26).[37]

The musculature which acts on the spine is complex (Figure 8.27), and combinations of muscles acting to mobilize the trunk, along with cocontractions of others for stability during movement, result in the application of axial compressive and shear forces as well as flexion–extension, lateral bending, and axial torsional moments to the spine. From myoelectric muscle signal analysis and modelling, Schultz et al[38] estimated the magnitudes of compressive forces at L3 to range from 340 N (sitting, holding no weight) to 2350 N (standing flexed 30° forward, arms out and holding an 8 kg weight), (Figure 8.28). During walking, the lumbar spine is estimated to support about 1.2 times body weight, and moments of about 15 N m.[39]

The shear force between two vertebrae in the lower lumbar spine can be considerable because

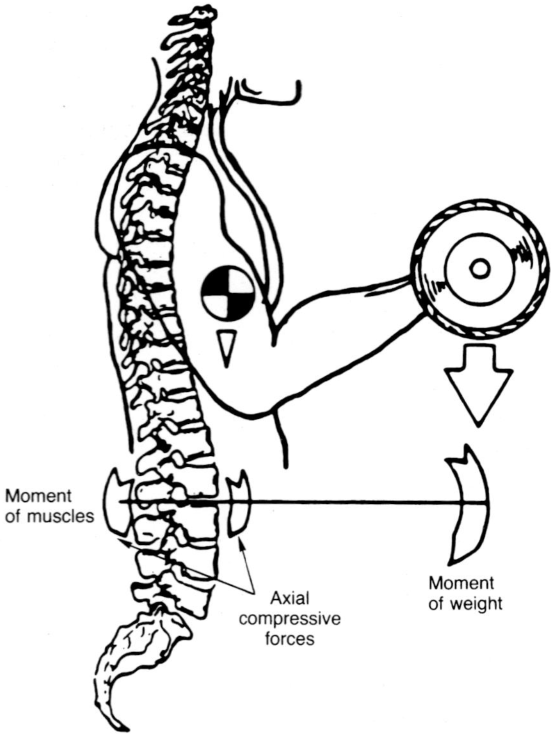

Figure 8.26

In a simple two dimensional representation of the trunk in the sagittal plane, the small moment arms of the spinal musculature require that large axial forces be generated to produce moments to counteract the weight of the upper body and external loads. (From Ref 37 with permission.)

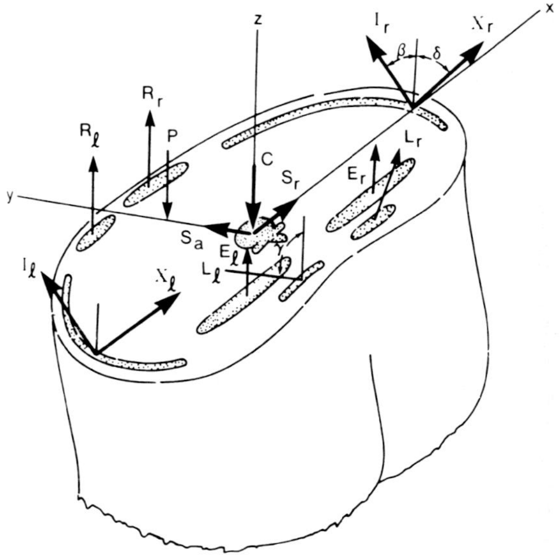

Figure 8.27

Schematic diagram of a model trunk cross section used to calculate forces on the lumbar spine (R_l, R_r, rectus abdominis; X_l, X_r, external obliques; I_l, I_r internal obliques; E_l, E_r, erector spinae; L_l, L_r latissimus dorsi). (From Ref 38 with permission.)

of the large axial force applied and the lordotic shape of the lower lumbar spine. As shown in Figure 8.29, the external axial load can be broken into two components: one acting perpendicular to the disc and one parallel. In the example of Figure 8.29, a 1900 N load acts on the spine and results, with an inclination of the disc of 15°, in a 490 N shear load.[37]

The effects of spinal injury on spinal stability

As was discussed in the section on the cervical spine, the type and degree of injury can influence the stability achieved by a fixation system and its ability to resist external loads. Posner et al[40] investigated the effects of soft tissue injuries on the stability of the lumbar spine. There was a progressive increase in flexion angulation with a flexion moment of 10.5 N m, due to progressive sectioning of soft tissue from posterior to anterior. Failure (at this load level) occurred in most specimens after all posterior elements had been sectioned (posterior ligaments, facets, and the posterior longitudinal ligament). In extension loading, loss of the anterior longitudinal ligament and the disc was sufficient to cause failure of the motion segment.

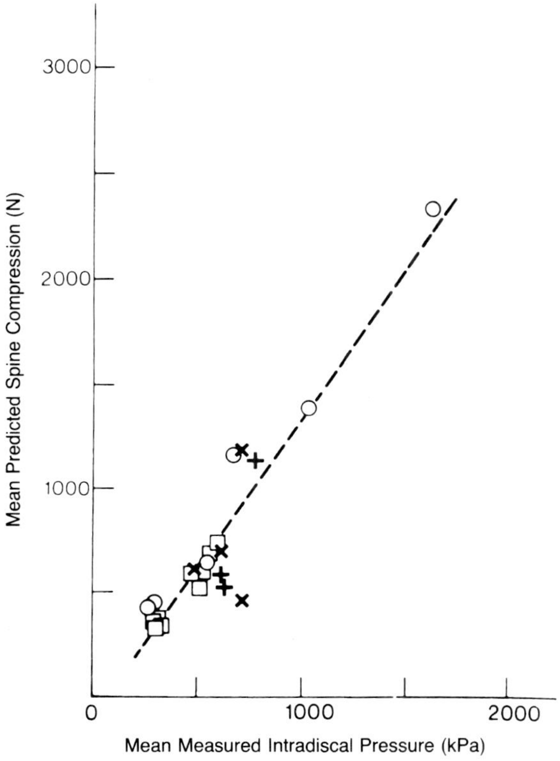

Figure 8.28

Predicted compressive force on the third lumber vertebra for different tasks, and its relation to measured intradistal pressure. Standing: ○, weight holding; ×, horizontal force resistance. Sitting: □, weight holding; +, horizontal force resistance. (From Ref 38 with permission.)

Denis[41] introduced the concept of the three "columns" of the spine in order to assist in visualizing the mechanical effects of injury. As shown in Figure 8.30, the anterior column consists of the anterior part of the disc and anterior longitudinal ligament, the middle column comprises the posterior part of the disc and the posterior longitudinal ligament, and the posterior column, the facets and posterior ligaments. Haher et al[42] demonstrated how injury to the different columns affects the center of rotation of the injured spine in flexion–extension. As shown in Figure 8.31, in the intact spine, the instant center of rotation in flexion is located in the anterior part of the disc, and posterior muscle forces balance the weight of the trunk, which acts through its center of gravity, located anterior to the spine. With loss of the anterior column (anterior longitudinal ligament and anterior half of the disc) (Figure 8.32), the center of rotation moves posteriorly, to the region of the facets, increasing the moment arm of the trunk weight and decreasing that of the posterior muscles. When both anterior and middle columns are compromised (Figure 8.33), the center of rotation moves posterior of the spinal musculature, and there is no effective way for muscle forces to counteract the trunk moment. Destruction of the posterior column, with the anterior and middle columns intact, shifts the

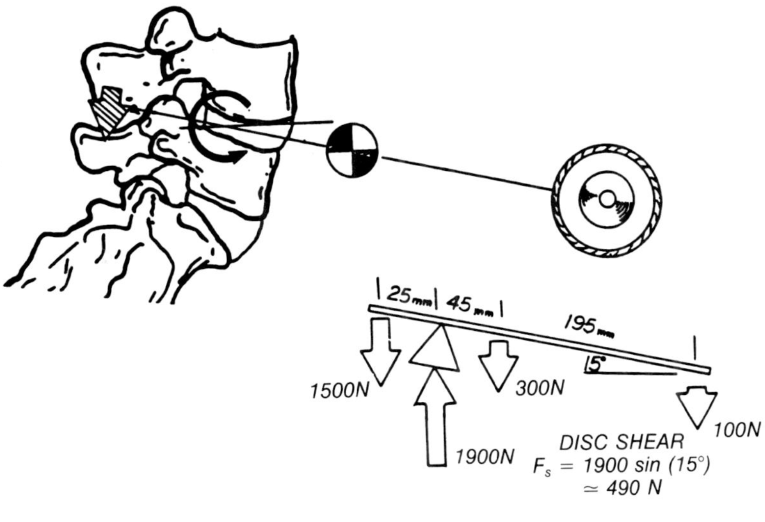

Figure 8.29

In the case where a body weight of 300 N acts 45 mm from the fulcrum (center of flexion–extension of the vertebra) and an external weight of 100 N acts 240 mm anteriorly, the erector spinae muscles must generate a counteracting force of 1500 N in order to balance the flexion moment produced by the anterior loads. The 1900 N load acting on the vertebral body, inclined at 15°, results in a 490 N shear force F_s at the disc. (From Ref 37 with permission.)

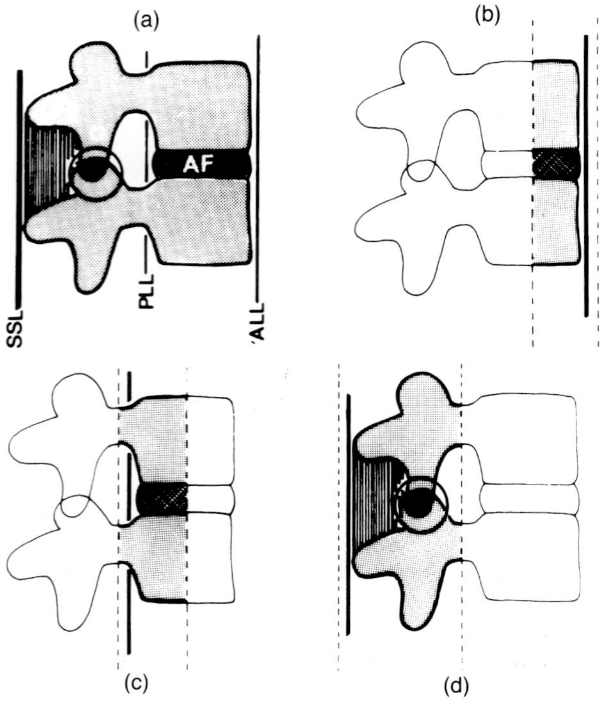

Figure 8.30

Concept of the three columns of the spine. (a) The intact spine motion segment. (b) the anterior column consists of the anterior half of the disc and the anterior longitudinal ligament (ALL). (c) The middle column consists of the posterior half of the disc and the posterior longitudinal ligament (PLL). (d) The posterior column consists of the facet joints and the posterior ligaments (SSL). (From Ref 41 with permission.)

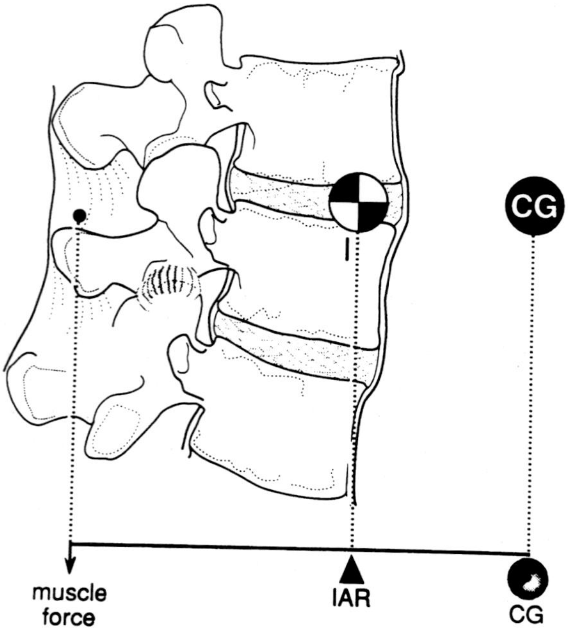

Figure 8.31

Sagittal plane view of a lumbar motion segment, showing the location of the flexion–extension axis of rotation (IAR) in the intact (I) spine and the balance between muscle forces and body weight acting through the center of gravity (CG) of the upper body. (From Ref 42 with permission.)

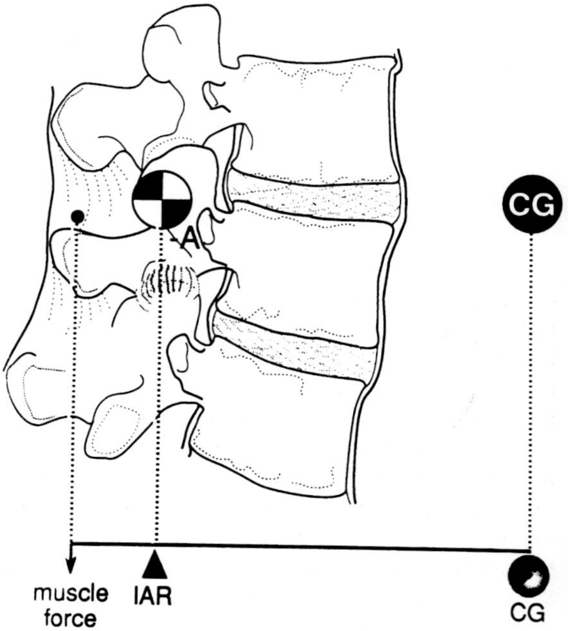

Figure 8.32

Sagittal plane view of a lumbar motion segment, showing the location of the flexion–extension axis of rotation (IAR) in the spine after loss of the anterior column (—A) (loss of the anterior half of the disc and the anterior longitudinal ligament). (From Ref 42 with permission.)

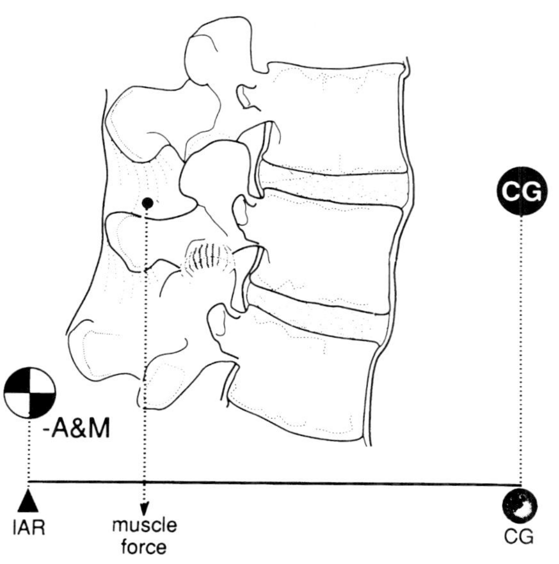

Figure 8.33

Sagittal plane view of a lumbar motion segment, showing the location of the flexion–extension axis of rotation (IAR) in the spine after loss of the anterior and middle columns (−A&M) (loss of the disc or vertebra and the anterior and posterior longitudinal ligaments). The center of rotation is shifted posterior to the line of action of the posterior musculature; therefore there is no counteracting moment to that produced by the weight of the trunk. (From Ref 42 with permission.)

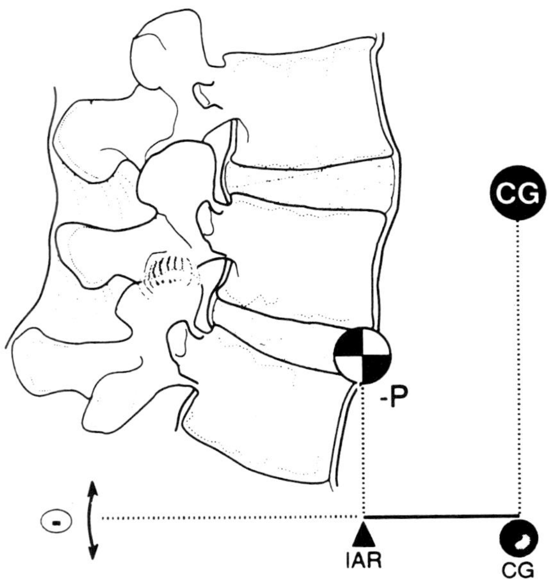

Figure 8.34

Sagittal plane view of a lumbar motion segment, showing the location of the flexion–extension axis of rotation (IAR) in the spine after loss of the posterior column (−P) (loss of the posterior ligaments and facets). (From Ref 42 with permission.)

center of flexion–extension to the anterior border of the vertebra (Figure 8.34). Understanding these basic mechanical principals can help in providing effective stabilization to the injured region, as will be discussed in the next section.

Haher et al[43] also demonstrated the effect of injury on the location of the axis of axial rotation of the lumbar motion segment, due to torsional loading. Both the facet joints and the disc affect the position of the axis of axial rotation (Figure 8.35). Loss of the facets moves the axis to the midpart of the disc. Conversely, injury to the disc and facets shifts the axis posterior to the facets, to a point that is approximately the location of the intersection of the perpendiculars from the surfaces of the facet joints. If the axis of rotation changes, the effective moment arms of muscles, soft tissue stabilizers, and any applied instrumentation are altered as well. Of most importance is maximizing the moment arms of the forces applied by spinal instrumentation in order to lower the forces they must exert to maintain stability of the injured spine. Lower forces in the instrumentation results in lower stresses on implant components and at the bone/implant interface.

Since the spine is subjected to loads in three dimensions, it is imperative to define the three dimensional instability of the spine. Ching et al[44] liken the mechanical stability of the spine conceptually to a ball in a flat bottom dish. As shown in Figure 8.36, the ball may move freely within a neutral equilibrium zone, which is equivalent to the normal mobility of the spinal intervertebral

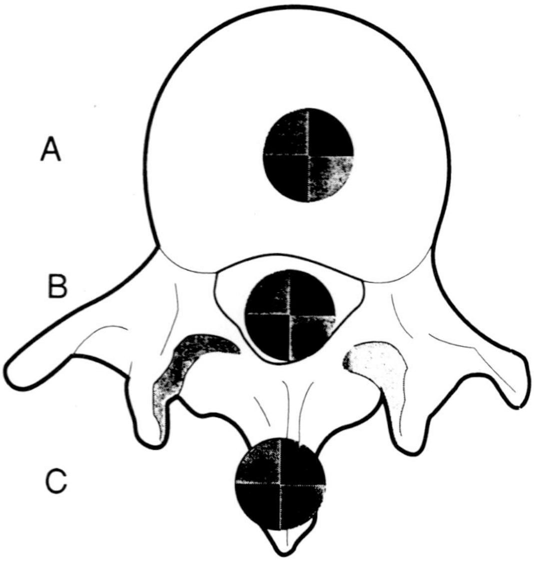

Figure 8.35

Coronal plane view of a lumbar vertebra showing the locations of the axes of axial rotation of the spine, due to axial torsion. A, facet joints injured; B, intact spine; C, facet joints and annulus injured. (From Ref 43 with permission.)

joint. If displaced excessively in any direction, the ball rises up the side of the dish, and when the load is released, returns to the neutral zone. This simulates the restraining effects of the disc and ligaments at the ends of the range of motion. If an injury occurs, a part of the dish is broken, increasing the range of the neutral zone. Although the spine may still be able to support external load, its range of mobility is abnormally large, resulting in clinical problems such as excessive kyphosis or occlusion of the spinal canal. A spinal implant therefore restores (or even reduces) the neutral zone range of motion.

Typical neutral zone plots are shown for three common types of thoracolumbar injuries. The plot shows the boundaries of the flexion–extension and lateral bending ranges plotted as a two dimensional map for comparative purposes. It was constructed by applying a load to an injured motion segment, in a cadaver experiment, then releasing it and recording the final position of the vertebra. As Figure 8.37 shows, a compressive (non bursting) injury with ligaments intact results

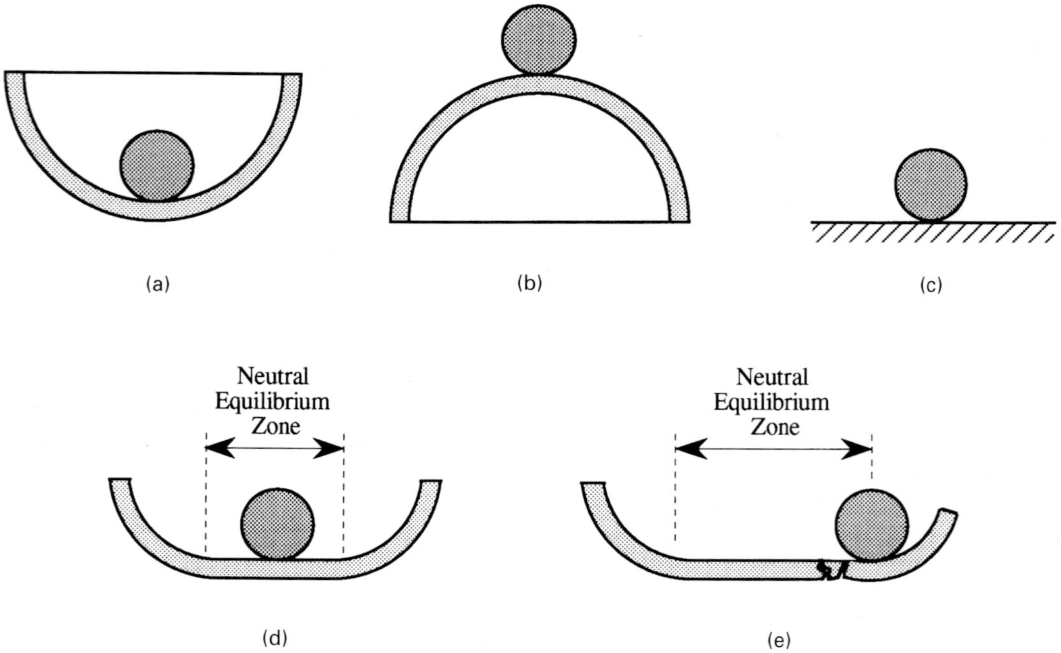

Figure 8.36

Conceptual model of stability with reference to the injured spine. Concepts of stability: (a) stable equilibrium; (b) unstable equilibrium; (c) neutral equilibrium. (d) The intact spinal motion segment, like a ball within a dish, allows a normal range of mobility but if this is exceeded, the soft tissue stabilizers return the vertebra to its neutral zone. (e) In the case of a fracture, the neutral zone is enlarged because the soft tissue stabilizers have been injured. (From Ref 45.)

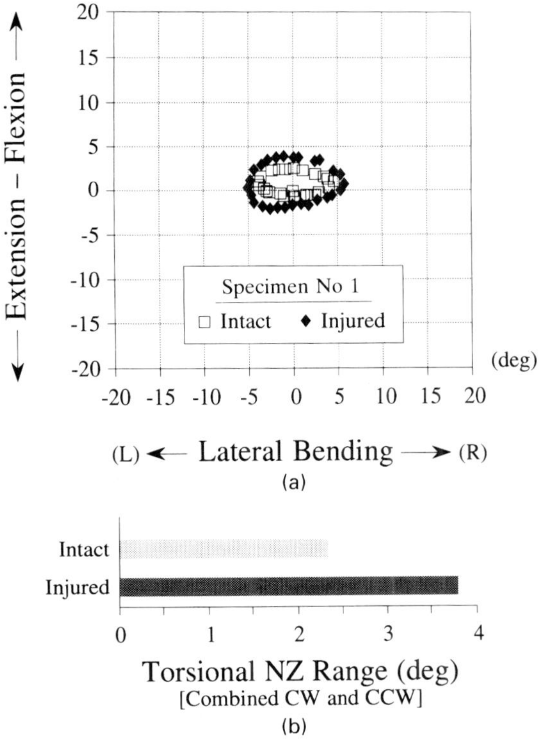

Figure 8.37

A "neutral zone" plot of a specimen with a thoracolumbar compression fracture. (a) This plot of the flexion–extension–lateral bending range of motion (a load is applied and released and the final position of the specimen is recorded; this is repeated in different directions) shows that the intact and injured specimens are similar. (b) The torsional range is increased after fracture. (From Ref 45.)

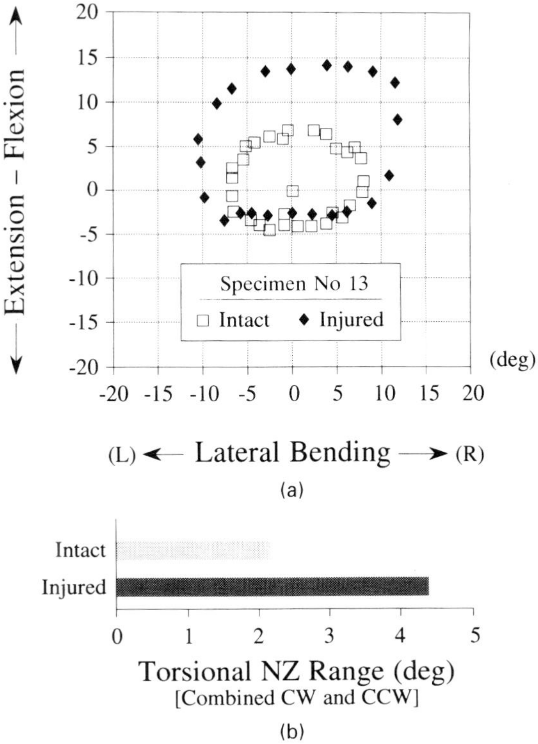

Figure 8.38

Example of the increase in neutral zone (a) in flexion and lateral bending and (b) in axial torsion, in a spine specimen with a bursting injury. (From Ref 45.)

in no difference in neutral zone compared with the intact spine, except in torsional loading. With a burst fracture (see Chapter 3) (Figure 8.38), the flexion and lateral ranges are increased, while a flexion–distraction injury results in a large increase in the flexion range only (Figure 8.39).[45]

It is interesting to note that although the neutral zone is enlarged in fracture, the intact and injured spine have similar flexion load–displacement behavior once the vertebra moves to a position where it can support load.[46] This is due to the ability of the remaining uninjured structures to support the applied loads. It should also be noted that preliminary studies indicate that the decrease in height of the vertebral body[44] (Figure 8.40) or the distance between vertebrae adjacent to the injured one at the anterior surface[47] are potential indicators of residual stability of the injured spine.

Summary

The three column concept of the spine is useful in visualizing the effect of injured structures on

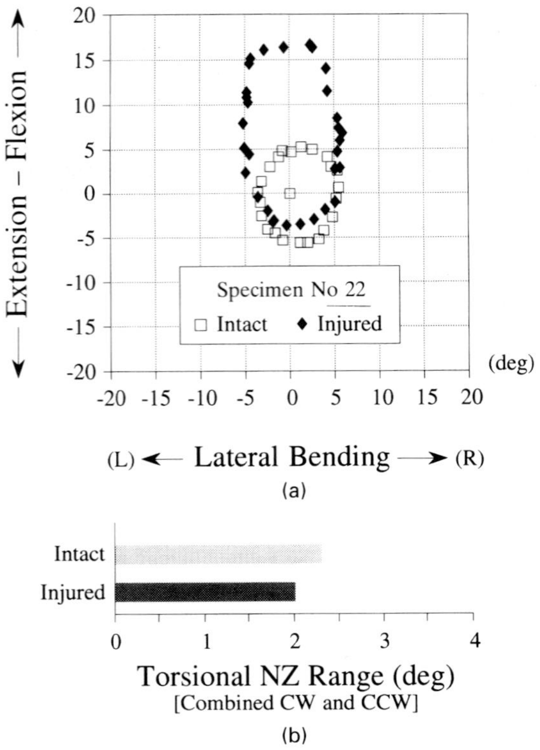

Figure 8.39

Example of the neutral zone ranges of motion of a specimen that sustained a flexion distraction injury. (a) Flexion–extension–lateral bending neutral zone. (b) Torsional range of motion. (From Ref 45.)

flexion–extension motions, and determining the effects of fixator placement. Loss of anterior column structures shifts the axis of rotation posteriorly to a position near the facets. With loss of anterior and middle columns, the axis shifts posterior to the spinal musculature. When the posterior column is injured, the axis shifts anterior to its location in the intact spine, which is in the central–posterior part of the disc.

The neutral zone is a useful way of representing the effect of injury on the mechanical behavior of the spine. The mechanical behavior of the injured spine can be explained in terms of the loss of contributions of the damaged components. In a pure compressive injury, the vertebral body height is decreased but soft tissue structures remain intact, allowing load bearing. With bursting, fracture of the facets and a greater loss in body height create ligamentous laxity and loss of facet contributions to flexion and lateral bending, increasing the neutral zone. A flexion–distraction injury disrupts the posterior elements, thereby increasing the flexion, but not the lateral bending or torsional neutral zones. These concepts are shown graphically in Figure 8.41.

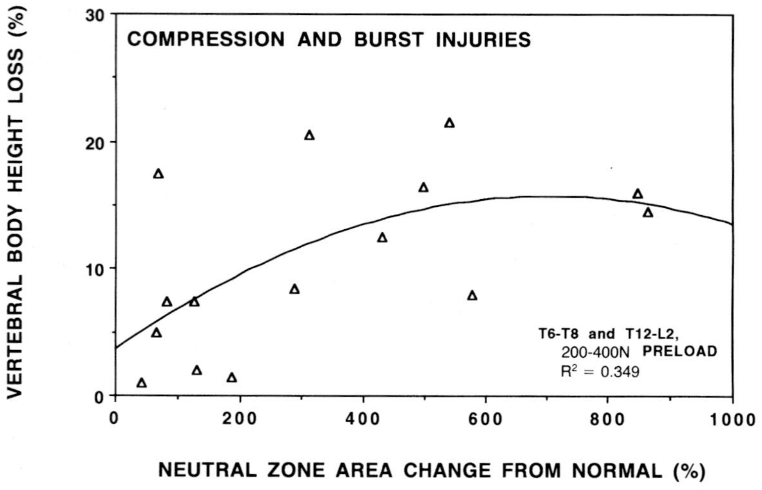

Figure 8.40

Plot of the percentage increase in neutral zone motion in flexion, lateral bending, and torsion (in degrees) versus percent height loss of the injured vertebral body. (Adapted from data in Ref 45.)

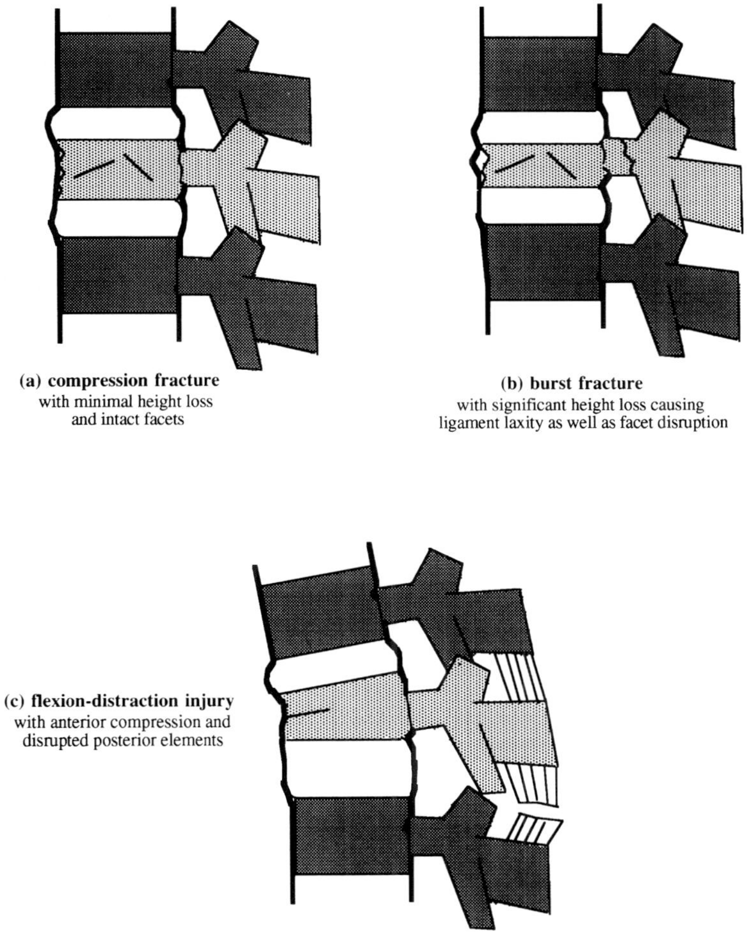

Figure 8.41

(a) A compression fracture does not disrupt the major soft tissues. (b) A bursting injury creates ligamentous laxity and facet disruption, which increase the neutral zone range of motion. (c) A flexion–distraction injury increases the flexion neutral zone.

8.7 The thoracolumbar bone/implant interface

The ability of an implant to transfer load depends upon the strength of the bone/implant interface. With posterior instrumentation, the lamina, transverse process, or (in the case of pedicle screw attachment) the vertebral body bone, are the sites at which load is transferred.

Hook and wire fixation

Pullout or direct posterior loading is considered to be a primary mechanism by which failure can occur in some instrumentation systems. This is due to the flexion moment acting on the spine, as shown in Figure 8.42. The thoracic lamina are quite weak in distractive loading (tension along the longitudinal axis of the spine), with failure loads reported to be in the range of 195–293 N.[48] The maximum pullout strength of a vertebral lamina increases from a mean of 1403 N in the upper thoracic spine (T1–T4), to 1348 N for T5–T8, 1793 N for T9–T12, and 3253 N for lumbar vertebrae.[49] Single sublaminar wires tend to cut through the lamina, failing at a mean of 850 N, while double wires or bands reduce cutting into laminar bone and increase failure loads to a mean of 1100 N.[50] Cotrel–Dubousset (C–D) hooks situated sublaminarly fail in pullout at a mean of 827 N compared with 595 N when they are

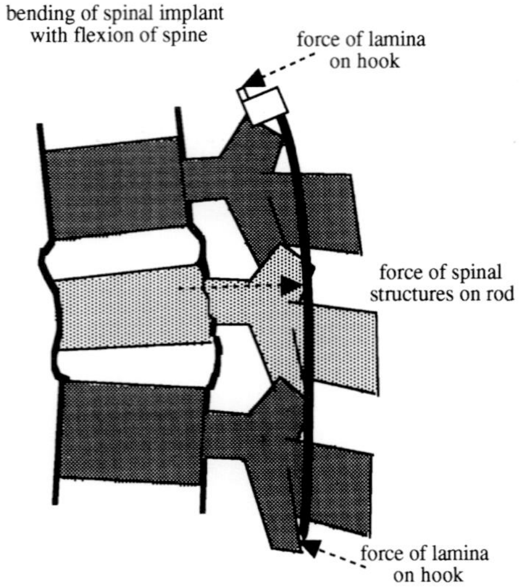

Figure 8.42

Flexion moment produces bending of a posterior implant and posterior pullout force at the spine/implant interface.

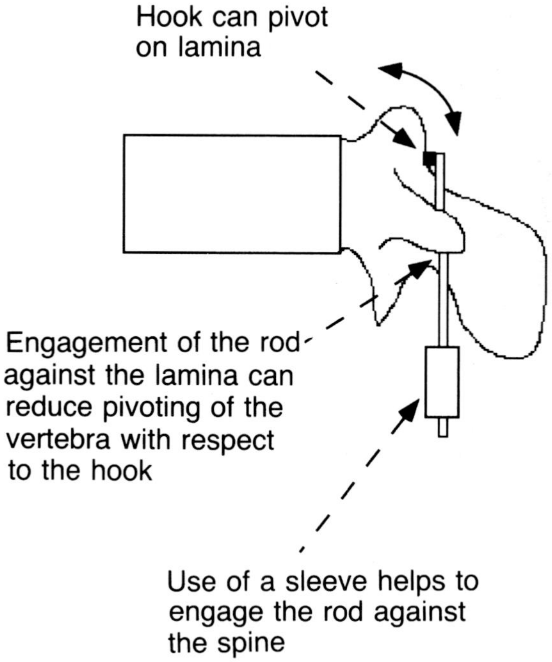

Figure 8.43

Using a hook to couple the instrumentation to bone allows rotation at the hook/lamina interface, reducing control of flexion–extension motion. If the rod engages the posterior laminar wall, or a sleeve is used, this effect can be reduced.

located on the pedicle inferiorly and the transverse process superiorly (in calf spines).[51] Wire pullout in spinous processes requires a mean 783 N tensile load.[52]

The lamina is the strongest purchase site in the posterior thoracolumbar spine, and, significantly, is less affected by osteoporotic bone loss than the trabecular bone within the pedicle and vertebral body, the site of the pedicle screw.[53] The hook/lamina interface is a connection that transfers load only in compression between the bone and hook material. This provides resistance to posterior pull and axial compression or distraction forces. Pivoting occurs between the hook and lamina, so that flexion rotation of the vertebra is not directly controlled by the hook. However, interaction of the rod with the lamina does block flexion rotation, as shown in Figure 8.43. Sublaminar wiring is not effective in transmitting axial load to the rods, and slippage of wire on the rod can result during lateral bending, flexion, and compression loading.[53]

The pedicle screw

The pedicle screw presents an alternative to fixation by hooks or wires. This type of implant permits the transmission of moments in all directions, except about the axis of the screw, along with the ability to resist loads transverse to and along that axis. The pullout strength of pedicle screws, as with other bone screws, depends upon several parameters (see Chapter 6). A most important controllable parameter is the diameter of the screw, since the bending strength, cyclic fatigue strength (Figure 8.44),[54] and pullout strength[55,56] increase significantly with increasing diameter. A number of studies have documented the minimum sagittal and transverse widths of the

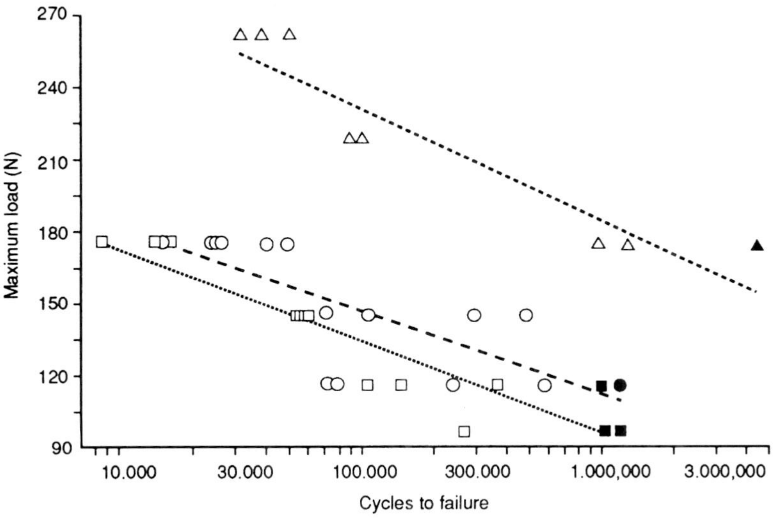

Figure 8.44

Number of cycles to failure for modified AO cancellous 6.5 mm lag screw (○), 5.5 mm (□) and 7.0 mm (△) diameter Steffee pedicle screws loaded in bending. (From Ref 54 with permission.)

pedicles in order to permit appropriate sizing of screws. Figure 8.45 shows a comparison of the results of several investigations. In general the minimum pedicle diameter ranges from about 5 to 7 mm in the thoracic spine, but increases rapidly towards the distal end of the lumbar spine, to between 15 and 18 mm at L5.[56–60]

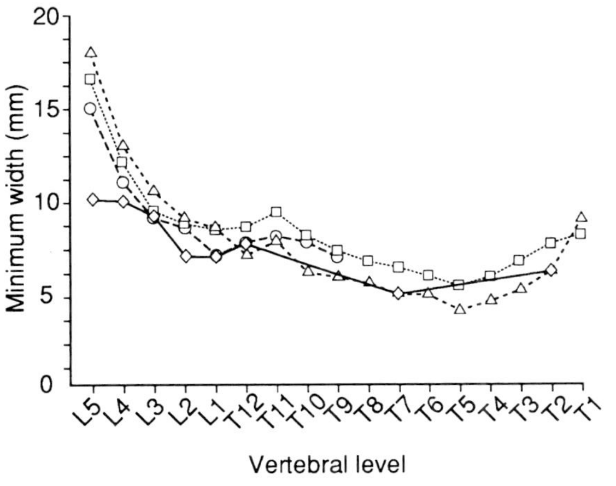

Figure 8.45

Comparison of mean minimum pedicle diameters at different vertebral levels as reported in several studies: Ref 54 (◇); Ref 55 (△); Ref 56 (○); Ref 57 (□). (From Ref 54 with permission.)

A second important parameter in determining the pullout strength of pedicle screws is the shear strength of the material into which they are embedded, i.e. the shear strength of cancellous bone. Pedicle screw purchase in the spine is correlated to bone mineral density, a measure of shear strength (see Chapter 6) (Figure 8.46).[61–64] In addition, bone density varies within the vertebra itself, being greatest near the endplates and cortical shell and least in the midplane. Wu et al[65] showed that pedicle screws placed close to the endplates provide the best overall stabilty.

The contributions of some other factors to the mechanical performance of the pedicle screw have been studied. Altering hole preparation technique (3 mm K wire probe versus 4 mm drill bit),[54,66] screw thread shape ("V" or buttress, shallow or deep thread),[54,57,62] or depth of insertion into the vertebral body (50% of vertebral diameter versus to anterior cortex)[59] produce little or no gain in screw pullout strength. However, screw depth of penetration (50% of vertebral diameter versus 80%) does increase the moment required to cut the screw laterally through the vertebral wall.[56] Also, screws pulled out at a mean

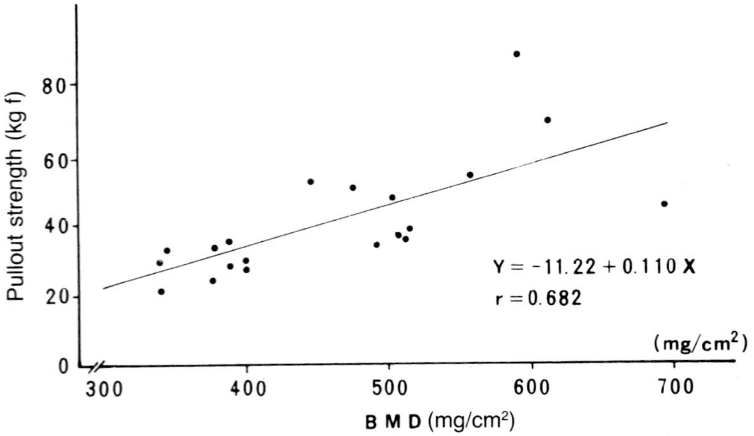

Figure 8.46

The correlation between vertebral bone mineral density (BMD) and the pullout strength of AO 6.5 mm cancellous pedicle screws. (From Ref 61 with permission.)

load of 903 N when positioned to the anterior vertebral cortex and 1186 N when they engaged the anterior cortex.[59]

When pedicle screws are loaded in a caudocephalad direction (i.e. transverse to their long axis), a "toggle" type of displacement can result.[59,67] This occurs because, as shown in Figure 8.47, the narrowest part of the pedicle is its base. The screw is therefore sized to fit the base of the pedicle, which becomes a fulcrum about which it can rotate when load is applied transverse to the axis of the screw.[67] Wittenburg et al[62] showed that if a controlled displacement of ± 2 mm is applied to the end of a screw in a caudocephalad direction, the initial load drops from about 200 N to less than half that value in fewer than 10 000 load cycles (Figure 8.48). The "butterfly" pattern of widening of the pedicle screw hole due to this type of loading is clearly seen in Figure 8.49, and can be reduced by, for example, capturing the head of the screw so that it cannot displace. With this method, rotation of the screw is eliminated by adding a second point of fixation to the screw (Figure 8.47c).[67] Alternately, applying screws so they are not parallel and then crosslinking them can reduce this effect.

Ashman et al[68] described an event that results in breakage of the screw instead of loosening, when adequate purchase is obtained in bone. If the instrumentation is applied posteriorly and there is little resistance to flexion in the stabilized spine (i.e. no graft is placed anteriorly to buttress the spine against flexion) anteriorly then the screws are loaded in bending, as shown in Figure 8.50. Under these conditions, the tensile stresses (caused by the cantilever bending) at the base of the screw can exceed the endurance limit tensile stress for stainless steel at axial load levels below 150 N, which is well below the expected physiological load (Figure 8.51). If the endurance limit stress magnitude is exceeded, the implant is potentially liable to fail by fatigue. Protection against fatigue failure requires reducing the load experienced by the implant, or increasing the minor diameter of the screw. Screws can also be unloaded by eliminating the rigid plate/screw connection (which reduces the bending moment on the screw), distributing the load among a greater number of screws, ensuring that an anterior vertebral body graft is well located to minimize flexion moments, and protecting the surgical site against excessive repetitive stresses.

Summary

The bone/implant interface is a critical component of the spinal fixation system, and is the location of many fixation failures. The lamina is the strongest region, and is less affected by osteoporotic bone

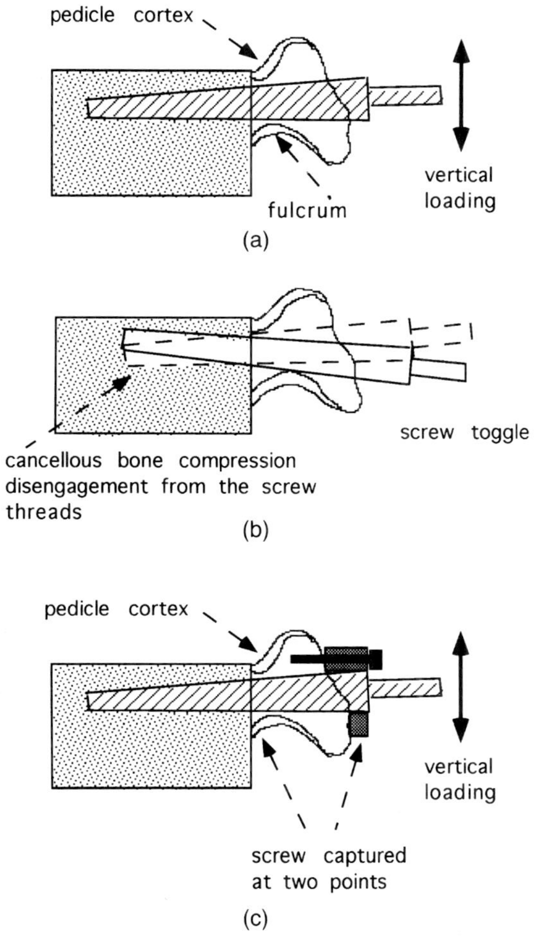

Figure 8.47

(a) A mechanism by which the pedicle screw can toggle and ultimately loosen with caudocephalad loading. (b) In this system, the base of the pedicle, being the most rigid region (there is the least cancellous bone for the screw to engage), becomes the fulcrum, and the screw can toggle and loosen. (c) If the head of the screw is prevented from moving, this toggle is greatly diminished. (From Ref 67.)

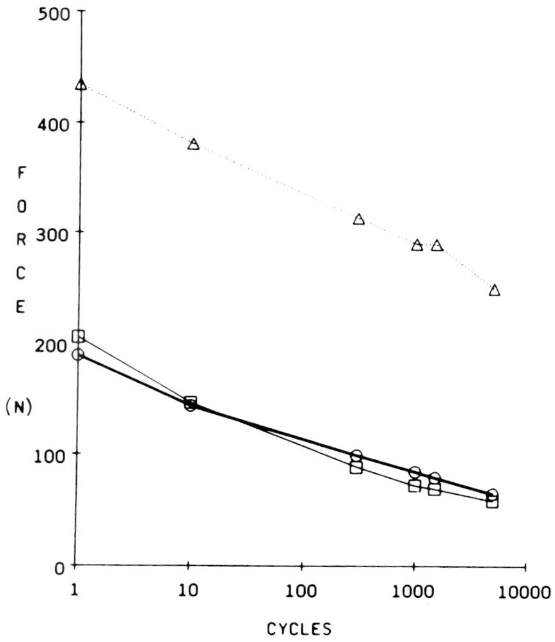

Figure 8.48

Decrease in resisting force with number of load cycles in a pedicle screw placed in a vertebra, in response to a caudocephalad displacement of ± 2 mm —□—, Kluger screw (human specimens); —○—, Steffee (human); --△--, Steffee (calf). (From Ref 62 with permission.)

loss than is the trabecular bone of the vertebra. Hooks placed in the lamina can transmit loads in directions where they are forced against bone, but cannot resist rotation about the lamina, unless the rod to which they are engaged is blocked from rotation by interference with posterior bony structures. Pedicle screws are an alternate form of fixation, but their purchase is governed by the same parameters that control other screws. In particular, purchase is decreased when they are placed into osteoporotic bone of the vertebral body. They can be susceptible to loosening due to caudocephalad loading, where they can pivot around the base of the pedicle and open a butterfly shaped depression in the vertebral body.

8.8 General considerations in applying thoracolumbar spinal fixation

Long versus short rods

Krag[53] outlines some important considerations when applying spinal constructs. In general,

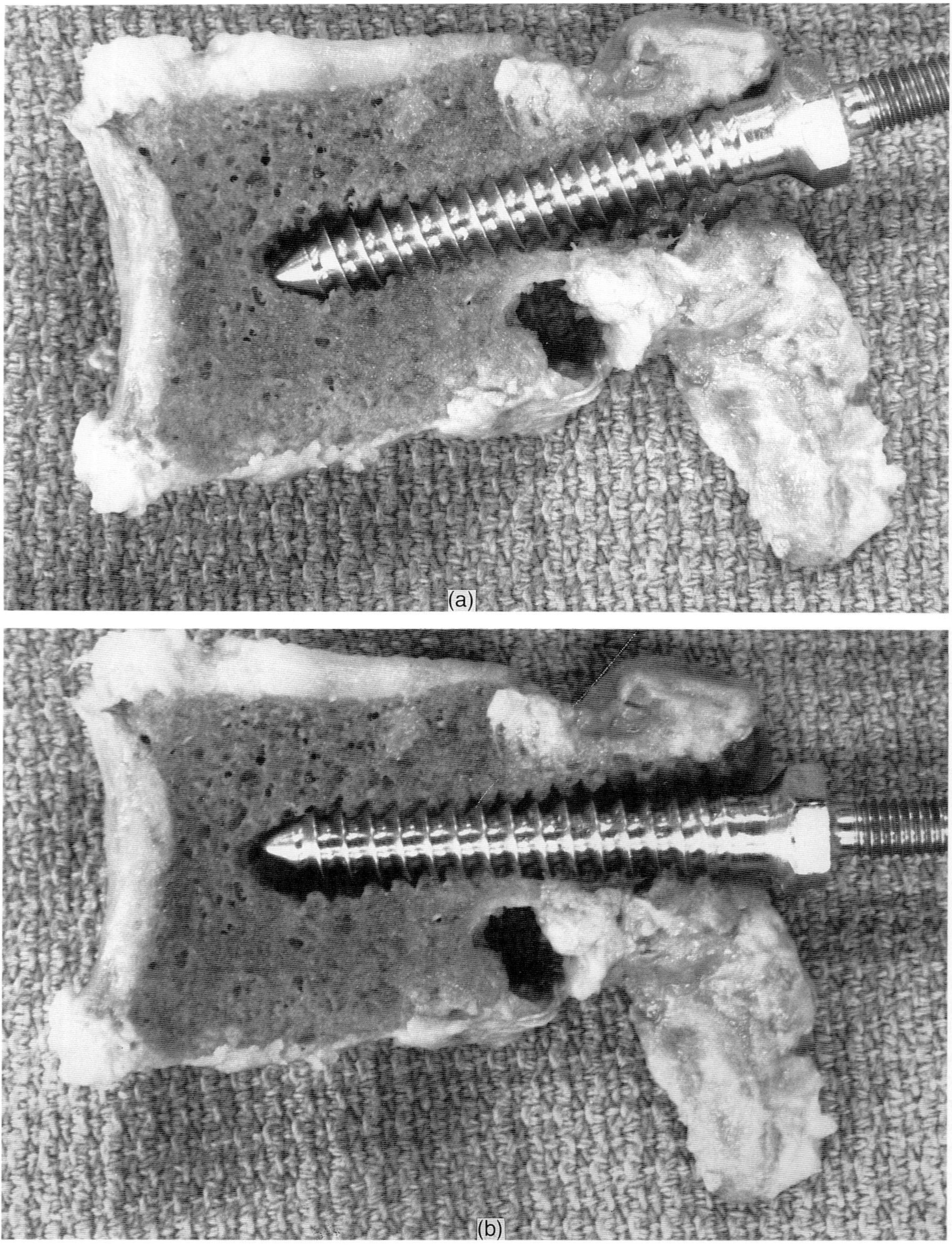

Figure 8.49

Photographs showing the positions of a screw in (a) maximum caudal and (b) maximum cephalad loading, demonstrating the cancellous bone that has been crushed during loading, causing the screw to loosen. (From Ref 67 with permission.)

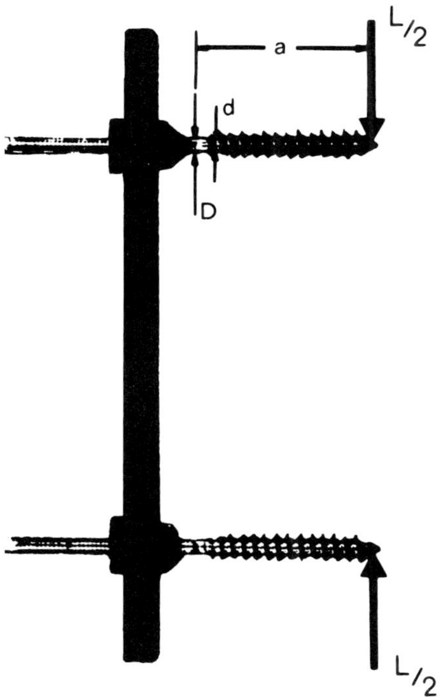

Figure 8.50

Forces acting on a pedicle screw fixation system with the screws rigidly attached to the plate. The loads applied to the screws through engagement with the vertebral body bone (*L*/2) bend the screws and plate. The screw acts as a cantilever beam, with the maximum stresses occurring at its base (the junction with the plate). (From Ref 68 with permission.)

because of the location of the center of gravity of the torso anterior to the lower lumbar spine, flexion is a predominant mode of loading, along with compression (see Figure 8.31). For the same applied moment, a construct in which the rod is applied over a larger number of spinal motion segments will produce smaller forces in the rod hooks, because the larger moment arm of the rod reduces the magnitude of forces required at the rod/implant interface to generate a moment able to resist an externally applied flexion moment (Figure 8.52).

Anterior strut graft

The mechanical function of an anterior graft is illustrated in Figure 8.53. With fixation to the vertebra above the injured one in a fracture with the anterior column compromised, the moment generated by a short segment pedicle screw implant to counteract the externally applied flexion moment is equal to the force in the screw times the length of the moment arm (distance from the axis of the screw to the fulcrum of the system). Screw forces can be reduced by either increasing the length of the moment arm, distributing the forces over a greater number of screws, and/or using an anterior strut graft. The compressive force from a well fitted anterior graft, times its distance from the fulcrum of the system, results in an additional moment to counteract the external flexion moment, thereby reducing forces in the implant.

Posterior spinal instrumentation biomechanics

A distraction type of instrumentation, such as a Harrington rod system (hooks on lamina of vertebrae above and below injury site and a ratcheted connecting rod that allows separation of the hooks), applies axial tension (distraction) to the immobilized segment in order to regain height in the injured area and also to maintain the positions of the hooks on the lamina. With this type of instrumentation, viscoelastic creep (continued tissue elongation under load; see Chapter 1) of the soft tissues of the spine will decrease the distractive force over a period of time, resulting in lower hook purchase forces at the lamina. Nachemson and Elfstrom[69] demonstrated this, using in vivo measurements of the axial force in Harrington rods applied for scoliosis. As shown in Figure 8.54, the axial force in the rod decreased sharply after initial application of the implants and more gradually thereafter, so that by 18 days postoperatively the axial force of distraction was only about 25% of that applied initially. It is important, when using soft tissue as a counterforce to distraction applied by the implant, to check the distractive force at a later time during the procedure.

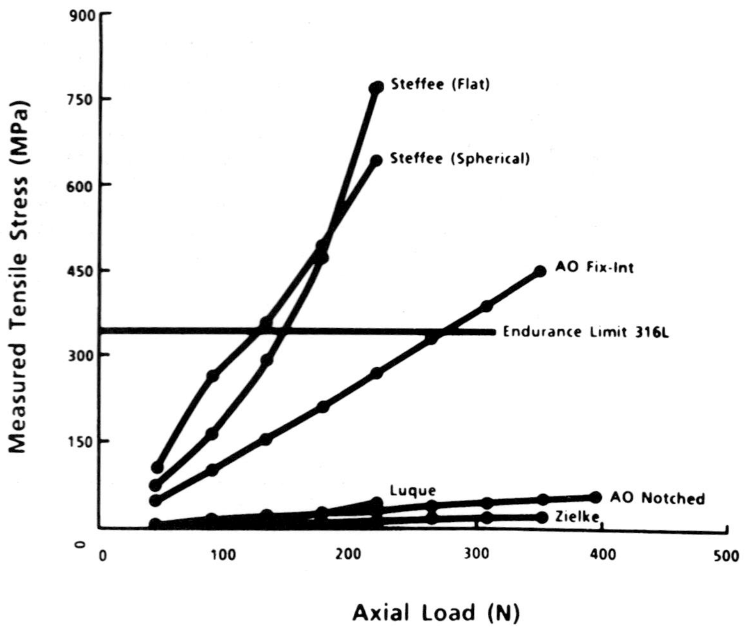

Figure 8.51

Tensile stress measured from strain gages at the bases of various pedicle screws as a function of the axial load applied to the implant. (From Ref 68 with permission.)

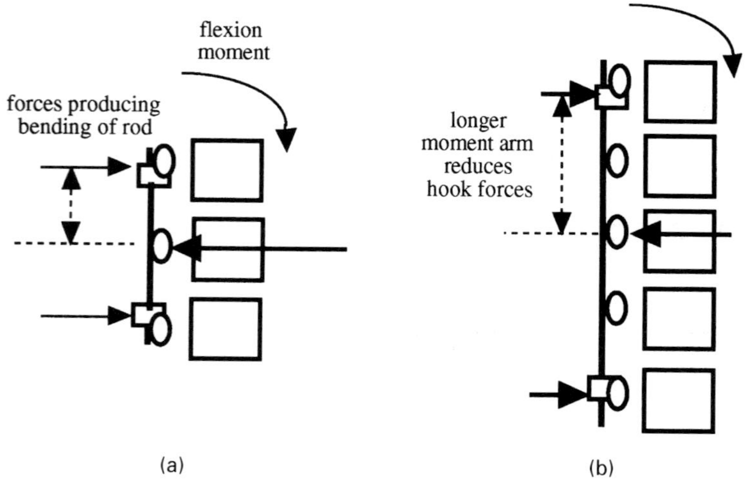

Figure 8.52

Biomechanical comparison of long and short posterior rodding of the spine. For the same externally applied flexion moment: (a) the short rodded segment produces a resisting moment in the rod equal to the force at the hook site times the distance of the force to the center of the rod; (b) if the rod is longer, the center of the rod to hook site distance is greater; therefore, to counteract the same moment, the hook site force is smaller. (Adapted from Ref 53.)

The loading on a posterior spinal instrumentation with different types of injury should be distinguished. In the case of posterior element injury (loss of the posterior column), where the motion segment can still maintain resistance to compression through intact discs (anterior and middle columns), the flexion center of rotation has shifted anteriorly (see Figure 8.34) and the flexion neutral zone has enlarged (Figure 8.39). Distractive force applied by the implant adds to the external flexion moment (Figure 8.55a). In order for the implant to contribute to resisting flexion of

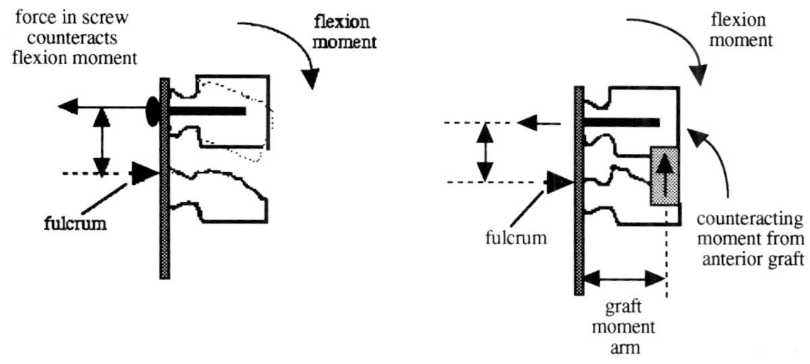

Figure 8.53

The mechanical role of an anterior strut graft. (a) Without an anterior graft, a moment is generated in the implant by screw forces due to the external flexion moment. The large force may cause screw toggle within the vertebra or high stresses in the screw. (b) An anterior graft produces a moment counteracting the external flexion moment, reducing force in the implant. (Adapted from Ref 53.)

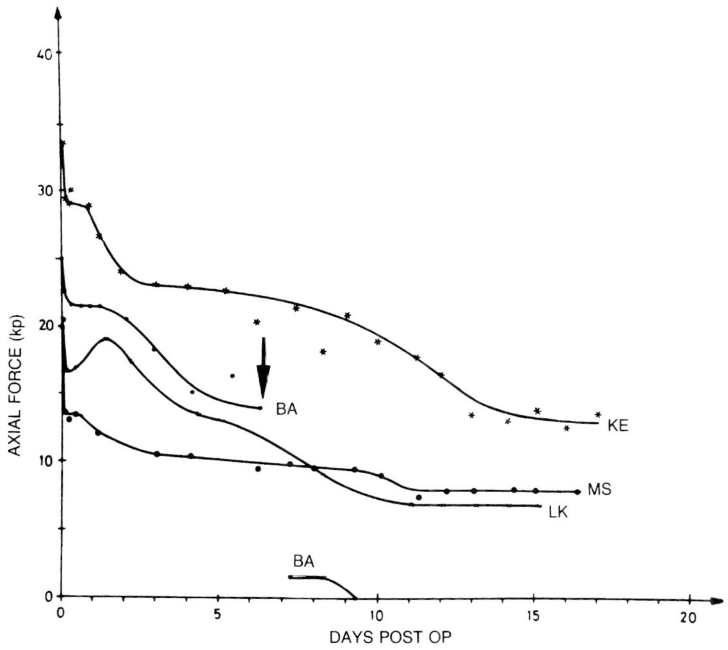

Figure 8.54

Decline in the axial force in the Harrington distraction rod with time post surgery due to creep in the soft tissues of the spine. (From Ref 69 with permission.)

the spine, either the implant must be converted so that it applies compression to the spine, or the flexion displacement of the spine must be converted into bending in the implant. A sleeve placed between the implant and the lamina results in bending and resistance to flexion, even while distraction is applied by the implant (Figure 8.55b).

If the anterior column is disrupted, the flexion–extension center of rotation moves posteriorly (Figure 8.32), close to the facets and the implant. The moment arm (distance from axis of rotation to axis of implant rod) and hence the resulting moment are small because the implant axis is close to the flexion–extension center (Figure 8.56). In this situation, bending of the implant is a

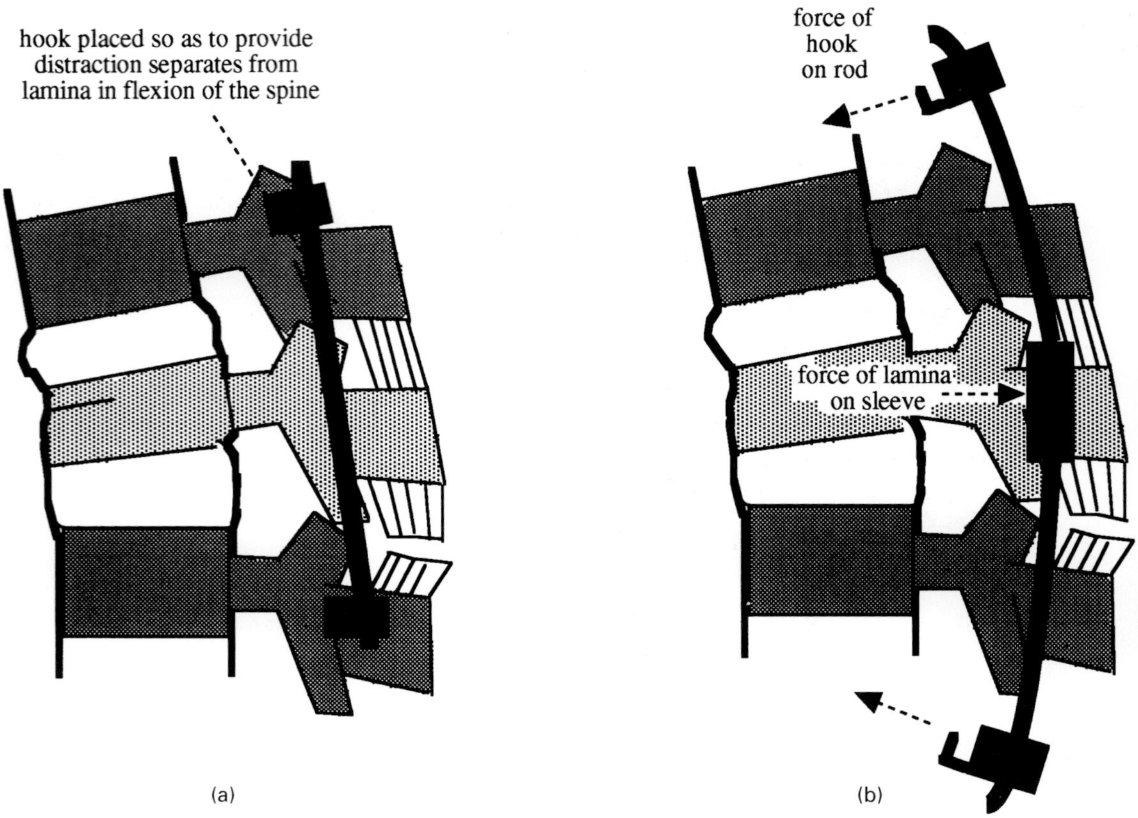

Figure 8.55

(a) In the case of posterior element disruption, the flexion–extension axis shifts anteriorly. A distraction instrumentation contributes to the external flexion moment applied to the spine instead of resisting it. A compression instrumentation counteracts the flexion moment. (b) Placing a sleeve between the lamina and the implant produces bending in the implant when a flexion moment is applied, allowing a distraction instrumentation to resist flexion.

primary mechanism for resisting flexion deformity, as opposed to compressive force generated through the hooks. If both the anterior and middle columns are disrupted, the center of flexion–extension moves posterior to the facets (Figure 8.33). With the center of rotation in this position, a distractive force from the implant now opposes the external flexion moment applied to the spine (Figure 8.57), in contrast to the case of posterior column disruption. The implant must, however, be able to support direct compressive forces as well as bending in this very unstable situation.

A bursting injury with disruption of the facets was shown to be unstable in lateral bending and torsion (Figure 8.38). If an implant is applied that has separate rods or plates as the longitudinal members, and fixed by screws as shown in Figure 8.58, the system can act as a four bar mechanism, which allows the injured motion segment to displace laterally, providing little resistance to

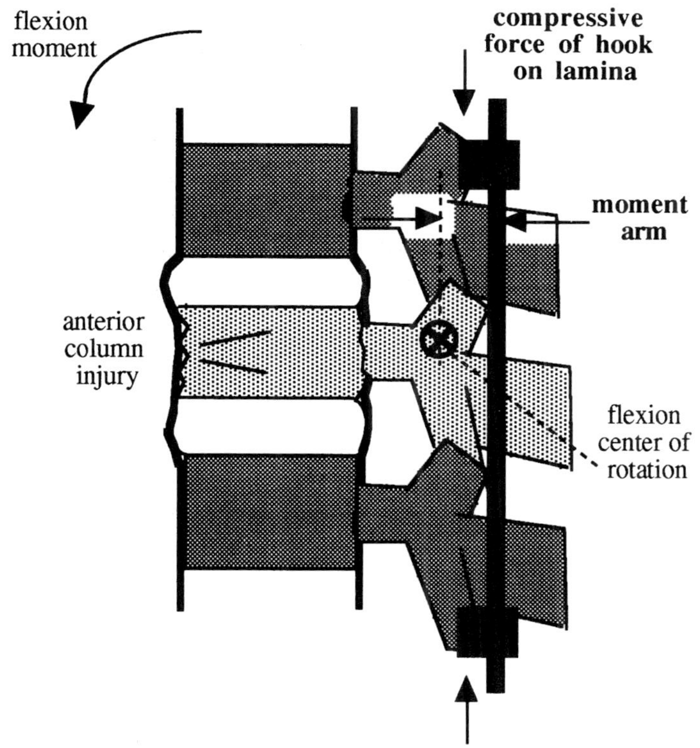

Figure 8.56

With anterior column disruption, the flexion–extension center of rotation shifts posteriorly, near to the axis of the implant, decreasing the moment arm. Therefore compressive force in the implant contributes little to opposing the external flexion moment, and bending of the device is necessary.

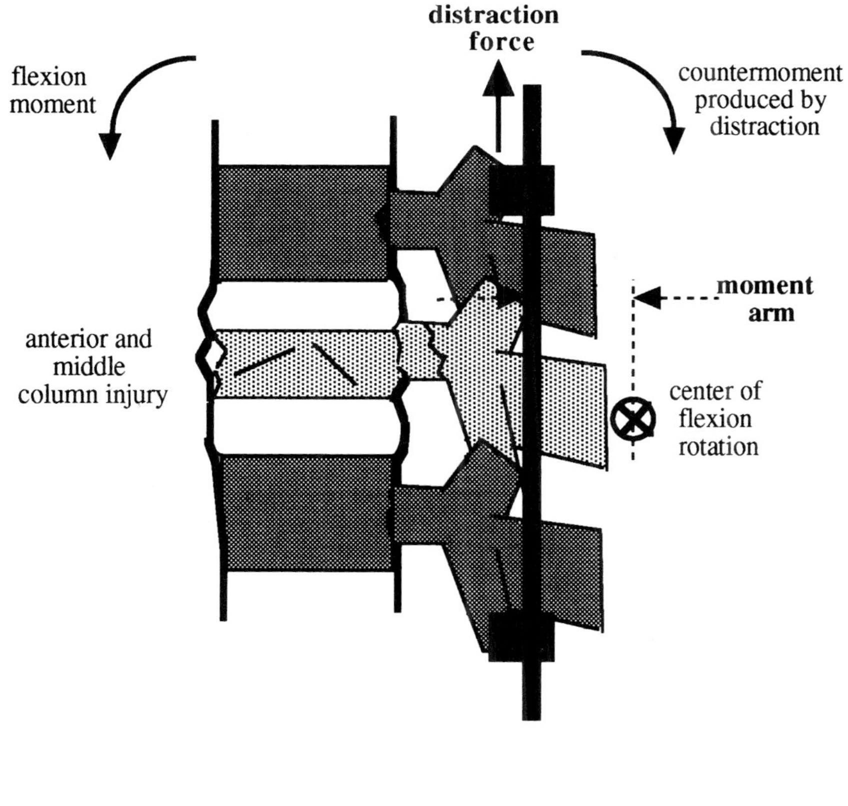

Figure 8.57

When both the anterior and middle columns are disrupted, the flexion–extension center of rotation shifts posterior to the implant, so that distractive force from the implant also counteracts flexion.

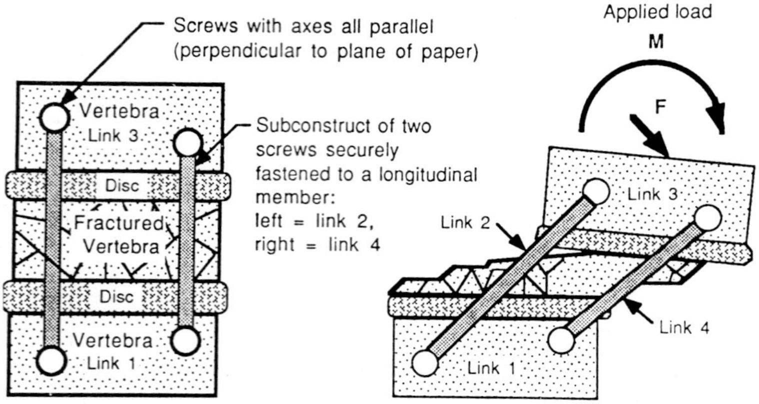

Figure 8.58

A fixation system arranged with parallel bars and parallel pedicle scews allows lateral displacement, which makes the construct less rigid in lateral bending and torsion. Addition of a coupler bar between the rods, creating an "H" configuration, or angling the screws towards each other, prevents this motion. (From Ref 70 with permission.)

torsion and lateral bending.[70] A coupler bar that connects the rods, making an "H" configuration, is a very effective method for increasing lateral bending and torsional stability.

Distraction of the injured spine to regain normal height is a very important aspect of the fixation procedure. Not only does it aid in returning retropulsed bone fragments in the spinal canal to their anatomic position,[71] but recreating the normal anatomic distances between vertebrae also retensions the ligamentous interconnections between vertebrae, which aids in restoring mechanical stability to the spine.[45]

Summary

Some general biomechanical principles can be defined related to the application of posterior fixation for unstable spinal injuries. Using fixation with hooks or screws placed further apart above and below the fracture decreases the force at the bone/implant interface, since the moment arm of the screw or hook force increases. An anterior strut graft also decreases implant forces by generating a moment that counteracts the external flexion moment acting on the spine. Posterior instrumentation applied in distraction in injuries that damage the posterior or posterior and middle columns does not counteract the external flexion moment. To generate resistance to deformity, the implant must bend, which can be accomplished by placing a sleeve on the rod that is in contact with the spinal lamina.

8.9 Performance of spinal fixation in thoracolumbar spinal injuries

A large number of studies have appeared comparing the stability offered by different forms of spinal constructs. It should be emphasized that the type and degree of injury play a large part in determining the stabilizing potential of various devices.[72] Therefore direct comparisons of the mechanical performance of various types of devices is given in the context of the type of injury that the implant is required to stabilize, and the discussion is limited to studies which simulate a realistic bone/implant interface.

Posterior column (flexion–distraction) injury

Shea et al[73] considered several configurations of three types of instrumentation systems: the Hartshill rectangle (with sublaminar wires at L2 and L5), the Dick fixateur interne (with pedicle screws at L3, L4 or L2, L5),[74] and the Steffee plate (with pedicle screws at L2, L5, or L3, L4, or L2, L3, L4, L5),[75] shown in Figure 8.59. The model was a posterior column injury (posterior ligaments disrupted, see Figures 8.34, 8.39, and 8.41), which can support compression, lateral bending, and axial rotation, but is unstable in flexion. All constructs, as would be expected, were similar in stiffness under compressive loading, which ranged from approximately 66.9 to 91.5% of the stiffness of intact spines. In flexion, as shown in Figure 8.60, the three constructs when attached to L2 and L5 produced stiffnesses from 265% to 174% of that of the intact spine, while if attached to shorter segments (L3, L4), stiffness ranged from 95.3% to 100% of intact. This demonstrates that the biomechanical advantage of applying an implant over a longer spinal segment overshadows individual differences between devices.

Performance of fixation systems for a posterior–middle column injury

This injury disrupts the posterior elements and the posterior half of the disc. The injured spine is unstable to loads in flexion, compression, lateral bending, and rotation, and therefore places high demands on the instrumentation. The axis of flexion–extension rotation is anterior to its normal location (Figure 8.34); therefore devices placed posteriorly and able to resist separation of the posterior part of the motion segment (i.e.

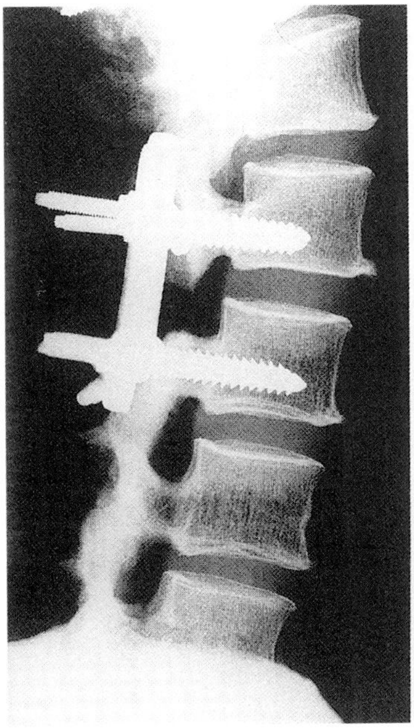

(a)

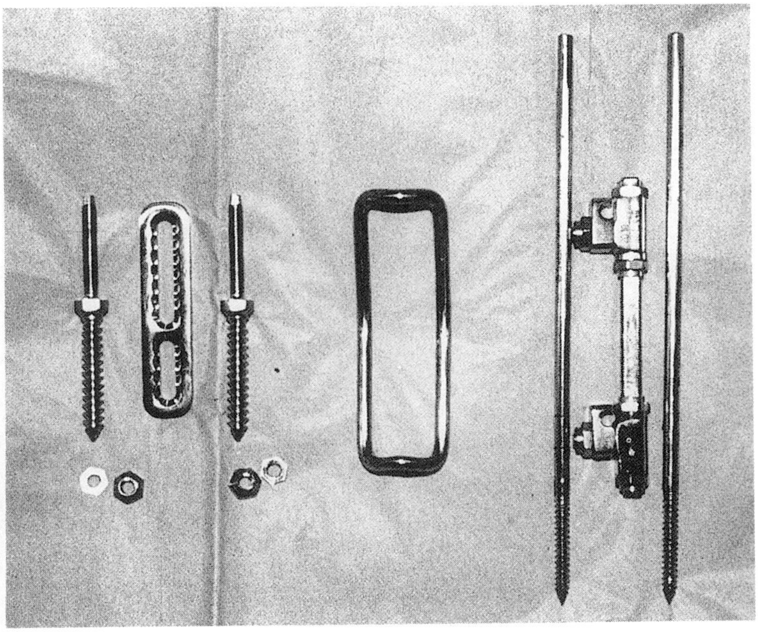

(b)

Figure 8.59

(a) Steffee plates and screws in situ. (b) Three implants tested in a posterior column injury model: (from left) Steffee plate, Hartshill rectangle, and Dick fixateur interne. (From Ref 73 with permission.)

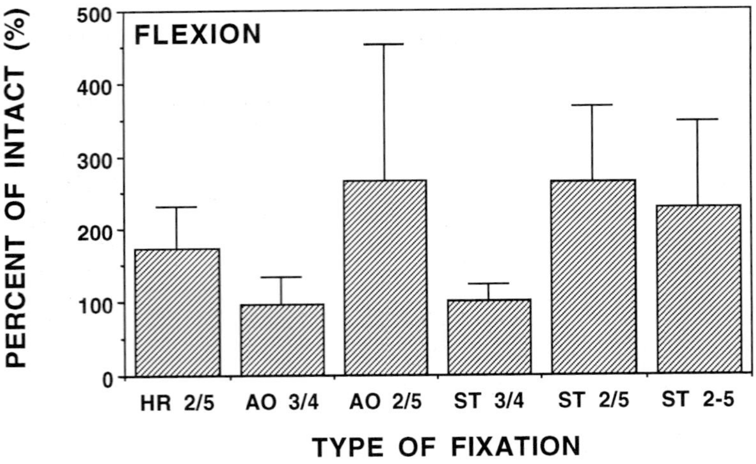

Figure 8.60

Relative stiffnesses in flexion compared with intact, of various posterior constructs with a posterior column injury (posterior elements only disrupted): HR2/5, Hartsfield rectangle with sublaminar wires at L2 and L5; AO3/4, fixateur interne with screws at L3, L4; AO2/5, fixateur interne with screws at L2, L5; ST3/4, Steffee plate with screws at L3, L4; ST2/5, Steffee plate with screws at L2, L5; ST2-5, Steffee plate with screws at L2, L3, L4, L5. (Data adapted from Ref 73.)

spreading of the lamina) have the greatest resistance to flexion and lateral bending loads.

Panjabi et al[76] compared the biomechanical properties of a number of constructs applied in this injury pattern, including the anterolaterally placed Dunn device, Harrington rods placed in distraction, compression, combined distraction and compression, or distraction with Edwards sleeves, and Luque rods, rectangle or short rectangle fixed with sublaminar wires (Figure 8.61). From Figure 8.62, in flexion, the Dunn device (note that this is the only device placed

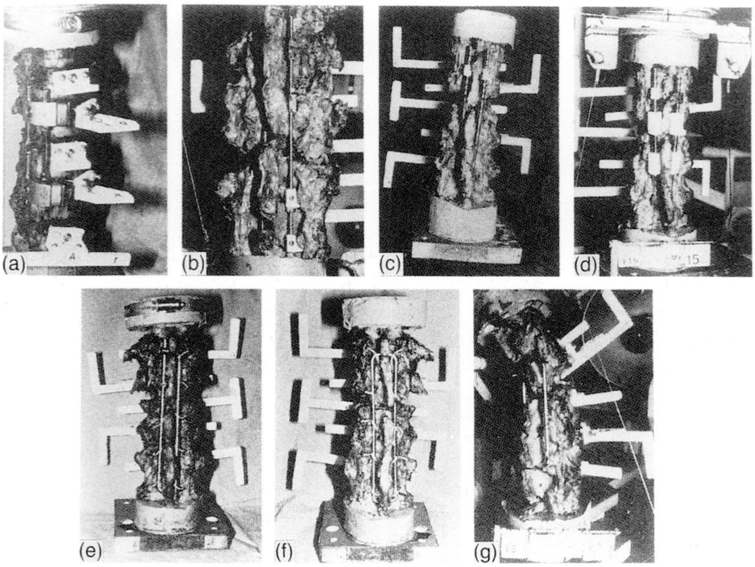

Figure 8.61

Spinal implant constructs for a posterior–middle column spinal injury: (a) Dunn device; (b) Harrington compression rods; (c) Harrington distraction rods; (d) Harrington distraction rods with sleeves; (e) Luque rod; (f) Luque rectangle; (g) Luque short rectangle. (From Ref 76 with permission.)

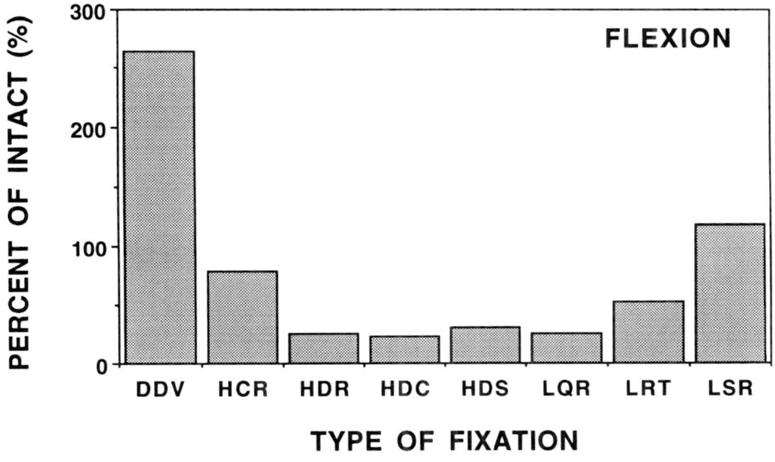

Figure 8.62

Motion allowed in flexion, as a percent of intact spinal motion, of some constructs in a spine posterior–middle column injury: DDV, Dunn anterior device; HCR, Harrington compression rods; HDR, Harrington distraction rods; HDC, Harrington distraction rods and compression rods; HDS, Harrington distraction rods with sleeves; LQR, Luque rod; LRT, Luque rectangle; LSR, Luque short rectangle. (Data adapted from Ref 76.)

anteriorly on the vertebral body) permits 265% of intact motion, the Luque short rectangle 118%, the Harrington compression rods 79%, and the other constructs (Harrington distraction and compression rods) from 52% to 23%. Clearly, the ineffectiveness of placing an anterior device in a posterior–middle column injury is demonstrated by these results. The Harrington compression rods, being threaded and of smaller diameters than the distraction rods, are less rigid in bending and probably flex more under load, while the Luque short rectangle is not long enough to develop an effective moment arm.

In lateral bending, the least effective fixation was the Luque short rectangle (181% of intact), and the most stabilizing were the Dunn device and Luque rod (72% of intact). The devices with distraction hooks cannot prevent the lamina on the side away from the direction of bending from lifting off the hook. The short Luque rectangle again has insufficient length and attachment points, and sliding of the wires on the rod makes the transmission of force to the rod difficult. The most stability is gained by the long Luque rod with multiple wiring sites, which transforms the lateral moment into bending in both rods. In extension, the Dunn device was least stable (208% of intact) and the Harrington distraction rods with (35%) and without sleeves (13%) were the most stable constructs. Since the spine lamina directly load the distraction hooks in extension, the superiority of distraction instrumentation in this loading mode is not unexpected. In torsion (Figure 8.63), no construct was able to reproduce the stiffness of the intact motion segment, with motion (compared to the intact spine) ranging from 447% (Harrington compression rods) to 219% (Luque rods). The main problem with most constructs in resisting torsion is the lack of a central coupler bar to prevent the implant from acting like a linkage (Figure 8.58).

Performance of fixation systems for an anterior–middle column (bursting) injury

An anterior–middle column injury shifts the flexion–extension center of rotation posteriorly, behind the instrumentation itself (Figure 8.33), and is highly unstable to compression, flexion, lateral bending, and torsion (Figure 8.38). Gurr et al[77] compared the stiffnesses of several anterior and posterior constructs applied in this situation. Figure 8.64 shows examples of strut grafting alone and the Kaneda device[78] applied anteriorly. Posterior fixation devices included Harrington distraction rods, Cotrel–Dubousset instrumentation (CD) with 5 mm pedicle screws,

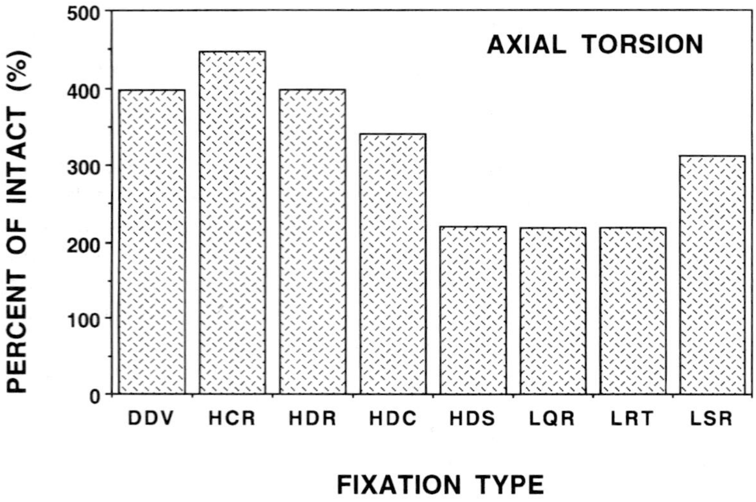

Figure 8.63

Motion in torsion, compared with the intact spine, of some constructs in a spine posterior–middle injury: DDV, Dunn anterior device; HCR, Harrington compression rods; HDR, Harrington distraction rods; HDC, Harrington distraction and compression rods; HDS, Harrington distraction rods with sleeves; LQR, Luque rod; LRT, Luque rectangle; LSR, Luque short rectangle. (Data adapted from Ref 76.)

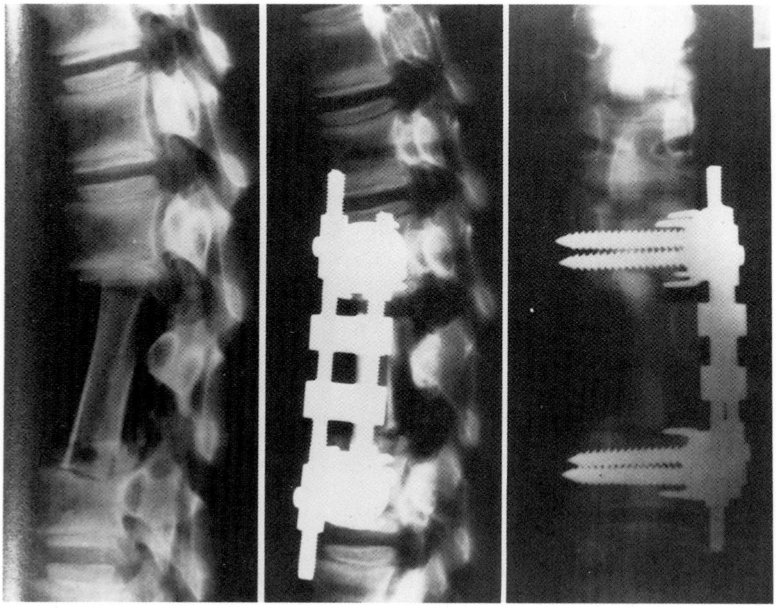

(a) (b) (c)

Figure 8.64

Examples of fixation of a spine fracture with anterior–middle column loss. (a) An iliac crest strut graft alone. (b) Lateral and (c) anterior–posterior views of the Kaneda device. (From Ref 77 with permission.)

Steffee plates and screws, and the Luque rectangle. All the posterior devices were fixed between the first and fifth levels with an anterior strut graft to replace the damaged vertebra.

In direct axial compression, the Kaneda (anterior), CD and Steffee plate systems produced constructs with displacements greater than that of the intact spine, the Harrington rodded construct 238% of intact, the Luque 302%, and the iliac graft alone 398%. These results demonstrate the need for rigid fixation with either pedicle or vertebral screws in addition to the anterior strut graft to control the displacement produced by compressive force in this injury pattern. In flexion (Figure 8.65), the three implants with screw attachments were most effective in limiting angulation, although the stiffest constructs had displacements that were still nearly the same as that of the intact spine. This result shows the difficulty in controlling flexion when the middle column is injured. Also of note is the fact that the strut graft alone does little by itself to control flexion angulation. Its function as a buttress is important, but possibly only at larger loads.

In torsion (Figure 8.66), the implants fixed with screws were again able to produce constructs with stiffnesses greater than that of the intact spine (122–137%). This extremely unstable model demonstrates the need for rigidity at the bone/implant interface with screws that are able to support bending, as opposed to hooks or wires, which permit rotation about the lamina (Figure 8.25). Further testing of other posterior pedicle screw constructs using Zielke,[79] fixateur interne,[74] AO notched plate, or Luque pedicular fixation[80] has shown no significant differences between them in axial compression or torsional rigidity for this injury type.[68] In this fracture, as shown in Figure 8.51, the screws may be highly loaded, especially if they are constrained so as not to be able to rotate with respect to the plate or rod to which they are attached.[68]

Performance of fixation systems for an anterior–middle–posterior column injury

This type of injury is the most severe, with all structures damaged and the spine unable to support any loads at all. Ferguson et al[71] compared spine fracture constructs using Harrington rods with sublaminar wires, C-rods (crossed segmentally wired "C" shaped rods), Jacobs rods,[81] the Vermont fixator,[56] and Roy-Camille plates fixed with pedicle screws[82] (Figure 8.67). In flexion, stiffnesses of the constructs ranged from 33.4% of intact (Vermont fixator) to 139% (Roy-Camille plate), which are values similar to those reported for anterior–middle spine injury constructs. These constructs were extremely stiff in extension (426–1399% of intact), especially the Roy-Camille plate with its multiple screws and stiff plates. The Roy-Camille plate was similarly stiff in lateral bending, while in torsion, stiffnesses ranged from 11.8% of intact for the J rod construct to 144% for the Roy-Camille plate.

The effectiveness of pedicle screw fixation systems in producing rigid constructs in severe spinal injuries is shown also in the study by Gaines et al,[70] who ranked constructs produced by various instrumentation systems by their ability to limit angular and linear displacements

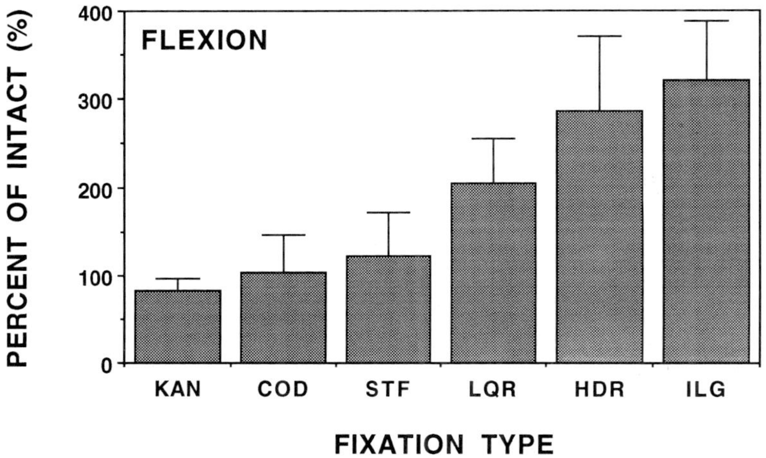

Figure 8.65

Comparison of motion, compared to the intact spine, of anterior and posterior devices in stabilizing an anterior–middle column injury to the spine with flexion loading: KAN, Kaneda device; COD, Cotrel–Dubousset posterior fixation with pedicle screws; STF, Steffee posterior plates and screws; LQR, Luque rectangle with posterior wires; HDR, Harrington distraction rods; ILG, illiac strut graft alone, applied anteriorly. (Data adapted from Ref 77.)

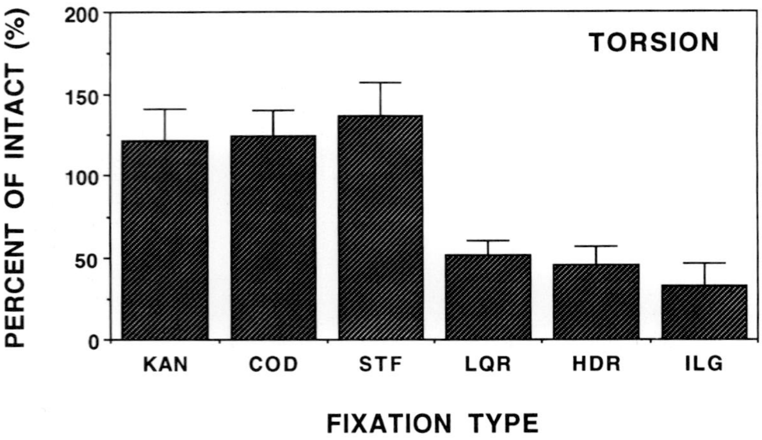

Figure 8.66

Torsional stiffness, compared to the intact spine, of anterior and posterior devices in stabilizing an anterior–middle column injury to the spine with torsion loading: KAN, Kaneda device; COD, Cotrel–Dubousset posterior fixation with pedicle screws; STF, Steffee posterior plates and screws; LQR, Luque rectangle with posterior wires; HDR, Harrington distraction rods; ILG, iliac strut graft alone, applied anteriorly. (Data adapted from Ref 77.)

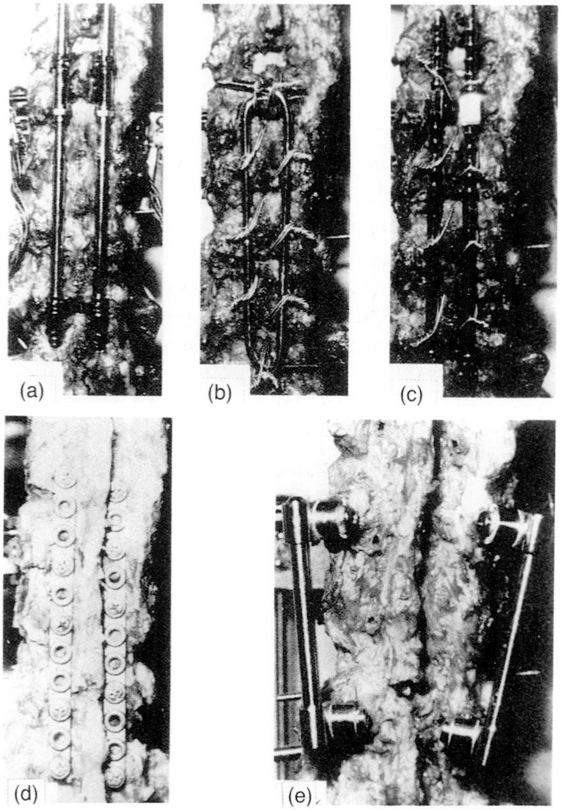

Figure 8.67

Some alternative methods for fixation of an anterior–middle–posterior column injury of the thoracolumbar spine: (a) Jacobs rods; (b) sublaminarly wired C rods; (c) sublaminarly wired Harrington distraction rods; (d) Roy-Camille plate with pedicle screws; (e) Vermont fixator. (From Ref 72 with permission.)

in various directions. The Steffee plate produced the highest rank construct, and the Harrington rods alone the lowest (Figure 8.68).

Summary

Fixation of fractures of the thoracolumbar spine is complex because of the variety of loads that the implant must bear and the variable contribution of the injured spine to load bearing. Posterior column injuries will retain some stability to compression, lateral bending, and torsion loading, especially with intact facets, so the main objective should be to install a construct capable of resisting flexion. The Harrington distraction system is more effective in resisting flexion moments when sleeves are located between the rods and the lamina because spine flexion is converted into bending in the rods. A more severe injury (either anterior–middle or anterior–middle–posterior) requires that the implant be able to sustain lateral bending, torsion, and compression loads as well as flexion moments. In these cases, posterior pedicle screw devices have demonstrated the ability to produce the most rigid constructs. However, rigidity may still be only slightly greater than that of the intact spine. Because high loads can be expected in the

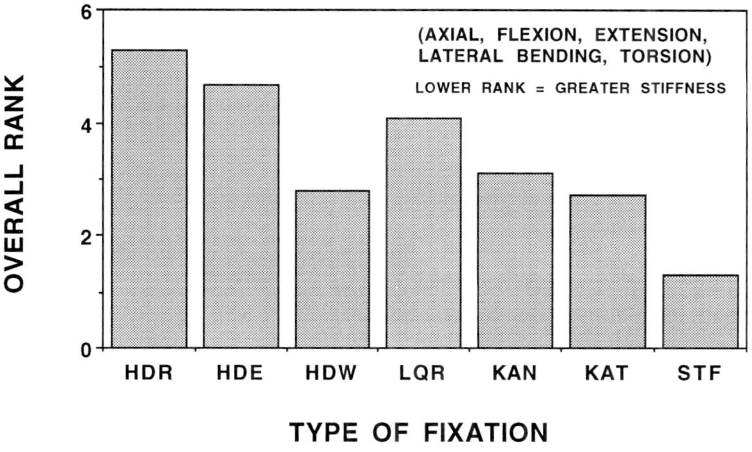

Figure 8.68

Overall ranking of seven methods of fixation of the anterior–middle–posterior column lumbar spinal injury. Rank 1: linear displacement < 1.3 mm, angular < 1°. Rank 5: 6.4 mm linear, 5° angular. HDR, Harrington rods; HDE, Harrington rods with Edwards sleeves; HDW, Harrington rods with sublaminar wiring; LQR, Luque rod; KAN, Kaneda device; KAT, Kaneda device with transverse fixator; STF, Steffee plate. (Data adapted from Ref 70.)

instrumentation in these situations, with screw stresses above the endurance limit in some cases, strategies to decrease implant stresses, such as placement of an anterior strut graft or increasing the length of the fixation, can be used to decrease implant stresses (see Section 8.8).

8.10 Lumbosacral junction fixation

Loading conditions

Fixation of the lumbosacral spine presents probably a greater challenge in some respects than thoracolumbar fixation. Although the degree of injury to the spine may be less severe, the lumbosacral junction will experience compression loads equivalent to those in the lumbar spine, as discussed in Section 8.6, as well as greater shear forces because of the greater angulation of the L5–S1 junction (see Figure 8.29). However, the most difficult aspect of fixation in this region is obtaining good screw purchase in the sacrum.

Sacral screw purchase

A major difficulty with sacral screw placement is locating sites with adequate purchase that are clinically safe. As shown by Licht et al[83] placement of sacral screws oblique to the ala puts the L5 nerve root at risk, while locating them directly posterior to anterior may result in penetration of the iliac veins or the sympathetic chain, and at S2 or S3, the rectum. A safe zone for screw placement was defined in the midline of the sacrum, as shown in Figure 8.69.

Zindrick et al[55] showed that the pullout strengths of screws located in the S2 pedicle were considerably lower than those of screws located at the S1 level. The strengths of screws placed from posterior to anteromedial versus to anterolateral, as shown in Figure 8.70, have been compared. Screws placed posterior to anteromedial, through the promontory, had greater maximum load capacity than those located anterolaterally (Figure 8.71).[55,84] In addition, when the screw is constrained against sagittal plane rotation (extension), as shown in Figure 8.72, greater force of failure can be developed. This is because, in the semiconstrained condition, a component of the applied load acts along the axis of the screw to produce pullout as the screw

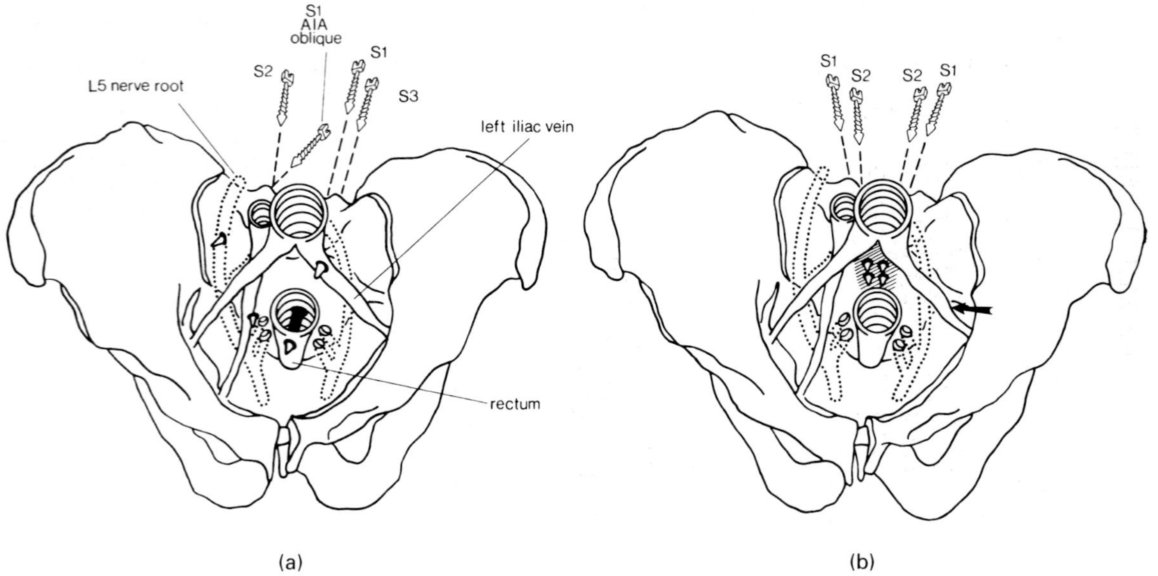

Figure 8.69

(a) Anatomical structures in danger of penetration due to placement of sacral screws. (b) Midline safe zone sacral screws. (From Ref 83 with permission.)

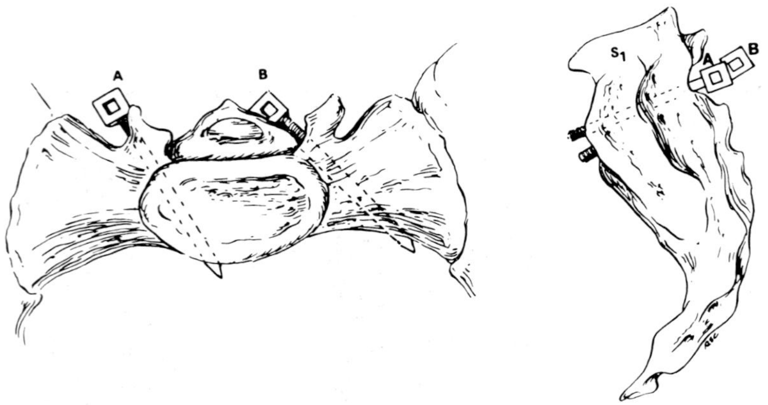

Figure 8.70

Alternative placement of sacral screws at the S1 level of the sacrum. (From Ref 84 with permission.)

angulates. The maximum load capacity of sacral screws increases significantly with increasing bone density (a mean of 2 N for every 1 mg/cm^3 increase in bone density). Also, there is only a 5% gain in strength with placement of screws bicortically (Figure 8.73).[85] Therefore the optimum location of sacral scews, for strength of purchase and safety, is medially towards the promontory at the S1 level, but without penetrating the anterior cortex of S1.

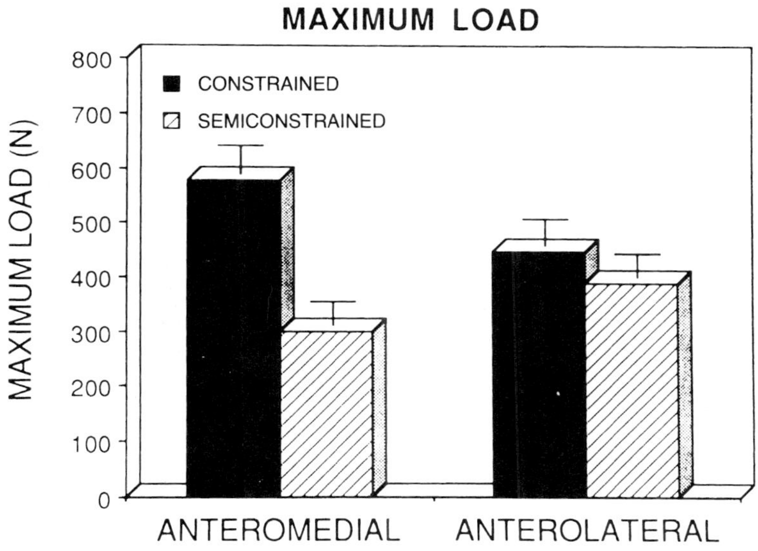

Figure 8.71

Maximum vertical load (transverse to the axis of the screw) sustained by sacral screws placed from posterior to anteromedially into the promontory of the sacrum as opposed to anterolaterally into the ala, at S1. (See Figure 8.72 for the definition of constrained and semiconstrained loading.) (From Ref 84 with permission.)

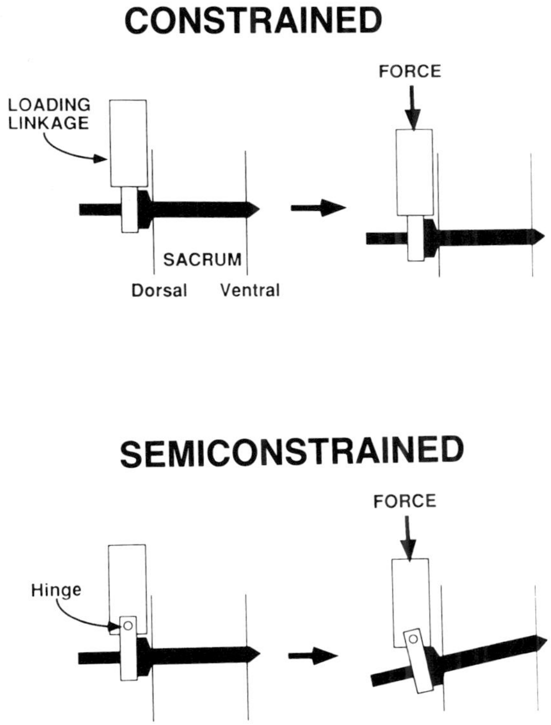

Figure 8.72

Vertical (along the long axis of the spine) loading of a screw "constrained" and "semiconstrained". The semiconstrained screw can rotate in the sagittal plane. (From Ref 84 with permission.)

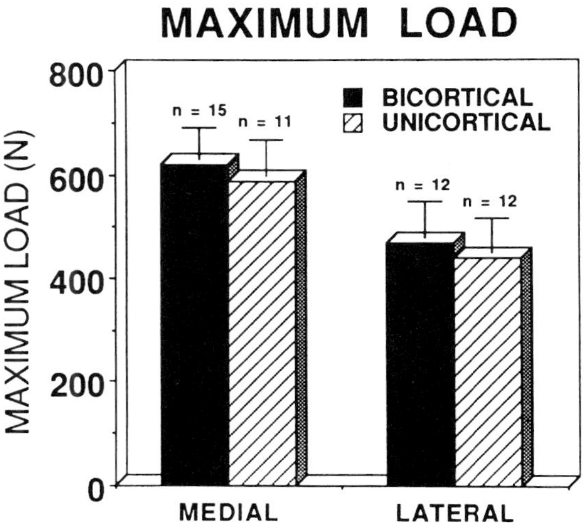

Figure 8.73

Maximum load capacity in vertical loading (transverse to the axis of the screw) of sacral screws placed unicortically or bicortically, medially (into the promontory) or laterally (into the ala). (From Ref 85 with permission.)

Comparison of sacral fixation constructs

As with thoracolumbar spinal instrumentation, the number of alternative methods for fixing lumbosacral spinal injuries has increased significantly recently. McCord et al[86] recently studied the performance of 10 different methods of fixation in the lumbosacral joint in flexion to failure. This study provided a comparison between five fundamentally different methods of load transfer between the sacrum and the implant: sacral wiring, sacral screws, sacral hooks, iliac screws, and rods embedded into the ilium.

The specific implants studied (Figure 8.74) were the Galveston technique (rods embedded into the ilia[87]) with the ISOLA system using $\frac{1}{4}$ in diameter

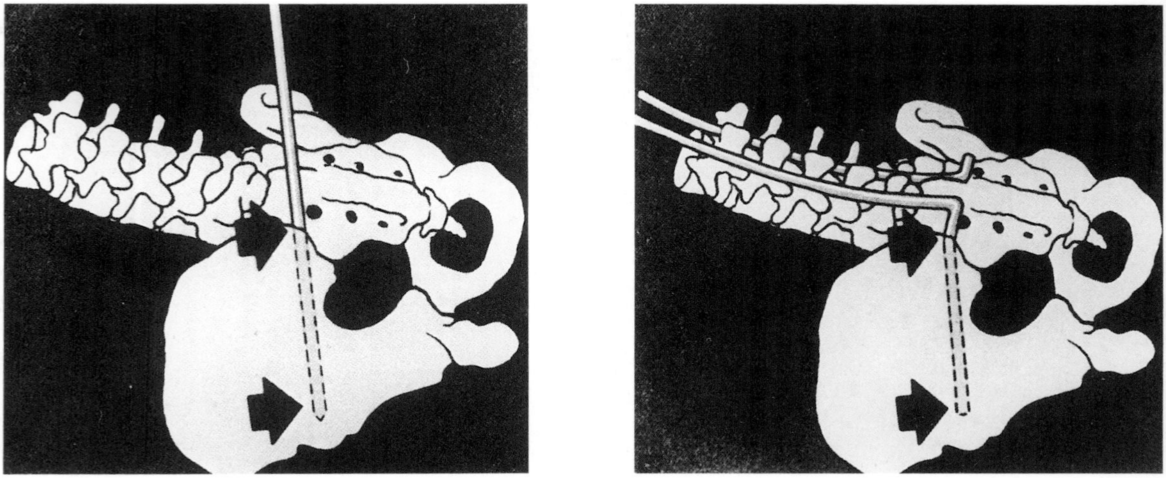

(a)

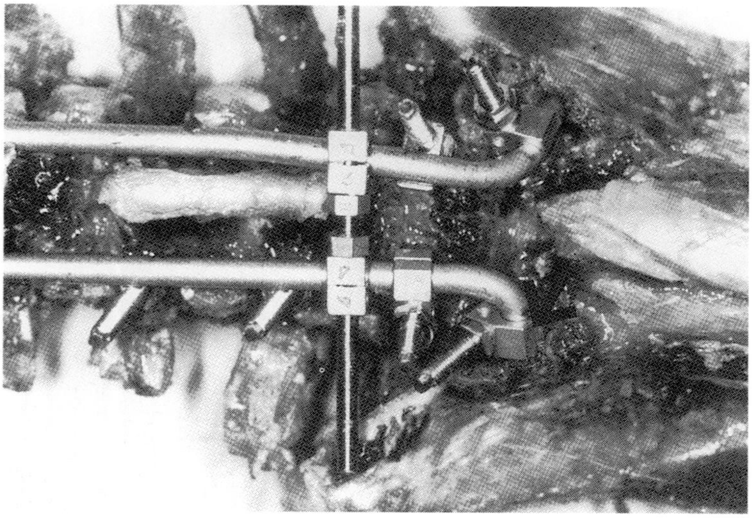

(b)

Figure 8.74

Some methods of fixation of the lumbosacral junction. (a) Galveston Luque rod technique (from Ref 87 with permission). (b) ISOLA Galveston configuration, partly assembled. (c) Cotrel–Dubousset butterfly plate. (d) Cotrel–Dubousset sacral screws (from Ref 85 with permission).

(*Continued next page*)

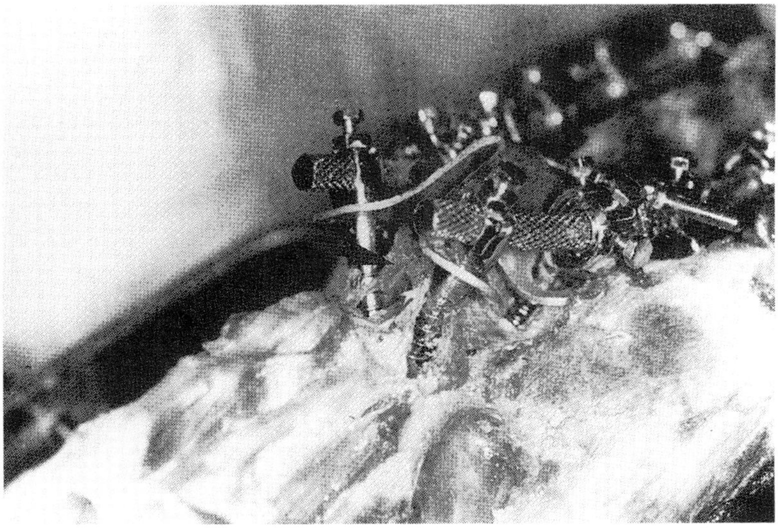

(c)

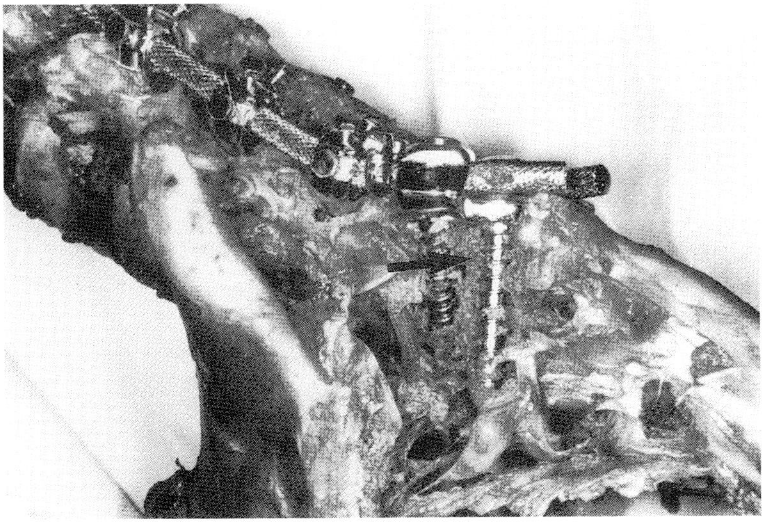

(d)

Figure 8.74

(Continued)

rods, the ISOLA system with iliac screws, Cotrel–Dubousset rods with iliosacral screws, Kirschner sacral plates, Cotrel–Dubousset butterfly plates Cotrel–Dubousset Chopin block, ISOLA hooks, Harrington distraction rods, Luque rods,[88] and Steffee plates.[75] Table 8.4 identifies the type of instrumentation tested in this experiment and the attachment method of each to the sacrum.

The results of the flexion testing demonstrate, as shown in Figure 8.75, that fixation into the ilia provides a clear advantage over other methods in developing a construct resistant to flexion. The

Table 8.4 Instrumentation used in lumbosacral fixation with type of attachment to the sacrum. (From Ref 86 with permission.)

Systems	*Group*	*S1*	*S2*	*Iliac*
ISOLA Galveston	1	Screw	—	Rod
ISOLA iliac screw	1	Screw	—	Screw
CD iliosacral screw	1	Screw	—	Screw
Kirschner sacral plate	1	Screw	Screw	Screw
CD Chopin block	2	Screw	Screw	—
CD butterfly plate	2	Screw	Screw	—
ISOLA sacral hook	2	Screw	Hook	—
Harrington rods	3	Hook	—	—
Luque	3	Wire	—	—
Steffee plate	3	Screw	—	—
Control	4	—	—	—

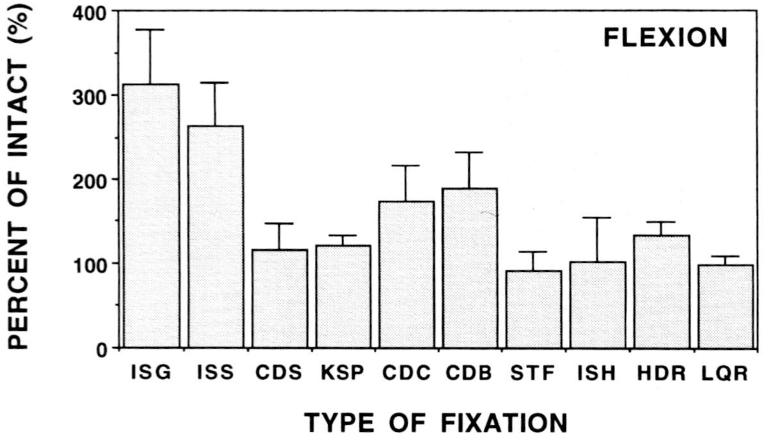

Figure 8.75

Comparison of the stiffness of various constructs in flexion loading compared with the intact lumbosacral joint. ISG, ISOLA Galveston; ISS, ISOLA iliac screw; CDS, Cotrel–Dubousset iliosacral screws; KSP, Kirschner sacral plate; CDC, Cotrel–Dubousset Chopin block; CDB, Cotrel–Dubousset butterfly plate; STF, Steffee plate; ISH, ISOLA sacral hook; HDR, Harrington distraction rods with sacral hooks; LQR, Luque rods with sublaminar wires. (Data adapted from Ref 86.)

Galveston construct was 313% as rigid as the intact lumbosacral joint, followed by the ISOLA iliac screw (263%). The rigidity of plated constructs varied from 189% of intact (CD Butterfly) to 90% (Steffee). Hook devices construct stiffnesses ranged from 132% to 102% of intact, and sublaminar wiring yielded 99% of intact. Further, the constructs using iliac rod fixation failed at significantly greater loads than those with plate and screw fixation. The greater rigidity of fixation to the ilium can be attributed to the longer lever arm of the anchoring mechanism of the iliac rod compared with the sacral screw. As shown in Figure 8.76, the lumbosacral fixation acts as a complex lever. With flexion loading, rotation in the fixation system may occur at the screw or rod and bone interface, at the screw/rod or screw/plate junction, and by bending of the rod or plate. The longer lever arm of the iliac fixation reduces bone/implant motion.

As with other spinal motion segments, the lumbosacral junction must resist loads in other planes. Puno et al[89] compared several techniques, including Galveston fixation,[87] Luque segmentally

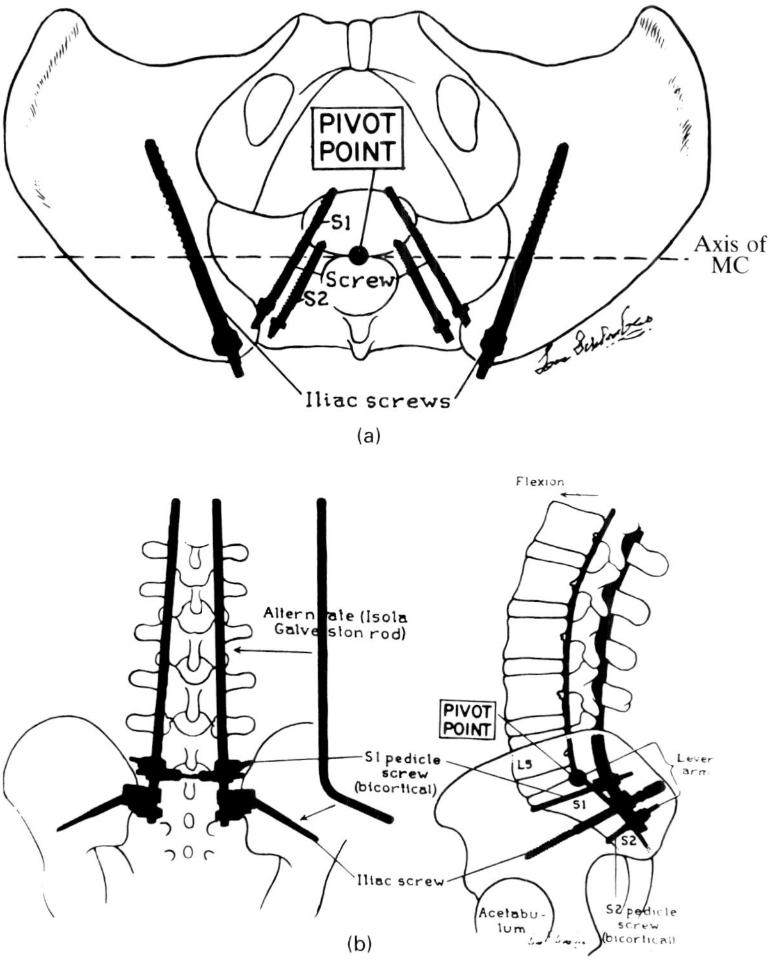

Figure 8.76

(a) A coronal view demonstrates the greater moment arm of iliac fixation with rods compared with sacral screws, with the axis of flexion rotation of the injured joint near the posterior wall of the vertebra. (b) Posterior and sagittal views demonstrate the differences in lever arm of the two fixation methods with flexion of the spine. (From Ref 86 with permission.)

wired ring fixation,[88] and Steffee plates,[75] with and without fixation to S2, in several loading directions, in otherwise intact specimens. (Note that in the previously discussed experiment, the Steffee plate was fixed only at S1.) In compression, all implants produced constructs with stiffnesses between 90% and 110% of intact, except for the Galveston–Luque technique (66% of intact). In torsion and lateral bending (Figure 8.77), the Steffee plate constructs were most rigid, while extension loading produced almost identical results regardless of instrumentation (140–168% of intact). It is interesting to note the contribution of the S2 screw, which improves fixation stiffness moderately in most loading modes, but significantly in flexion (82% without to 129% with the S2 screw). Although the S2 purchase site is weak,[55] the gain in moment arm length between the S1 and S2 screws is such that a considerable additional resisting moment to flexion is generated in the instrumentation with the S2 screw in place.

Summary

The lumbosacral junction presents a most challenging area in which to gain biomechanical stability, because of a combination of the large

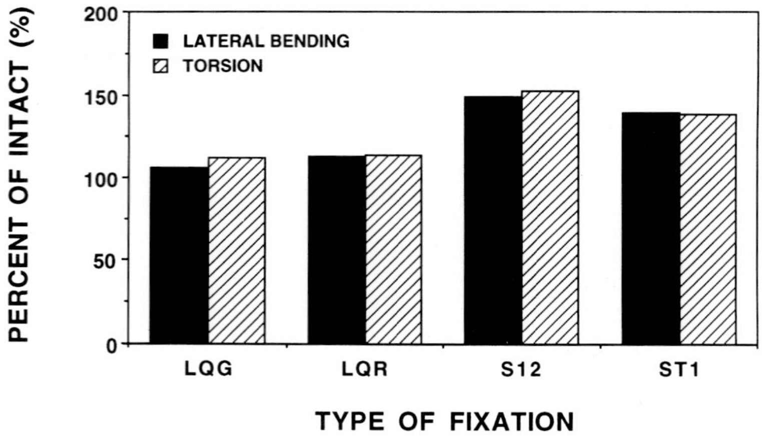

Figure 8.77

Comparisons of the fixation stiffnesses of various lumbosacral constructs in torsion and lateral bending loading: LQG, Luque rods with Galveston iliac fixation; LQR, Luque segmentally wired ring; S12, Steffee plate with S1 and S2 screws; ST1, Steffee plate with S1 screws only. (Data adapted from Ref 89.)

loads acting on, and the relatively poor screw purchase sites within the sacrum. Screws angled medially into the promontory at the level of S1 provide the greatest purchase of any location in the sacrum. Fixation systems that use rods embedded into the ilia provide the greatest rigidity to flexion loading, because of the long lever arm provided by the iliac fixation. In lateral bending and torsion, plated constructs provide the greatest rigidity. Also, a second screw located below the primary sacral screw, even if its purchase is relatively weak, can be beneficial in increasing flexion stiffness of plated fixation.

8.11 Pelvic fracture fixation

Loading conditions

The pelvis can be considered mechanically to be the base of the spine, as well as the connection point for the lower extremities. Major loads acting on the pelvis from the spine consist of the weight of the trunk, and the muscle forces that control bending and rotational motions of the spinal column. Forces acting on the pelvis also include those generated by the muscles that control the position of the femur and the joint reaction force from the femoral head acting through the acetabulum.

Typical physiological loads from the spine and trunk are estimated to be in the range of 1000–2000 N in axial compression, 500 N in anterior shear (because of the inclination of the lumbosacral junction), and 10 N m in flexion and lateral bending.[90] In addition, femoral head joint reaction forces range from two to four times body weight.[91] The specific magnitudes of muscle forces that balance these applied loads have not been determined; however, Figure 8.78 shows the lines of action of some major muscle groups acting on the pelvis.[92] In the most simple view, one can expect the joint reaction force of the femoral head to rotate the ilium into extension with respect to the sacrum, and conversely the sacrum to be rotated into flexion because of spinal loads. Asymetrically applied loads from the femora, such as those occurring in walking, must cause vertical shearing and separation at the symphysis pubis, and muscle forces will bend the hemipelvis laterally. Therefore fixation of the pelvis must accomplish several goals. At the symphysis pubis, both separation and vertical shearing should be prevented. At the sacroiliac (SI) joints, flexion of the sacrum (or extension of the ilia) and gapping between the sacrum and ilium must be counteracted.

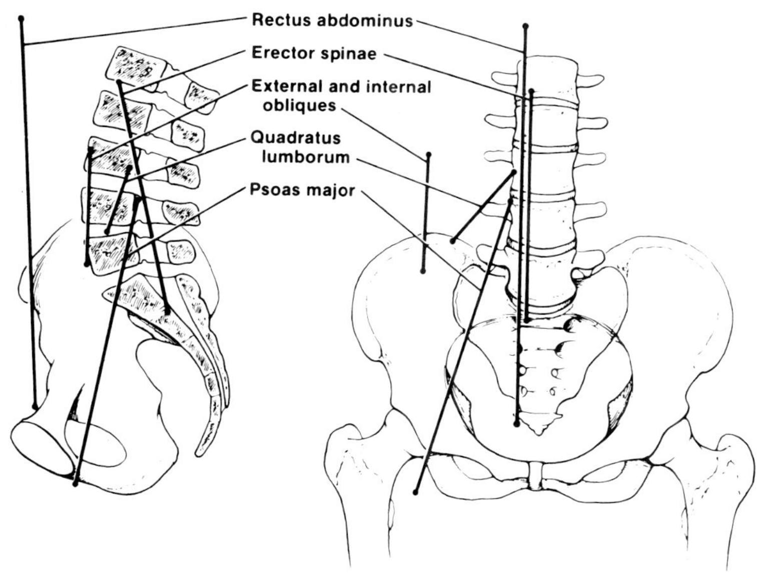

Figure 8.78

Lines of action of some muscle forces acting on the pelvis. (From Ref 92 with permission.)

Mechanical functions of the pelvic joints

The SI joints are considered to be highly stable, since the wedge shaped sacrum, being wider superiorly, requires that the ilia spread to allow downward displacement of the sacrum. Also, the SI joint surfaces are narrower posteriorly, which prevents posterior displacement of the sacrum. The SI joint surfaces are large and irregular while the SI ligaments are dense, further adding to mechanical stability.

It is important to appreciate that the pelvis is a complex structure of multiple components and that damage to one of its connections can significantly affect the others. With both SI joints intact and the ilia prevented from separating, measured SI joint translations ranged from 0.1 to 0.53 mm under a 294 N load, and only 1.94° of rotation with a 42 N m moment. However, with one SI joint disrupted, as would occur in a typical injury, translations in the other intact side were considerable, especially when loading was directed posteriorly (Figure 8.79). Rotations ranged from 2.7° in flexion to 6.2° in torsion due to a 42 N m moment.[93] Therefore disruption of one SI joint also has an effect on the other (intact) side, since the sacrum is now supported asymmetrically. As shown by Simonion et al,[94] if a compressive load is applied to the L5 vertebral body, gapping at the symphysis pubis (SP) occurs when the SP ligament is disrupted. However, disrupting the SP ligament also permits greater flexion of the sacrum, because the SP helps to hold the SI joints together (Figure 8.80). The sacrospinal (SS) and sacrotuberal (ST) ligaments have relatively little effect on the SI and SP joints.

Strength of screw sites about the pelvis

The relative screw purchase strengths at sites about the pelvis have been investigated. In general, as for any screw, the screw pullout strength correlates to bone thickness, and in particular to the thickness of the cortex.[95] In particular, considering five possible screw insertion sites (Figure 8.81), the medial side of the ilium and anterior side of the sacrum provided greater

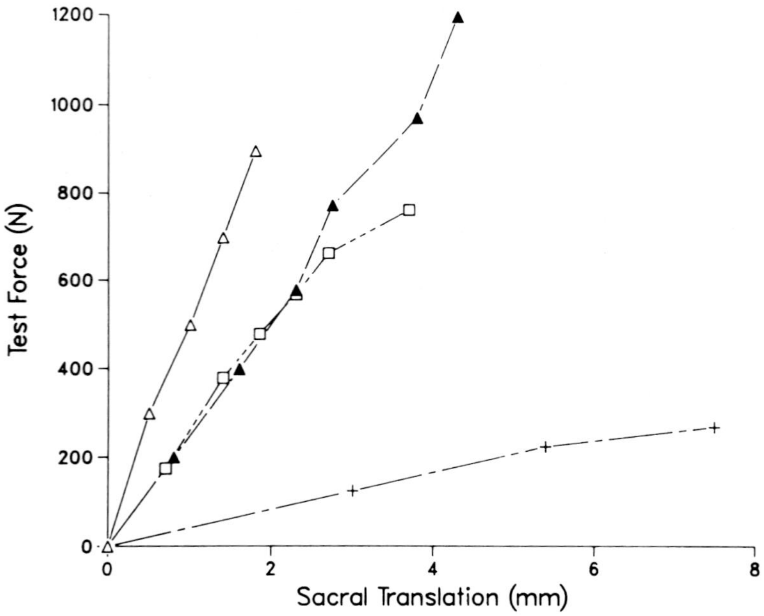

Figure 8.79

Load–displacement relationship of the sacrum with respect to the ilium at the sacroiliac joint, loaded in various directions. Test direction: (specimens 1 and 2) △, inferior 1, ▲, inferior 2; □, anterior; +, posterior. (From Ref 93 with permission.)

resistance to pullout than did sites on the lateral posterior aspect of the ilium (Figure 8.82).[96]

External fixation versus combined internal/external fixation or totally internal fixation of the pelvis

The primary objective of a fixation system should be to stabilize the fractured region so that physiological forces can be applied and the patient can be mobilized safely as soon as possible. Rubash et al[97] compared the load bearing properties of external fixation frames with combined external/internal and totally internal fixation methods, some of which are shown in Figure 8.83. External fixation systems, because of the long lever arms of the components (particularly the pins), tend to allow slip (defined as allowing 0.5 mm of vertical displacement at the fracture) at axial loads below 140 N, and fail at loads below 300 N, well under those that would be encountered in ambulation. Slip and failure loads using combined internal and external fixation (such as the Slatis frame placed anteriorly, combined with the internal cobra plate posteriorly) significantly increased the loads at which slip and failure occurred, to values of about 375 and 766 N respectively. These values were also achieved by internal fixation plates applied anteriorly and posteriorly.

Anterior plating of the pubis symphysis

Sacral bar fixation[100] combined with either external fixation or SP plating[101] is another method for achieving stability of the pelvis with SI joint disruption or sacral fracture. Using anterior external fixation only on an SI joint disruption results in rigidity (load/displacement at the SI joint) and maximum load capacity equal to 5% of intact. Adding posterior sacral bars increases these values to 34% and 43% respectively. Using sacral

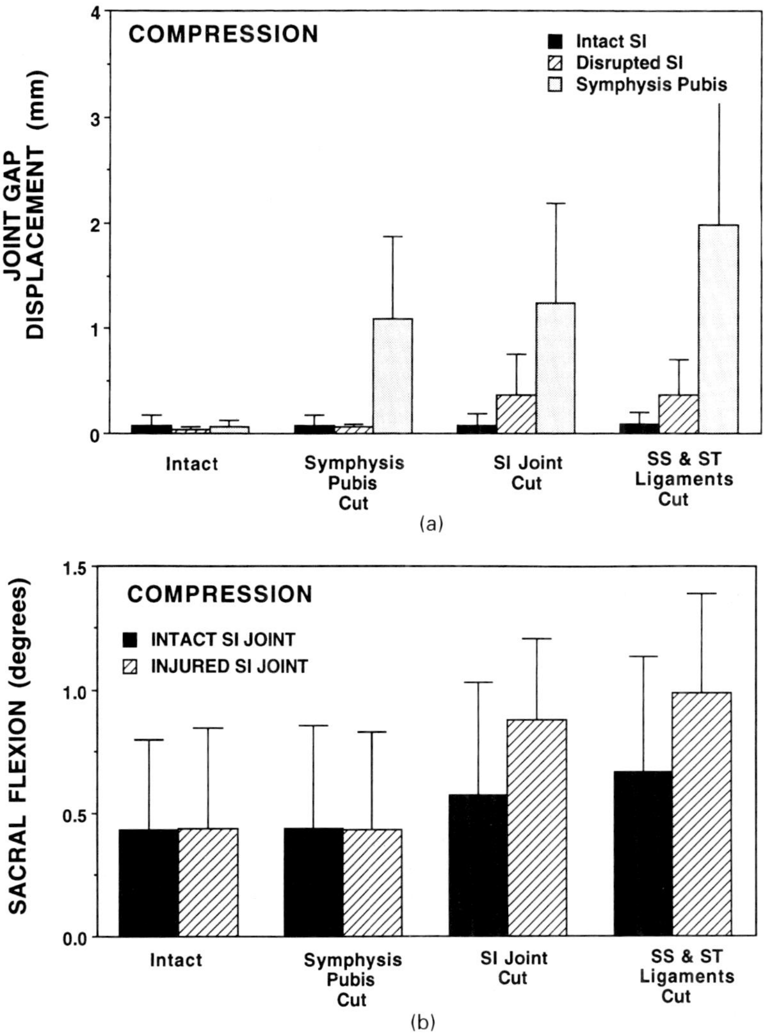

Figure 8.80

Transverse gap and sacral flexion in the pelvis with intact sacroiliac (SI) and pubis symphysis (SP) joints, after sectioning the SP ligament, and after sectioning one SI joint with the SP sectioned (SS, sacrospinal; ST, sacrotuberal ligaments). (a) Joint gapping under load. (b) Sacral flexion with respect to the ilium on either side. (From Ref 94.)

bars and either single or double symphysis plates results in nearly the same performance (rigidity, 38% of intact; load to failure, 49.5% of intact).[102] Figure 8.84 illustrates the displacement of the SP under load when fixed anteriorly by an external frame and posteriorly with sacral bars. Stocks et al[102] noted that the use of two symphysis plates reduced the separation of the SP joint from 30.9 to 15.7 mm at failure load compared with an anterior external frame.

Anterior plating with posterior percutaneous screws

Leighton et al[103] compared the rigidities and load capacities achieved with an SI plate (Figure 8.83) or three percutaneous screws for fixation of the SI joint, in combination with anterior plating. As shown in Figure 8.85, the greatest construct rigidity (39.3% of intact) was achieved using three posterior screws and two SP plates,

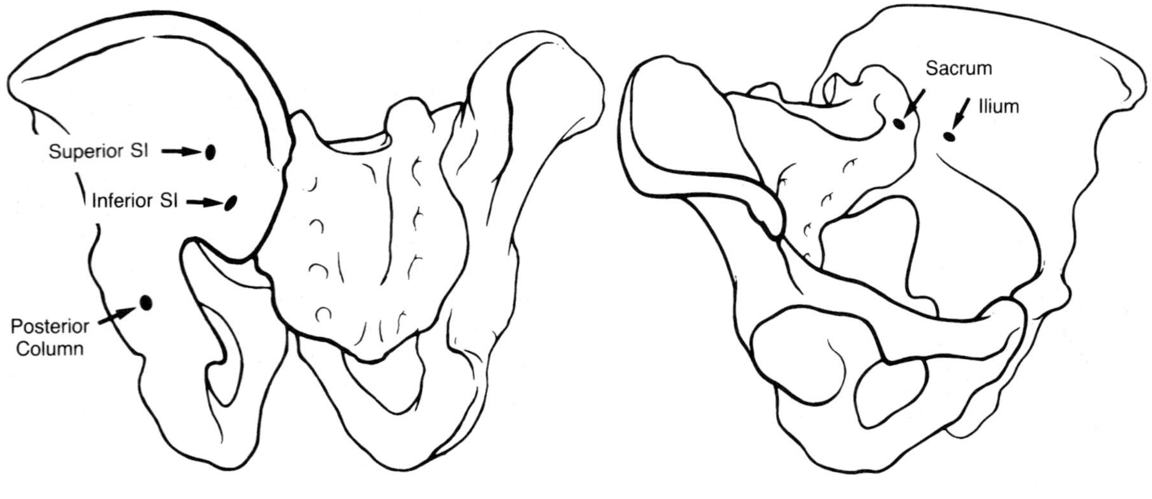

Figure 8.81

Schematic drawing of some tested screw fixation sites about the pelvis. (From Ref 96 with permission.)

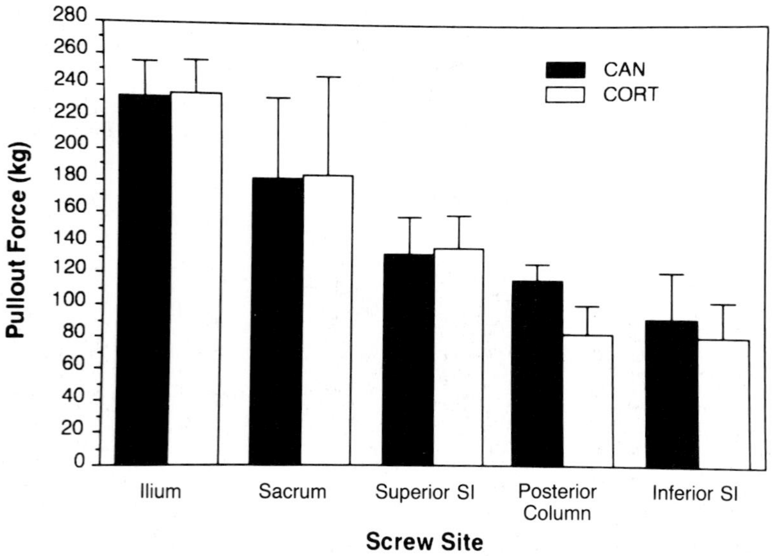

Figure 8.82

Pullout strengths of 4.5 mm diameter cortical and 6.5 mm cancellous screws at various sites about the pelvis (see Figure 8.81). (From Ref 96 with permission.)

followed by an SI plate and two SP plates (33.9% of intact). The load capacities of the two constructs are equivalent, about 52% of that of the intact pelvis.

As well as increasing load capacity, a fixation system should control motion and gapping at the injury site to permit healing in an undisplaced position. Simonion et al[94] compared the total motion across the injured and intact SI joint and the SP, along with flexion of the sacrum under various types of loads, using various combinations of the devices described above. Total motion

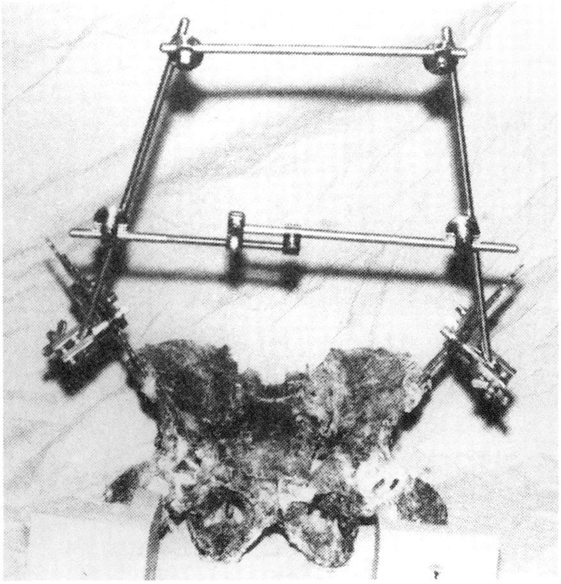

(a)

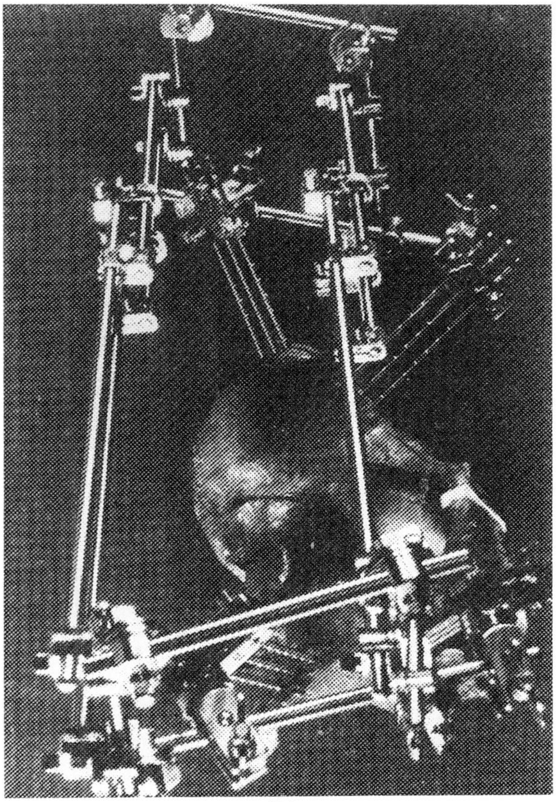

(b)

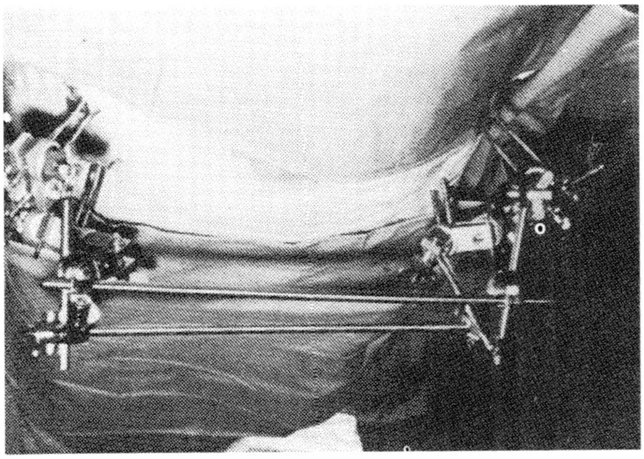

(c)

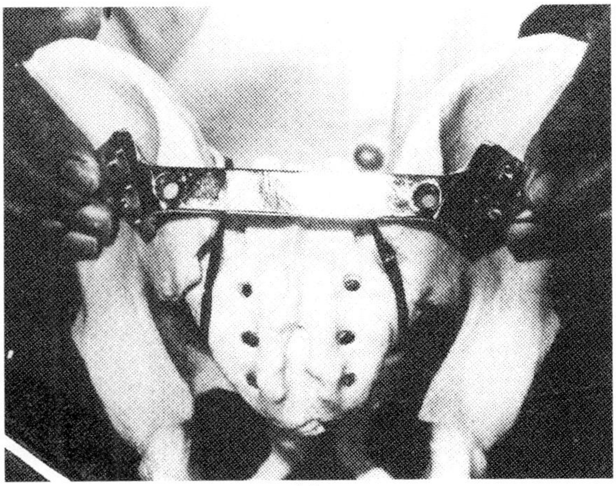

(d)

Figure 8.83

Some configurations of external and internal fixation of the pelvis: (a) Slatis frame;[98] (b) anterior and posterior quadrilateral frame with through pins;[99] (c) triangular frame;[97] (d) posterior cobra plate;[97] (e) symphysis pubis plate;[97] (f) sacral bars.[100] (All with permission.)

(*Continued over the page*)

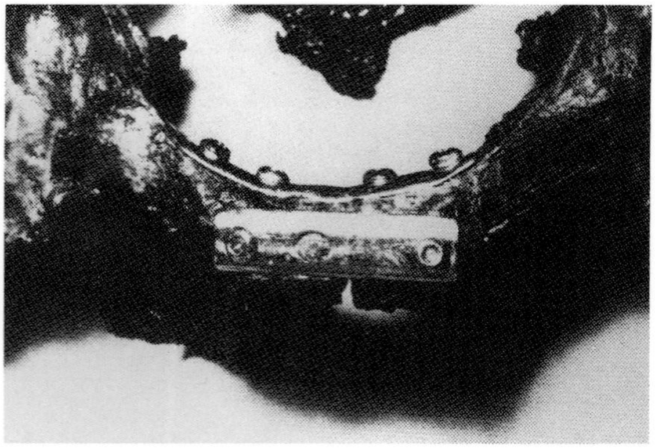

(e)

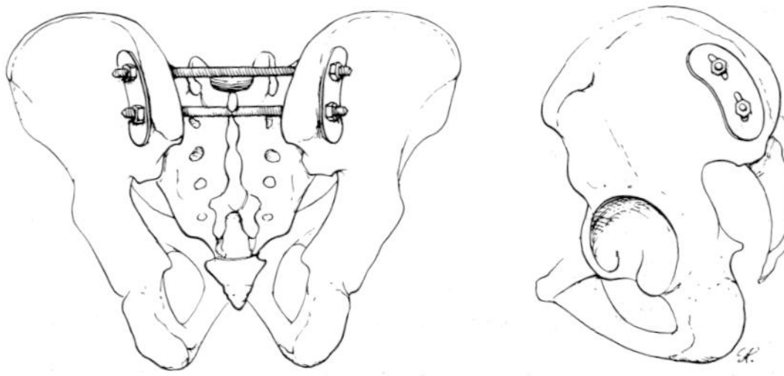

(f)

Figure 8.83

(Continued)

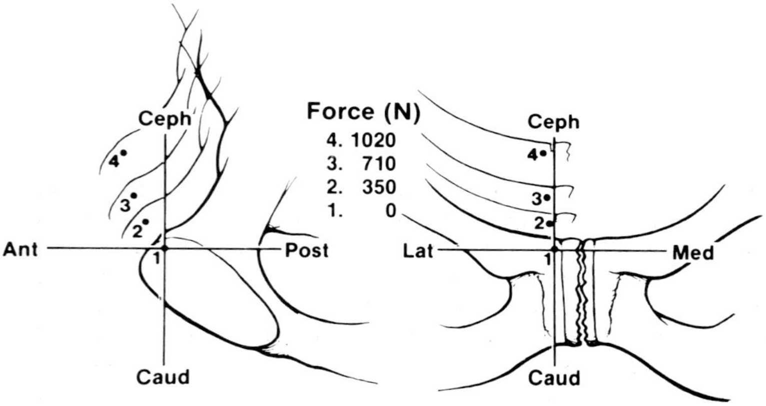

Figure 8.84

Motion of points on the symphysis pubis under increasing vertical loading of the sacrum, in a simulated fracture of the sacroiliac joint and the pubis symphysis fixed with an external frame anteriorly and sacral bars posteriorly. (From Ref 102 with permission.)

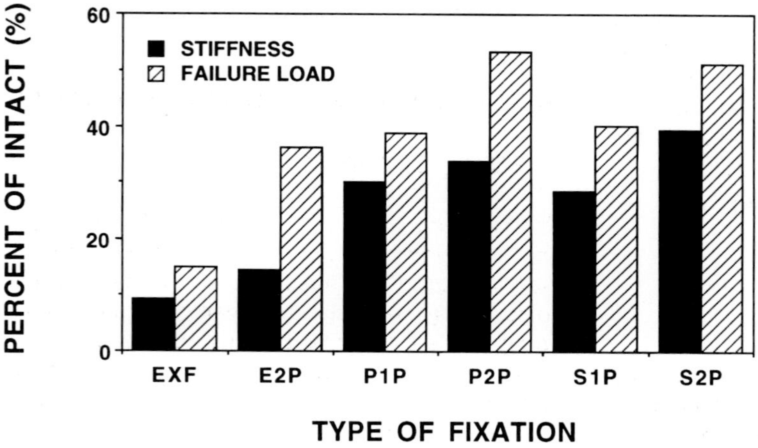

Figure 8.85

Rigidity (load/vertical deformation of the SI joint) and maximum load achieved using various types of pelvic fixation methods: EXF, anterior external fixation; E2P, anterior external fixation and anterior symphysis pubis (SP) plate; P1P, sacroiliac (SI) plate and one SP plate; P2P, SI plate and two SP plates; S1P, three posterior screws and one SP plate; S2P, three posterior screws and two SP plates. (Data adapted from Ref 103.)

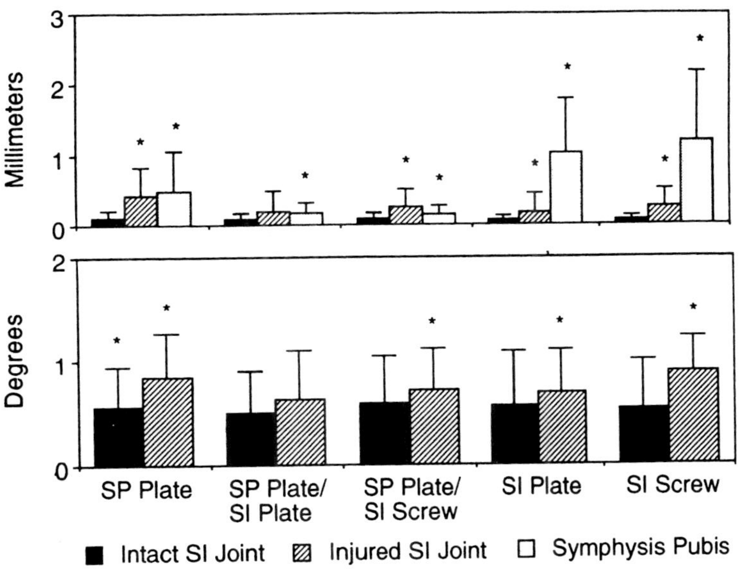

Figure 8.86

Total motion, including (lower) rotation and (upper) separation of the intact sacroiliac (SI) joint, the disrupted SI joint, and the symphysis pubis (SP) joints, with various combinations of fixation, under combined compression and lateral bending loading. (From Ref 94.)

includes both shearing and gapping or opening of the joint space. In direct vertical compressive loading, both combinations of SP plating with SI plates or SI screws controlled gapping equivalently, and provided significantly greater stability than either anterior or posterior fixation applied alone. In lateral bending/compression and torsion, the symphysis plate was found to be the key fixation component for controlling SP gapping, as shown in Figure 8.86. The biomechanical importance of the SP plate is as follows. With posterior fixation alone, the loads from the femora through the acetabula create upward motion of the ilia and extension rotation relative to the sacrum at the SI joints. With one SI joint intact and the other injured, this motion will not be the same on either side, creating shearing and separation of the SP joint. An SP plate is necessary to control this motion.

Summary

Biomechanical studies have shown the necessity of using both anterior and posterior fixation for disruptions of the pelvis ring that involve disruption of the SI joints or sacrum, and the SP, in order to gain adequate mechanical stability. External fixation does not provide adequate strength and rigidity for stabilizing these injuries, nor does posterior internal fixation alone. The most rigid fixation is provided by double anterior (SP) plates in combination with posterior SI screws or SI plates. Both of these posterior devices are biomechanically equivalent.

8.12 Acetabular fracture fixation

Loading conditions

The hip joint, being a low friction ball and socket, delivers primarily a uniform compressive load to the cartilage of the acetabulum. The pelvic bone surrounding the acetabulum can be thought of as being divided into anterior and posterior columns, shown in Figure 8.87. Therefore if the anterior column is fractured, joint loading will cause it to displace upward and outward.[103]

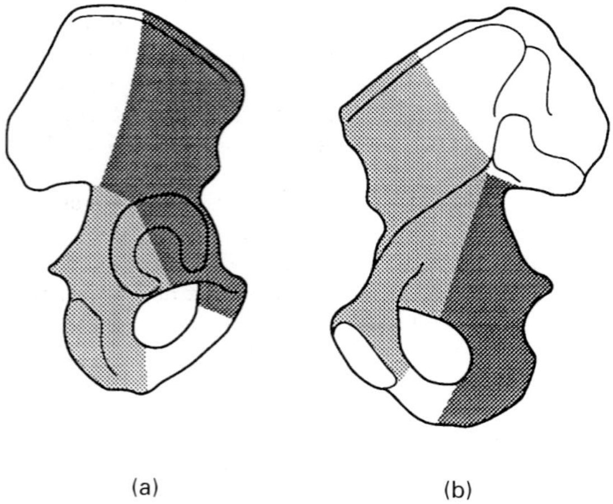

Figure 8.87

(a) Lateral and (b), medial views of the pelvis, showing the concept of anterior (light shading) and posterior (dark shading) columns supporting the joint reaction force through the acetabulum. (From Ref 104 with permission.)

Fixation of acetabular fractures

In transverse posterior wall fractures of the acetabulum, Mason et al[105] found greater fracture site stiffness with a reconstruction plate and screws than with screws alone (Figure 8.88), while no difference was noted in sagittal fracture constructs using either reconstruction plates alone or with accessory hook plates. The most important objective in fixation of these fractures is providing direct bony contact and compression to achieve stability.

8.13 References

1. Nachemson A, Morris JM, In vivo measurements of intradiscal pressure, *J Bone Jt Surg* (1964) **46A:** 1077–91.
2. Brinckmann P, Frobin W, Hierholzer E, Horst M, Deformation of the vertebral endplate under axial loading of the spine, *Spine* (1983) **8:** 851–6.
3. Seroussi RE, Krag MH, Muller DL, Pope MH,

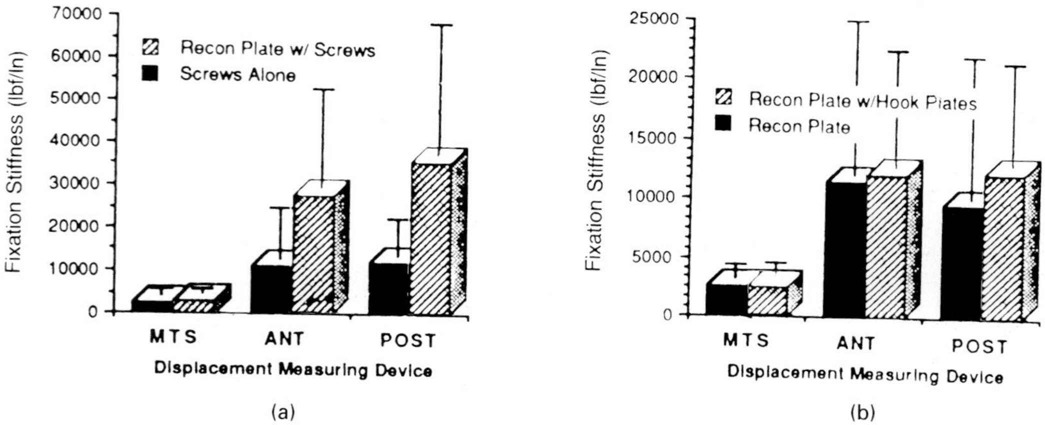

Figure 8.88

Comparison of the fixation stiffness achieved in two fractures of the acetabulum. (a) Transverse fracture of the posterior column. (b) Sagittal fracture of the posterior column. The data show stiffness derived from motions across the fracture line at its anterior and posterior edges in the acetabulum for a given load. Recon Plate, Reconstruction Plate; w/Hook Plates, with accessory hook plates; MTS, materials tester measured displacement; ANT, gauge across fracture line, anterior; POST, gauge across fracture line, posterior. (From Ref 105 with permission.)

4. Panjabi MM, Krag MH, Chung TQ, Effects of disc injury on the three dimensional viscoelastic behavior of the human spine, *Spine* (1984) **9**: 707–13.
5. Tencer AF, Ahmed AM, Burke DL, Some static mechanical properties of the lumbar intervertebral joint, intact and injured, *J Biomech Eng* (1982) **104**: 193–201.
6. Adams MA, Hutton WC, The mechanical function of the lumbar apophyseal joints, *Spine* (1983) **8**: 327–30.
7. Panjabi MM, Goel VK, Takata K, Physiologic strains in the lumbar spinal ligaments, *Spine* (1982) **7**: 192–203.
8. Moroney SP, Schultz AB, Miller JAA, Analysis and measurement of neck loads, *J Orthop Res* (1988) **6**: 713–20.
9. Panjabi MM, Oda T, Crisco III JJ, Oxland TR, Katz L, Nolte LP, Experimental study of atlas injuries I, Biomechanical analysis of their mechanisms and fracture patterns, *Spine* (1991) **16**: S460–5.
10. Crisco III JJ, Oda T, Panjabi MM, Bueff HU, Dvorak J, Grob D, Transections of the C1–C2 joint capsular ligaments in the cadaveric spine, *Spine* (1991) **16**: S474–9.
11. Panjabi MM, White III AA, Johnson RM, Cervical spine mechanics as a function of transection of components, *J Biomech* (1975) **8**: 327–36.
12. Panjabi MM, Duranceau JS, Oxland TR, Bowen CE, Multidirectional instabilities of traumatic cervical spine injuries in a porcine model, *Spine* (1989) **14**: 1111–15.
13. Podolsky S, Baraff LJ, Simon RR, Hoffman JR, Larmon B, Ablon W, Efficacy of cervical spine immobilization methods, *J Trauma* (1983) **23**: 461–4.
14. Wolf Jr JW, Johnson RM, Cervical orthoses. In: Sherk HH, ed, *The cervical spine* (The Cervical Spine Research Society, JB Lippincott: New York 1989) 33–103.
15. Lind B, Sihlbom H, Nordwall A, Forces and motions across the neck in patients treated with halo-vest, *Spine* (1988) **13**: 162–7.
16. Anderson PA, Budorick TE, Easton KB, Henley MB, Salciccioli GG, Failure of the halo vest to prevent in vivo motion in patients with injured cervical spines, *Spine* (1991) **16**: S501–5.
17. Whitehill R, Richman JA, Glaser JA, Failure of immobilization of the cervical spine by the halo vest, *J Bone Jt Surg* (1986) **68A**: 326–32.
18. Walker PS, Lamser D, Hussey RW, Rossier AB, Farberov A, Dietz J, Forces in the halo vest apparatus, *Spine* (1984) **9**: 773–7.
19. Mirza S, Anderson PAA, Tencer AF, Biomechanical factors controlling intervertebral motion in cervical spine injuries fixed with a halo vest (unpublished data).
20. Krag MH, Beynnon BD, A new halo-vest: rationale, design and biomechanical comparison to standard halo-vest designs, *Spine* (1988) **13**: 228–35.
21. Wang GJ, Moskal JT, Albert T, Pritts C, Schuch CM, Stamp WG, The effect of halo-vest length on stability of the cervical spine, *J Bone Jt Surg* (1988) **70A**: 357–60.
22. Gallie WE, Fractures and dislocation of the cervical spine, *Am J Surg* (1939) **46**: 495–9.
23. Brooks AL, Jenkins EB, Atlanto-axial arthrodesis by the wedge compression method, *J Bone Jt Surg* (1978) **60A**: 279–84.
24. Grob D, Magerl F, Dorsale Spondylodese der Halswirbelsäule mit der Hakenplatte, *Orthopäde* (1987) **16**: 55–61.
25. Magerl F, Spondylodesen an der oberen halswirbelsäule, *Acta Chir Austr* (1986) Supp 43: 69–71.
26. Tucker HH, Technical report: method of fixation of subluxed or dislocated cervical spine below C1–C2, *Can J Neurol Sci* (1975) **2**: 381–2.
27. Grob D, Crisco III JJ, Panjabi MM, Wang P, Dvorak J, Biomechanical evaluation of four different posterior atlantoaxial fixation techniques, *Spine* (1992) **17**: 480–90.
28. Amevo B, Aprill C, Bogduk N, Abnormal instantaneous axes of rotation in patients with neck pain, *Spine* (1992) **17**: 748–56.
29. Pelker RR, Duranceau JS, Panjabi MM, Cervical spine stabilization, a three dimensional biomechanical evaluation of rotational stability, strength, and failure mechanisms, *Spine* (1991) **16**: 117–22.
30. Rogers WA, Fractures and dislocations of the cervical spine: an end result study, *J Bone Jt Surg* (1957) **39A**: 341–76.
31. Callahan RA, Johnson RM, Margolis RN, Keggi KJ, Albright JA, Southwick WO, Cervical facet fusion for control of instability following laminectomy, *J Bone Jt Surg* (1977) **59A**: 991–1002.
32. Fairbank TJ, Spinal fusion after laminectomy for cervical myelopathy, *Proc Roy Soc Med* (1971) **64**: 634–6.
33. Orozco Delclos R, Llovet Tapies R, Osteosíntesis en las lesiones traumáticas y degenerativas de la columna vertebral, *Revista Traumatol Cirurg Rehabil* (1971) **1**: 45–52.
34. Magerl F, Grob D, Seeman P, Stable dorsal fusion of the cervical spine (C2–Th1) using hook plates. In: Kehr P, Weidner A, eds, *Cervical spine I* (Springer-Verlag: Berlin 1987) 217–21.
35. Ulrich C, Woersdoerfer O, Kalff R, Claes L, Wilke H-J, Biomechanics of fixation systems to the cervical spine. *Spine* (1991) **16**: S4–9.
36. Tencer AF, Comparison of posterior cervical plating techniques in cyclic loading, *Report to Synthes Ltd, Paoli, PA* (July 1992).
37. Smith TJ, Fernie GR, Functional biomechanics of the spine, *Spine* (1991) **16**: 1197–203.

38. Schultz A, Andersson G, Ortengren R, Haderspeck K, Nachemson A, Loads on the lumbar spine, validation of a biomechanical analysis by measurements of intradiscal pressures and myoelectric signals, *J Bone Jt Surg* (1982) **64A**: 713–20.
39. Cromwell R, Schultz AB, Beck R, Warwick D, Loads on the lumbar trunk during level walking, *J Orthop Res* (1989) **7**: 371–7.
40. Posner I, White III AA, Edwards WT, Hayes WC, A biomechanical analysis of the clinical stability of the lumbar and lumbosacral spine, *Spine* (1982) **7**: 374–88.
41. Denis F, The three column spine and its significance in the classification of acute thoracolumbar injuries, *Spine* (1983) **8**: 817–31.
42. Haher TR, Bergman M, O'Brien M, Felmly WT, Choueka J, Welin D, Chow G, Vassiliou A, The effect of the three columns of the spine on the instantaneous axis of rotation in flexion and extension, *Spine* (1991) **16**: S312–18.
43. Haher TR, Bergman M, O'Brien M, Felmly WT, Welin D, Perrier G, Choueka J, Devlin V, Vassiliou A, Chow G, Instantaneous axis of rotation as a function of the three columns of the spine, *Spine* (1992) **17**: S149–54.
44. Ching RP, Tencer AF, Anderson PA, Residual stability of the thoracolumbar spine after injury, *J Orthop Res* (in press).
45. Ching RP, Residual stability in thoracolumbar spine fractures: a biomechanical study, *PhD dissertation, The University of Washington, Dept of Mechanical Engineering* (1991).
46. Slosar Jr PJ, Patwardhan A, Lorenz M, Havey R, Nixon R, Seymour S, Sartori M, The three dimensional instability patterns of the thoracolumbar burst fracture, *Trans 38th Orthopedic Research Society Meeting* (1992) **17**: 67.
47. Lin RM, Oxland TR, Functional radiographs of acute thoracolumbar burst fractures: a biomechanical study, *Trans 38th Orthopedic Research Society Meeting* (1992) **17**: 66.
48. Waugh TR, The biomechanical basis for the utilization of methylmethacrylate in the treatment of scoliosis, *J Bone Jt Surg* (1971) **53A**: 194–5.
49. Tencer AF, Self J, Allen Jr BL, Drummond D, Design and evaluation of a posterior laminar clamp spinal fixation system, *Spine* (1991) **16**: 910–18.
50. McNeice G, Biomechanics research of fracture fixation: application to the thoracolumbar spine, *Biomechanics Laboratory Research Report, University of Texas Medical Branch, Galveston* (1983).
51. Errico TJ, Paonessa K, McHenry T, Casar R, The strength of a C–D claw: a comparison of thoracic sub-laminar hook claw to pedicle/transverse process hook claw, *Trans 38th Orthopedic Research Society Meeting* (1992) **17**: 463.
52. Drummond D, Guadagni J, Keene JS, Breed A, Narechania R, Interspinous process segmental spinal instrumentation, *J Pediatr Orthop* (1984) **4**: 397–404.
53. Krag MH, Biomechanics of thoracolumbar spinal fixation. A review, *Spine* (1991) **16**: S85–98.
54. Moran JM, Berg WS, Berry JL, Geiger JM, Steffe: transpedicular screw fixation, *J Orthop Res* (1989) **7**: 107–14.
55. Zindrick MR, Wiltse LL, Widell EH, Thomas JC, Holland WR, Field BT, Spencer CW, A biomechanical study of intrapeduncular screw fixation in the lumbosacral spine, *Clin Orthop* (1986) **203**: 99–112.
56. Krag MH, Beynnon BD, Pope MH, Frymoyer JW, Haugh LD, Weaver DL, An internal fixator for posterior application to short segments of the thoracic, lumbar or lumbosacral spine. Design and testing, *Clin Orthop* (1986) **203**: 75–98.
57. Saillant G, Anatomical study of vertebral pedicles, surgical application, *Rev Chir Orthop* (1976) **62**: 151–60.
58. Olsewski JM, Simmons EH, Kallen FC, Mendel FC, Severin CM, Berens DL, Morphometry of the lumbar spine: anatomical perspectives related to transpedicular fixation, *J Bone Jt Surg* (1990) **72A**: 541–9.
59. Zindrick MR, Wiltse LL, Doornik A, Widell EH, Knight GW, Patwardhan AG, Thomas JC, Rothman SL, Fields BT, Analysis of the morphometric characteristics of the thoracic and lumbar pedicles, *Spine* (1987) **12**: 160–6.
60. Misenhimer GR, Peek RD, Wiltse LL, Rothman SLG, Widell EH, Anatomic analysis of pedicle canal and cancellous diameter related to screw size, *Spine* (1989) **14**: 367–72.
61. Yamagata M, Kitahara H, Minami S, Takahashi K, Isobe K, Moyira H, Tamaki T, Mechanical stability of the pedicle screw fixation systems for the lumbar spine, *Spine* (1992) **17**: S51–4.
62. Wittenberg RH, Shea M, Swartz DE, Lee KS, White III AA, Hayes WC, Importance of bone mineral density in instrumented spinal fusions, *Spine* (1991) **16**: 647–52.
63. Coe JD, Herzig MA, Warden KE, McAfee PC, Load to failure of spinal implants in osteoporitic spines — A comparison study of pedicle screws, laminar hooks, and spinous process wires, *Trans 35th Orthopedic Research Society Meeting* (1989) **14**: 71.
64. Mann KA, Bartel DL, A structural analysis of the fixation of pedicle screws to vertebrae, *Trans 36th Orthopedic Research Society Meeting* (1990) **15**: 611.
65. Wu S-S, Edwards WT, Zou D, Ordway NR, Fay LA, Yuan HA, Transpedicular vertebral screws in human vertebrae: effect on screw–vertebra interface stiffness, *Trans 38th Orthopedic Research*

Society Meeting (1992) **17:** 459.
66. George DC, Krag MH, Johnson CC, van Hal ME, Haugh LD, Grobler LJ, Hole preparation techniques for transpedicle fixation. Effects on pullout strength from human cadaveric vertebrae, *Spine* (1991) **16:** 181–4.
67. Law M, Tencer AF, Anderson PA, Mechanism of loosening of pedicle screws, *Spine* (in press).
68. Ashman RB, Galpin RD, Corin JD, Johnston CE, Biomechanical analysis of pedicle screw instrumentation in a corpectomy model, *Spine* (1989) **14:** 1398–405.
69. Nachemsen A, Elfstrom G, Intravital wireless telemetry of axial forces in Harrington distraction rods in patients with idiopathic scoliosis, *J Bone Jt Surg* (1971) **53A:** 445–65.
70. Gaines RW, Carson WL, Satterlee CC, Groh GI, Experimental evaluation of seven different fracture internal fixation devices using non failure stability testing, *Spine* (1991) **16:** 902–9.
71. Anderson PA, Harrington R, Budorick TE, Hoyt J, Tencer AF, Biomechanics of indirect reduction of an anterior mass protruding into the spinal cord, *Spine* (1993) **18:** 692–9.
72. Ferguson RL, Tencer AF, Woodard PL, Allen Jr BL, Biomechanical comparisons of spinal fracture models and the stabilizing effects of posterior instrumentations, *Spine* (1988) **13:** 453–60.
73. Shea M, Edwards WT, Clothiaux PL, Crowell RR, Nachemson AL, White III AA, Hayes WC, Three dimensional load displacement properties of posterior lumbar fixation, *J Orthop Trauma* (1991) **5:** 420–27.
74. Dick W, The "fixateur interne" as a versatile implant for spine surgery, *Spine* (1987) **12:** 882–900.
75. Stefee AD, Biscup RS, Sitkowski DJ, Segmental spine plates with pedicle screw fixation. A new internal fixation device for disorders of the lumbar and thoracolumbar spine, *Clin Orthop* (1986) **203:** 45–53.
76. Panjabi MM, Abumi K, Duranceau J, Crisco JJ, Biomechanical evaluation of spinal fixation devices: II. Stability provided by eight internal fixation devices, *Spine* (1988) **13:** 1135–40.
77. Gurr KR, McAfee PC, Shih C-M, Biomechanical analysis of anterior and posterior instrumentation systems after corpectomy, *J Bone Jt Surg* (1988) **70A:** 1182–91.
78. Kaneda K, Kuniyoshi A, Masanori F, Burst fractures with neurologic deficits of the thoracolumbar spine. Results of anterior decomposition and stabilization with anterior instrumentation, *Spine* (1984) **9:** 788–95.
79. Dank R, Zielke K, Harms J, Hack HP, *Surgical treatment of post-traumatic kyphosis: a followup study of 66 patients* (Scoliosis Research Society: Vancouver, BC 1987).
80. Luque ER, Rapp GF, A new semirigid method for interpedicular fixation of the spine, *Orthopedics* (1988) **11:** 1445–50.
81. Jacobs RR, Schlaepter F, Mathys R, Nachemson A, Perren SM, A locking hook spinal rod system for stabilization of fracture–dislocations and corrections of deformities of the dorsolumbar spine, *Clin Orthop* (1984) **189:** 168–177.
82. Roy-Camille R, Saillant G, Marie-Anne S, Mamoudy P, Behardlung von wibelfrakturen und luxation am thorako-lumalen übergang, *Orthopäde* (1980) **9:** 63–8.
83. Licht NJ, Rowe DE, Ross LM, Pitfalls of pedicle screw fixation in the sacrum, *Spine* (1992) **17:** 892–6.
84. Carlson GD, Abitbol JJ, Anderson DR, Krag MH, Kostuik JP, Woo SL-Y, Garfin SR, Screw fixation in the human sacrum, *Spine* (1992) **17:** S194–203.
85. Smith SA, Abitbol JJ, Anderson DR, Carlson GD, Taggart KW, Garfin SR, The effects of depth of penetration, screw orientation, and bone density on sacral screw fixation, *Trans 38th Orthopedic Research Society Meeting* (1992) **17:** 462.
86. McCord DH, Cunningham BW, Shono Y, Myers JJ, McAfee PC, Biomechanical analysis of lumbosacral fixation, *Spine* (1992) **17:** S235–42.
87. Allen Jr BL, Ferguson RL, The Galveston technique of pelvic fixation with Luque rod instrumentation of the spine, *Spine* (1984) **9:** 388.
88. Ogilvie JW, Bradford DS, *Lumbar and lumbosacral fusion with segmental fixation* (Scoliosis Research Society: Orlando, FL 1984).
89. Puno RM, Bechtold JE, Byrd III JA, Winter RB, Ogilvie JW, Bradford DS, Biomechanical analysis of transpedicular rod systems. A preliminary report, *Spine* (1991) **16:** 973–80.
90. Scholten PJM, Schultz AB, Luchies CW, Miller JAA, Motions and loads within the human pelvis: a biomechanical model study, *J Orthop Res* (1988) **6:** 840–50.
91. Paul JP, Approaches to design, force actions transmitted by joints in the human body, *Proc Roy Soc London* (1976) **B192:** 163–72.
92. Stocks GW, Gabel GT, Noble PC, Hanson GW, Tullos HS, Anterior and posterior internal fixation of vertical shear fractures of the pelvis, *J Orthop Res* (1991) **9:** 237–45.
93. Miller JAA, Schultz AB, Anderson GBJ, Load–displacement behavior of sacroiliac joints, *J Orthop Res* (1987) **5:** 92–101.
94. Simonion P, Harrington RM, Mayo KA, Routt Jr ML, Seuft DC, Tencer AF, Pelvic ring fixation: analysis of new techniques, presented at the 60th Meeting, American Academy of Orthopaedic Surgeons, San Francisco, 1993.
95. Daum WJ, Tencer AF, Cartwright TJ, Simmons DJ,

Woodward PL, Koulisis CW, Pull-out strengths of bone screws at various sites about the pelvis—A preliminary study, *J Orthop Trauma* (1988) **2**: 229–33.

96. Daum WJ, Patterson RM, Carwright TJ, Viegas SF, Comparison of cortical and cancellous screw pull out strengths about the posterior column and sacroiliac joint, *J Orthop Trauma* (1991) **5**: 34–7.
97. Rubash HE, Brown TD, Nelson DD, Mears DC, Comparative mechanical performances of some new devices for fixation of unstable pelvic ring fractures, *Med Biol Eng Computing* (1983) **21**: 657–63.
98. Slatis P, Karaharju EO, External fixation of the pelvic girdle with a trapezoidal compression frame, *Injury* (1975) **7**: 53–6.
99. Mears DC, Fu FH, Modern concepts of external fixation of the pelvis, *Clin Orthop* (1980) **151**: 65–72.
100. Shaw JA, Mins DE, Warner FW, Murray DG, Posterior stabilization of pelvic fractures by use of threaded compression rods, *Clin Orthop* (1985) **192**: 240–54.
101. Tile M, *Fractures of the pelvis and acetabulum* (Williams & Wilkins: Baltimore 1984).
102. Stocks GW, Gabel GT, Noble PC, Hanson GW, Tullos HS, Anterior and posterior internal fixation of vertical shear fractures of the pelvis, *J Orthop Res* (1991) **9**: 237–45.
103. Leighton RK, Waddell JP, Bray TJ, Chapman MW, Simpson L, Martin RB, Sharkey NA, Biomechanical testing of new and old fixation devices for vertical shear fractures of the pelvis, *J Orthop Trauma* (1991) **5**: 313–17.
104. Sawaguchi T, Brown TD, Rubash HE, Mears DC, Stability of acetabular fractures after internal fixation, *Acta Orthop Scand* (1984) **55**: 601–5.
105. Mason DJ, Goulet JA, Rouleau JP, Goldstein SA, Comminuted posterior wall fractures of the acetabulum: a study of fixation stability, *Trans 37th Orthopedic Research Society Meeting* (1991) **16**: 144.

CHAPTER 9

Lower extremity fixation

This chapter deals with fixation of the lower extremity. Topics include femoral neck fixation, as well as fixation of subtrochanteric, midshaft, and distal femur fractures. In the tibia, the biomechanics of tibial plateau fixation, and tibial shaft fixation using external fixation or unreamed nails is discussed. Information is also provided related to fixation of the tibiofibular syndesmosis.

9.1 Fixation of the proximal femur

Loading conditions

Forces acting on the hip joint have been determined from force plate studies to range from a minimum of about body weight during midstance to nearly eight times body weight near toe off in fast walking (Figure 9.1). The orientation of the applied force through the hip varies during the gait cycle, but at maximum magnitude ranges from 12.5° to 21° from the vertical (Figure 9.2).[1] Since the joint reaction force is not perpendicular to the femoral neck, there is a component that can contribute to maintaining the stability of a fixed fracture by creating compression of the fracture components.

The hip joint reaction and hip abductor forces combine to generate large stresses on the femur. Apart from direct compression along the shaft, bending stresses are considerable, as shown in Figure 9.3.[2] Bending in the femoral neck and shaft results from the hip joint reaction force being applied through the head, which is offset with respect to the shaft of the femur. Also, the abductors pull from the tensile (lateral) side of the bone. It should be noted that the stresses in the subtrochanteric region of the femur are particularly large. From strain gages mounted to nail plates installed in patients, bending moments on fixation implants have been shown to range from 13 to 30 N m in the sagittal plane, relative to the nail, and from 2 to 12 N m horizontally (in the anterior–posterior direction).[3]

Factors affecting fixation

In fixation of femoral neck fractures, the femoral shaft and the intact part of the subtrochanteric region act as a load supporting buttress. It is a major benefit for the bone to support as much of the applied loads as possible so that loading of the implant, particularly at the bone/implant interface (i.e. at the threads of screws), is reduced. Bone can support compressive load across the fracture line if cortical contact exists (i.e. there is an absence of comminution). Compressive loading across the fracture line is created by physiological forces as well as through the

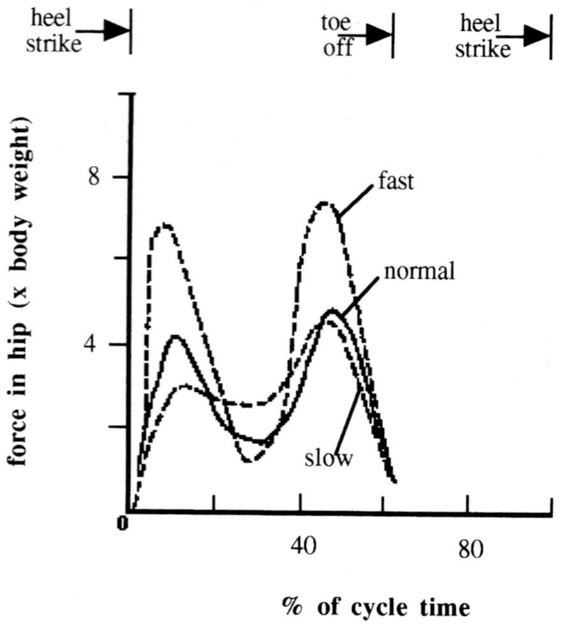

Figure 9.1

Joint reaction force magnitude in the hip joint, in terms of multiples of body weight, for different parts of the gait cycle. (From Ref 1 with permission.)

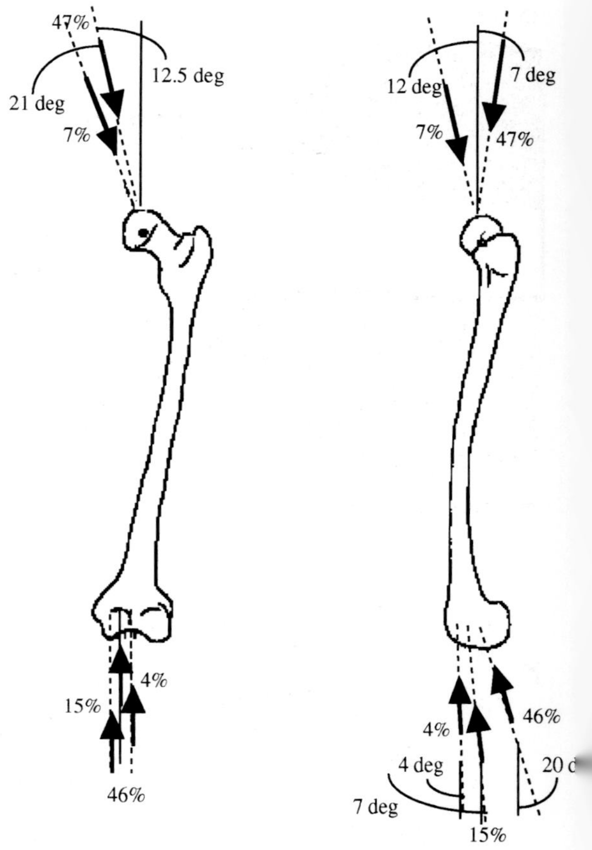

Figure 9.2

Orientation of the joint force acting through the hip and knee during gait. The percentage values refer to the location within the gait cycle where this orientation occurs. (From Ref 1 with permission.)

compression mechanism of the implant itself. With increased compression, the shear resistance (resistance to slip along the fracture line), which depends upon the frictional force at the fracture interface, and interdigitation of the fragments, is enhanced. Shear resistance is important in preventing inferior displacement of the femoral head.[4] These concepts are illustrated in Figure 9.4.

In an in vivo study, Ragnarsson et al[5] demonstrated that the distal migration of the femoral neck and head was linearly, though very weakly, correlated to Pauwel's angle (the fracture line/femoral shaft angle) (Figure 9.5). Apart from the orientation of the fracture line, several other factors, as shown in Figure 9.6, affect the stability of a femoral neck fracture fixed with cancellous screws. From observations of the average axial force and the maximum sustainable force on fixed femoral specimens subjected to 10 000 cycles of combined axial and torsional loading at a magnitude of 2.2 times body weight, other factors that affect the success of fixation include the density of the cancellous bone into which the screws are embedded, the degree of comminution at the inferior surface of the fracture,[5,6] and the moment arm of the joint load.[6] The moment

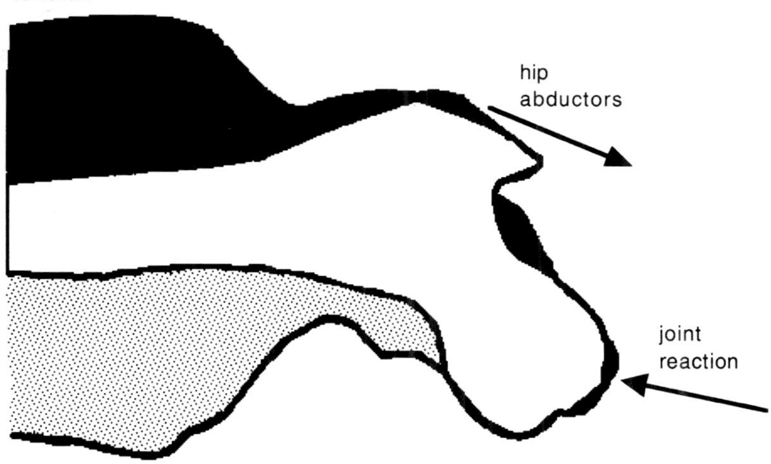

Figure 9.3

Relative stresses in the proximal third of the femur due to joint reaction and hip abductor forces: black = tension; dotted = compression; magnitude = distance of area border from bone at any particular location. (Adapted from Ref 2.)

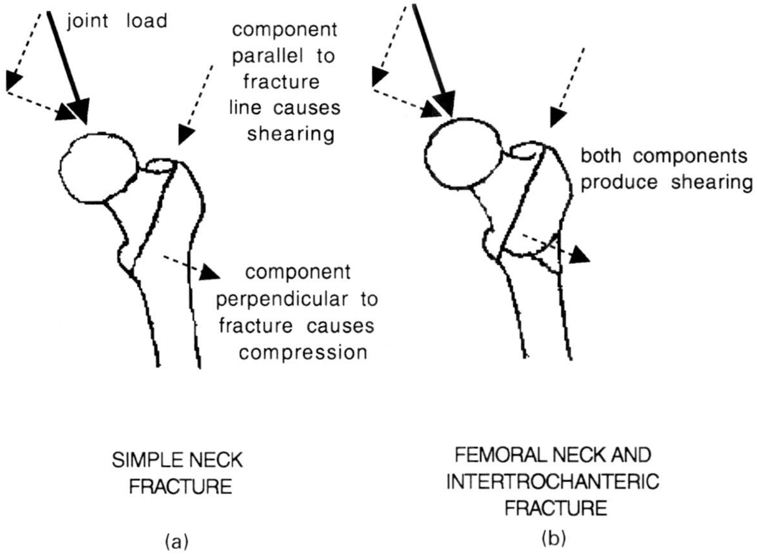

Figure 9.4

Loads acting parallel and perpendicular to the fracture line, and resulting shear resistance for two typical types of proximal femoral fractures: (a) simple trochanteric; (b) combined trochanteric and subtrochanteric fractures. (Adapted from Ref 4.)

arm magnitude is determined by the length of the femoral neck and the neck/shaft angle.

As shown in Figure 9.7, a femoral neck/head cancellous bone density of 1250 CT units (computed tomography density units) in combination with less than 30% comminution of the inferior half of the fracture surface is a good indicator of "success of fixation" (the ability to support the defined load in the experimental situation). It should also be noted that from comparison of plain films and direct measurements, plain film measurements overestimate the degree of comminution by a factor of nearly two.[6] Swiontkowski et al[7] showed that two other methods of

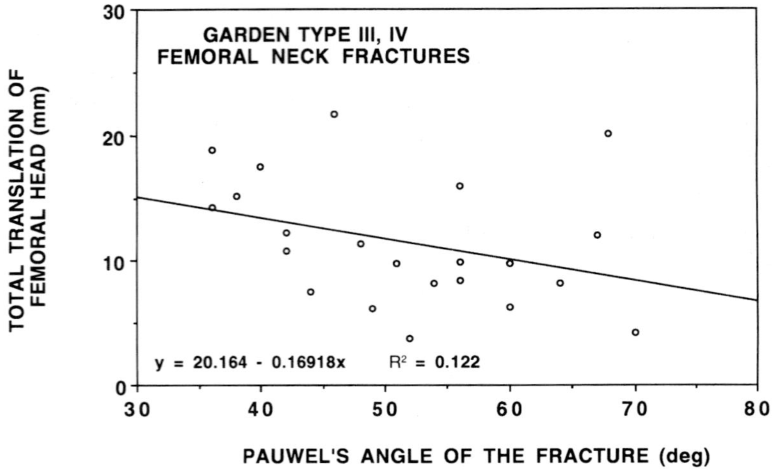

Figure 9.5

Relationship between the in vivo distal translation of fixed proximal femoral fractures and the femoral fracture line/femoral shaft angle. (Adapted from Ref 5.)

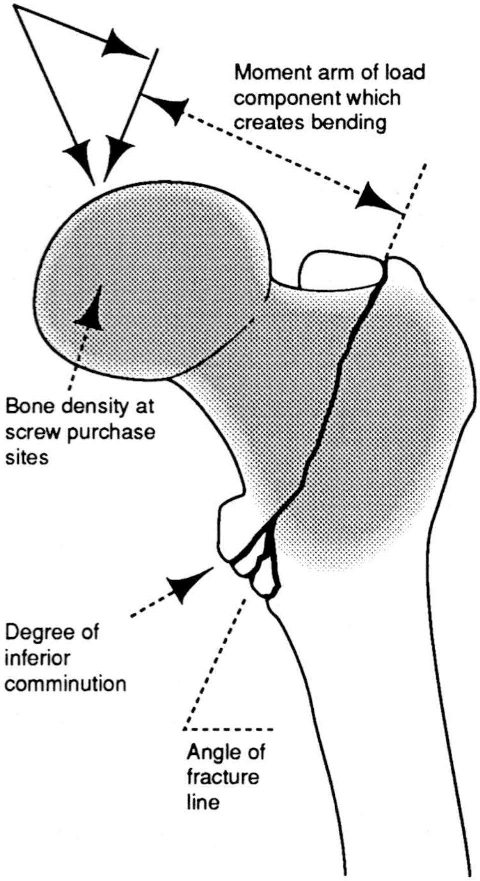

Figure 9.6

Several factors that may contribute to the success of fixation of a femoral neck fracture.

determining femoral bone density also correlated with success of fixation. These were a Singh index[8] of 3.8 or greater, and a fixation screw insertion torque of greater than 18.9 N m.

Considering the importance of bone density in fixation, it would be of benefit to locate the fixation screws in the densest region of the femoral head. Crowell et al[9] showed that the pullout strength of hip screws is related to the square of bone density in the femoral head. The greatest mean bone density was located in the center of the head, followed by lateral (both posterior and anterior) and medial locations (Figure 9.8). Other factors dictate the position of the fixation screws as well; however, bone density should be considered when selecting the locations of screws.

Alternative methods of fixation

A review publication by the American Academy of Orthopaedic Surgeons lists 79 devices for use in fixation of fractures of the proximal end of the femur.[10] In terms of their generic biomechanical function, the Jewett nail[11] is an example of a device in which the load bearing part of the nail replaces the structure of the neck, acting as a rigid beam in bending. The hip joint reaction load is transferred from the part of the nail in the femoral neck to a sideplate fixed to the femoral shaft. A

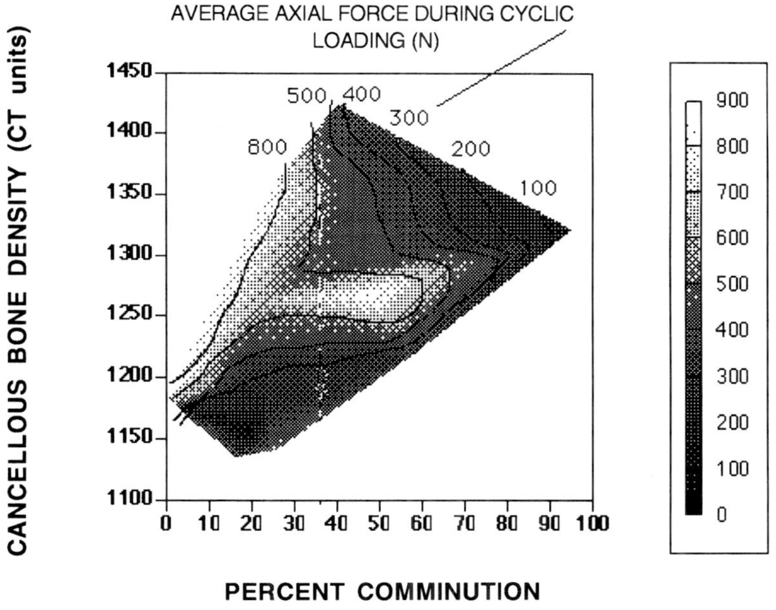

Figure 9.7

The effects of comminution and femoral head trabecular density on the average load supported during cyclic testing of femoral fixation.[6]

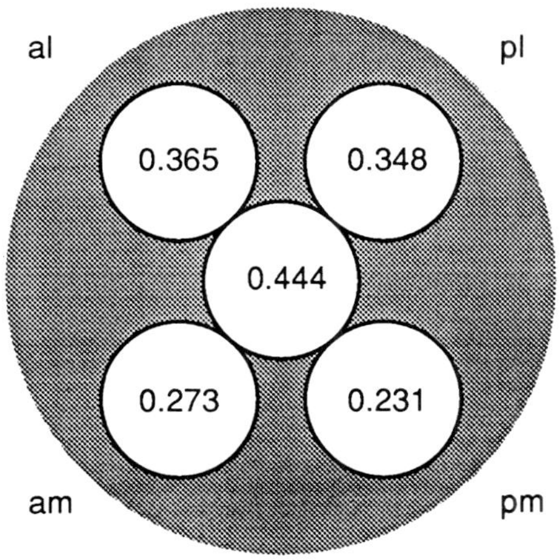

Figure 9.8

Mean bone density in the femoral head: a, anterior; p, posterior; l, lateral; m, medial. (From Ref 9 with permission.)

second type, exemplified by the compression hip screw,[12,13] functions partly to transfer joint load to the sideplate similar to the Jewett nail. However, it also allows the proximal part of the fracture to impact the distal part, which permits transfer of some load across the fracture line (Figure 9.9a,d).

More recently, intramedullary nails[14] have been used to replace the sideplate as a method for transferring load to bone. In an equivalent situation, the bending moment transferred to the IM nail will be smaller than that to the sideplate, because the moment arm distance (distance from the joint load to the intersection of the hip screw and plate or rod) is smaller. Further, the greater length of the IM nail produces a larger counteracting moment arm, thereby reducing the force along the nail/bone interface. The force is distributed to the lateral endosteal surface of the medullary canal along its entire length (at least where there is nail/bone contact), in contrast to the compression hip screw, where the sideplate screws provide discrete load transfer points and can be under higher stress (Figure 9.9b).

Multiple pins[15] can be used when the trochanteric part of the femur is intact (Figure 9.9c). When this implant is used, direct compression of the fracture surfaces is created by the lag effect of the screw (i.e. the screw having a thread on one end and a smooth surface on the other pulls the bone fragments together; see Chapter 6), and the compression created along with the bending resistance of the screws is important in maintaining stability.

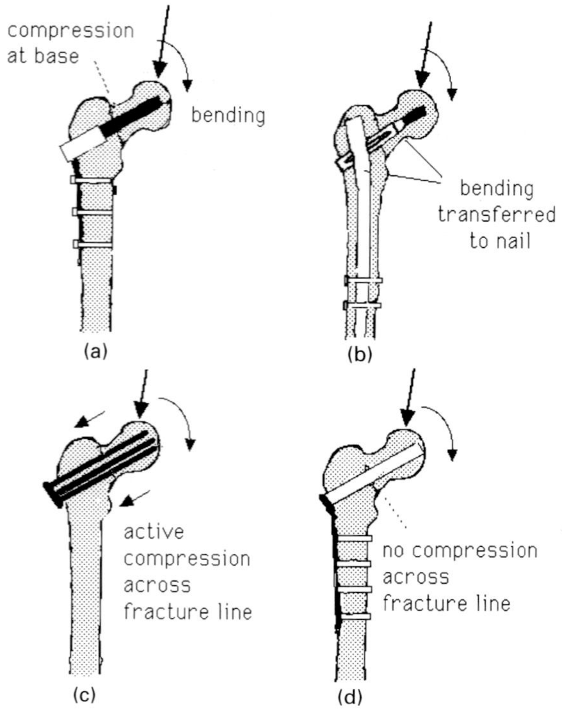

Figure 9.9

Differences in the mechanics of load transfer across a femoral neck fracture with different types of fixation implants. (a) The compression hip screw permits the fracture components to slide together and impact. This allows the femur to partly support the compressive component of the applied load, as well as resisting shear parallel to the fracture line. The shear component is supported due to impaction, which increases friction at the fracture surface. Also, the bending moment is supported by fracture component contact in the inferior region of the fracture surface. (b) A reconstruction nail supports the applied bending moment, which is transferred to the IM nail and is resisted by contact of the nail against the intramedullary canal of the femoral shaft. (c) Pins apply active compression across the fracture site, which allows transfer of axial compressive and shear loads and bending moments, similarly to the compression hip screw fixation. However, the implants themselves do not transfer load to the femoral cortex. (d) The Jewett nail acts as a rigid beam, transferring joint load to the femoral cortex, with no impaction of the fracture components.

Compression hip screw versus triflanged nail

Comparing the ultimate strength of fixation, Kaufer et al[16] found that femoral fractures fixed with the Jewett nail failed at a mean of 4.07 times body weight, compared with the compression hip screw at 5.53 times. From strain gages mounted at the inner and outer surfaces of the nail/plate or screw barrel/plate junction and on bone under the implant, it has been demonstrated that for the same applied loads, the tensile strain in the sideplate of the Jewett nail is greater than in the hip screw device. This result indicates that greater load was being borne by the implant in the case of the Jewett nail. The compressive load was shared by both bone and the implant, with the greatest bone loads recorded when the hip screw was set to act as a compression device, followed by the hip screw set in sliding mode, and then the Jewett nail (Figure 9.10).[17] These data confirm the difference in biomechanical function of these implants. Comparative testing of devices that allow sliding but utilize a screw or triflanged nail for fixation into the femoral head demonstrate that both devices cut out of bone at similar shear load magnitudes (i.e. transverse to the axis of the implant), but the resistance of the screw to failure when loaded parallel to its long axis is 4.23 times that of the triflanged nail.[18]

Compression hip screw versus lag screws or pins

The mechanical differences between sliding hip screws and cancellous lag screws have been the subject of several investigations. No differences were found in the biomechanical properties of femoral fracture constructs utilizing screws or the compression hip screw.[19] Screw or sliding nail plate fixed specimens loaded through the femoral head, with the load vector at 15° from the vertical, fail at a mean load of 40.3% of intact, and do so by progressive migration of the screw in the femoral head, as shown in Figure 9.11. Pins, whether three, five or seven, fail at a slightly higher load, 43.2% of intact, and do so by bending of the pins (Figure 9.12).[20] Several recent studies have independently demonstrated that the type of

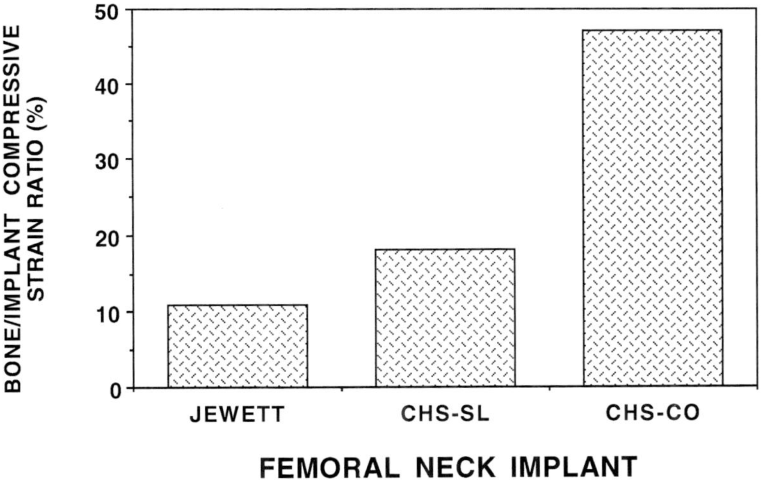

Figure 9.10

Comparison of the ratios of compressive strain (femoral cortex/plate) for the Jewett nail, the hip screw with the screw sliding (CHS-SL), and the hip scew with the screw in compression (CHS-CO). (Adapted from data of Ref 17.)

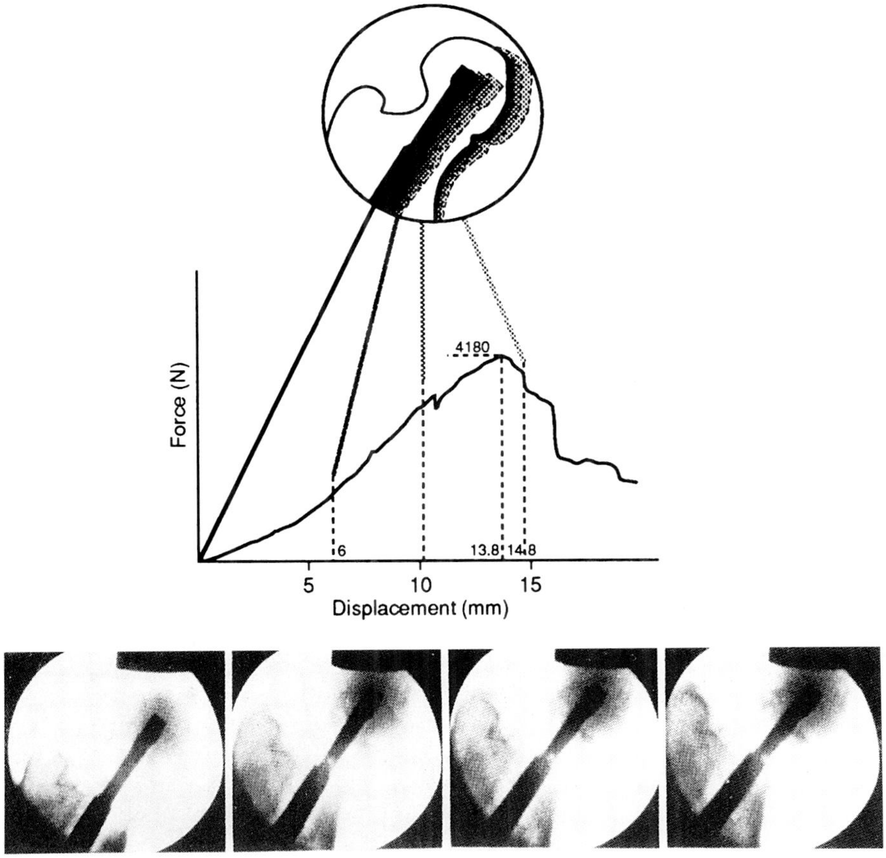

Figure 9.11

Progressive failure of a compression hip screw under load, showing positions of the screw within the head and the corresponding point in the load–deformation curve. (From Ref 20 with permission.)

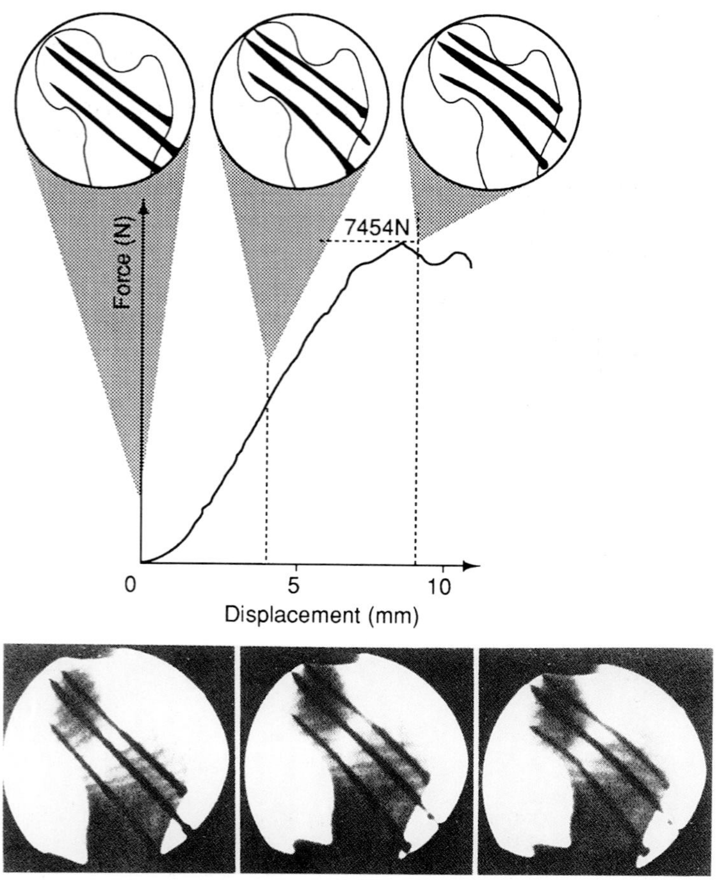

Figure 9.12

Progressive failure of fixation pins under load, showing positions of the pins within the head and the corresponding point in the load–deformation curve. (From Ref 20 with permission.)

implant, whether pins or compression hip screw, yield fixation of equivalent stiffness and strength.[7,19,20] The number of pins used does not significantly increase fracture stability. The important factors in increasing fixation stability and strength are

- the orientation of the fracture line with respect to the axis of the screws (screws more perpendicular to fracture yields greater impaction)[21]
- bone density[6,7]
- a more horizontal fracture surface[5,21]
- the degree of comminution[6,22]
- the moment arm of the applied load.[6]

Intramedullary devices

Intramedullary nail devices have been introduced for use in femoral neck fracture fixation. In a comparison of the cortical strain produced in the calcar under load with fixation using the Gamma nail or the sliding hip screw for femoral fracture fixation, Rosenblum et al[23] found that with the hip screw, calcar compressive strain increases to between 130% and 155% of intact, because of impaction and the fact that load is supported mainly by the medial cortex (Figure 9.13). The locked IM device significantly unloads the cortex (2–7% of intact strain), because the implant itself resists the applied bending moment and it may be resistant to sliding of the hip screw. The actual effect of these changes from physiological strain

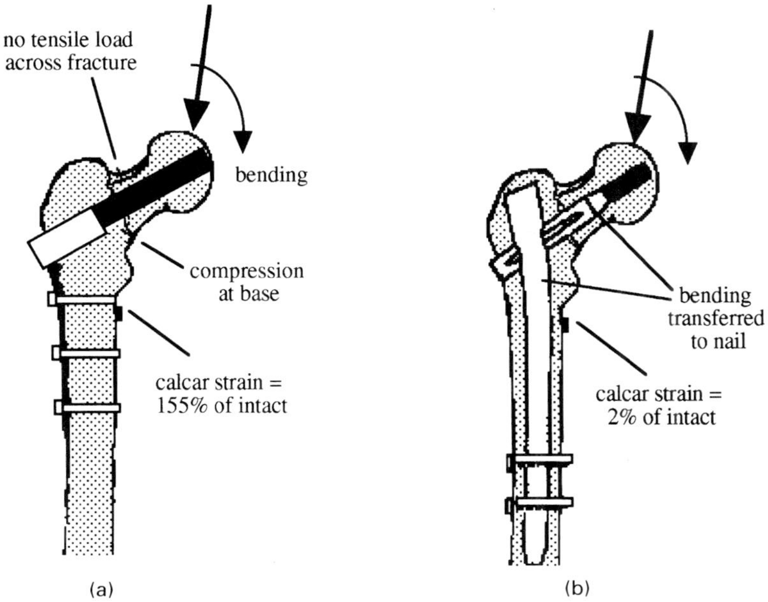

Figure 9.13

Differences in load transfer between (a) a sliding hip screw and (b) a Gamma nail fixed femur fracture, and resulting strains on the femoral shaft. (Data from Ref 23.)

on fracture healing is at this point unclear, but this study does demonstrate the differences in how the devices support and transfer the loads applied to the femoral head. Comparisons of the reconstruction IM nail show that fractures fixed with this device are 76% stiffer in torsion and 37% in bending than the compression hip screw. In comparison with multiple pin fixation, the increases in fixation stiffness were 53% and 140% respectively (Figure 9.14).[24]

Biomechanical aspects of the sliding hip screw

The hip screw is a unique device, because it acts as a mechanism allowing sliding and impaction of the fracture components, as well as a fixation (structural) device. In order for the device to function as intended, it is critical that sliding occurs between the screw and barrel. Kyle et al[25] showed that sliding of the screw depends on two factors. The first is the angle between the barrel and the sideplate. For a greater barrel/sideplate angle (i.e. 150° instead of 135°), the screw is more closely aligned with the applied joint force. Therefore the component of the joint force acting parallel to the screw (i.e. the component that assists sliding) is greater, and conversely the component perpendicular to the axis of the screw (i.e. the component that resists sliding) is smaller, as shown in Figure 9.15. The ratio of force available to produce sliding to the force resisting sliding (ratio of parallel to perpendicular force components) is about 2 in a 135° device, and more than 4 in a 150° device.

A second important consideration in enhancing the sliding characteristics of the hip screw is the ratio of the length of the screw within the barrel to that extending out of the barrel. As shown in Figure 9.16, the fulcrum of this system can be considered to be the proximal edge of the barrel, since the screw will rotate about this point under load. Multiplying the magnitude of the component of the applied joint force perpendicular to the barrel by the length from the point of application to the fulcrum results in the magnitude of the moment that rotates the proximal end of the

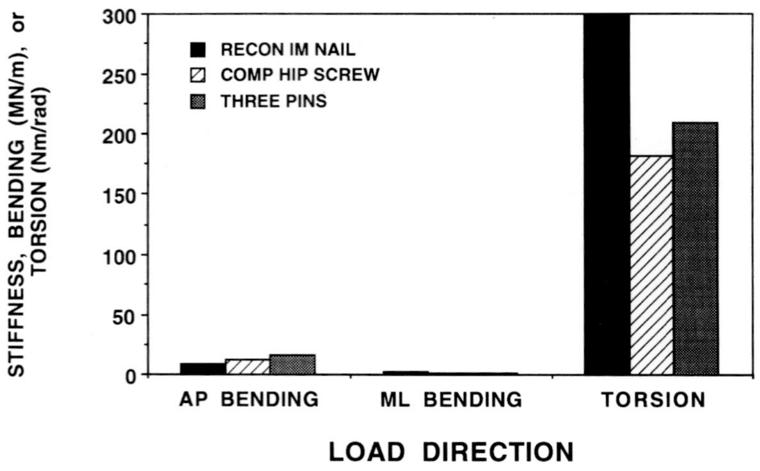

Figure 9.14

Comparison of the stiffness of femoral neck fractures in bending and torsion fixed by different implants: RECON IM NAIL, reconstruction intramedullary nail; COMP HIP SCREW, compression hip screw. (Data adapted from Ref 24.)

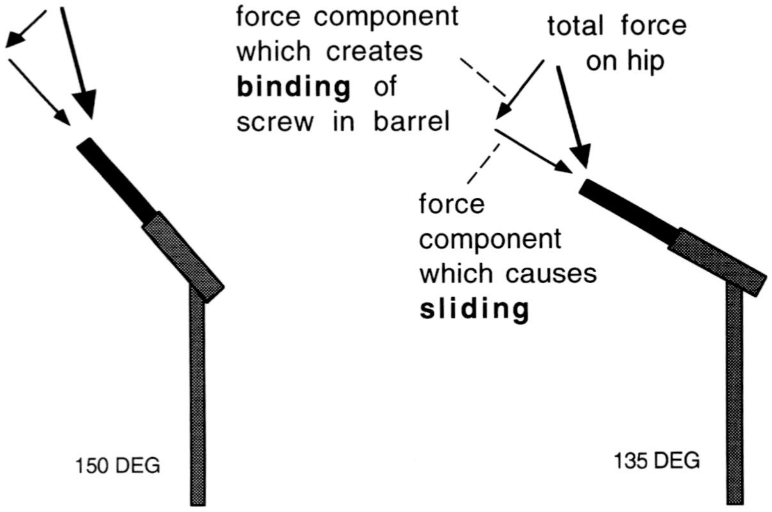

Figure 9.15

Effect of the barrel/side plate angle on the force components acting parallel and perpendicular to the long axis of the sliding screw. The parallel component aids in sliding and the perpendicular component produces resistance to sliding by creating friction between the screw and the barrel.

screw inferiorly. This must be counteracted by a moment arising from the force of interaction between the barrel and the screw. If the screw extends further out of the barrel, the proximal end moment arm is larger, so the applied moment is increased. At the same time, the moment arm of the screw/barrel force decreases. Therefore the internal force of contact between the screw and barrel must become larger, and, with it, the frictional resistance to sliding. Kyle et al[25] showed a relationship between this apparent frictional coefficient (a measure of the frictional resistance to sliding) and the ratio of the length of the screw extended to the length within the barrel. As shown in Figure 9.17, when the length of the screw within the barrel is equal to the length outside ($L_n/L_b = 1$), the coefficient of friction is about 0.65. When the length of the screw outside the barrel is 3.5 times the length within, the frictional coefficient increases to about 1.75. This

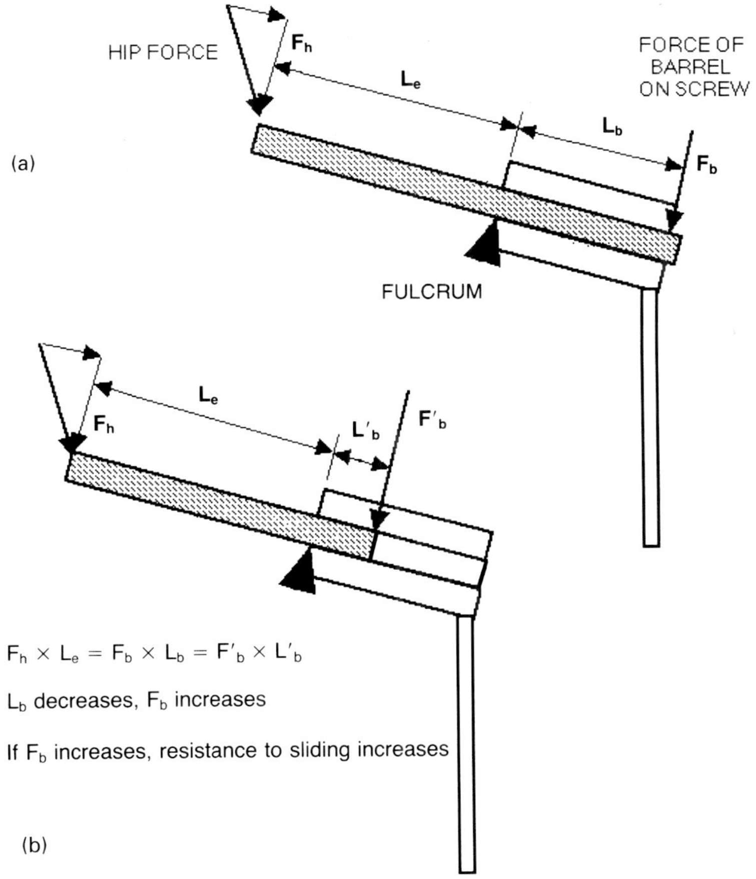

Figure 9.16

The joint force creates a moment, $F_h \times L_e$ acting at the fulcrum, which is located at the lower edge of the proximal end of the barrel. (a) When the screw extends through the barrel, the moment resisting the joint moment is $F_b \times L_b$. (b) If L_b decreases to one third of its previous length, the force F_b must increase by three times to generate the same moment. This increase in F_b also increases the screw/barrel frictional force which increases the resistance of the screw to sliding within the barrel.

implies that the force needed to overcome the frictional resistance to sliding increases by 1.75 times. The ultimate force to failure is unaffected by the length of screw outside to that within the barrel; however, the stiffness of fixation does tend to increase (though not statistically significantly).[26]

Summary

The proximal femur represents a difficult area for fracture fixation because of the large bending moment produced at the base of the femoral neck by the joint reaction force acting through the femoral head. In addition, the fixation must resist shearing at the fracture line. Although a number of methods have been advocated for fixation, one major biomechanical difference between them is the ability to create compression across the fracture site. This may occur passively (the sliding compression hip screw) or actively (cancellous lag screws), or it may be resisted (Jewett nail). Compression allows the bone to share load with the implant and also helps to prevent distal displacement of the proximal femur due to shear slip at the fracture line. The most

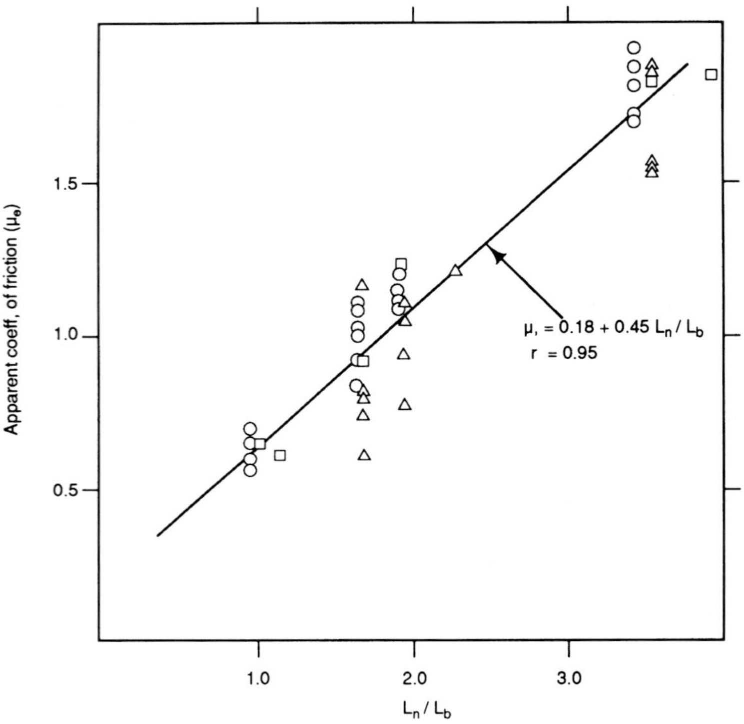

Figure 9.17

Measured increase in the apparent frictional coefficient between the screw and the barrel with increasing length of the screw outside the barrel (L_n) to the length of screw within the barrel (L_b). 316L stainless steel sliding hip screw devices: OEC (□); Richards (○); Zimmer (△). (From Ref 25 with permission.)

important biomechanical factors in maintaining stable fixation are the density of bone into which the fixation device is implanted, the degree of inferior comminution at the fracture site, the angle of the fracture line with respect to the femoral shaft, and the moment arm of the joint reaction force, which increases with both a longer femoral neck and one that is oriented more horizontally. The differences between the hip screw and triflanged nail are significant; however, there are no differences in strength and load transfer between the hip screw and cancellous lag screws or pins. In order to obtain the best sliding characteristics from a compression hip screw, one with a higher shaft barrel angle should be selected. Also, the screw should be inserted as completely as possible within the barrel.

9.2 Fixation of the femoral shaft

Loading conditions

The physiological loads applied to the femur were described in the previous section. Michel et al[27] have recently reported on the in vivo loads encountered in an intramedullary nail implanted in a patient with a comminuted diaphyseal fracture of the femur. The nail was locked both proximally and distally. Figure 9.18 shows the axial load in the nail at various post operative time periods. It decreases from about 320 to 180 N as healing progresses and the callus takes more load. The increase at 17 weeks represents a change in activity level and the application of greater muscle forces. Therefore the peak load in

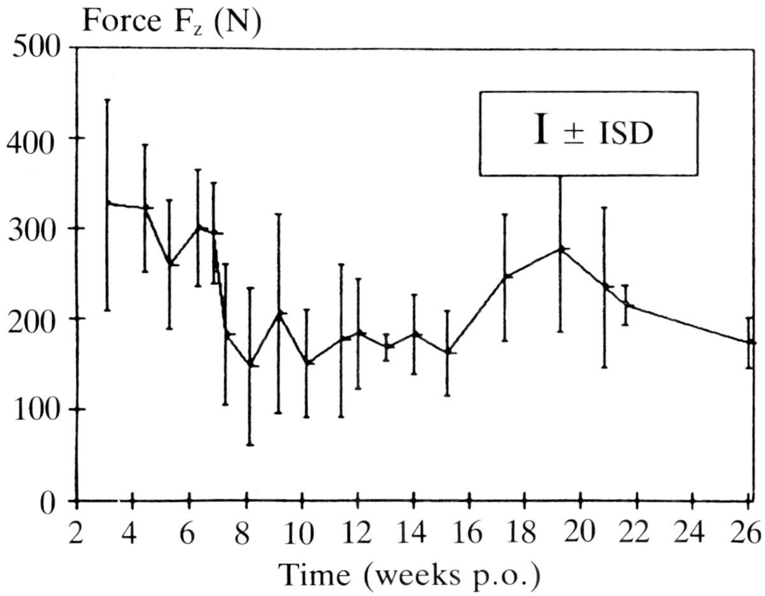

Figure 9.18

Axial load recorded in an interlocked nail applied in a comminuted fracture of the femur, in vivo, versus time post implantation. (From Ref 27 with permission.)

the nail (but not the total load applied to the femur) is about 46% of body weight.

The major load on the femur is usually considered to be that due to body weight acting on the femoral head. However, the abductor muscles and the tensor fasciae latae play important roles in the strains generated in the femoral cortex of the subtrochanteric region of the femur. With load applied directly to the femoral head, as shown in Figure 9.19, the ratio of tensile (lateral cortex) to compressive (medial cortex) strain is 0.59. With the body weight load placed to simulate its position at the center of the trunk, and the abductors loaded to counteract the moment produced, the ratio of tensile to compressive strain increases to 0.89, and the strain magnitudes increase by a factor of 5.3. Increasing the force exerted by the tensor fasciae latae decreases the tension/compression strain ratio to 0.36 and the cortical strains to about 2.3 times those of the simple loading case.[28] These measurements demonstrate clearly the effects of musculature and the importance of the tensor fasciae latae in the resulting strains (and stresses) in the subtrochanteric region of the femur.

Mechanics of the IM nail

The mechanical properties of the intramedullary (IM) nail are important because factors such as bending stiffness and curvature of the implant affect the force required to insert it and its ability to generate frictional force against the medullary canal, thereby stabilizing the fracture. The cross sectional shapes of commonly used IM nails for the femur are substantially the same (Figure 9.20); therefore their bending stiffnesses (Figure 9.21) and strengths are similar. The principal factor that alters bending stiffness is nail diameter. A 16 mm diameter nail is 2.5 times as stiff as a 12 mm nail, and 1.5 times as stiff as a 14 mm nail. The slot in the nail (note that the Russell–Taylor nail has no slot while the others in this comparison do) has little effect on its bending stiffness. However, a nonslotted nail, such as the Russell–Taylor device,[14] is more than 40 times stiffer in torsion than nails of the same diameter with a longitudinal slot (Figure 9.22).[29]

Fatigue of the IM nail is of concern, especially at the distal locking hole sites. A 6 mm diameter hole transversely placed through a 13–16 mm

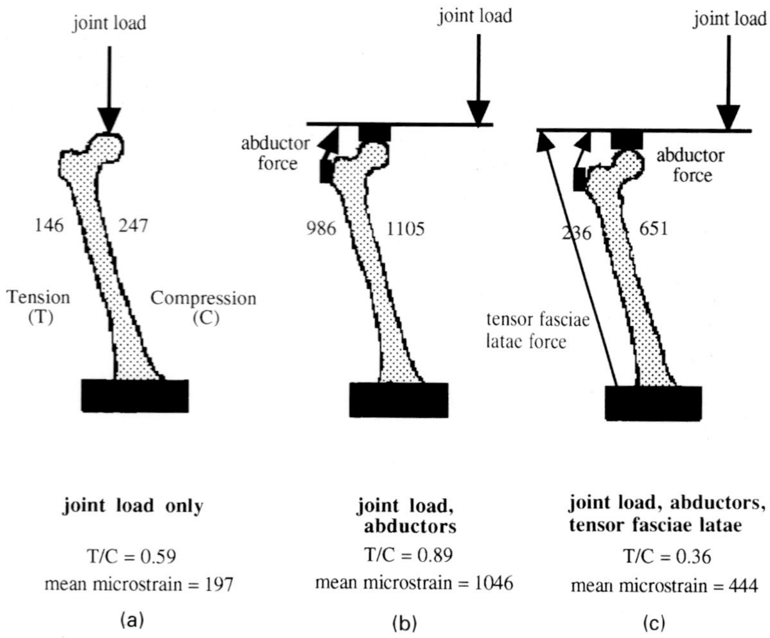

Figure 9.19

Strains (in microstrain) and strain ratio (tension/compression, *T/C*) in the femur in different loading conditions. (a) Joint load applied directly on the femoral head. (b) Body weight acting at the center of gravity of the trunk, and a counteracting moment from the abductor muscles. (c) Body weight, abductor muscle load, and tensor fasciae latae load, which helps to counteract the body weight moment and thereby reduces the subtrochanteric cortical strains. (Adapted from Ref 28.)

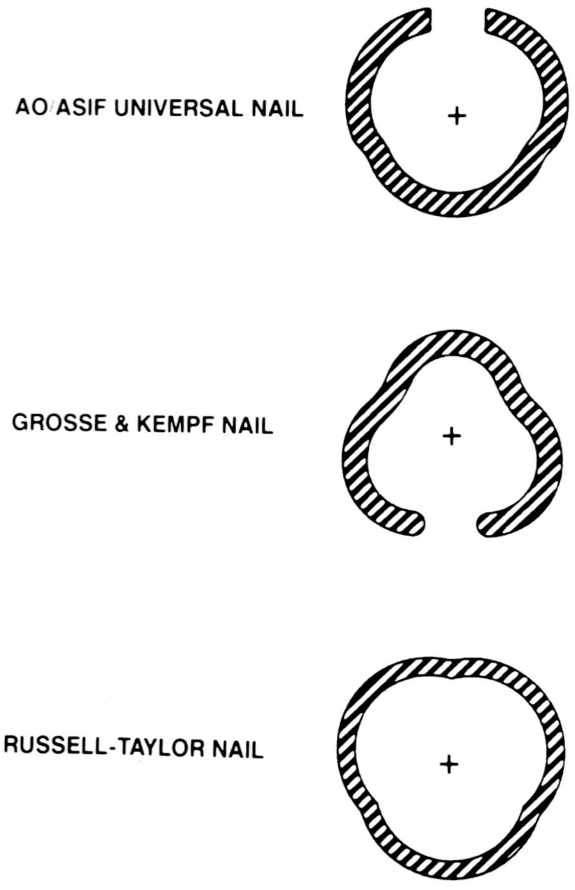

Figure 9.20

A comparison of the cross sectional shapes of three commonly used IM rods for femur fracture stabilization. (From Ref 29 with permission.)

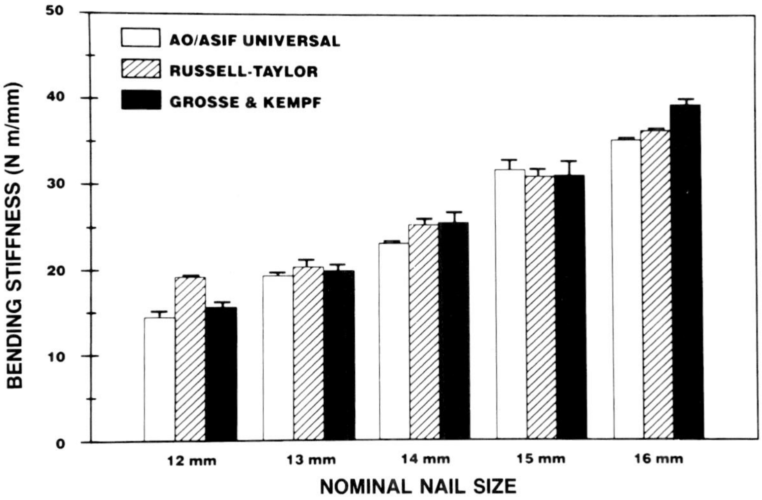

Figure 9.21

A comparison of the bending stiffnesses of three femoral IM rods of different diameters. (From Ref 29 with permission.)

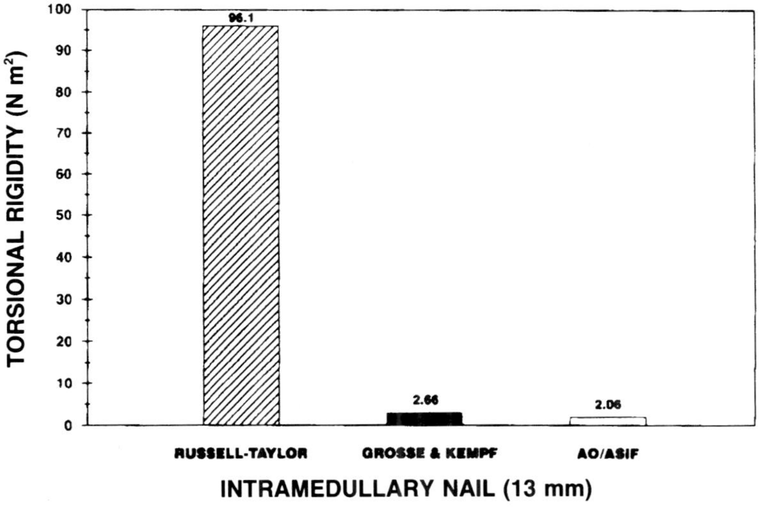

Figure 9.22

A comparison of the torsional rigidities of the three femoral IM rods. (From Ref 29 with permission.)

diameter rod (38–46% of nail diameter) acts as a significant stress riser. Coupling the stress riser effect of the hole with the tendency to nick its perimeter during the distal locking procedure, the potential for fatigue fracture becomes a possibility. Bucholz et al[30] showed that if the femoral fracture site is located within 5 cm of the most proximal of the distal locking screws, the peak stress around the hole may exceed the endurance limit of the metal (the stress level above which fatigue fracture can occur) (Figure 9.23). The large distal stresses result from the nail being loaded as a cantilever beam. If the length of support around the nail is reduced, which occurs in a more distally located fracture, the stresses in the nail itself will be higher (Figure 9.24).

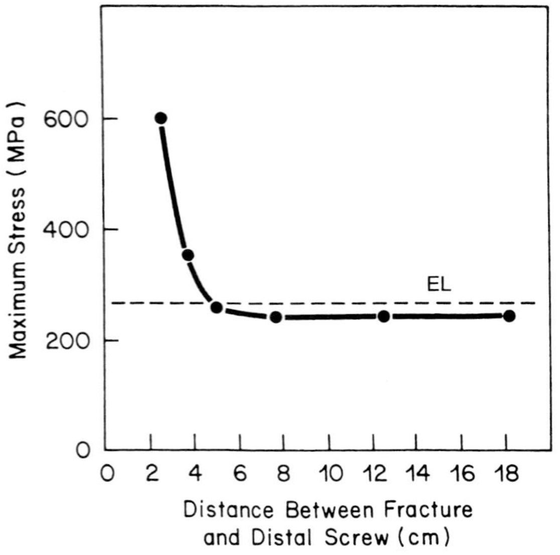

Figure 9.23

Stress around the perimeter of the most proximal of the distal locking screws of an IM nail as a function of the distance between the screw hole and the fracture site. (From Ref 30 with permission.)

Biomechanics of nail insertion

The IM nail and the femur have different radii of curvature, defined in Figure 9.25 for the nail. For a sample of femora, the mean value was found to be 1020 mm.[32] IM nails are manufactured with a bow that is meant to conform to that of the femur when fully inserted (Figure 9.26). As shown in Figure 9.27, an axial force is required to insert a nail into the femur, because it must bend to conform to the curve of the medullary canal. The force of nail insertion, when the nail is used to fix a subtrochanteric fracture, is maximum at about three-quarters of the insertion length, and decreases thereafter as the deformation in the nail decreases. The bending deformation decreases because, as the nail comes to its fully inserted position, it conforms more closely to the shape of the femur.

The force of insertion generates hoop stress in the bone. This is a circumferential expansion stress, similar to that supported by the hoops of a barrel. The greater the insertion force, the larger is the hoop stress (Figure 9.28). Excessively large hoop stresses can cause splitting of the femur,

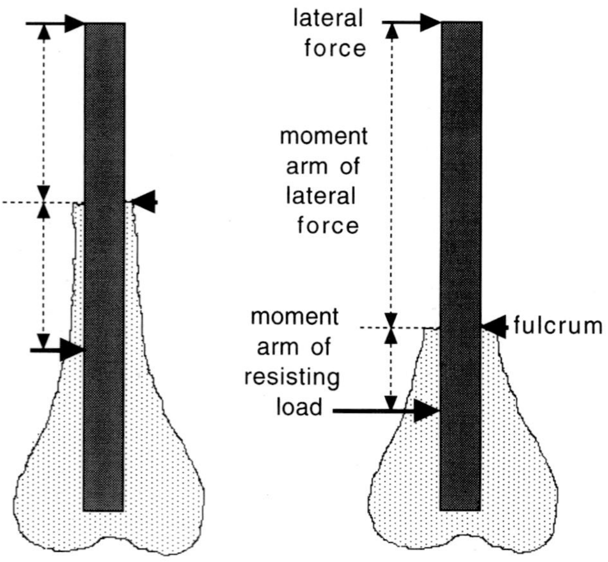

Figure 9.24

The stress in the distal part of the interlocking IM nail increases when the fracture line is closer to the screw hole because the bone support of the rod in bending is decreased, resulting in a smaller moment arm.

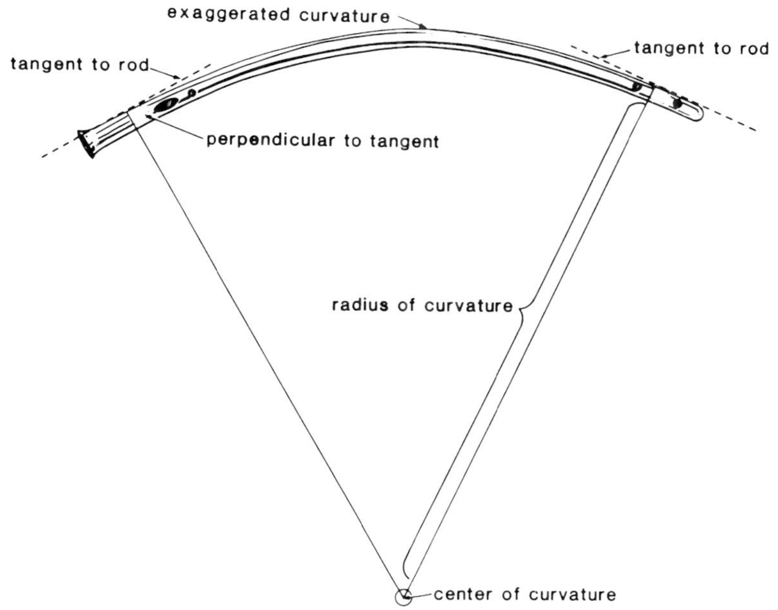

Figure 9.25

Definition of the radius of curvature of an intramedullary nail. (From Ref 31 with permission.)

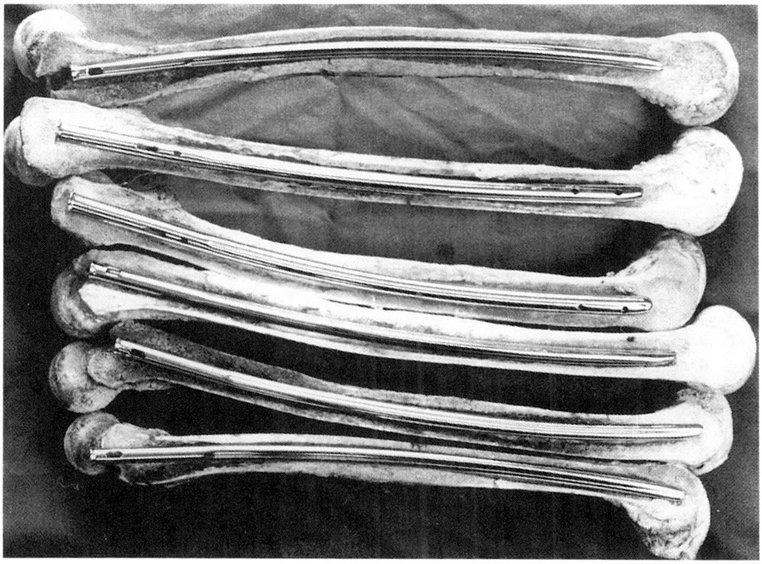

Figure 9.26

Sections through femora of varying anterior bows, showing the fit of the nail in the medullary canal. (From Ref 32 with permission.)

turning a relatively simple transverse fracture into one having subtrochanteric or intertrochanteric components. Several factors control the hoop stresses produced. The choice of a nail that more closely conforms to the particular femur being fixed and the use of a more flexible IM rod decrease hoop stress. Overreaming the entry hole, even by 0.5 mm, significantly decreases

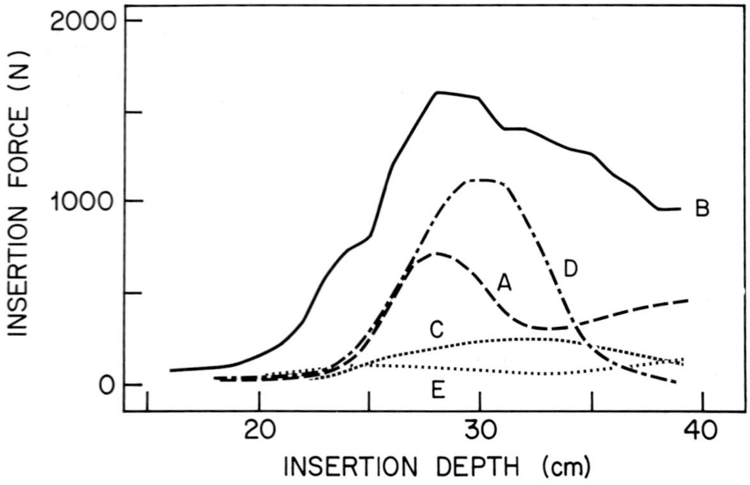

Figure 9.27

Insertion force (force along the longitudinal axis of the nail) versus depth of insertion for nails of the same diameter but different curvatures and bending stiffnesses, inserted into femora with a simulated subtrochanteric fracture (letters refer to the type of nail tested). (From Ref 33 with permission.)

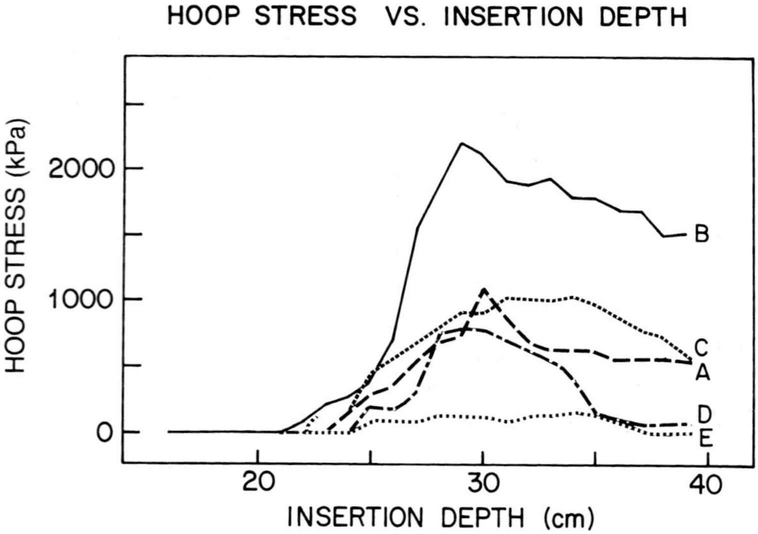

Figure 9.28

Hoop stresses (internal expansion stresses against the medullary cortex) generated in the femoral cortex during insertion of intramedullary nails (letters refer to the type of nail tested). (From Ref 33 with permission.)

insertion force and hoop stress (Figure 9.29). Similarly, the shorter the length of the fracture component, the less the nail must deform to pass through the canal, resulting in lower insertion force and hoop stress (Figure 9.30).[33]

A most important parameter is appropriate selection of the starting hole for the nail. As Figure 9.31 shows, the anterior bow of the femur dictates that the ends of the nail should be more posterior than the midpoint of the femoral canal, when fully inserted. If the starting hole is anterior to the central axis of the femur, the nail is excessively deformed, leading to high hoop stresses and the potential for bursting the femur. An example of this is shown in Figure 9.32. Typically, placement of the starting hole more than 6 mm anterior to the central axis of the medullary canal of the femur results in a high

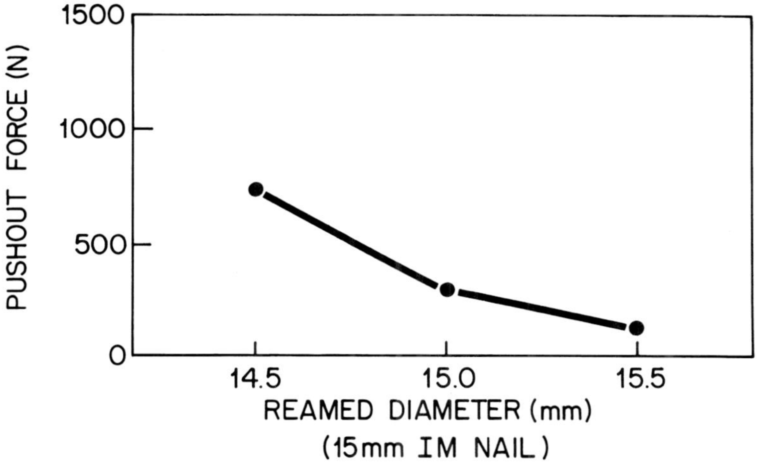

Figure 9.29

The force of IM nail insertion decreases with increased reamed diameter of the medullary canal. (From Ref 33 with permission.)

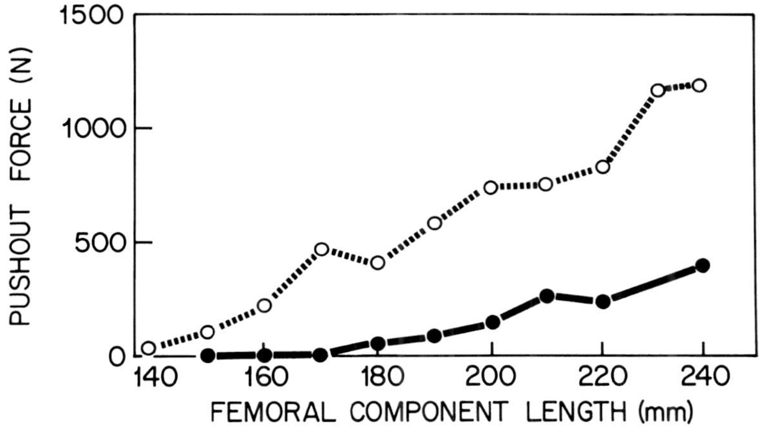

Figure 9.30

Change in the axial insertion force with length of the fracture component in the femur: ○, proximal; ● distal. (From Ref 33 with permission.)

potential for bursting the femur.[33] An excessively posterior starting point can produce the same effect. In the medial–lateral plane, the starting hole should be at the junction of the femoral neck and the greater trochanter.[34]

Stability of subtrochanteric fractures

As previously discussed, the subtrochanteric region of the femur experiences large bending stresses (Figure 9.3). Therefore the ability of a fixation device to support these loads should be an important factor in considering which device to employ. Figure 9.33 shows four alternative methods of fixation that can be used. In bending tests where fixations were implanted in femora with simulated transverse subtrochanteric fractures, all devices except Enders' pins provided a construct stiffness in the range of 69–92% of the intact femur. The Enders' pins fixed femora were considerably less stiff. The compression hip screw and nonslotted nail produce constructs of

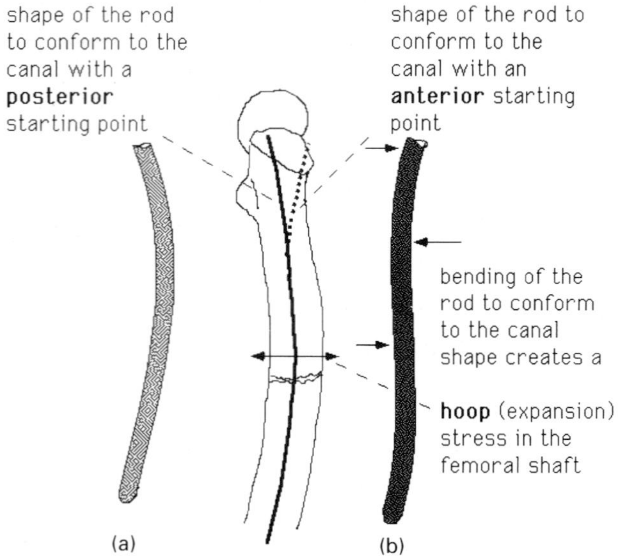

Figure 9.31

The anterior bow of the femur dictates that the proximal end of the nail should be located posterior to the midline of the medullary canal in the anterior–posterior plane. (a) Deformed shape of a nail when fully inserted, placed with a posterior starting hole. (b) Deformed shape of the nail when placed with an anterior starting hole. The anterior starting position causes more deformation of the nail, which results in greater insertion force and resultant hoop stress.

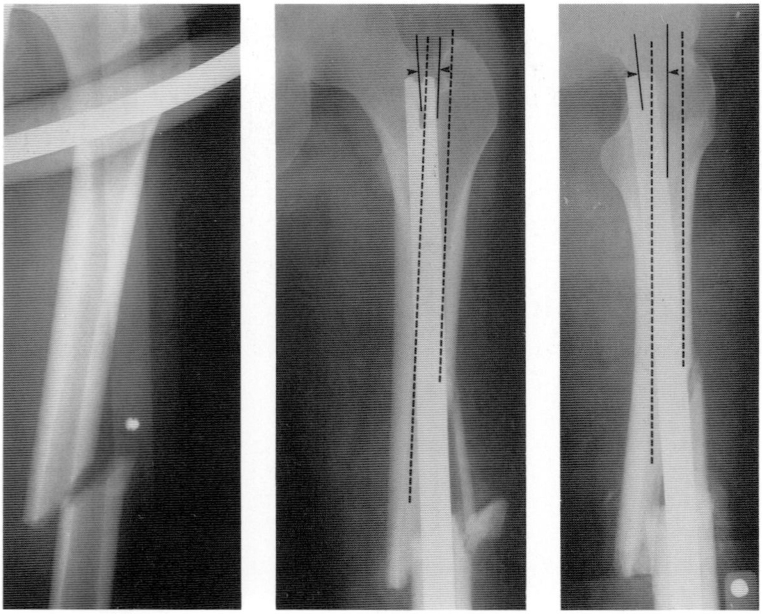

Figure 9.32

Clinical example of the position of the starting hole of an IM nail and resulting fracture of the femur during insertion. (a) The fracture before nail insertion. (b,c) Bursting of the femur. The dotted lines indicate the position of the medullary canal, the solid lines the midline of the canal and the nail. (From Ref 33 with permission.)

about 50% of intact femoral torsional stiffness.[39] In torsion, slotted intramedullary nail fixed fractures are about 3% as stiff as the intact femur.[39] It should be emphasized that this is in the worst case condition, with no cortical contact or load sharing across the fracture site. When a compressive load is applied in addition, the torsional stiffness of IM rod constructs can

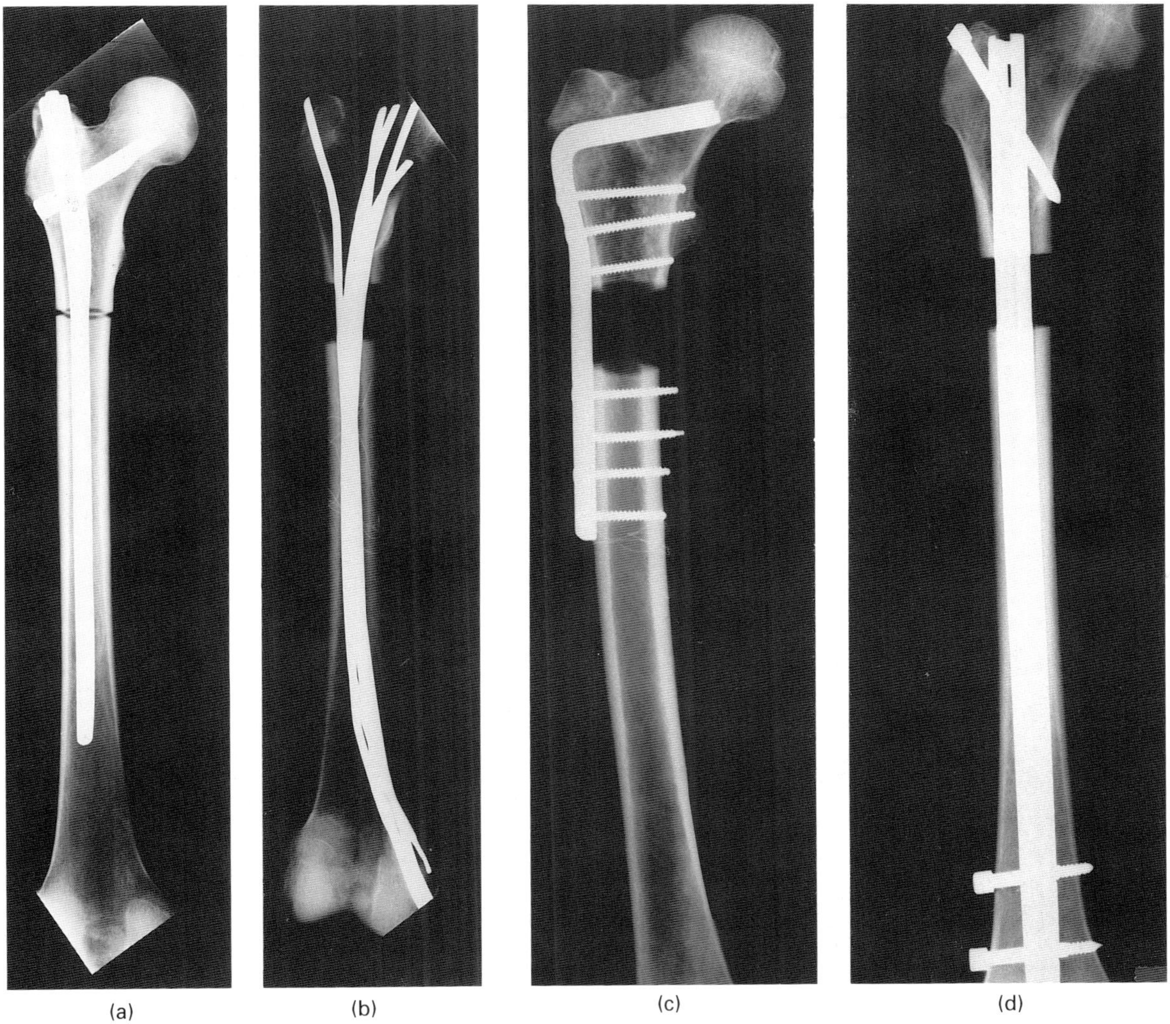

Figure 9.33

Four alternative methods of fixation of a subtrochanteric fracture of the femur: (a) Zickel nail;[35] (b) Enders' pins;[36] (c) angled blade plate;[37] (d) interlocked intramedullary nail.[38] (From Ref 39 with permission.)

increase to as much as 20% of intact.[40] An increase in stiffness occurs because loading the rod axially causes it to bow. This increases contact with the medullary canal, reducing bone/implant slip and the "working length" of the rod (Figure 9.34).

As shown in Figure 9.35, interlocked nail fixed constructs support about 3.5–4 times body weight in axial loading before failure, which is considerably greater than blade plate, compression hip screw, or Enders' pins fixed fractures. Again, these values represent the worst case

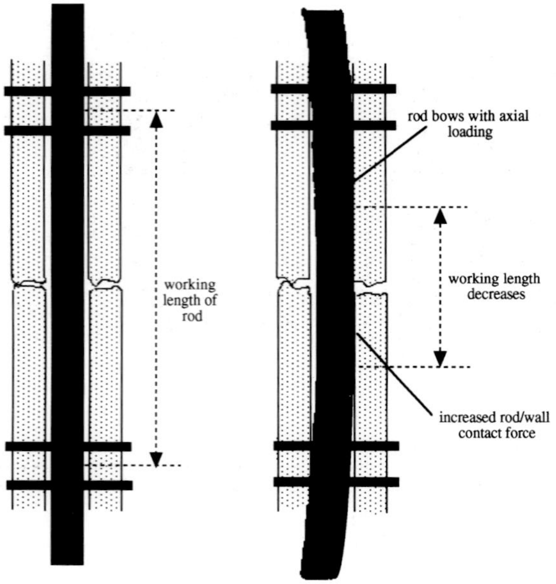

Figure 9.34

An interlocking nail used in a femur fracture transfers torque from the distal femoral component through the locking screws into the nail, through the proximal locking screws, and into the proximal femoral component. An axial load increases the bow in the femur, forcing it into contact with the medullary canal, and effectively shortens the "working length" or the section of the rod that actually deforms. This increases its torsional stiffness.

situation, without cortical contact.[31,39] Failure of locked nail fixed fractures in axial loading may occur by bending of the rod at the fracture site, splitting of the greater trochanter, or pushing out of the nail and locking screws through the trochanteric bone, as demonstrated in Figure 9.36.[31]

Fixation of the femoral shaft

Interlocking IM nails used in femoral midshaft fractures perform similarly biomechanically to subtrochanteric constructs in torsion, with torsional stiffnesses of less than 3% of the intact femur (slotted nails). A major influence on torsional stability of the construct used in a midshaft fracture is the applied axial load, as shown in Figure 9.34, which can increase torsional stiffness by a factor of seven.[40] In addition to low stiffness, the friction between the rod and the endosteal cortex inhibits the rod from completely recovering its original untwisted shape after release of a torsional load. Thimsen et al[41] termed the angle recovered after being torsionally deformed, the "springback angle," and compared the effects of various combinations of locking screw configurations as well as the length

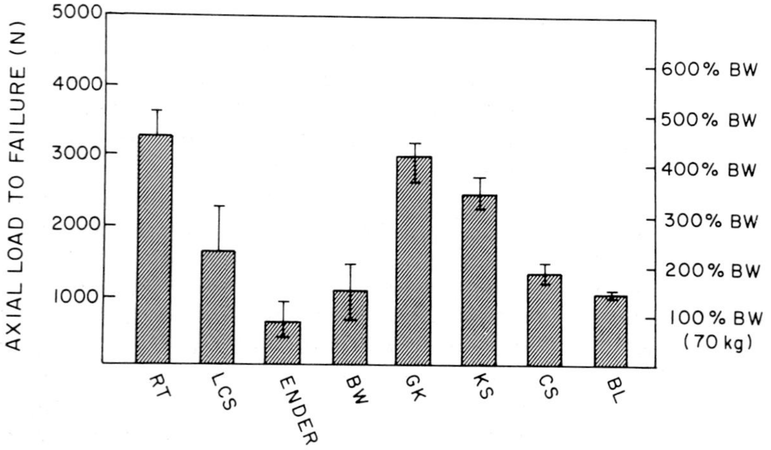

Figure 9.35

Axial load capacity of some devices in subtrochanteric fracture fixation without cortical contact: RT, Russell–Taylor; LCS, compression screw; ENDER, Enders' pins; BW, Brooker–Wills nail; GK, Grosse–Kempf nail; KS, Klemm–Schellman nail; CS, compression hip screw; BL, blade plate. All nails are 16 mm diameter and locked both proximally and distally. (From Ref 31 with permission.)

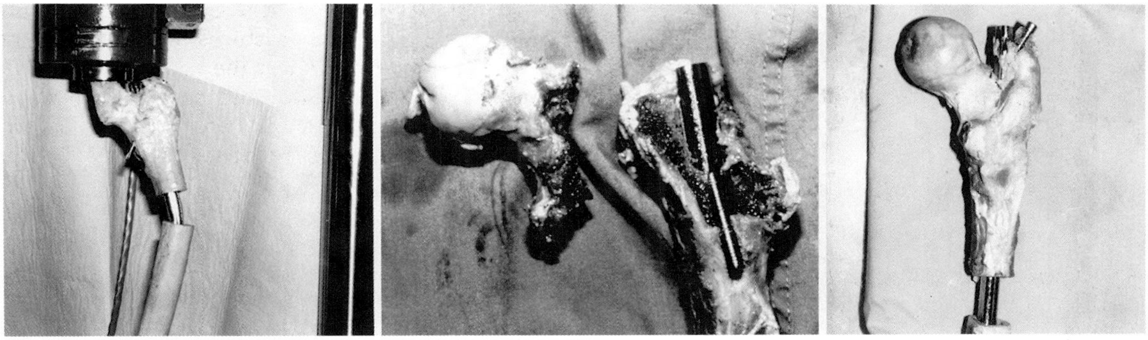

(a) (b) (c)

Figure 9.36

Examples of different modes of failure of locked intramedullary rod fixed fractures in axial loading. (a) Bending of the rod at the fracture site. (b) Splitting of the trochanter. (c) Proximal pushout of the rod and locking screws.

of the defect on the ability of the nail to recover to its original shape. This is an important point clinically, because a small springback angle implies that a large residual malrotation deformity can result from torsional loading after load release. They showed that both proximal and distal locking screws must be in place to recover most of the torsional deformation, and that recovery increases when a larger segmental defect is present (Figure 9.37).

Bending stiffnesses of femora fixed with interlocking rods decrease significantly with increasing length of the midshaft defect (Figure 9.38). With a 3 cm defect, construct stiffnesses range from 55% to 70% of intact bending stiffness, while with an 8 cm defect, this decreases to about 20% of the stiffness of the intact femur. Stiffness of midshaft femoral fractures fixed with femoral rods is similar in axial loading to that of subtrochanteric constructs. However, the angle of the proximal locking screw can, as shown in Figure 9.39, affect the load capacity of the device. The more vertical the locking bolt, the less bone there is between the screw and the rod, and the more likely that failure will occur by pushout of the rod through the trochanter, at a lower load.[42]

Fixation of distal femoral fractures

The distal locking screws provide resistance to axial and torsional loading; however, they also help to prevent toggling of the rod in the femoral canal. Gleis et al[43] showed that the amount of rod toggle in the anterior–posterior direction is directly related to the length of the distal femoral component, and the location and number of locking screws that are used (Figure 9.40). They recommend the use of two distal screws if the fracture is located less than 60% of the length from the distal end to midshaft of the femur.

Fixation of distal fractures of the femur is challenging for several reasons. The fracture site is close to the distal locking screws, which places greater stress on the implant.[30] Purchase in the femoral condyles may be poor, especially if there is significant distal comminution or the bone is osteoporotic. Two types of IM nail implants that permit distal locking are shown in Figure 9.41. The nonlocked nail relies only on frictional contact with bone. The Brooker–Wills nail uses retractable blades acting against cancellous bone to prevent axial settling and torsional angulation, and the interlocking nail depends on direct transverse

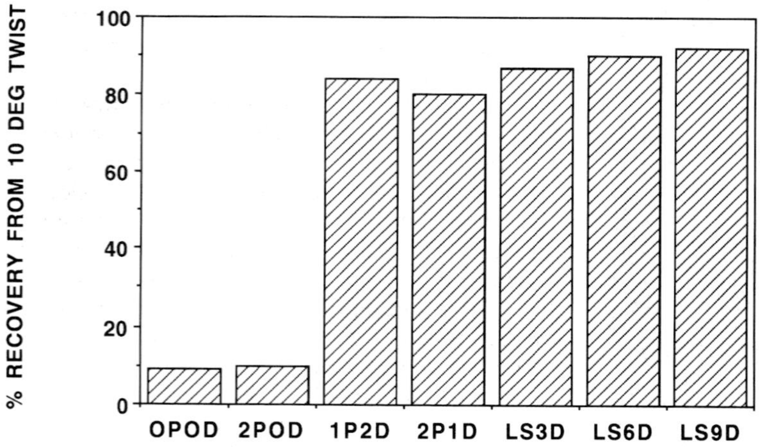

Figure 9.37

Springback angle or angle of recovery after twisting an osteotomized cadaver femur with an implanted Grosse–Kempf interlocking IM nail to 10° and releasing the torque. OPOD, no proximal or distal screws; 2POD, two proximal and no distal screws; 1P2D, one proximal and two distal screws; 2P1D, two proximal and one distal screw; LS3D, all locking screws and 3 cm midshaft defect; LS6D, all locking screws and 6 cm midshaft defect; LS9D, all locking screws and 9 cm midshaft defect. (Data adapted from Ref 41.)

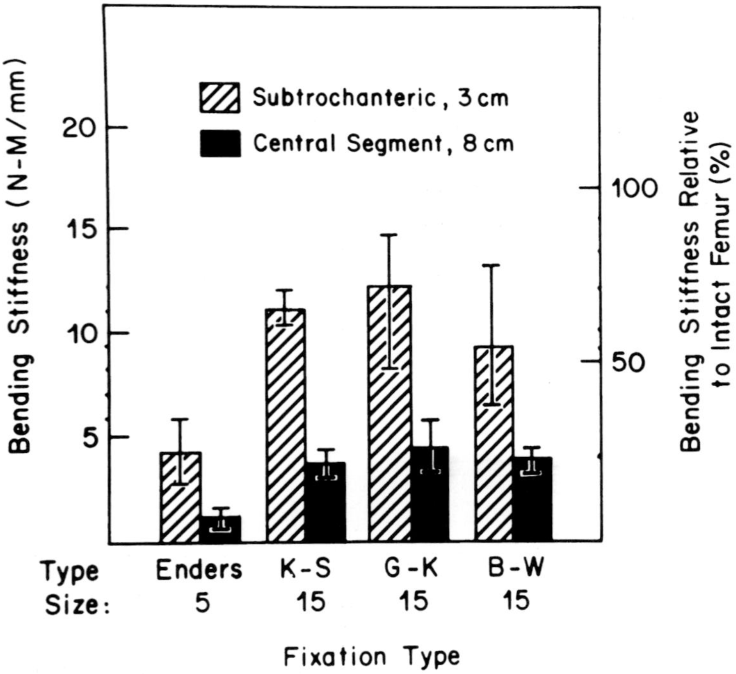

Figure 9.38

Bending stiffness of constructs with various intramedullary devices having either a 3 cm subtrochanteric or an 8 cm midshaft defect. Enders, five Enders' pins; K-S, Klemm–Schellman 15 mm diameter locked nail; G-K, Grosse–Kempf 15 mm diameter locked nail; B-W, Brooker–Wills 15 mm diameter nail with proximal locking bolt and distal blades. (From Ref 42 with permission.)

fixation of the rod by screws through cortex. Testing shows that the interlocking nail is superior to the other devices in terms of resistance to both compression and torsional loads.[44] Locked nails, which rely on cortical purchase of the screws, are less affected by increasing osteoporosis of the bone into which they are implanted. The Brooker–Wills nail, which transfers load to the cancellous

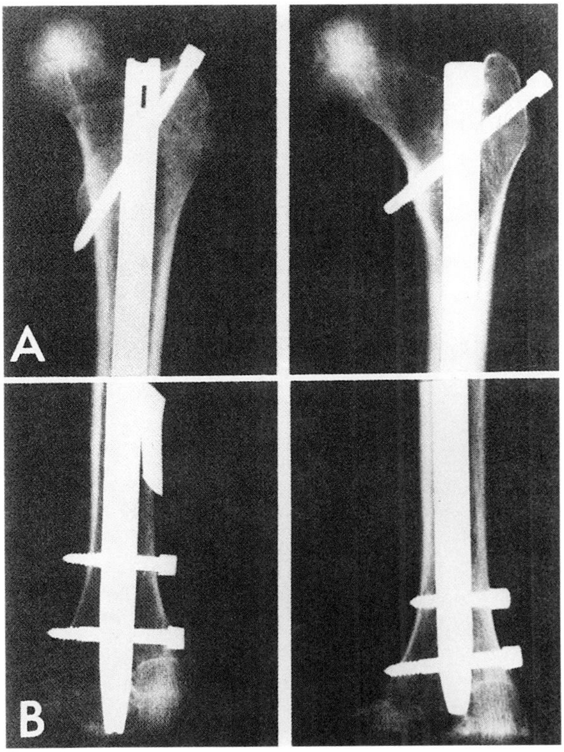

Figure 9.39

A comparison of the proximal locking hardware of two different IM locking nails, demonstrating the differences in locking screw/nail angle. (From Ref 42 with permission.)

bone of the distal femur, is significantly affected by osteoporosis, losing the ability to spring back after a torque is applied.[45]

In order to gain purchase in more distal fractures, it may be possible to locate the locking screws more distally. However, the effect on the load capacity of the screws must be considered. Considering that the main method of load transfer between bone and screw comes from the support of the screw by the cortices, the screw is in effect loaded in four point bending when an axial load is applied through the rod (Figure 9.42). Since the distal femur flares rapidly towards the joint, the unsupported span of the screw increases when screws are placed more distally. This significantly decreases the stiffness (by the cube of the span) and ultimate strength of the screw in four point bending.

Fixation of supracondylar fractures

Several implants can be used for fixation of supracondylar fractures of the femur. Biomechanical study shows that the key factor in producing rigidity of fixation is maintaining cortical contact so that load transfer occurs across the

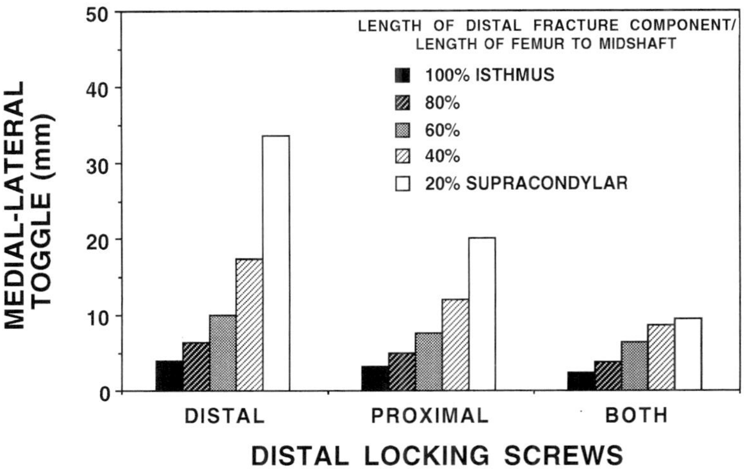

Figure 9.40

Medial–lateral toggle of an IM rod located in the distal half of the femur as a function of the location of the fracture relative to the length of the distal half of the femur, and the number of screws used. (Data adapted from Ref 43.)

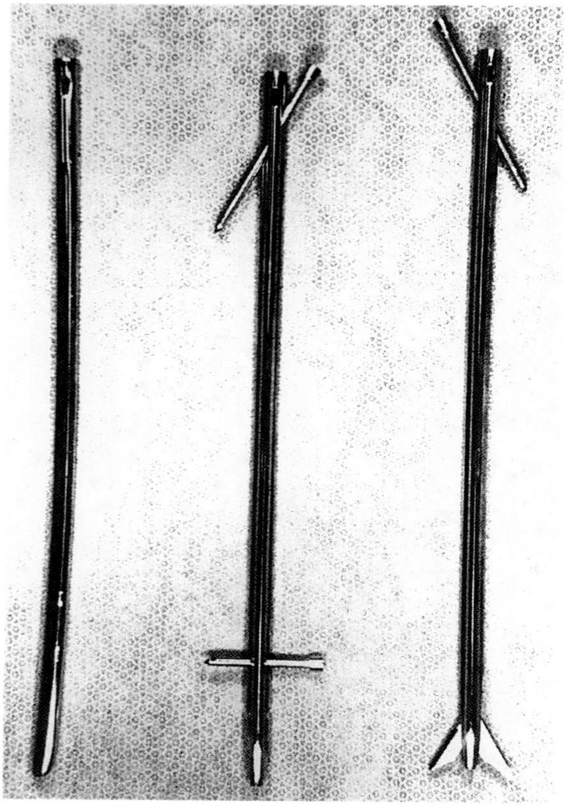

(a) (b) (c)

Figure 9.41

Three alternative methods for fixation of the distal end of the femur using an intramedullary device: (a) standard Kuntscher nail; (b) interlocking nail; (c) Brooker–Wills nail. (From Ref 44 with permission.)

fracture. Constructs without cortical contact were found to be only about 20% as stiff those with contact. A plate with lag screw, which creates compression across the fracture site, provided the greatest construct rigidity to loading when cortical contact was present. Without contact, all devices (condylar plate, plate and lag screw, and blade plate) provided equivalent resistance to deformation.[46]

Summary

Currently, intramedullary rodding is the technique of choice for fixation of most femoral shaft fractures. Rod stabilized fractures result in constructs with about 70% of the bending stiffness of the intact bone and the ability to support about four times body weight. Torsional stiffness of these constructs varies from about 3% for slotted rods to 50% for nonslotted tubular rods. Insertion of the rod can lead to complications such as splitting of the femur if the geometry of the situation is not appreciated. Since the femur has a bow such that the apex is anterior to the ends, the rod, which is also bowed, must be inserted in the same manner. This requires a posterior starting point for insertion. Other factors can reduce the stresses in the femur associated with insertion. These include increasing the diameter of the reamed canal, or using a more flexible rod or one with a curvature closer to that of the femur. In addition, the shorter the length of the fracture component, the lower the insertion stresses. Distal fractures must be protected, since the stresses on the distal end of the rod can increase to a point where the endurance limit of the material is exceeded and fatigue failure becomes a possibility.

9.3 Fixation of the patella

Loading conditions

The patella is a key component in producing a moment that permits extension of the lower leg. As shown in Figure 9.43, in free extension of the lower extremity, the weight of the lower limb produces a moment that flexes the knee. The quadriceps musculature produces a countermoment that raises the leg (i.e. extends the knee). The result of these forces is a reaction force that tends to compress the patella into the femur. Therefore the patella is subjected to tension on its anterior surface (through the quadriceps force, Figure 9.44), and compression at the patellofemoral articulation (Figure 9.45), both of which vary with knee flexion angle.[47] Therefore bending of the patella with tension on the anterior surface is a major loading mode that

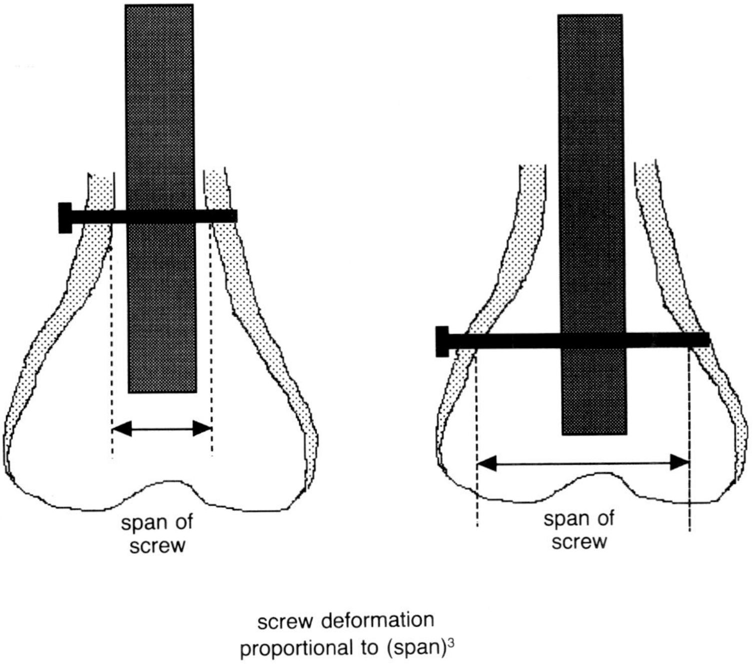

Figure 9.42

The effect of locating the distal locking screws more distally is to increase the distance between support points (span) of the screw. This decreases the stiffness and strength of the screw in resisting four point bending generated by axial loading through the rod.

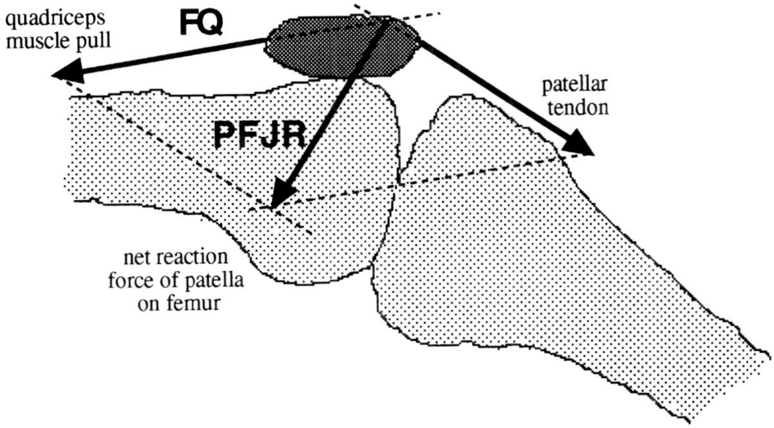

Figure 9.43

A free body diagram of the knee joint, showing the external forces and major loads acting on the patella and the patellofemoral joint. FQ, force of quadriceps; PFJR, patellofemoral joint reaction. (Adapted from Ref 47.)

must be considered in fixation of patellar fractures.

Fixation of patellar fractures

A variety of techniques have been used in fixation of patellar fractures.[48–53] The fixation should be applied as a tension band to counteract the tensile force and moment resulting from quadriceps tension, and prevent gapping of the anterior side of the fracture. Of several wiring methods shown in Figure 9.46, Magnusson wiring[49] produced the least fracture gapping during loading from flexion to extension of the knee. This straightforward method places the wire within the central plane of the patella, so that it is aligned with and directly

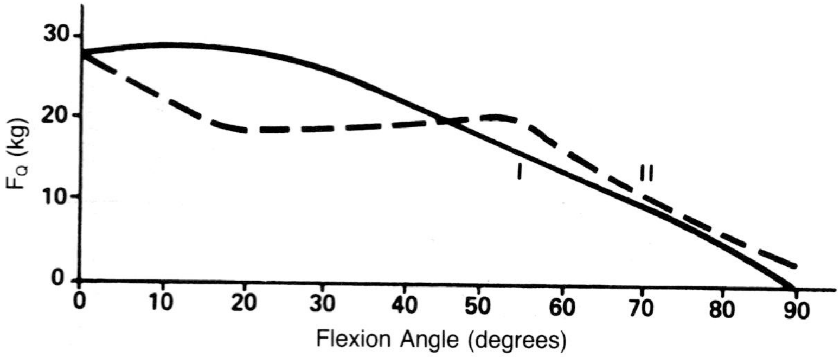

Figure 9.44

Quadriceps force F_Q acting on the patella in free extension (i.e. not against resistance) of the knee joint. (From Ref 47 with permission.)

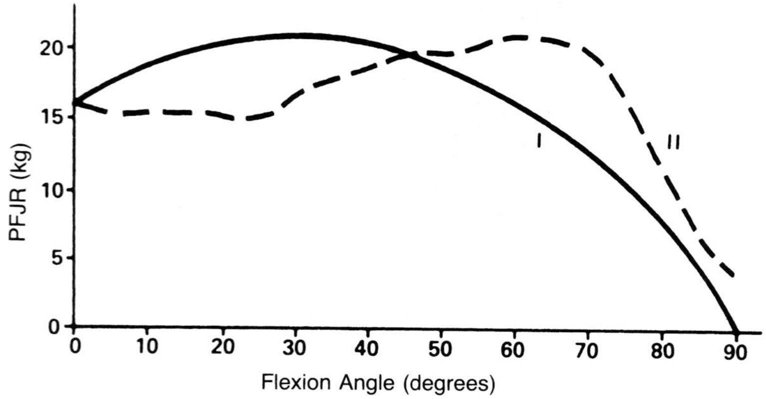

Figure 9.45

Patellofemoral joint reaction force (PFJR) in free extension of the knee joint. (From Ref 47 with permission.)

resists the tensile force created by the quadriceps tendon. It is important to note that tension band wiring, which places the wire over the anterior surface of the patella, tends to cause the posterior surface of the patella to gap during loading, as shown in Figures 9.47 and 9.48.[51]

The application of cancellous screws[52] is an alternative method for gaining compression at the fracture site. Screws provide a significantly greater mechanical advantage and so result in greater compression across a fracture gap than does wiring. As wire is bent around a corner, friction and permanent deformation in it reduce the tensile force and fracture site compression it can transmit. A disadvantage to screw fixation is that the screws rely on cancellous bone within the patella for purchase, whereas wiring transfers load to cortex. Therefore in mechanical testing, with failure of fixation defined as the load required to produce 3 mm of fracture gapping, wiring has been found to withstand greater quadriceps force than screw fixation.[52]

Another technique of patellar fixation is the use of a load sharing cable to partially unload force transmitted to the patella (Figure 9.46a).[53] Since some of the force carried by the patellar tendon is transferred to a cable placed parallel to the tendon and inserted in bone tunnels in the patella and tibial tubercule, the fracture site and its fixation should be partially unloaded. An additional advantage to use of the cable is its significantly increased resistance to fatigue compared with

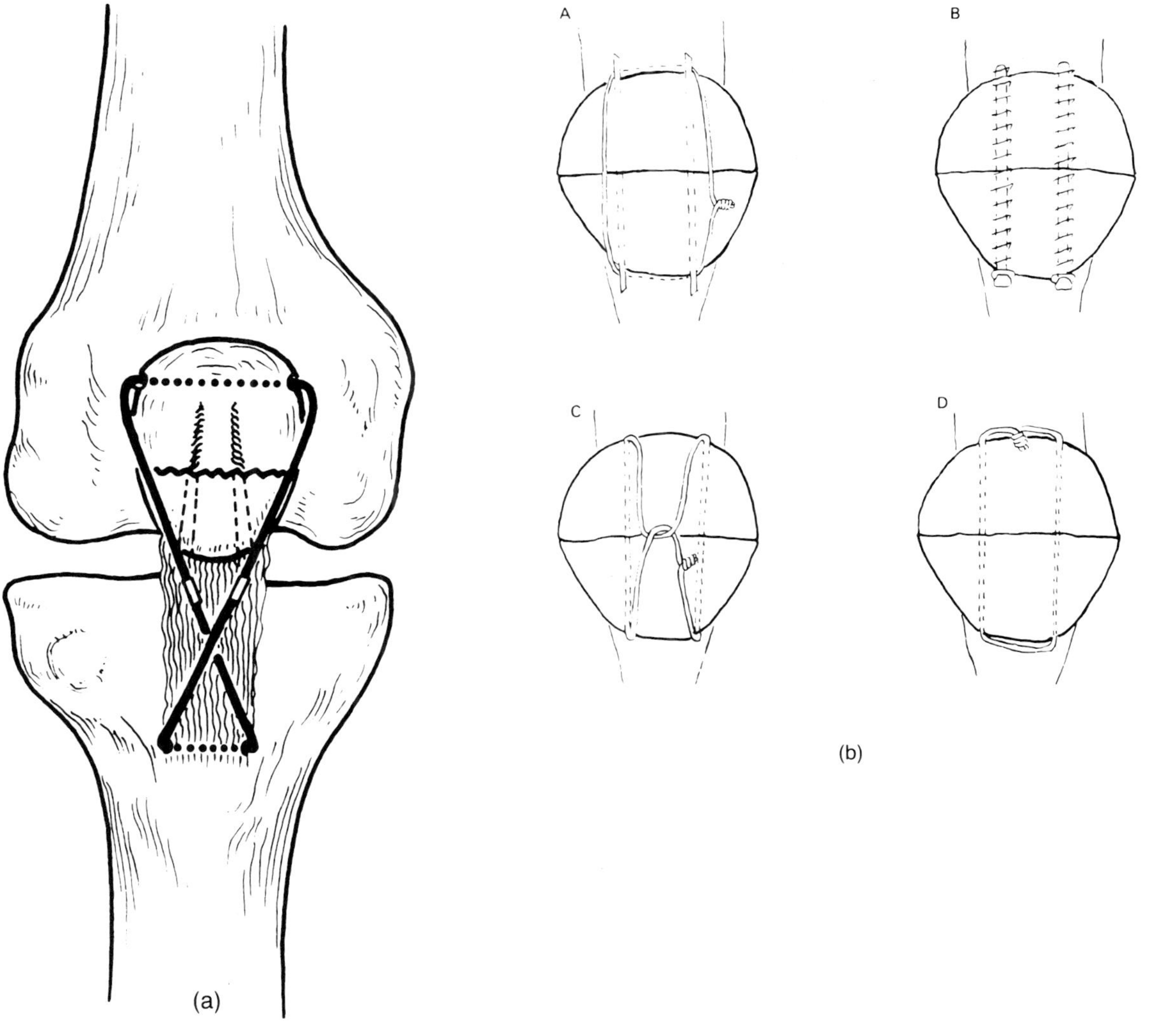

Figure 9.46

Some alternative methods of patellar fixation. (a) Load sharing cable (from Ref 53 with permission). (b): A, Magnusson;[49] B, screw fixation;[52] C, modified tension band;[51] D, circumferential[48] (from Ref 52 with permission).

wire (see Chapter 6). Perry et al[53] showed that in specimens cycled from 0° to 90° of flexion, with a fracture gap fixed by screws or wires alone, fatigue of fixation and fracture site gapping occurred rapidly. In contrast, augmentation with a load sharing cable resulted in no failure of fixation with cyclic loading.

Summary

Modified tension band wiring appears to be the fixation method of choice biomechanically, since this simple wire configuration with 90° corners permits the maintenance of tension in the wire, which results in compression across the fracture

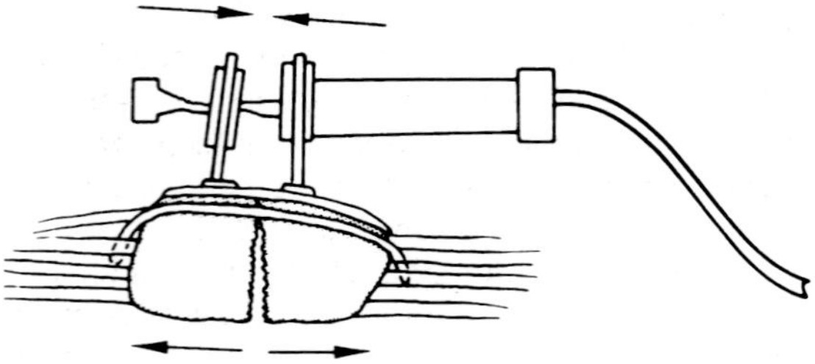

Figure 9.47

Gapping of a patellar fracture at the base (posterior side) of the patella, with fixation applied over the anterior surface of the bone. (From Ref 51 with permission.)

site. Alternatively, if bone stock is adequate and comminution not excessive, cancellous screws can provide greater fracture site compression. A cable arranged in parallel with the patellar ligament can be used to share load with the ligament and significantly improve the resistance of the fixation to fatigue during flexion/extension.

9.4 Fixation of tibial fractures

Loading conditions

The loads applied through the tibia due to gait can reach magnitudes of between three and four times body weight (Figure 9.49).[1] Because the tibiofemoral joint load has a posteriorly directed component in some parts of the gait cycle (Figure 9.2), and the quadriceps musculature generates anterior bending in the tibia while the hamstrings produce posterior bending, the tibia is subjected to a complex loading pattern. In addition, rotation about the vertical axis of the tibia averages 19° during gait.[54] Laurence et al[55] estimated that the maximum bending moment imposed by straight leg raising is 10 N m, by walking 80 N m, and by resisted torsion 20–29 N m. Therefore fixation systems that are designed to permit load bearing should accommodate axial loading, bending in two planes, and torsion.

Fixation of tibial plateau depressions

Buttress plates, either "T" or "L" shaped, or parallel cancellous screws can be used to support

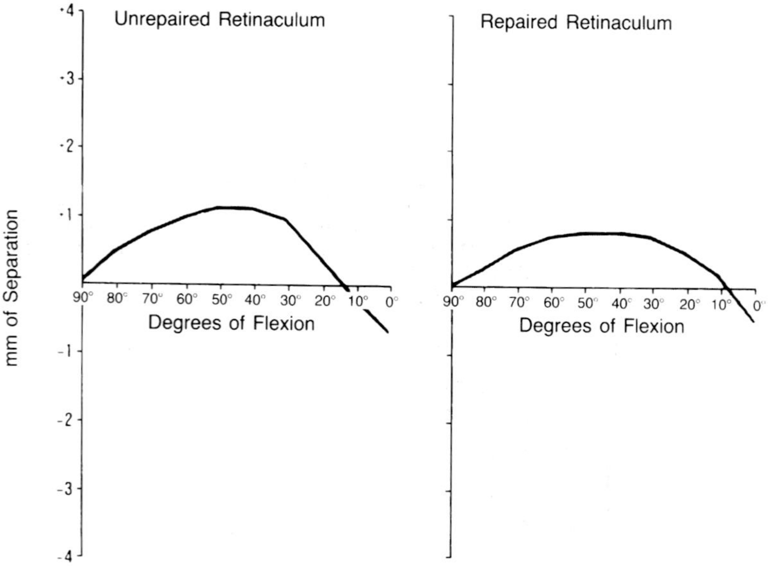

Figure 9.48

Angle of knee flexion versus fracture gap (mm of separation) for modified tension band wiring (see Figure 9.46). (From Ref 52 with permission.)

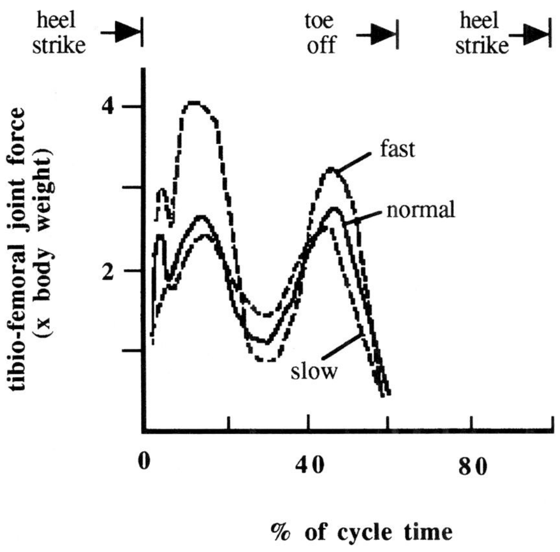

Figure 9.49

Force at the tibiofemoral joint during gait at various speeds between heel strike and toe off. (From Ref 1 with permission.)

a split and depressed lateral tibial plateau fracture, as shown in Figure 9.50. Testing by application of a direct axial load to the fixed plateau fracture component showed that buttress plate fixation is significantly stronger than screw fixation alone, and that T plates support the largest loads (Figure 9.51).[57] Plate fixation is superior to screws, because the load in a buttress plate fixed fracture is transferred to cortex while the screws rely on cancellous bone purchase (Figure 9.52).

For more localized plateau depressions, a K wire cluster may be employed to provide support beneath the cartilage and subchondral bone after repositioning the depressed region and placing bone graft below it. Although no fixation method produced stiffness (resistance of the depressed region to displacement under load) greater than 30% of intact (Figure 9.53), clusters of four or more K wires did produce stiffnesses that were significantly greater than that of bone grafting alone.[58] The greater the number of wires, the more effectively they can distribute the load from the injured region to the intact trabecular bone surrounding the injury.

Nonoperative fixation of tibial shaft fractures

Tibial shaft fractures have been treated by a variety of methods, depending on the severity of the injury to bone and the surrounding soft tissues. Alternatives include casting or cast bracing, internal fixation by cerclage wiring,

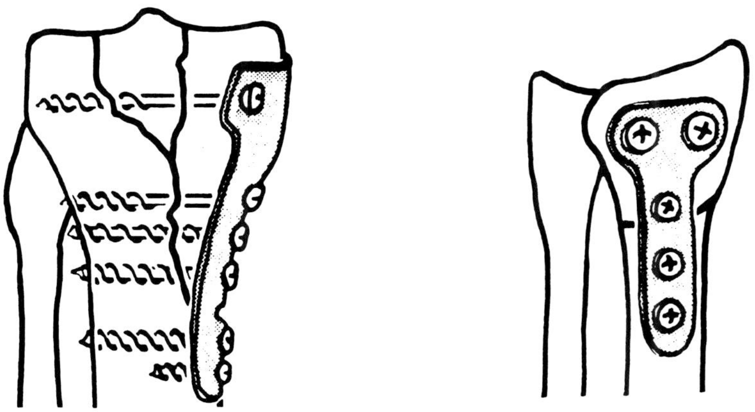

Figure 9.50

Examples of buttress plate fixation of a depressed fracture of the lateral tibial plateau. (From Ref 56 with permission.)

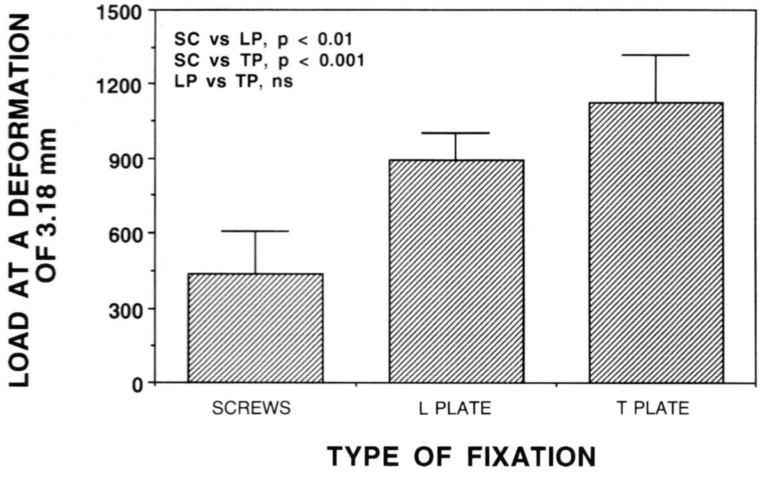

Figure 9.51

Comparison of the magnitudes of axial load supported by a simulated tibial plateau fracture at a relative fracture component distal displacement of 3.18 mm for three types of tibial plateau fixation. (Data adapted from Ref 57.)

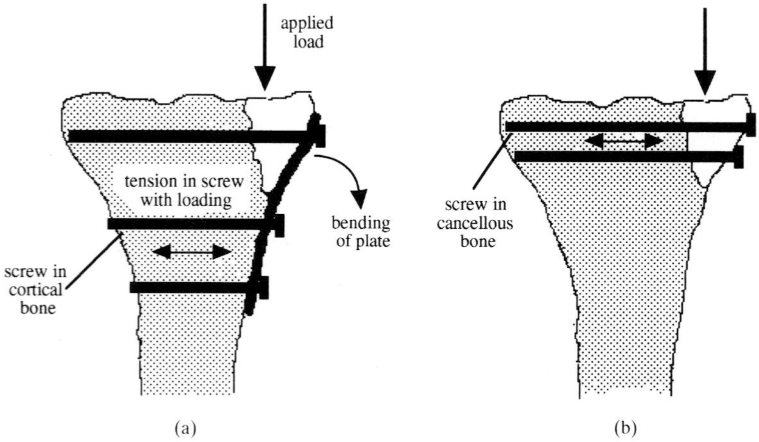

Figure 9.52

(a) The load transferred to a buttress plate is transferred to bending of screws embedded in cortical bone. (b) In comparison, cancellous screw fixation relies on the purchase of the screw in trabecular bone.

screws, plates and screws, intramedullary rodding, or external fixation using a variety of devices and configurations. The specific biomechanics of some of these devices will be discussed later.

Closed, low energy injuries to the tibia with minimal comminution are usually treated by casting, functional braces[59] or custom fabricated braces. Zagorski et al[60] compared the axial, angular, and torsional stability of external devices, and found, as shown in Figure 9.54, that no cast or brace was able to effectively control shortening under axial loading. However, all devices reduced angulation under load to below 5°, compared with greater than 30° for the unstabilized injured tibia. The greatest resistance to torsional rotation was provided by the short leg functional cast.

External fixation results in significantly lower fracture site displacement compared with casting. In an oblique fracture with cortical contact, fracture bracing permits about 4 times as much axial motion at the fracture site, 10 times the

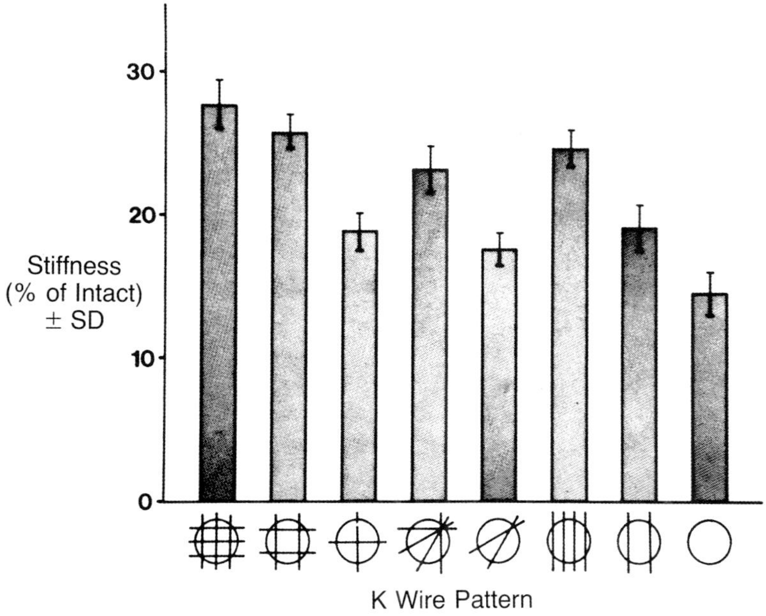

Figure 9.53

A comparison, in terms of percent of intact stiffness of the tibial plateau, provided by various K wire configurations used to support a depressed region of the plateau. (From Ref 58 with permission.)

anterior posterior displacement, and from 3 to 10 times as much angulation as does a unilateral external fixator (Figure 9.55).[61] The greater motion with functional bracing is due to loads having to be transmitted to the brace from the tibia through the flexible muscle and skin interface. This will inevitably permit more motion than the rigid mechanical connection that the bone–pin–external fixator bar allows.

Internal fixation of tibial fractures

Direct mechanical fixation of the tibia can be performed, depending on the severity and type of fracture, by dynamic compression (DC) plating, external fixation (EXFIX), or intramedullary rodding (IM).[62] In some applications, lag screws without plates may be employed. Recently, with concern about the effect of the undersurface of the plate on periosteal blood flow,[63] low and noncontact (NC) places have been proposed as alternative methods to DC plating (Figure 9.56).[64] A comparison of some typical fixation systems demonstrates the relative stiffness of the construct that results from the use of each method. It must be noted that the stiffness of a fixation system can be altered by its configuration, size, material, and position on the tibia. The examples given here are clinically representative of some common methods currently in use. A more detailed discussion of the factors affecting construct stiffness for noncontact plates, cerclage wires, IM rods, and external fixators is given in following sections.

Figure 9.57 shows that in the case of spiral fractures with cortical contact, direct lag screw fixation produces 50–70% of intact bending stiffness,[66] while DC plates, NC plates and EXFIX provide from 82% to 160% of intact stiffness,[65] depending on the plane of bending and the orientation of the fixation. In axial compression, plates and EXFIX provide 90–115% of intact stiffness,[65] while IM rods generate 69–117%.[62] In torsion, these values are 9% of intact for lag screw fixation,[66] 40–64% for plates and EXFIX,[65] and 6.5% for IM rods.[62] These data show that for bending and axial loading, any of the above mentioned

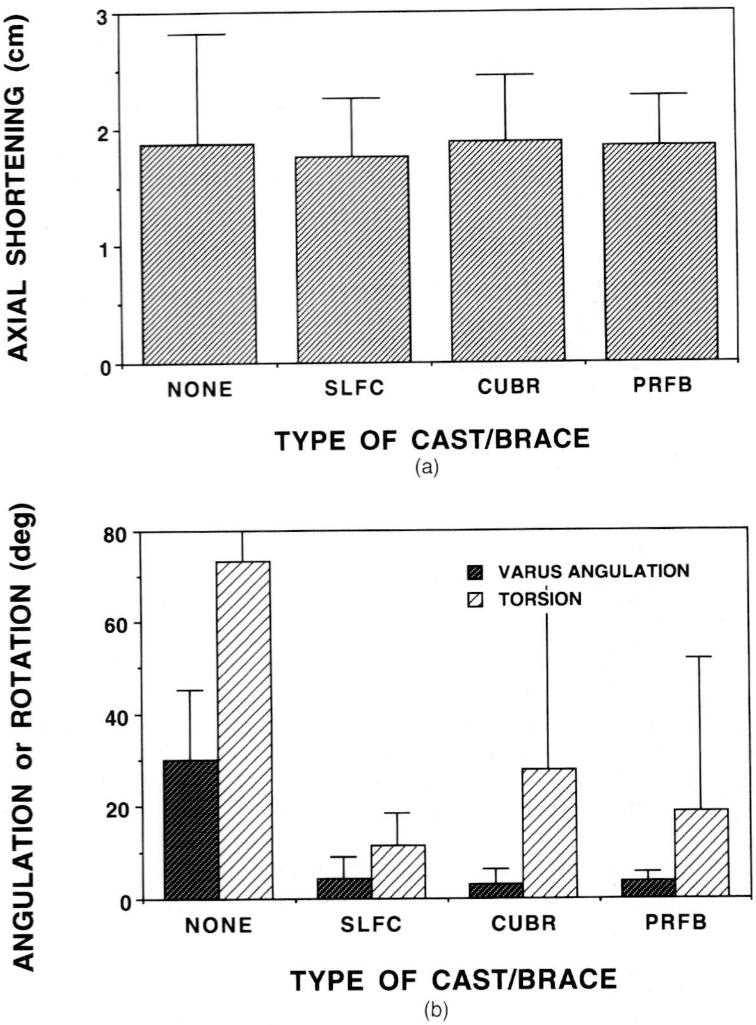

Figure 9.54

Comparison of (a) the axial shortening and (b) the angulation and torsional rotation, with fixation in a closed tibial fracture by various external casts and braces: NONE, no device on injured leg; SLFC, short leg functional cast; CUBR, custom brace; PRFB, prefabricated brace. (Data adapted from Ref 60.)

methods provide constructs of adequate rigidity, providing that cortical contact exists to share load. In torsion, as expected, IM rodding produces constructs of considerably lower stiffness.

The loss of cortical contact decreases stiffness most significantly in axial loading and bending, as shown in Figure 9.58. For example, the stiffness of the tibia/external fixator construct drops from 90% of intact with contact to 34% without. The IM rod fixed constructs decrease from 117% to 55% of intact axial stiffness with loss of contact. As has been found in other fracture fixation situations, cortical contact is a key element in increasing the rigidity of fixation and reducing stress on the implant.

Summary

A number of alternatives are available for fixation of tibial fractures. Cast or functional brace

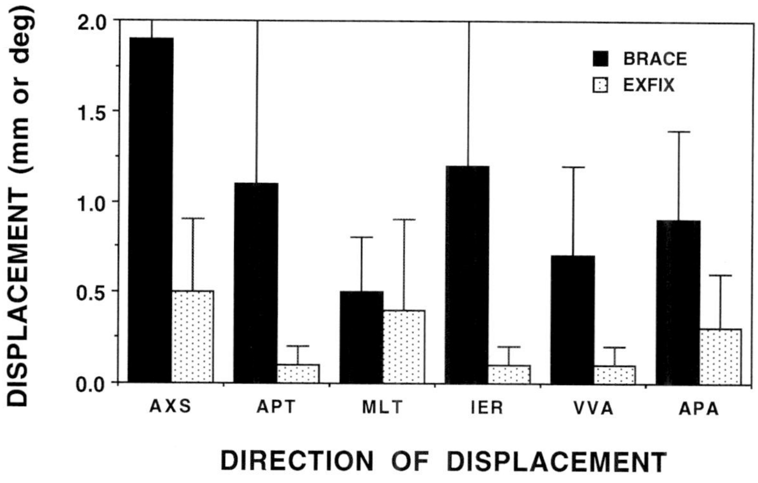

Figure 9.55

Comparison of tibial fracture site relative motion (i.e. between fracture components) in six directions using a functional fracture brace or a single plane external fixator in a stable oblique fracture pattern: AXS, axial shortening; APT, anterior–posterior translation; MLT, medial–lateral translation; IER, internal–external rotation; VVA, varus–valgus angulation; APA, anterior–posterior angulation. (Adapted from Ref 61.)

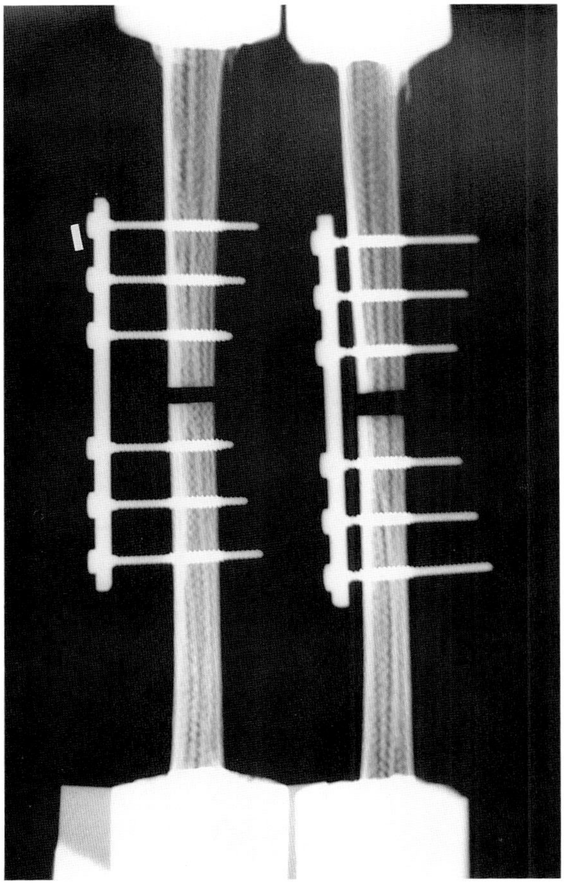

Figure 9.56

Example of fixation of the tibia using a noncontact plate set at (a) 20 mm from the bone surface; (b) 5 mm.[65]

immobilization does not provide control of shortening, but does reduce angulation deformity. Bracing permits considerably greater fracture site motion than does direct fixation; therefore it should be considered primarily for stable fractures with cortical contact. External fixators, plates, lag screws (with cortical contact) and IM rods all provide adequate and nearly equivalent fixation stiffness in bending and (except for the IM nail) in torsion. For noncontacting plates, the distance of the plate from bone is important in determining the stiffness of the construct.

9.5 Biomechanics of tibial fixation devices

The noncontact plate

Kowalski et al[65] studied the mechanics of a noncontact plate system, shown in Figures 9.56 and 9.59. This system uses platform screws that support the plate at a fixed distance from the periosteal surface of the tibia. The distance can be varied by choosing different lengths of screws. After the screws are positioned, the plate is placed on them, with the stems of the screws protruding through it. The plate is secured by placing nuts on the screw stems. This system permits compression of the fracture components. Two configurations were tested with and without cortical

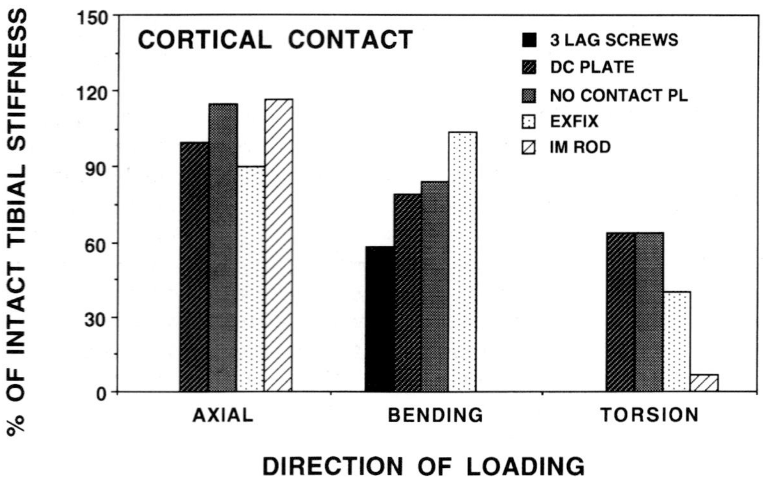

Figure 9.57

Comparison of the stiffness of tibial constructs fixed with various devices, and having cortical contact at the fracture site. (DC PLATE, dynamic compression plate, six hole, 4.5 mm, stainless steel; NO CONTACT PL, noncontact plate, six hole, 4.5 mm, stainless steel, set 5 mm above the periosteal surface; EXFIX, external fixator, single plane, 5 mm Schanz screws, double tubes; IM ROD, intramedullary rod, solid, 9 mm diameter, stainless steel, proximally and distally interlocked with double 3.9 mm diameter screws). (Data adapted from Refs 62, 65, 66.)

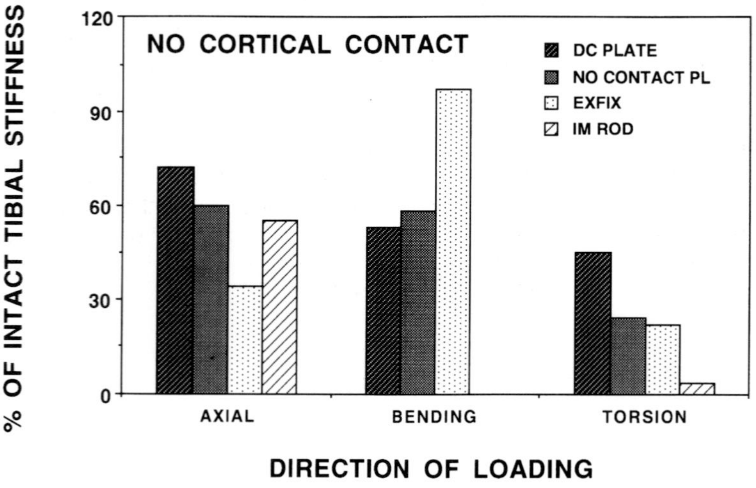

Figure 9.58

Comparison of the stiffness of tibial constructs fixed with various devices, and having no cortical contact at the fracture site (DC PLATE, dynamic compression plate, six hole, 4.5 mm, stainless steel; NO CONTACT PL, noncontact plate, six hole, 4.5 mm, stainless steel, set 5 mm above the periosteal surface; EXFIX, external fixator, single plane, 5 mm Schanz screws, double tubes; IM ROD, intramedullary rod, solid, 9 mm diameter, stainless steel, proximally and distally interlocked with double 3.9 mm diameter screws). (Data from Refs 62, 65.)

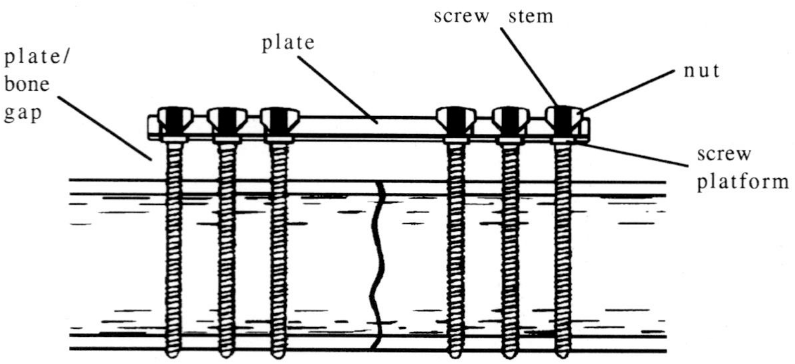

Figure 9.59

Schematic diagram of a noncontact plating system.[65]

contact; having the plate located 5 or 20 mm from the surface of bone. As shown in Figure 9.60, with cortical contact, the directions most affected by displacing the plate away from the bone surface are bending and torsion. With loss of cortical contact, axial loading is also affected by positioning the plate further from bone. This demonstrates the load sharing role of bone in axial loading when cortical contact is maintained.

The tibial intramedullary nail

Using strain gages bonded to the interior surface of a slotted tubular intramedullary nail, Pfister and Frigg[67] demonstrated how a reamed tibial nail deforms during insertion from an anterior starting position near the tibial tubercle to its final position in the medullary canal. Bending is initiated as the inserted nail encounters the posterior wall of the medullary canal, and gradually reaches a peak when the tip of the nail reaches the distal third of the tibia. Bending strains decrease as the nail reaches the fully inserted position. Also, there is initially opening and later closing of the slot in the nail, shown in Figure 9.61.

Several design parameters can affect the performance of an unreamed tibial nail, apart from the material of which it is composed, and its overall dimensions. The proximal locking screw holes are in some nails oriented parallel and in others obliquely to each other. While this does not affect the stiffness of the nail construct in axial compression or torsion, the resistance to motion in varus–valgus bending is affected. Figure 9.62 shows that parallel proximal locking screws allow significantly greater medial–lateral translation of the proximal fracture component in varus–valgus bending loading. This results from the fracture component being able to slide on parallel screws when loaded in this direction.[62]

A second important consideration in tibial nails is the location of the bend in the nail with respect to the location of the fracture. Shown in Figure 9.63 is a proximal fracture that was reduced. However, with insertion of the nail, the distal component has been displaced posteriorly. This could result from the bend in the nail being located such that when it is inserted it lies within the distal fracture component, as shown in Figure 9.64. In this position, it can impinge on both the anterior cancellous bone and the posterior cortex, acting like a wedge and blocking further insertion. Then, driving the nail produces posterior and distal translation of the distal component into which it is wedged.[62]

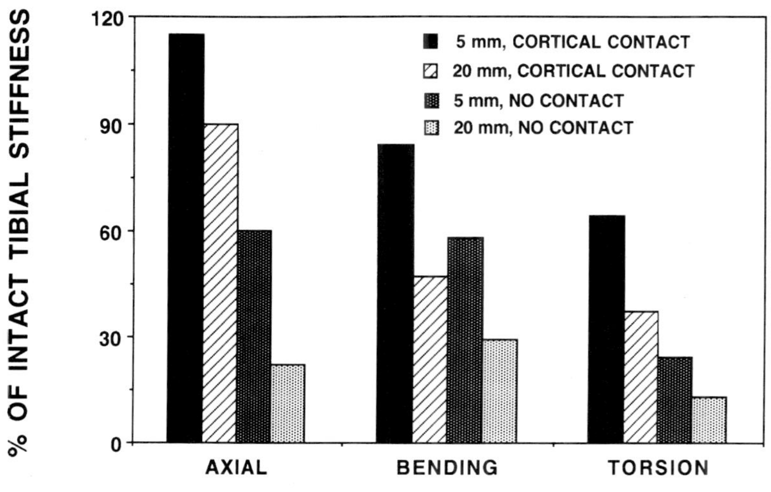

Figure 9.60

Comparison of construct stiffnesses in bending, axial compression and torsion, with and without cortical contact, for a noncontact plate set either at 5 mm or 20 mm from the periosteal surface. (Note that the bending stiffness is a mean of stiffnesses in anterior, posterior, medial, and lateral bending directions.) (Data adapted from Ref 65.)

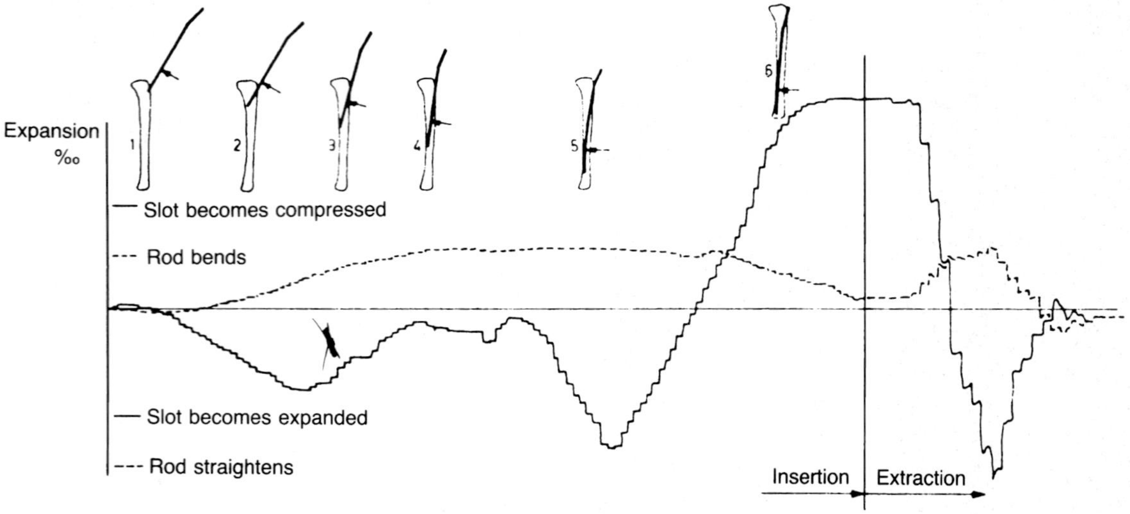

Figure 9.61

Typical deformations of a reamed slotted tubular IM tibial nail during insertion, with reaming to the same diameter as the nail. (From Ref 67 with permission.)

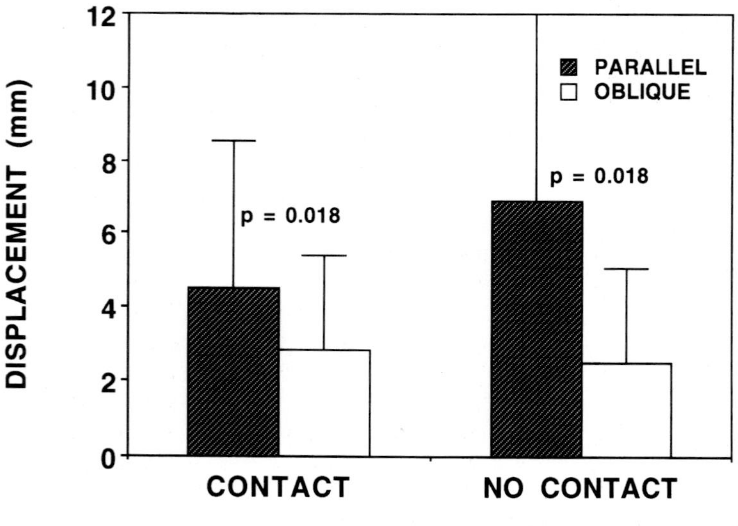

Figure 9.62

Varus–valgus translation of the proximal with respect to the distal fracture component, due to a varus–valgus bending moment of 11.75 N-m applied to the proximal fracture component of a tibia fixed with an unreamed locked tibial nail. Proximal locking screws are either parallel or oblique to each other, and with or without fracture component contact. (From Ref 62 with permission.)

Cerclage wiring

Cerclage wiring is commonly used in fracture fixation. A number of methods and materials have been suggested for gaining compression and maintaining the positions of the wired fracture components. Cheng et al[68] compared six methods of wire knot ties using 18 gage stainless steel wire, and showed that the "hairpin knot" generated significantly greater compression of the fracture

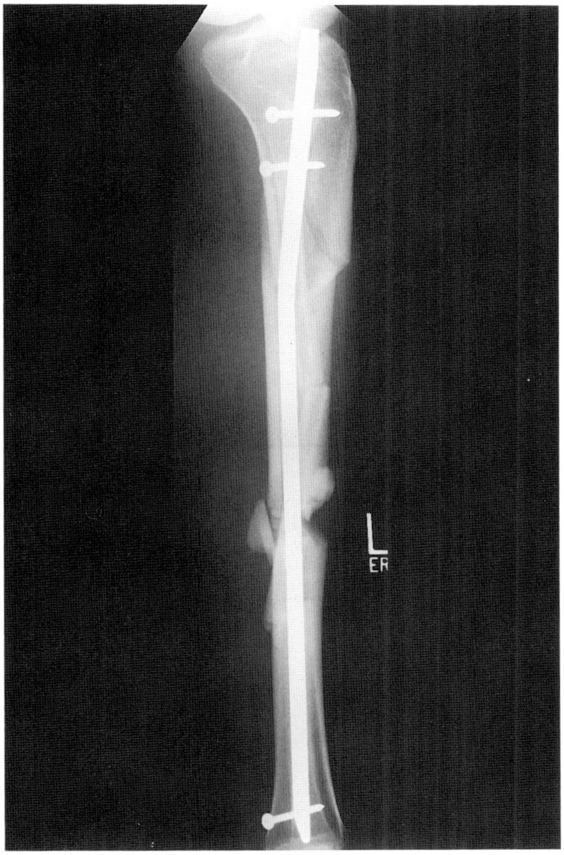

Figure 9.63

Clinical example of a high proximal tibial fracture fixed with an unreamed tibial nail. The initially reduced distal component of the fracture has been displaced posteriorly, with full insertion of the nail. (From Ref 62 with permission.)

fragments and failed at higher tensile loads than other common methods (Figure 9.65). As described by the authors, this knot is formed by a wire bent upon itself into the shape of a hairpin or a U, and passed around the bone. One free end is passed through the loop of the hairpin. A single throw is made with the two ends, and a twist knot is tied using the Harris knotter. Shaw and Daubert[69] showed that the greatest fracture site compression and ultimate tensile strengths were achieved using Parham bands, or titanium cable, followed by 18 gage stainless steel wire (47% of the compressive force and 77% of the tensile strength of Parham bands). Mersilene tape, nylon or polypropylene cable ties produced much lower values (34% of compressive force and 30% of tensile strength).

External fixation, failure of pins or interface loosening

The external fixator is a versatile device which finds use in many applications in fracture fixation. A number of mechanical factors control the rigidity of the fixation, as shown in Figure 9.66; however, a stable pin/bone interface is critical in maintaining fixator performance and preventing pin loosening. The design of the pin tip in self tapping external fixator (EXFIX) pins has been shown to affect heat generation within the pin and in cortex near the insertion hole. Some pins, shown in Figure 9.67, generated temperatures significantly greater than 50°C in the entry cortex during insertion,[70] a temperature above which thermal necrosis becomes significant.[71] In addition, microcracking was noted in cortex around all pins tested.[70] This process may initiate loosening.

When the fractured tibia is loaded in bending or axial compression, the pins are loaded primarily as cantilever beams, with the load at the bone/pin interface oriented transverse to the longitudinal axis of the pin. In a half pin fixator, this creates a stress distribution as shown in Figure 9.68, with the highest stresses at the cortical surface where the pin exits.[72] The stresses that act on bone are compressive because there is no mechanism (such as bonding of bone to the pin) that permits the transfer of tensile stress. Armstrong et al[73] showed that, with no cortical contact, in a fixator assembly with 5 mm diameter pins, the yield strength of the cortex was exceeded when a 550 N load (about 78% of body weight) was applied.

Thermal necrosis and microcracking during pin insertion coupled with high pin/bone interface stresses during functional use suggest a mechanism that explains pin loosening. Bone stresses can be reduced by decreasing the sidebar separation from bone, and increasing pin diameter, as shown in Figure 9.69. If the sidebar/bone distance is decreased, the bending moment acting on the pin

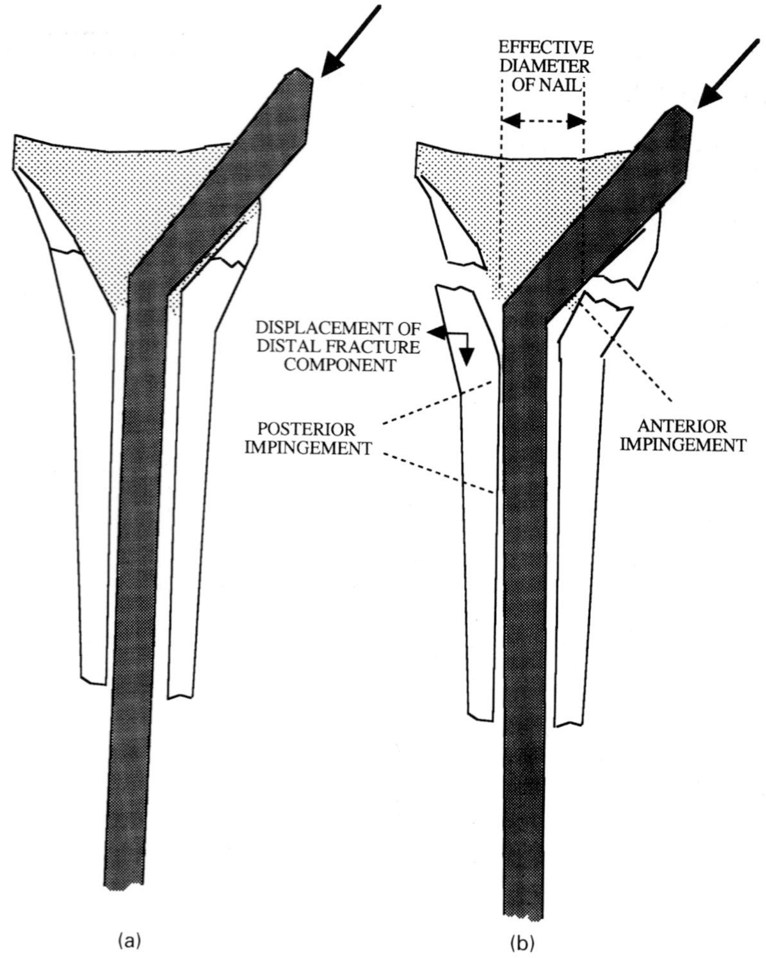

Figure 9.64

Schematic diagram of a mechanism that may cause malpositioning of the distal component of a tibial fracture. (a) When the bend in the nail is superior to the fracture line, the nail displaces down the canal. (b) When the bend is distal to the fracture line, the nail in effect becomes wider above the bend, and may impinge on both the anterior and posterior walls of the canal. In this case, it becomes wedged so that further insertion of the nail tends to carry the distal component posteriorly and distally. (From Ref 62 with permission.)

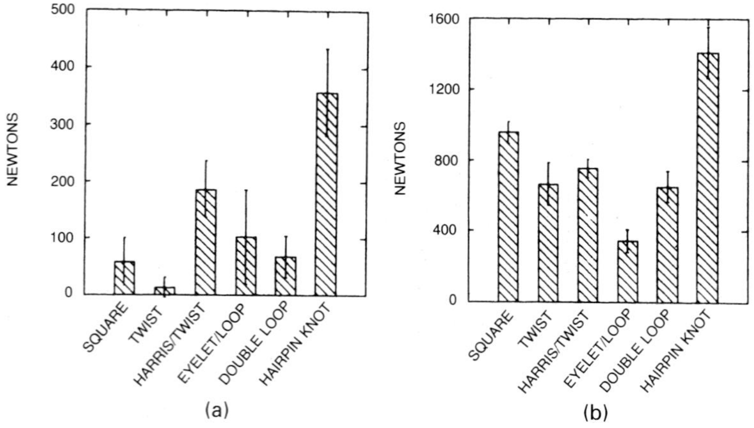

Figure 9.65

Comparison of the properties of a bone fracture fixed using various methods of cerclage wiring. (a) Compression at the fracture site. (b) Ultimate tensile strength. (From Ref 68 with permission.)

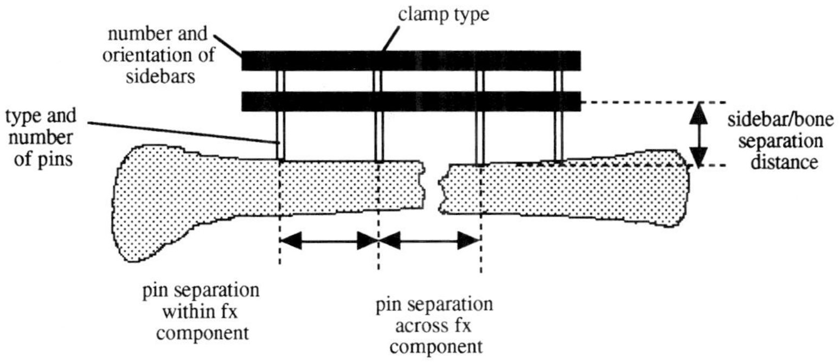

Figure 9.66

Factors controlling the stiffness of an external fixation frame.

1

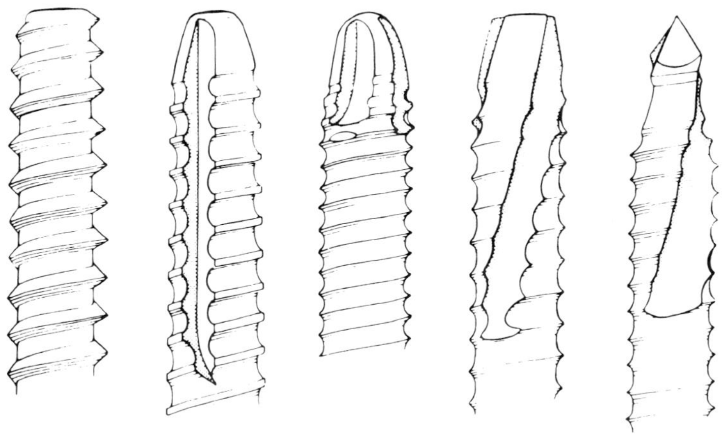

(a)

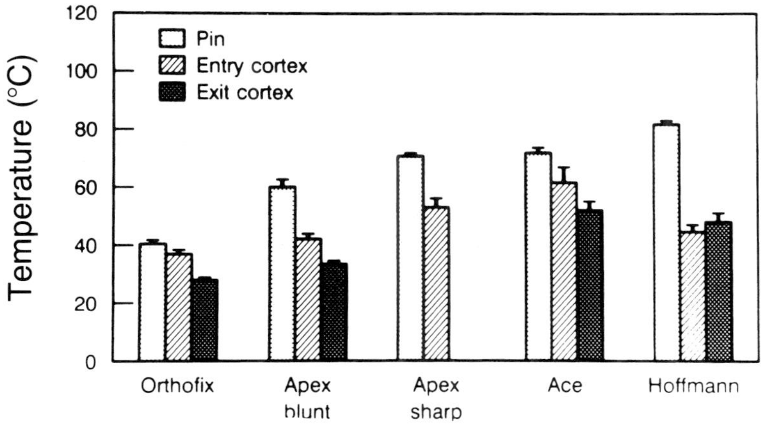

(b)

Figure 9.67

(a) Five types of external fixation pins. (b) Peak temperatures recorded at the entry cortex, at the exit cortex, and within the pin itself during insertion. (From Ref 70 with permission.)

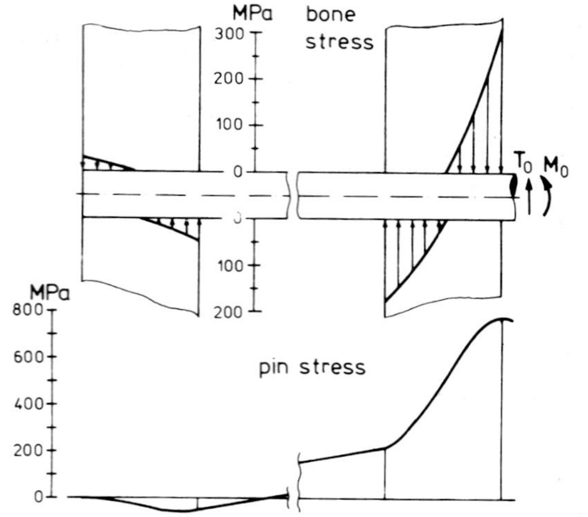

Figure 9.68

(a) Compressive stresses in bone generated at the interface with an external fixation pin acting to resist bending and loading transverse to its longitudinal axis. The pin exits to the right. (Magnitude and direction of stress given by vertical arrows.) (b) Plot of stress in the pin along it. (From Ref 72 with permission.)

will be smaller, because the distance from the location of the applied force (i.e. through the sidebar) to the base of the cantilever (i.e. the pin/bone interface) is shorter. Increasing the pin diameter has the effect of distributing the stresses over a larger area, which also decreases stress. Similarly, spreading the load over a larger number of pins will decrease local pin/bone stresses (Figure 9.70).[72]

Another mechanism for pin loosening in bone has been described by Perren et al.[74] As shown in Figure 9.71, if the pin is the same diameter as the hole in bone, micromotion induces bone resorption at the pin/bone interface. If the hole for the pin is drilled 0.3 mm in diameter undersize, the yield stress of bone is exceeded when the pin is inserted, and mechanical destruction of bone occurs. If the hole is less than 0.1 mm undersize, the bone is prestressed and the pin/bone interface becomes stabilized. It is clear that bone requires some stress at the interface in order to remain viable; however, the combination of prestress (by

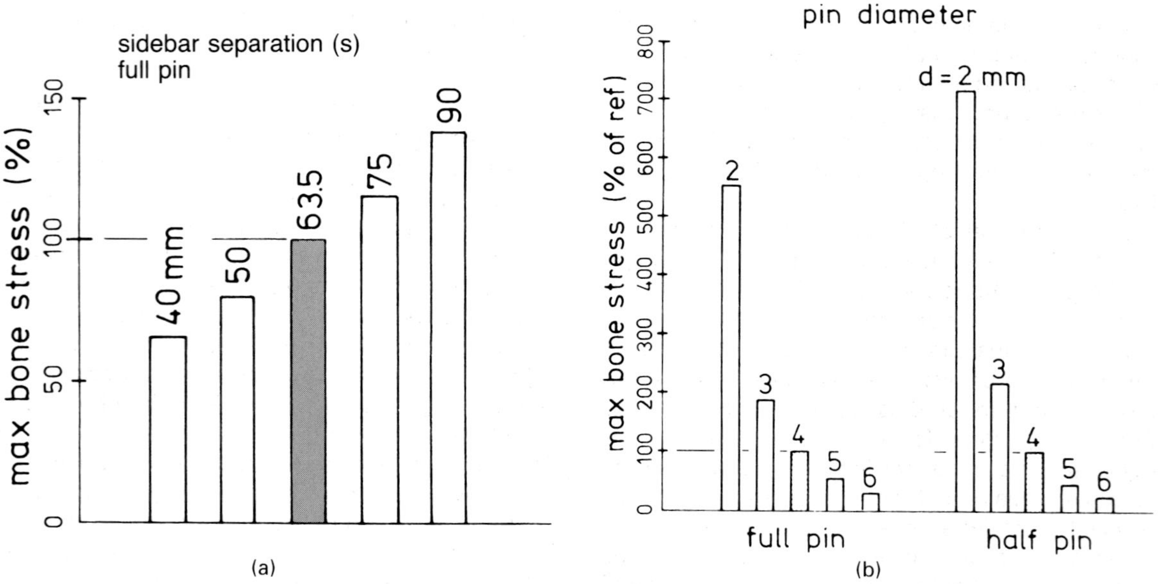

Figure 9.69

The effects of two parameters on external fixator pin/bone interface stresses. (a) Separation of the sidebars from the bone surface (in mm). (b) Pin diameter, for both half and full pins. (From Ref 72 with permission.)

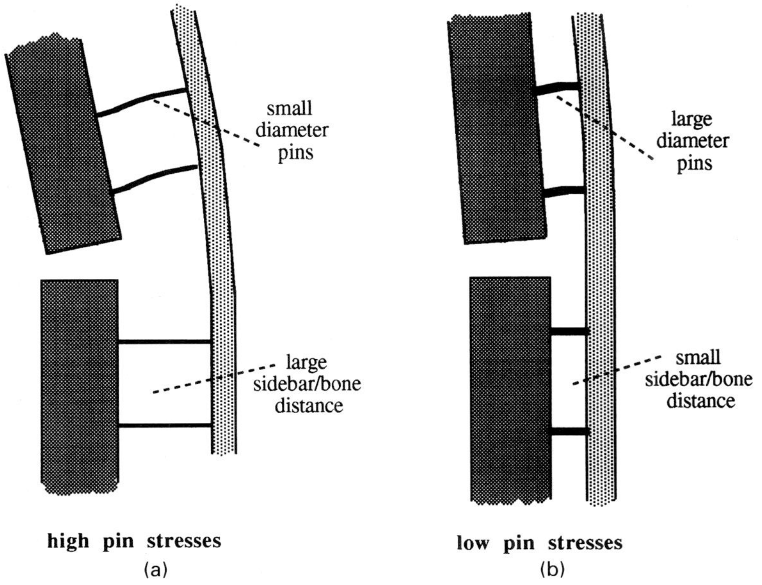

Figure 9.70

External fixation factors that produce (a) high pin/bone interface stresses; (b) lower stresses.

undersizing the hole) and functional stress (by the actions of muscle and gravity loads) may create stresses exceeding the yield strength of bone. Therefore if prestressing is considered, the fixation should probably be protected until callus at the fracture site begins to share load with the fixator.

Further sources of failure of external fixator pins include direct pullout and fatigue. Pullout strength of the pin in bone has been shown to increase with a greater outer and smaller inner (minor) diameter of the pin, and to not be affected by thread profile or pitch[75] – a conclusion similar to those found in studies of screw design (see Chapter 6). Pins fatigue within the threads because this is a region of reduced cross sectional area (i.e. higher stresses) and stress concentrators (the thread/root junction). Shallower threads and those formed by rolling as opposed to machining are less likely to fatigue.[76] Note that the desire for shallower threads or a larger minor diameter to prevent fatigue is in opposition to the requirement for a smaller minor diameter to improve pin pullout strength.

External fixation, factors affecting stiffness

As shown in Figure 9.66, a number of factors affect the rigidity of an external fixation fracture construct. Among these are the geometry of the frame and the materials used for its components. The stiffness of an external fixation sidebar is directly related to its cross sectional moment of inertia and material properties. Recently carbon fiber sidebars have become popular because they are radiolucent, allowing excellent viewing of the injured region on radiographs. A comparison of the bending stiffnesses of solid carbon fiber rods of 11 mm diameter and stainless steel tubes (11 mm outer and 9 mm inner diameters) shows a significant difference in their properties (Figure 9.72). Initially, both rods are equivalently stiff in bending; however, after loading to about 33% of failure strength, the stainless tube begins to yield, whereas the carbon fiber rod maintains the same stiffness until failure, although they both ultimately fail at about the same load.[77] The difference between them is that the stainless

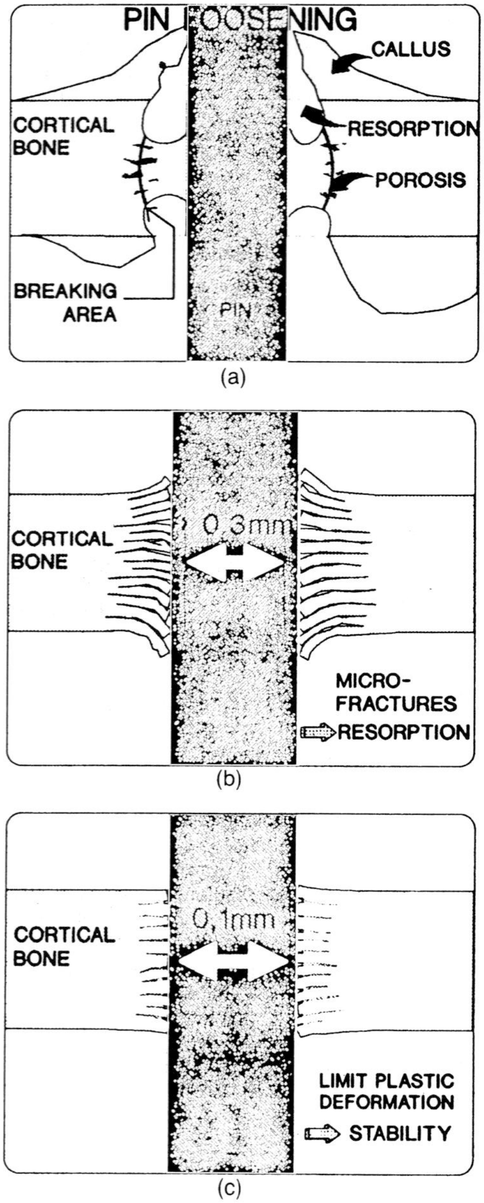

Figure 9.71

An alternate mechanism for loosening at the external fixation pin/interface. (a) If the pin is the same size or smaller than the hole, micromotion and bone resorption occur. (b) If the hole is more than 0.3 mm in diameter undersize compared with the diameter of the pin, bone may fail locally. (c) At 0.1 mm undersize, the pin is stable in bone. (From Ref 74 with permission.)

steel bar allows considerably greater deformation before failure. Therefore at low loads, frames constructed with the different bars would have similar properties; however, the frame with the carbon fiber bars would maintain the same rigidity as load increases.

A second factor governing frame rigidity is the distance of the sidebar from the surface of the bone, as shown quantitatively in Figure 9.73(b) and schematically in Figure 9.74(a). In the case of a unilateral half pin fixator applied in the anterior plane of the tibia, sidebar separation most significantly affects axial loading and anterior–posterior (AP) bending. In both cases, the pins are subjected to cantilever bending moments, so the shorter the length of the pin (i.e. the closer the sidebar to bone), the less it will deflect for the same applied load, and the more rigid will be the fixator.

Several other factors also affect fixator stiffness. Increasing the separation of the pins across the fracture site affects mainly the bending stiffness of the fixator. This occurs because the span of the sidebar between the pins increases as they are separated, creating a less rigid structure (Figures 9.73a, 9.74b). As the number or diameter of pins increases, fixator stiffness is increased in all loading directions (Figure 9.73c). When the distance between the innermost pins (i.e. those across the fracture site) is fixed, but the pin to pin distance within a fracture component is increased, the bending stiffness of the frame increases (Figure 9.73d). Further, using a partly threaded pin with the thread buried in bone significantly increases the bending stiffness of the pin and frame compared with a fully threaded pin or one with threads exposed.[78,79] An alternative method for changing fixator stiffness consists in separating the pins so that they are not all in the same plane. The maximum bending stiffness decreases as the pins are moved out of alignment. Most importantly, the torsional stiffness of the frame is increased by a factor of 280 with a pin angle of 90° compared with 0° (all pins aligned) (Figure 9.75).[80]

Most common external fixator configurations have sufficient rigidity to withstand physiological loading. With two coupled unilateral four pin frames (set in the anterior and medial planes, 120° apart, and using 5 mm Schanz pins, a sidebar/bone separation distance of 4–6 cm, a pin separation distance of 9.75–12 cm within the fracture component and 3–6 cm across the

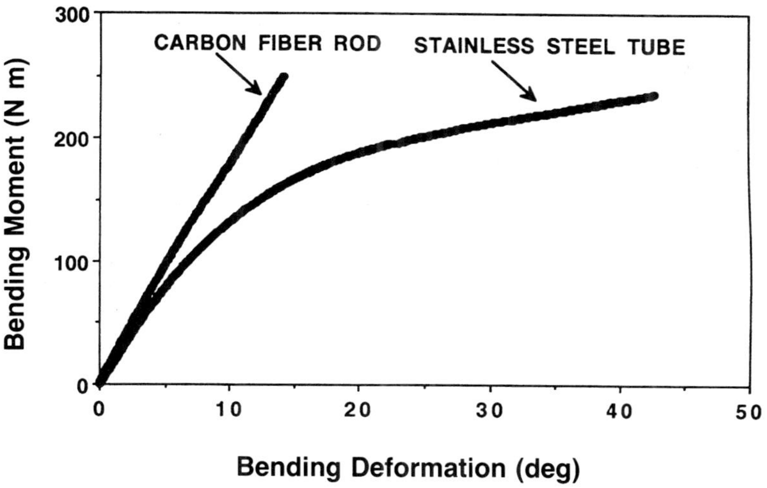

Figure 9.72

Plot of bending moment versus deformation, comparing the performance of carbon fiber and stainless steel rods used in external fixation sidebars.[77]

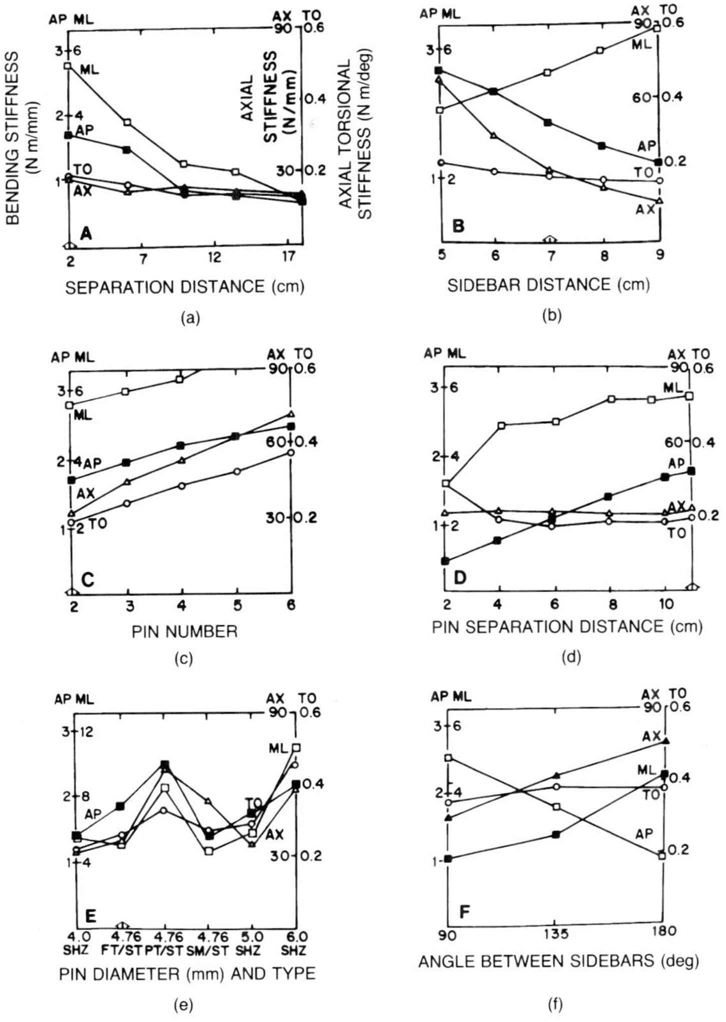

Figure 9.73

The effects of six external fixation structural factors on its mechanical stiffness under various loads (AP, anterior–posterior bending; ML, medial–lateral bending; AX, axial compression; TO, axial torsion). (a) Pin separation distance across the fracture site; (b) sidebar distance from center of bone; (c) pin number in a fracture component; (d) pin separation distance within a fracture component; (e) pin diameter and type (SHZ, Schanz screw; FT, full thread; ST, Steinmann pin; PT, partly threaded, 2.54 cm; SM, smooth); (f) angle between sidebars of a triangulated frame. (From Ref 78 with permission.)

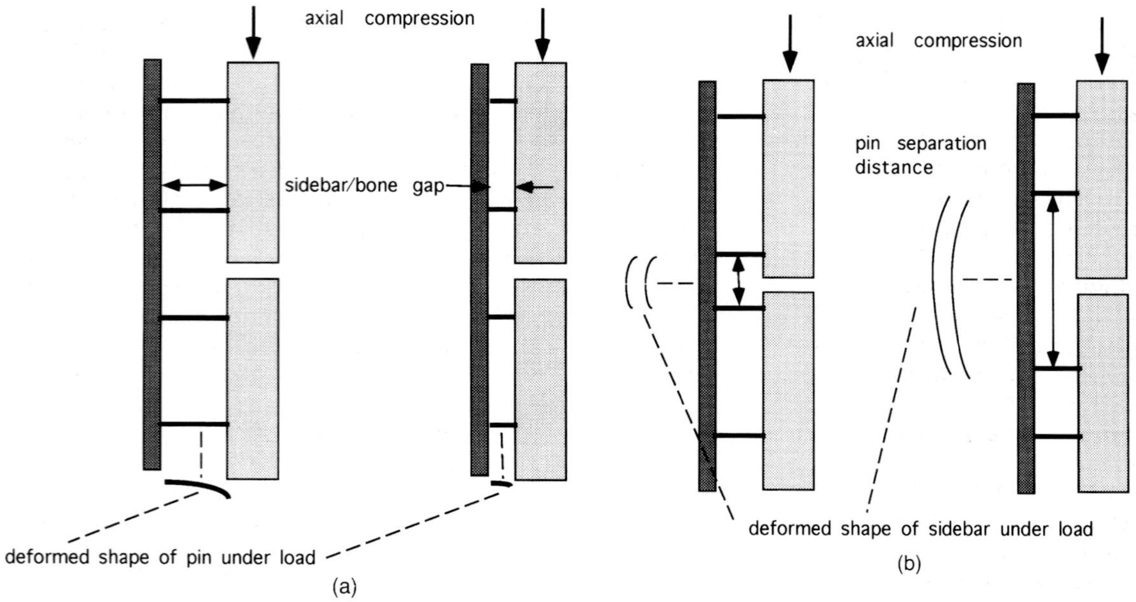

Figure 9.74

The effects of various parameters on the stiffness of an external fixator applied to the tibia. (a) Increasing the sidebar/bone distance increases the length of the pin and decreases its rigidity. (b) Separating the pins across the fracture increases the span length of the sidebar, and decreases its bending rigidity.

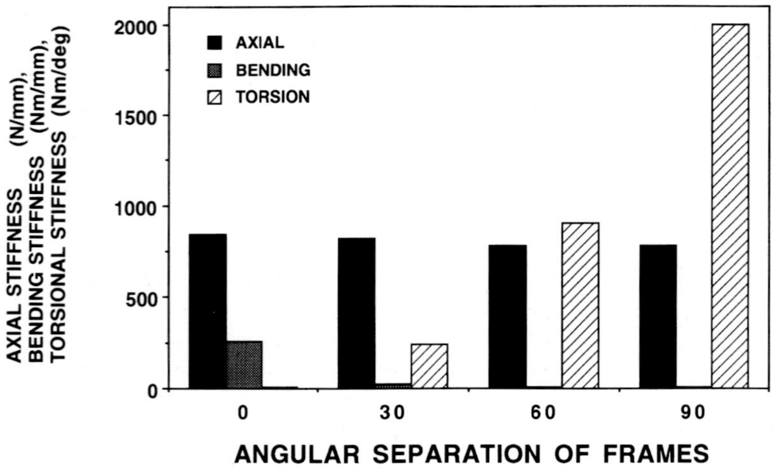

Figure 9.75

Effect of pin separation angle between unilateral frames on construct stiffness in bending and torsion. (Data adapted from Ref 80.)

fracture gap, with no bone/bone fracture site contact), the fixator reaches 66% of AP bending, 95% of ML bending, 65% of axial compressive, and 51% of torsional stiffness compared with the intact tibia.[78] In comparison, a unilateral fixator with double anterior sidebars and no medial frame is 91% as rigid as intact bone in AP bending, 60% in ML bending, and 68% in axial loading.[81] With a single sidebar, the values are 70%, 49%, and 47% respectively. The relative effects of sidebar configuration are shown in Figure 9.76.

Kristiansen et al[82] compared the axial stiffnesses of some configurations of commonly used fixators. As shown in Figure 9.77, the stiffest configuration in axial loading was produced by the EBI Orthofix (57.5% of the intact tibia), followed by the AO with stacked bars, the Richards unilateral, and several bilateral frames, which ranged from 22.7% to 46.5% of intact. The unilateral Hoffman frame produced the least stiffness (18.6% of intact).

Fracture gap axial and shear motions under various types of bending and torsional loading correlated with the stiffness of the fixator itself in that loading direction. While the relationship between axial motion at the fracture gap and fracture healing has been explored to a certain extent,[83] the effect of shearing deformations on callus healing is unknown. An external fixation system that is rigid in axial compression and allows little axial deformation at the fracture site may permit considerable shearing in torsion if it is not rigid in this loading mode. The relationship between axial and torsional stiffnesses of a fixation device is not particularly strong, when comparing unilateral and bilateral frames (Figure 9.78). In torsional loading, the resisting moment of a unilateral frame comes from the twist of the sidebar. The center of rotation is at the sidebar, considerably away from the fracture site. In a double plane frame, the center of rotation is between the two frames, which would be nearer the fracture site. Therefore smaller fracture site shearing would be expected with a double plane frame (Figure 9.79). The deformation of a bilateral frame in axial compression or torsion depends to a large extent on the flexibility of the pins, while for a unilateral frame, it depends on both pin and sidebar deformations.

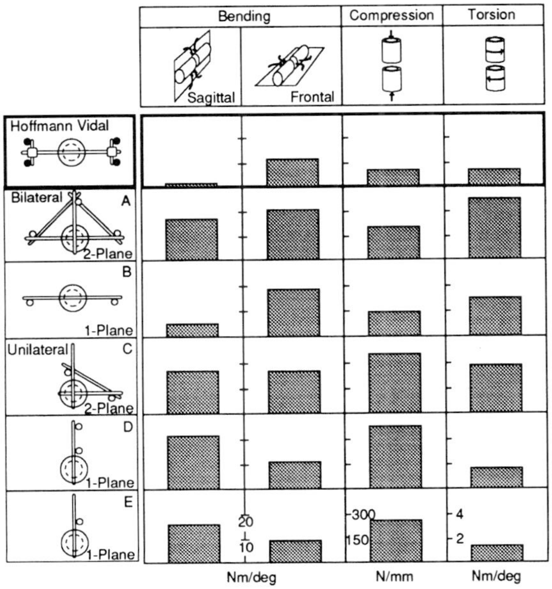

Figure 9.76

Relative stiffnesses of several external fixation frame configurations based on 5 mm pins and AO sidebars and clamps. (From Ref 81 with permission.)

Another type of fixator that has been adapted for fracture fixation is the Ilizarov system.[84] This device is characterized by the use of thin tensioned wires placed transversely through the fracture components instead of pins. They are mounted to full rings, which are then cross coupled, creating the frame structure (Figure 9.80). The most important factor governing rigidity of this frame is bone contact. The most flexible system (two 1.8 mm diameter smooth wires in each fracture component loaded to 110 kg in tension without bone contact) is only 6.1% as stiff in axial loading as the intact tibia. With cortical contact and compression, stiffness increases to 94.4% of intact. With eight wires and no bone contact, axial stiffness increases to 53.7% of intact (Figure 9.81a). While bone contact is the most important factor in gaining axial stiffness, the number of wires governs the torsional stiffness of the frame (Figure 9.81b).[85]

A new concept in external fixation is the pinless fixator.[86] This device uses C shaped clamps that fix to cortex without penetrating the medullary canal. The clamp employs a moveable pin on one end and a fixed pin on the other. The clamping force is derived from a device that drives the pins together, capturing the bone between them, at the same time bending the clamp. Therefore the holding power of the clamps depends on how deeply they penetrate cortex, and is limited by the

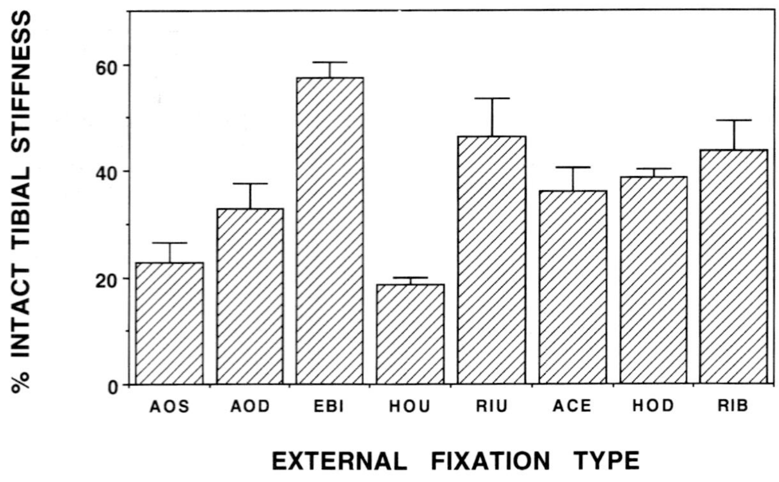

Figure 9.77

Comparison of the axial stiffnesses of various types of external fixators in common use. All fixators were set at 2.5 cm from the bone surface, and all used 5 mm pins except for the EBI device. AOS, AO unilateral, single anterior bar, four pins; AOD, AO unilateral, double anterior bars, four pins; EBI, EBI Orthofix, unilateral, four pins; HOU, Hoffman unilateral, six pins; RIU, Richards unilateral, six pins; ACE, Ace Fischer bilateral, eight pins; HOD, Hoffman delta bilateral, eight pins; RIB, Richards bilateral, eight pins. (Data adapted from Ref 82.)

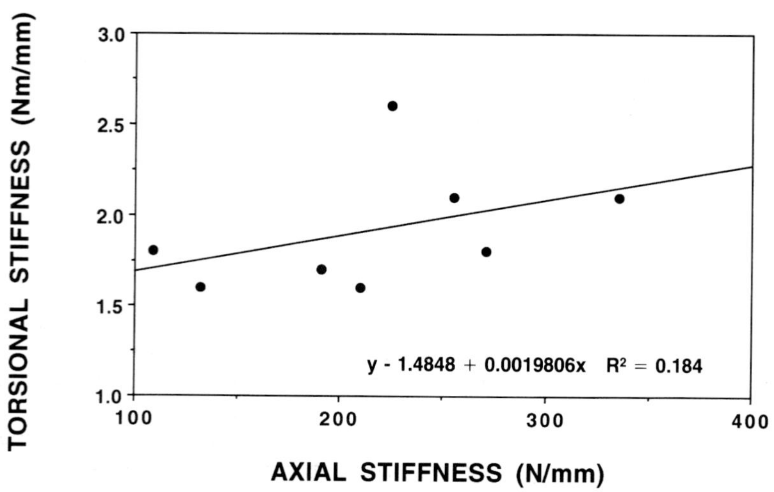

Figure 9.78

Relationship between the axial and torsional stiffnesses of external fixation frames. This demonstrates that the relationship is not strong, which implies that a fixator that is rigid in axial loading may permit considerable shearing because of low torsional stiffness. (Data adapted from Ref 82.)

rigidity of the clamp frame. Peak clamp pullout force transverse to the long axis of the bone has been found to reach 470 N.[87] The clamps can be used with standard AO bars and sidebar/pin clamps. Testing shows that, compared with a standard single sidebar, external fixator construct (unilateral, four 5 mm diameter Schanz pins, sidebar distance to bone of 5 cm), the pinless construct is 37% as stiff in axial loading, 65% as stiff in torsion, 39.4% as stiff in medial–lateral bending, and 30.2% as stiff in anterior–posterior bending. The decreases in stiffness of this device results from the relative flexibility of the clamps and the fact that the clamp pins can rotate at their cortical clamping sites.[87]

The effect of the fibula on tibial fixation

When the tibia is fractured and the fibula remains intact, Teitz et al[88] have shown that the intact fibula influences (i.e. distracts) the healing tibia.

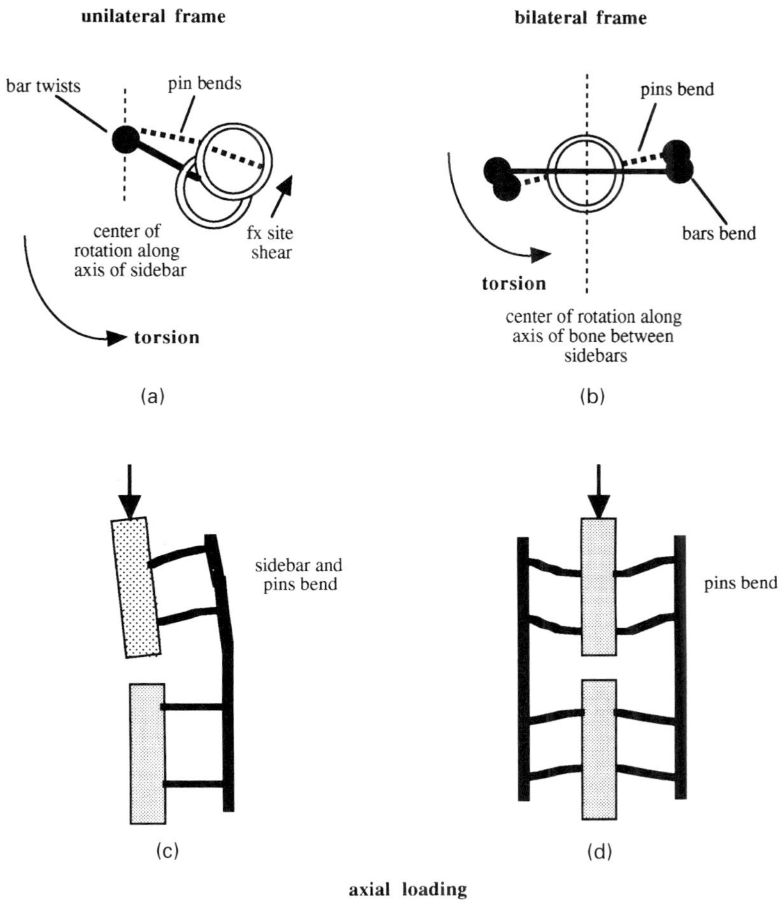

Figure 9.79

The different types of deformation exhibited by unilateral and bilateral external fixation frames. View down the axis of the bone: (a) unilateral frame; (b) bilateral frame subjected to torsion. (c) Unilateral frame and (d) bilateral frame deformations due to axial loading.

Alternatively, when both tibia and fibula are fractured, questions arise as to whether the tibia should be fixed as well. The load bearing role of the fibula has been demonstrated;[89,90] therefore it is reasonable to expect that an intact or reconstructed fibula can influence the stiffness of a fixed tibia. Gotzen et al[91] showed that fixing the fibula in addition to the tibia reduces tibial interfragmentary movement by 39% in axial loading, which is equivalent to an increase in axial stability of 160%. They consider the fibula to act as a buttress under compressive loading and a tension band when the axial load on the tibia is offset to the medial side of the joint (Figure 9.82). Considering these different views, it may be best to fix the fibula when good alignment and contact between the tibial fracture components is ensured, so that the fibula does not distract the tibia fracture.

Summary

Closed injuries to the tibial shaft can be treated by casting or functional bracing. It should be recognized that these methods cannot control axial shortening of the fracture; however they are able to control both angulation and torsional rotation effectively. Internal and external fixation

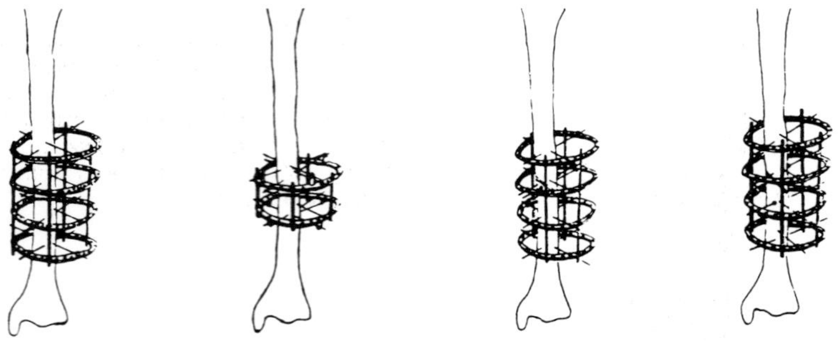

Figure 9.80

Different configurations of an Ilizarov external fixation frame used in fracture fixation. (From Ref 85 with permission.)

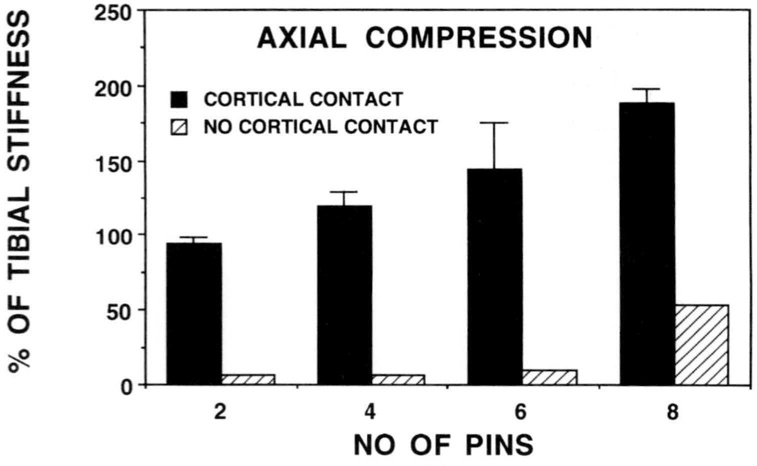

(a)

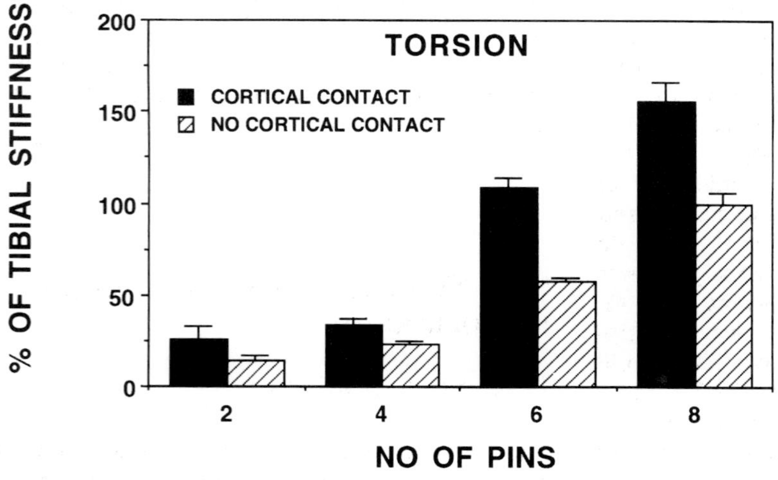

(b)

Figure 9.81

Comparison of the effects of the number of wires in the fracture component and cortical contact on stiffnesses of constructs using the Ilizarov frame: (a) axial compression; (b) axial torsion. (Data adapted from Ref 85.)

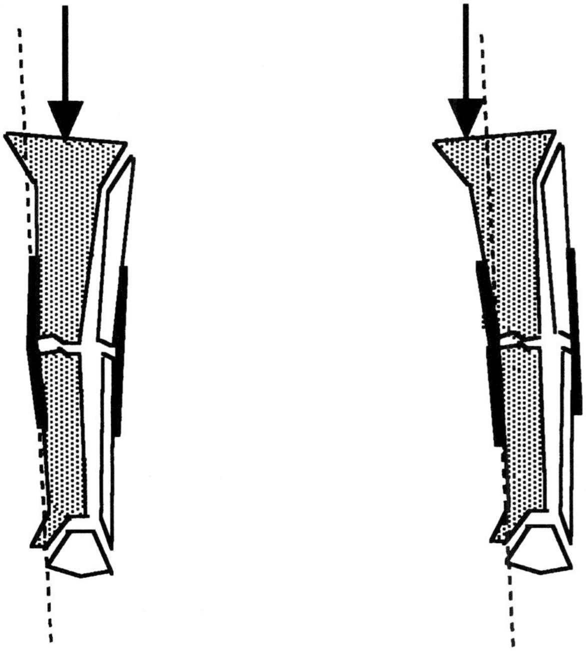

(a) (b)

Figure 9.82

The load bearing role of the fibula with a fractured tibia (a) as a buttress against compression with the joint load centered and (b) as a tension band when the medial side of the joint is loaded. (Adapted from Ref 91.)

devices provide stability to tibia fractures, with the major factor in axial compression and bending being contact of the fracture cortices. Intramedullary unreamed nails with proximal and distal interlocking screws provide appropriate fixation in axial and bending loading directions; however, they are quite flexible in torsion. Apart from the material from which the nail is made and its shape, the orientation of the locking screws and the location of the nail bend can affect its performance. Parallel proximal locking screws permit some sliding of the fracture fragment on the screw shafts resulting in medial–lateral translation during varus–valgus bending. Also, if the nail bend resides within the distal fracture component, it may wedge into the component and carry it distally and posteriorly during insertion. External fixators allow for great flexibility in setup of a mechanical system to control fracture site motion. The most important parameters affecting the rigidity of a frame are the number, diameter and separation of the pins across the fracture site, the material, diameter and distance of the sidebar from the bone, and the geometry of the fixator.

9.6 Fixation of the tibiofibular syndesmosis

Loading conditions

The fibula is accepted to be a weight bearing bone, supporting between 10% and 17% of the load acting through the lower extremity.[89–91] As shown in Figure 9.49, the peak load in the tibia is estimated to reach four times body weight.[1] Therefore the tibiofibular syndesmosis may be loaded to between 40% and 68% of body weight. Further, the disruption of this joint increases ankle drawer by 25% (mean of both anterior and posterior loading of the foot transverse to the long axis of the tibia), and tibiotalar motion by 11%.[92]

Fixation of the syndesmosis

Biomechanical testing, as shown in Figure 9.83, demonstrates that some motion occurs between the tibia and fibula during load bearing with plantar to dorsiflexion of the foot. In the normal joint, the fibula rotates externally to 2° and the joint gaps to 1.25 mm as the foot moves from plantar to dorsiflexion.[93] Fixation with a trans-syndesmotic screw (Figure 9.84a) limits both rotation and translation (Figure 9.83). Recently, the use of a flexible suture has been proposed (Figure 9.84c). This may permit more normal functioning of the joint, while providing adequate immobilization.[94]

9.7 Fixation of the metatarsal

Metatarsal osteotomy fixation

The stability of a corrective osteotomy of the metatarsal depends partly on the fixation used and partly on the orientation of the osteotomy cuts themselves. Osteotomies through the base of the metatarsal do not permit adequate purchase of the fixation, so are not capable of supporting load, regardless of the fixation used. Suture does not provide adequate load bearing capability, and

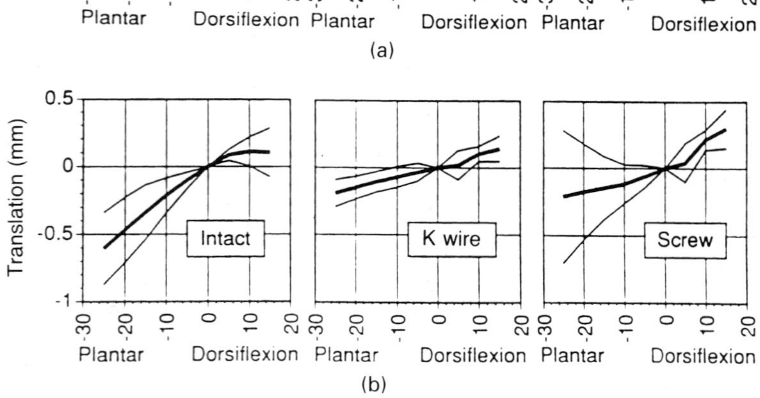

Figure 9.83

Motion of the fibula with respect to the tibia during movement of the foot from plantar to dorsiflexion with an axial load of 700 N applied through the tibia. (a) Rotation of the fibula with respect to the tibia (in degrees) (external rotation = positive; internal rotation = negative). (b) Translation of the fibula (lateral direction = positive; medial direction = negative). (The center line of each graph is the mean value; outer lines indicate ± standard deviation.) (From Ref 93 with permission.)

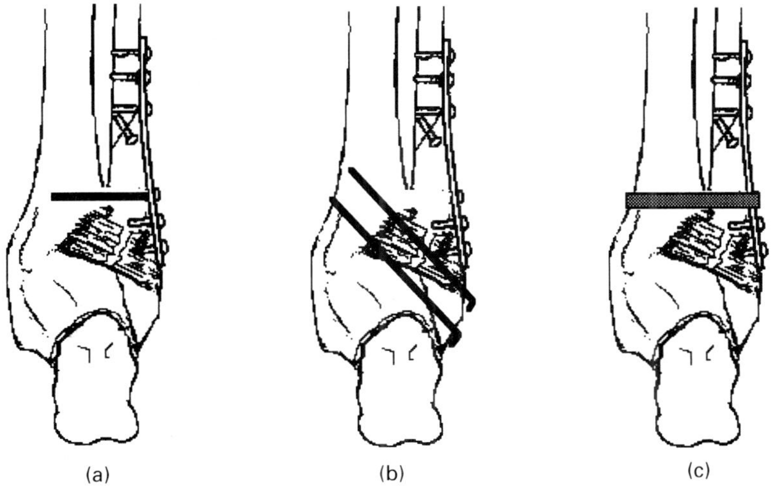

Figure 9.84

Examples of fixation of the tibiofibular syndesmosis by (a) screw, (b) K wire,[93] or (c) flexible suture.[94] (Adapted from Ref 94.)

tends to cut through bone. The most effective fixation in bending is provided by either crossed K wires or screws.[95]

9.8 References

1. Paul JP, Approaches to design, Force actions transmitted by joints in the human body, *Proc Roy Soc London* (1976) **B192**: 163–72.
2. Rybicki EF, Simonen FA, Weis Jr EB, On the mathematical analysis of stress in the human femur, *J Biomech* (1972) **5**: 203–15.
3. Brown RH, Burstein AH, Frankel VH, Telemetering in vivo loads from nail plate implants, *J Biomech* (1982) **15**: 815–23.
4. Boyd HB, Anderson LD, Management of unstable trochanteric fractures, *Surg Gynecol Obstet* (1961) **May**: 633–8.
5. Ragnarsson JI, Karrholm J, Stability of femoral neck fracture, *Acta Orthop Scand* (1991) **62**: 201–7.
6. Muthusamy R, Quaid G, Tencer AF, Schemitsch EH, Ching RP, Predictors of successful femoral neck fixation, *J Orthop Res* (submitted).
7. Swiontkowski MF, Harrington RM, Keller TS, Van Patten PK, Torsion and bending analysis of internal fixation techniques for femoral neck fractures: the role of implant design and bone density, *J Orthop Res* (1987) **5**: 433–44.
8. Singh M, Nagrath AR, Maini PS, Changes in the trabecular pattern of the upper end of the femur as an index of osteoporosis, *J Bone Jt Surg* (1970) **52A**: 457–67.
9. Crowell RR, Edwards WT, Hayes WC, Pullout strength of fixation devices in trabecular bone of the femoral head, *Trans 31st Orthopedic Research Society Meeting* (1985) **10**: 189.
10. Calandruccio RA, Graham RJ, Peltier LF, Urist MR, Weisman S, *Internal fixation devices for fractures of the proximal femur* (American Academy of Orthopaedic Surgeons, Committee on the History of Orthopaedic Surgery).
11. Jewett EL, One piece angle nail for trochanteric fractures, *J Bone Jt Surg* (1941) **23**: 803–10.
12. Massie WK, Functional fixation of femoral neck fractures: telescoping nail technique, *Clin Orthop* (1959) **12**: 230–55.
13. Ecker ML, Joyce JJ, Kohl EJ, The treatment of trochanteric hip fractures using a compression screw, *J Bone Jt Surg* (1975) **57A**: 23–7.
14. Russell TA, Taylor JC, Interlocking intramedullary nailing of the femur, *Seminars in Orthop* (1986) **1**: 217.
15. Knowles FL, Fractures of the neck of the femur, *Wisconsin Med J* (1936) **35**: 106–9.
16. Kaufer H, Matthews LS, Sonsegard D, Stable fixation of intertrochanteric fractures, a biomechanical evaluation, *J Bone Jt Surg* (1974) **56A**: 899–907.
17. Jacobs RR, McClain O, Armstrong HJ, Internal fixation of intertrochanteric hip fractures: a clinical and biomechanical study, *Clin Orthop* (1980) **146**: 62–70.

18. Hamm JT, Saha S, Lipka JM, Albright JA, A comparison of the triflanged nail vs screw fixations' resistance to migration in the femoral head, *Trans 34th Orthopedic Research Society Meeting* (1988) **13:** 400.
19. Goodman SB, Davidson JA, Locke L, Novotny S, Jones H, Csongradi JJ, A biomechanical study of two methods of internal fixation of unstable fractures of the femoral neck, *J Orthop Trauma* (1992) **6:** 66–72.
20. Van Audekercke R, Martens M, Mulier JC, Stuyck J, Experimental study on internal fixtion of femoral neck fractures, *Clin Orthop* (1979) **141:** 203–12.
21. Edwards WT, Lewallen DG, Hayes WC, The effect of pin number and fracture pattern on immediate mechanical fixation of a subcapital hip fracture model, *Trans 31st Orthopedic Research Society Meeting* (1985) **10:** 219.
22. Rubin R, Trent P, Arnold W, Burstein, A, Knowles pinning of experimental femoral neck fractures: a biomechanical study, *J Trauma* (1981) **21:** 1036–9.
23. Rosenblum SF, Zuckerman JD, Tam BS, Strain gauge analysis of the effects of the gamma nail on intertrochanteric fractures, *Trans 38th Orthopedic Research Society Meeting* (1992) **17:** 55.
24. Russell TA, Dingman CA, Wisnewski P, Mechanical and clinical rationale for femoral neck fracture fixation with a cephalomedullary interlocking nail, *Trans 38th Orthopedic Research Society Meeting* (1992) **17:** 177.
25. Kyle RF, Wright TM, Burstein AH, Biomechanical analysis of the sliding characteristics of compression hip screws, *J Bone Jt Surg* (1980) **62A:** 1308–14.
26. Yoshimine F, Latta LL, Milne EL, Fixation of unstable intertrochanteric hip fractures in osteopenic and normal femora—effects of screw–plate angle and barrel engagement, *Trans 37th Orthopedic Research Society Meeting* (1991) **16:** 450.
27. Michel MC, Schneider E, Genge M, Perren SM, Loading history of an interlocking femoral nail subsequent to fracture treatment, *Trans 37th Orthopedic Research Society Meeting* (1991) **16:** 141.
28. Cochran GVB, Zickel RE, Fielding JW, Stress analysis of subtrochanteric fractures; effect of muscle forces and internal fixation devices. In: Uhthoff HK, ed, *Current concepts of internal fixation* (Springer-Verlag: New York 1980) 211–27.
29. Russell TA, Taylor JC, LaVelle DG, Beals NB, Brumfield DL, Durham AG, Mechanical characterization of femoral interlocking intramedullary nailing systems, *J Orthop Trauma* (1991) **5:** 332–40.
30. Bucholz RW, Ross SE, Lawrence KL, Fatigue fracture of the interlocking nail in the treatment of fractures of the distal part of the femoral shaft, *J Bone Jt Surg* (1987) **69A:** 1391–9.
31. Johnson KD, Tencer AF, Mechanics of intramedullary nails for femoral fractures, *Unfallchir* (1990) **93:** 506–11.
32. Zuber K, Schneider E, Eulenberger J, Perren SM, Form und Dimension der Markhöhle menschlicher Femora in Hinblick auf die Passung von Marknagelimplantaten, *Unfallchir* (1988) **91:** 314–19.
33. Johnson KD, Tencer AF, Sherman MC, Biomechanical factors affecting fracture stability and femoral bursting in closed intramedullary nailing of femoral shaft fractures, with illustrative case presentations, *J Orthop Trauma* (1987) **1:** 1–11.
34. Harper MC, Carson WL, Curvature of the femur and the proximal entry point for an intramedullary rod, *Clin Orthop* (1987) **220:** 155–61.
35. Zickel RE, An intramedullary fixation device for the proximal part of the femur, *J Bone Jt Surg* (1976) **58A:** 866–72.
36. Chapman MW, Bowman WE, Csongradi JJ, Trafton PG, Bovill EG, The use of Enders' pins in extracapsular fractures of the hip, *J Bone Jt Surg* (1981) **63A:** 14–28.
37. Müller ME, Allgöwer M, Schneider R, Willenegger J, *Manual of internal fixation* (Springer-Verlag: Berlin 1979) 85–96.
38. Johnson KD, Johnston DWC, Parker B, Comminuted femoral shaft fractures. Treatment by: roller traction, cerclage wires and an intramedullary nail, or an interlocking intramedullary nail, *J Bone Jt Surg* (1984) **66A:** 1222–35.
39. Tencer AF, Johnson KD, Johnston DWC, Gill K, A biomechanical comparison of various methods of stabilization of subtrochanteric fractures of the femur, *J Orthop Res* (1984) **2:** 297–305.
40. McKellop H, Ebramzadeh E, Fortune J, Williams M, Brion W, Sarmiento A, Stability of subtrochanteric fractures fixed with intramedullary rods, *Trans 13th Society for Biomaterials Meeting* (1987) 101.
41. Thimsen DA, Hoeltzel DA, Kyle RF, A biomechanical analysis of the Grosse–Kempf interlocking intramedullary nail in torsion and 4-point bending, *Trans 30th Orthopedic Research Society Meeting* (1984) **9:** 70.
42. Johnson KD, Tencer AF, Blumenthal S, August A, Johnston DWC, Biomechanical performance of locked intramedullary nail systems in comminuted femoral shaft fractures, *Clin Orthop* (1986) **206:** 151–61.
43. Gleis GE, Frederick LD, Johnson JR, Biomechanical stability of distally blocked fractures: is one screw enough?, *Techniques Orthop* (1988) **3:** 6–8.
44. Bankston AB, Keating EM, Saha S, The biomechanical evaluation of intramedullary nails in distal femoral shaft fractures, *Clin Orthop* (1992) **276:** 277–82.
45. Zych GA, Greenbarg PE, Milne EL, Levi DM, Latta

LL, Mechanics of distal locking IM nail fixation in osteopenic and normal femora, *Trans 34th Orthopedic Research Society Meeting* (1988) **13**: 406.
46. Frankenburg EP, Robinson AP, Urquhart AG, Goulet JA, Supracondylar femur fractures: a biomechanical analysis of four fixation devices, *Trans 38th Orthopedic Research Society Meeting* (1992) **17**: 413.
47. Hungerford DS, Barry M, Biomechanics of the patellofemoral joint, *Clin Orthop* (1979) **144**: 9–15.
48. Anderson LD, Fractures. In: Crenshaw AH, ed, *Campbell's operative orthopedics*, 5th edn (CV Mosby: St Louis, MO 1971) 537–41.
49. McConnell BE, An operation for fractures of the patella using the temporary patellar tendon substitution technic, *Southern Med J* (1971) **64**: 87–9.
50. Müller ME, Allgöwer M, Willenegger H, *Manual of internal fixation* (Springer-Verlag: Berlin 1970).
51. Weber MJ, Janecki CJ, McLeod P, Nelson CL, Thompson JA, Efficacy of various forms of fixation of transverse fractures of the patella, *J Bone Jt Surg* (1980) **62A**: 215–20.
52. Benjamin J, Bried J, Dohm M, McMurtry M, Biomechanical evaluation of various forms of fixation of transverse patellar fractures, *J Orthop Trauma* (1987) **1**: 219–22.
53. Perry CR, McCarthy JA, Kain CC, Pearson RL, Patellar fixation protected with a load sharing cable: a mechanical and clinical study, *J Orthop Trauma* (1988) **2**: 234–40.
54. Levens AS, Inman VT, Blosser JA, Transverse rotation of the lower extremity in locomotion, *J Bone Jt Surg* (1948) **30A**: 859–72.
55. Laurence M, Freeman MAR, Swanson SAV, Engineering considerations in the internal fixation of fractures of the tibial shaft, *J Bone Jt Surg* (1969) **51B**: 745–68.
56. Gonza ER, Biomechanics of long bone injuries, In: Gonza ER, Harrington IJ, eds, *Biomechanics of musculoskeletal injury* (Williams & Wilkins: Baltimore 1982) 1–30.
57. Denny LD, Keating EM, Engelhardt JA, Saha S, A comparison of fixation techniques in tibial plateau fractures, *Trans 30th Orthopedic Research Society Meeting* (1984) **9**: 314.
58. Beris AE, Glisson RR, Seaber AV, Urbaniak JR, Load tolerance of tibial plateau depressions reinforced with a cluster of K-wires, *Trans 34th Orthopedic Research Society Meeting* (1988) **13**: 301.
59. Sarmiento A, A functional below-the-knee cast for tibial fractures, *J Bone Jt Surg* (1967) **49**: 855–75.
60. Zagorski JB, Latta LL, Finnieston A, Comparative tibial fracture stability in casts, custom and prefabricated braces, *Trans 29th Orthopedic Research Society Meeting* (1983) **8**: 217.
61. McKellop H, Hoffman R, Sarmiento A, Lu B, Ebramzadeh E, Comparison of tibial fracture motions for different fixation devices using a six-degree-of-freedom transducer, *Trans 37th Orthopedic Research Society Meeting* (1991) **16**: 451.
62. Henley MB, Meier M, Tencer AF, Influences of some design parameters on the biomechanics of the unreamed tibial intramedullary rod, *J Orthop Trauma* (1993) **7**: 311–19.
63. Swiontkowski MF, Senft D, Taylor S, Agnew SG, Santoro V, Plate design has an effect on cortical bone blood flow, *Trans 37th Orthopedic Research Society Meeting* (1991) **16**: 66.
64. Ramotowski W, Granowski R, Zespol: an original method of stable osteosynthesis, *Clin Orthop* (1991) **272**: 67–75.
65. Kowalski M, Schemitsch EH, Harrington RM, Chapman JR, Swiontkowski MF, Comparative biomechanical evaluation of different tibial fixation devices, *Trans 39th Orthopedic Research Society Meeting* (1993) **18**: 568.
66. Cox LG, Dahners LE, Gilbert JA, Internal fixation of spiral fractures: an in vitro biomechanical study, *Trans 32nd Orthopedic Research Society Meeting* (1986) **11**: 315.
67. Pfister U, Frigg R, Die Verklemmung des Marknagels in der Markhöhle der Tibia, *Akt Traumatol* (1980) **10**: 117–21.
68. Cheng SL, Smith TJ, Davey JR, A comparison of the stability and strength of six techniques of cerclage wire fixation for fractures, *Trans 37th Orthopedic Research Society Meeting* (1991) **16**: 143.
69. Shaw JA, Daubert HB, Fixation capabilities of cerclage systems: a biomechanical study, *Trans 34th Orthopedic Research Society Meeting* (1988) **13**: 403.
70. Wikenheiser MA, Lewallen DG, Markel MD, In vitro mechanical, thermal, and microstructural performance of five external fixation pins, *Trans 38th Orthopedic Research Society Meeting* (1992) **17**: 409.
71. Rouiller C, Majno G, Morphologische und Chemische Unterbuchungen an Knochen nach Hitzeeinwirkung, *Beitr Z Path Anat* (1953) **113**: 100–20.
72. Huiskes R, Chao EYS, Crippen TE, Parametric analyses of pin–bone stresses in external fracture fixation, *J Orthop Res* (1985) **3**: 341–9.
73. Armstrong RD, Finlay JB, Rorabeck CH, Pin–bone stresses in external fixation: a reflective photoelastic analysis, *Trans 32nd Orthopedic Research Society Meeting* (1986) **11**: 311.
74. Perren SM, Cordey J, Baumgart F, Rahn BA, Schatzker J, Technical and biomechanical aspects of screws used for bone surgery, *Int J Orthop Trauma* (1992) **2**: 31–48.
75. Halsey D, Fleming B, Pope MH, Krag M, Kristiansen T, External fixator pin design, *Clin Orthop*

(1992) **278**: 305–12.

76. Chao EYS, Kasman RA, Fatigue performance of external fixator pins, *Trans 30th Orthopedic Research Socity Meeting* (1984) **9**: 269.
77. Kowalski M, Schemitsch EH, Harrington RM, Chapman JR, Swiontkowski MF, Comparative biomechanical evaluation of different external fixation sidebars (stainless steel tubes versus carbon fiber rods), *J Orthop Trauma* (submitted).
78. Tencer AF, Claudi B, Pearce S, Bucholz RW, Johnson KD, Development of a variable stiffness external fixation system for stabilization of segmental defects of the tibia, *J Orthop Res* (1984) **1**: 395–404.
79. Huiskes R, Chao EYS, Guidelines for external fixation frame rigidity and stresses, *J Orthop Res* (1986) **4**: 68–75.
80. Egan JM, Shearer JR, Behavior of an external fixation frame incorporating an angular separation of the fixator pins: a finite element approach, *Clin Orthop* (1987) **223**: 265–74.
81. Behrens F, Johnson WD, Unilateral external fixation, methods to increase and reduce frame stiffness, *Clin Orthop* (1989) **241**: 48–56.
82. Kristiansen T, Fleming B, Reinecke S, Pope MS, Comparative study of fracture gap motion in external fixation, *Clin Biomech* (1987) **2**: 191–5.
83. Kenwright J, Goodship AE, Controlled mechanical stimulation in the treatment of tibial fractures, *Clin Orthop* (1989) **241**: 36–47.
84. Ilizarov GA, Deviatov AA, Operative elongation of the leg, *Ortop Travmatol Protez* (1971) **32**: 20–5.
85. Calhoun JH, Li F, Ledbetter BR, Gill CA, Biomechanics of Ilizarov for fracture fixation, *Trans 37th Orthopedic Research Society Meeting* (1991) **16**: 439.
86. Stene GM, Frigg R, Schlegal U, Swiontkowski M, Perren SM, In vitro and in vivo evaluation of the pinless external fixator, *Trans 38th Orthopedic Research Society Meeting* (1992) **17**: 56.
87. Tencer AF, Senft D, Swiontkowski MF, Mechanical studies of modified pinless external fixation system, *Report 003, Biomechanics Laboratory, Department of Orthopedics, University of Washington* (1991).
88. Teitz C, Carter DR, Frankel VH, Problems associated with tibial fractures with intact fibulae, *J Bone Jt Surg* (1980) **62A**: 770–6.
89. Lambert KL, The weight bearing function of the fibula, *J Bone Jt Surg* (1971) **53A**: 507–13.
90. Takebe K, Nakagawa A, Minami H, Kanazawa A, Hirohata A, Role of the fibula in weight-bearing, *Clin Orthop* (1984) **184**: 289–92.
91. Gotzen L, Haas N, Hutter J, Koller J, Die Bedeutung der Fibula für die Stabilität der Plattenosteosynthese an der Tibia, *Unfallheikunde* (1978) **81**: 409–16.
92. Scheidt KB, Stiehl JB, Skrade DA, Barnhardt T, Posterior malleolar ankle fractures: an in vitro biomechanical analysis of stability in the loaded and unloaded states, *J Orthop Trauma* (1992) **6**: 96–101.
93. Peter RE, Harrington RM, Henley MB, Effect of implants on the motion of the distal tibio-fibular syndesmotic joint. Comparison of screw versus K-wire fixation of Weber type "C" injuries, *Trans 38th Orthopedic Research Society Meeting* (1992) **17**: 264.
94. Seitz Jr WH, Bachner EJ, Abram LJ, Postak P, Polando G, Brooks DB, Greenwald AS, Repair of the tibiofibular syndesmosis with a flexible implant, *J Orthop Trauma* (1991) **5**: 78–82.
95. Kummer FJ, Sobel MA, Shereff MJ, Stability of metatarsal osteotomy fixation, *Trans 34th Orthopedic Research Society Meeting* (1988) **13**: 408.

INDEX

References in *italics* refer to illustrations. In many cases there are text references on these pages too.